Anatomic Basis
of Tumor Surgery

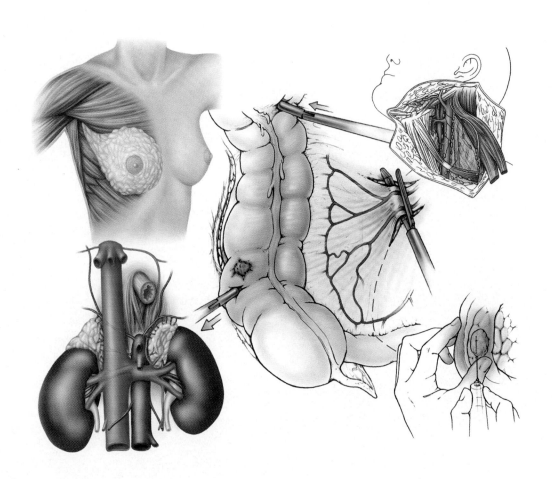

Anatomic Basis of Tumor Surgery

EDITED BY

William C. Wood, M.D.

The Joseph Brown Whitehead Professor and Chairman, Department
of Surgery, and Clinical Director, Winship Cancer Center, Emory University
School of Medicine; Chief of Surgery, Emory University Hospital,
Atlanta, Georgia

John E. Skandalakis, M.D., Ph.D.

The Chris Carlos Distinguished Professor and Director, Centers for
Surgical Anatomy and Technique, and Professor of Surgery, Emory University
School of Medicine, Atlanta; Clinical Professor of Surgery, The Medical
College of Georgia, Augusta; Clinical Professor of Surgery, Mercer University
School of Medicine, Macon; Senior Attending Surgeon, Piedmont Hospital,
Atlanta, Georgia

Illustrators
Alexandra Baker, C.M.I. • David L. Baker, C.M.I.
Sharon Harris, C.M.I. • Joel Harris, C.M.I.

Quality Medical Publishing, Inc.

ST. LOUIS, MISSOURI 1999

To

our best friends

Judy and **Mimi**

who bring joy to every day

This book presents current scientific information and opinion pertinent to medical
professionals. It does not provide advice concerning specific diagnosis and treatment of
individual cases and is not intended for use by the layperson. The authors, editors,
and publisher will not be responsible or liable for actions taken as a result of
the opinions expressed in the book.

The illustration on page 364 is adapted from Smith J, Shiu MH, Kelsey L, et al. Morbidity
of radical lymphadenectomy in the curative resection of gastric carcinoma. Arch Surg 126:1469, 1991;
copyright 1991, American Medical Association. The illustrations on pages 478 to 482,
485 to 488, and 490 are modified from Sugarbaker PA, Malawer MM. Musculoskeletal Surgery
for Cancer. New York: Thieme Medical Publishers, 1992.

PUBLISHER   Karen Berger
PROJECT MANAGEMENT   Katherine Spakowski
COPY EDITOR   GeorgeMary Gardner
ASSISTANT EDITOR   Esha Gupta
PRODUCTION   Accu-Color, Inc.
BOOK DESIGN   Diane M. Beasley, Susan Trail
COVER DESIGN   Diane M. Beasley

Quality Medical Publishing, Inc.
11970 Borman Drive, Suite 222
St. Louis, MO 63146
Telephone: 1-800-348-7808
Web site: http//www.qmp.com

LIBRARY OF CONGRESS CATALOGING-IN-PUBLICATION DATA
Anatomic basis of tumor surgery / edited by William C. Wood, John E.
    Skandalakis : illustrators, Alexandra Baker . . . [et al.].
        p.   cm.
    Includes bibliographical references and index.
    ISBN 1-57626-003-8
    1. Tumors—Surgery—Physiological aspects. 2. Anatomy, Surgical
and topographical. 3. Surgery, Operative. I. Wood, William C.,
1940- . II. Skandalakis, John Elias, 1920- .
    [DNLM: 1. Neoplasms—surgery. 2. Surgical Procedures, Operative—
methods. 3. Anatomy, Regional.   QZ 268 A535 1999]
    RD651.A73   1999
    616.99'2059—dc21
    DNLM/DLC   98-51163
    for Library of Congress   CIP

AC/D/D
5 4 3 2 1

Contributors

Albert J. Aboulafia, M.D.
Assistant Professor, Department of Orthopaedic Surgery, Emory University School of Medicine, Atlanta, Georgia

George Barnes, Jr., M.D.
Attending Surgeon, Department of Surgery, Kaiser Permanente Medical Group, Los Angeles, California

John Bostwick III, M.D.
Professor and Chairman, Division of Plastic, Reconstructive, and Maxillo-Facial Surgery, Department of Surgery, Emory University School of Medicine, Atlanta, Georgia

Gene Branum, M.D.
Assistant Professor, Department of Surgery, Emory University School of Medicine, Atlanta, Georgia

Grant W. Carlson, M.D.
Associate Professor, Department of Surgery, Emory University School of Medicine, Atlanta, Georgia

Gene Colborn, M.D., Ph.D.
Professor of Surgery and Anatomy, Department of Cellular Biology and Anatomy, and Director, Center for Clinical Anatomy, The Medical College of Georgia, Augusta, Georgia

George W. Daneker, Jr., M.D.
Assistant Professor, Department of Surgery, Emory University School of Medicine/Veterans Administration Medical Center, Atlanta, Georgia

John M. DelGaudio, M.D.
Assistant Professor, Department of Otolaryngology—Head and Neck Surgery, Emory University School of Medicine, Atlanta, Georgia

Rizk E.S. El-Galley, M.B., B.Ch., F.R.C.S.(Edin)
Chief Resident, Department of Urology, Emory University School of Medicine, Atlanta, Georgia

Roger S. Foster, Jr., M.D.
Wadley Glenn Professor of Surgery, Department of Surgery, Emory University School of Medicine, and Chief, Surgical Services, Crawford Long Hospital of Emory University, Atlanta, Georgia

Allen A. Futral III, M.D.
Applied Associate Clinical Faculty, Department of Urology, Emory University School of Medicine, Atlanta, Georgia

John R. Galloway, M.D.
Associate Professor, Department of Surgery, Emory University School of Medicine, Atlanta, Georgia

Sam D. Graham, Jr., M.D.
Urologist, The Virginia Center, Richmond, Virginia; former Louis McDonald Orr Professor of Urology, Department of Surgery, Emory University School of Medicine, Atlanta, Georgia

Ira R. Horowitz, M.D.
Associate Professor and Director, Gynecologic Oncology, Department of Gynecology and Obstetrics, Winship Cancer Center, Emory University School of Medicine, Atlanta, Georgia

John G. Hunter, M.D.
Professor and Vice Chairman, Department of Surgery, Emory University School of Medicine, Atlanta, Georgia

Thomas E. Keane, M.B., B.Ch., F.R.C.S.(Ire)
Associate Professor, Department of Urology, Emory University School of Medicine, Atlanta, Georgia

Robert B. Lee, M.D.
Cardiovascular Surgical Clinic, Jackson,
Mississippi; former Assistant Professor, Division
of Cardiothoracic Surgery, Department of
Surgery, Emory University School of Medicine,
Atlanta, Georgia

†William C. McGarity, M.D.
Professor Emeritus, Department of Surgery,
Emory University School of Medicine,
Atlanta, Georgia

David K. Monson, M.D.
Assistant Professor, Department of Orthopaedic
Surgery, Emory University School of Medicine,
Atlanta, Georgia

William S. Richardson, M.D.
Staff Surgeon, Department of General Surgery,
Ochsner Clinic, New Orleans, Louisiana

John E. Skandalakis, M.D., Ph.D.
The Chris Carlos Distinguished Professor and
Director, Centers for Surgical Anatomy and
Technique, and Professor of Surgery, Emory
University School of Medicine, Atlanta; Clinical
Professor of Surgery, The Medical College of
Georgia, Augusta; Clinical Professor of Surgery,
Mercer University School of Medicine, Macon;
Senior Attending Surgeon, Piedmont Hospital,
Atlanta, Georgia

Lee J. Skandalakis, M.D.
Clinical Associate Professor of Surgical Anatomy
and Technique, Centers for Surgical Anatomy
and Technique, Emory University School of
Medicine, Atlanta, Georgia

Panajiotis N. Skandalakis, M.D., M.S.
Clinical Associate Professor, Centers for Surgical
Anatomy and Technique, Emory University
School of Medicine, Atlanta, Georgia

C. Daniel Smith, M.D.
Assistant Professor, Department of Surgery,
Emory University School of Medicine,
Atlanta, Georgia

Hadar Spivak, M.D.
Head, Advanced Laparoscopic Unit,
Department of Surgery, Rabin Medical Center,
Petah-Tikva, Israel

Charles A. Staley, M.D.
Assistant Professor, Department of Surgery,
Emory University School of Medicine,
Atlanta, Georgia

Nikolas P. Symbas, M.D.
Resident, Department of Surgery,
Emory University School of Medicine,
Atlanta, Georgia

Panagiotis N. Symbas, M.D.
Professor, Division of Cardiothoracic Surgery,
Department of Surgery, Emory University
School of Medicine, Atlanta, Georgia

Collin J. Weber, M.D.
Professor, Department of Surgery,
Emory University School of Medicine,
Atlanta, Georgia

William C. Wood, M.D.
The Joseph Brown Whitehead Professor
and Chairman, Department of Surgery, and
Clinical Director, Winship Cancer Center,
Emory University School of Medicine;
Chief of Surgery, Emory University Hospital,
Atlanta, Georgia

†Deceased.

Preface

Although surgeons often defer to those colleagues whose technical expertise is flawless, it is nevertheless true that medical decision making based on sound anatomic precepts is the ultimate key to operative success. The best surgeons are those who draw on a reservoir of fundamental anatomic knowledge. It reflects a basic tenet for politicians and taxi drivers, as well as surgeons. In other words, "You have to know the territory." A thorough understanding of normal anatomy, anatomic variations, and the distortions caused by disease distinguishes the master surgeon from the journeyman.

There is no magic formula for mastering this knowledge, but an approach that co-mingles surgical techniques and anatomy can expedite this process. This atlas was developed with that goal in mind. We have entitled it *Anatomic Basis of Tumor Surgery* in deference to the critical role that anatomy plays in oncologic surgery today. Surgical oncology, one of the youngest branches of surgery, has developed in the last two or three decades as a solid body of knowledge. The surgical oncologist knows all too well that tumors respect no anatomic boundaries.

We believe that this book fills a void because the teaching of anatomy has all but disappeared from the medical school curriculum of today. We decided to give equal weight to anatomic knowledge and a contemporary understanding of the techniques of surgical extirpation of malignant tumors to help prevent the anatomic complications associated with surgical resection. Our contributors and bibliographic sources were carefully selected to ensure this balance.

Each chapter has been structured to include the anatomic entities related to the specific surgery of the organ involved with cancer. The basic characteristics of epithelial and nonepithelial malignant tumors, invasion, and metastasis are also emphasized.

The blood supply and lymphatics of each organ are presented in detail. We recall the wise dictum of Lord Moynihan, "The surgery of malignant disease is not the surgery of organs; it is the anatomy of the lymphatic system."[1] Although our understanding of the role of lymphatics in cancer is very different today, knowledge of lymphatic drainage is essential to clearance of local tumors for both staging and control. The regional lymph node–bearing areas are presented from a surgical-anatomic standpoint, rather than a physiologic perspective. This focus will aid the surgeon in the removal of involved regional lymph nodes.

The surgical resident, whose knowledge of anatomy is still evolving, will find this book extremely useful. Minimally invasive surgery techniques are included with the caveat that advances are being made in both technique and application and the final impact of these nascent techniques on outcomes has yet to be determined.

We hope that readers will find this unique fusion of anatomy, surgical technique, and tumor biology replete with numerous color illustrations to be particularly helpful.

Acknowledgments

We wish to thank the entire staff of Quality Medical Publishing, Inc. Karen Berger, the President of QMP, was personally involved in this book from its inception to its completion. Without her untiring efforts this book would still be in process.

We also would like to express our sincere gratitude to our four dedicated and talented medical illustrators. Alexandra and David L. Baker and Sharon and Joel Harris spent countless hours working with each of the contributors to provide artistic depictions of their surgical descriptions.

A final word of appreciation is due to our wonderful administrative assistants, Patricia McWhorter, Ali Bufkin, and Cyndi Painter, who together with Sean Moore, Phyllis Bazinet, and Carol Froman, editorial assistants, made the assembly and review of this book at all stages go as smoothly as possible.

William C. Wood
John E. Skandalakis

REFERENCE

1. Moynihan BGA. The surgical treatment of cancer of the sigmoid flexure and rectum. Surg Gynecol Obstet 6:463, 1908.

Contents

†Deceased.

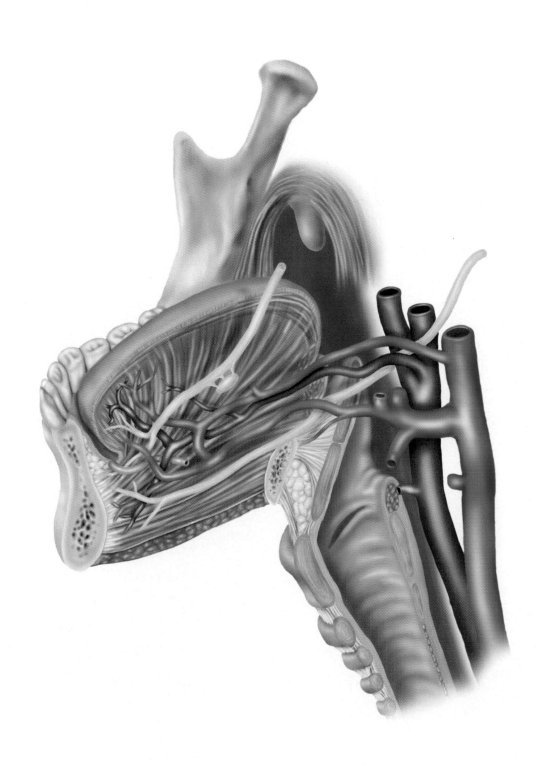

Chapter 1

Oral Cavity and Oropharynx

John M. DelGaudio, M.D.

Surgical Applications

Peroral Resection
Anterior Partial Glossectomy

Anterior Floor of Mouth Resection

Floor of Mouth Resection With Marginal Mandibulectomy

Soft Palate Resection

Tonsil Resection

External Approaches
Lip-Splitting Incision

Visor Flap

Mandibular Osteotomies
Lateral Mandibulotomy Approach to Tonsil Resection

Mandibular Swing Approach to Resection of Oropharyngeal Tumors

Total Glossectomy

Lateral Pharyngotomy for Resection of Oropharyngeal Tumors

Malignant tumors of the oral cavity and oropharynx are predominantly (greater than 90% to 95%) squamous cell carcinomas. Less common tumors include minor salivary gland tumors (especially on the hard palate), verrucous carcinomas, lymphomas, melanomas, and sarcomas. The most common risk factors are tobacco, smoked and smokeless, and alcohol abuse. Less common factors include poorly fitting dentures, poor dentition with irregular surfaces, poor oral hygiene, and papillomavirus. Malignancies of the oral cavity and oropharynx account for approximately 4% of all newly diagnosed nonskin malignancies, with a 2:1 male predominance. Approximately 30,000 new cases are diagnosed each year. Two thirds of these are in the oral cavity and one third are in the oropharynx. Oral cancer accounts for an estimated 8400 deaths yearly (Cancer Facts and Figures, 1997).

While oral cavity and oropharynx cancer accounts for only a small number of all new cancers, the functional problems created by these tumors and their treatment are significant. Oral cavity and pharyngeal dysfunction affects speech, oral competence, the first and second (oral and pharyngeal) phases of swallowing, and in some instances the ability to adequately protect the airway. Even small tumors may result in significant weight loss due to pain, dysphagia, and odynophagia, resulting in malnutrition. Dysarthria affects interpersonal communication and frequently results in withdrawal from public situations.

An important consideration in the treatment of oral cavity and oropharyngeal malignancies is the high incidence of second primary tumors. These tumors may be synchronous or metachronous, and occur in approximately 20% of patients. More than half of these second primary tumors are found in the upper airway and digestive tract, most commonly in the esophagus, larynx, oral cavity, and pharynx, as a result of the widespread carcinogenic effects of tobacco and alcohol. Second primary cancers of the lung are also common and for the same reasons. Pretreatment evaluation with chest radiography or computed tomography (CT), barium esophagography, and rigid laryngoscopy and esophagoscopy is advised to fully stage these tumors.

Staging of oral cavity and oropharyngeal tumors is based on the TNM staging system. Treatment options include surgery, radiation, and combined modality treatment. In general, early squamous cell carcinomas of the oral cavity and oropharynx (i.e., T1 and T2) are treated equally effectively with either surgery or radiation therapy. When deciding on the appropriate treatment modality the physician needs to take into account patient characteristics such as age, overall health, and whether the patient will continue using tobacco or alcohol. Those patients who will continue smoking and drinking are better served with surgical treatment, to reserve radiation therapy for possible future

Table 1-1 *Clinical Classification of Squamous Cell Carcinoma of the Oral Cavity*

Primary Tumor (T)		Regional Lymph Nodes (N)		Distant Metastases (M)		Stage
TX	Carcinoma in situ	NX	Unassessable	MX	Unassessable	I: T1 N0 M0
T1	Tumor ≤2 cm in greatest dimension	N0	No nodal metastases	M0	No nodal metastases	II: T2 N0 M0
		N1	Single ipsilateral node, ≤3 cm	M1	Distant metastases	III: T3, N0, M0, T1-3, N1, M0,
T2	Tumor 2 to 4 cm					
T3	Tumor >4 cm	N2a	Single ipsilateral nodes, 3-6 cm			IV: T4, any N or M0
T4	Tumor invades adjacent structures (through cortical bone, deep tongue musculature, maxillary sinus, skin)	N2b	Multiple ipsilateral nodes, none >6 cm			T1-3, N2 or N3, M0
		N2c	Bilateral or contralateral nodes, none >6 cm			Any T or N1, M1
		N3	Node >6 cm			

Modified from American Joint Committee on Cancer. Manual for staging of cancer, 4th ed. Philadelphia: JB Lippincott, 1992, p 29.

primary tumors or recurrent lesions. It is also important to consider the functional morbidity related to treatment (i.e., consequences of surgical resection or reconstruction). Advanced tumors, T3 or T4, or N+, are best treated with primary surgical resection and postoperative radiation therapy. Bone invasion mandates surgical resection because of the poor response of these tumors to radiation therapy. CT scanning is helpful in assessing the presence and degree of bony invasion. When cervical nodal metastases are present, neck dissection is indicated. Also, when the risk for occult metastases exceeds 30%, prophylactic treatment of the neck, whether with surgery or radiation therapy, should be included in the treatment planning.

There is no clearly defined role for chemotherapy in oral cavity and oropharynx squamous cell carcinoma. Chemotherapy is usually reserved as treatment for palliation of unresectable disease or as induction chemotherapy for advanced tumors when primary resection would result in extensive morbidity, such as advanced tongue base tumors with pre-epiglottic space involvement. Resection would necessitate total glossectomy and total laryngectomy. The role of chemotherapy continues to be evaluated.

SURGICAL ANATOMY

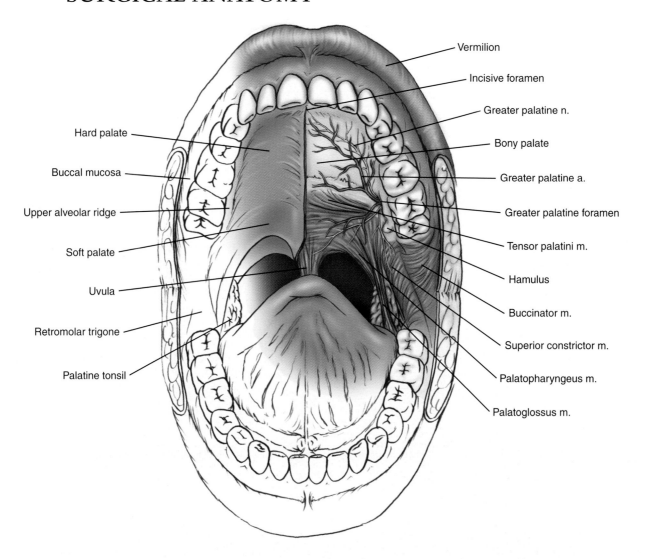

The oral cavity extends posteriorly from the lips to the junction of the hard and soft palates superiorly, the anterior tonsillar pillars laterally, and the line of the sulcus terminalis and circumvallate papillae of the tongue inferiorly. The oral cavity is subdivided into multiple entities: lips, oral tongue, floor of mouth, buccal mucosa, lower alveolar ridge, retromolar trigone, hard palate, and upper alveolar ridge.

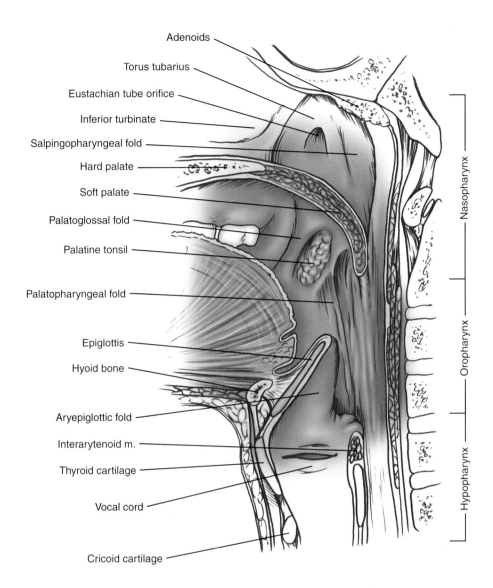

Adenoids

Torus tubarius

Eustachian tube orifice

Inferior turbinate

Salpingopharyngeal fold

Hard palate

Soft palate

Palatoglossal fold

Palatine tonsil

Palatopharyngeal fold

Epiglottis

Hyoid bone

Aryepiglottic fold

Interarytenoid m.

Thyroid cartilage

Vocal cord

Cricoid cartilage

Nasopharynx

Oropharynx

Hypopharynx

The oropharynx is a posterior continuation of the oral cavity and extends superiorly to the level of the soft palate and inferiorly to the level of the hyoid bone. The oropharynx is subdivided into multiple sites: the tonsils, soft palate, tongue base, valleculae, and posterior pharyngeal wall. Each component of the oral cavity and pharynx is discussed individually because each presents unique problems with regard to surgical resection and reconstruction.

ORAL CAVITY
Tongue

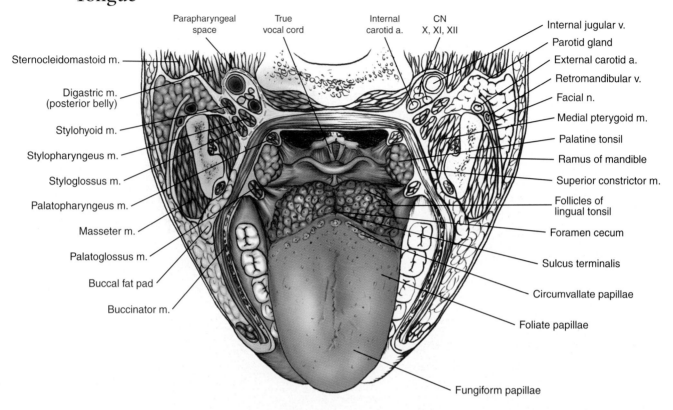

The tongue occupies portions of both the oral cavity and the oropharynx. The mobile anterior two thirds is part of the oral cavity and is referred to as the oral tongue. The fixed posterior third occupies the oropharynx and is referred to as the tongue base. The line of demarcation of the oral tongue and tongue base is at the sulcus terminalis, which is a V-shaped groove just behind the circumvallate papillae. The dorsum, or upper surface, of the tongue is velvety because it is covered by numerous filiform papillae, with interspersed larger fungiform papillae. Just anterior to the sulcus terminalis are a row of large circumvallate papillae, which contain taste buds. The foramen cecum, a small blind pit at the apex of the sulcus terminalis, represents the site of origin of the thyroid gland and may also be the site of ectopic thyroid tissue or a true lingual thyroid gland. The dorsum of the tongue base is covered by lymphoid tissue, which represents the lingual tonsils. The mucosa of the ventral tongue, or undersurface, is smooth and transitions into the floor of mouth mucosa anteriorly and laterally. Anteriorly the lingual frenulum attaches the tongue to the anterior floor of mouth. More posteriorly is the root of the tongue, which is the attached part of the tongue, through which the extrinsic muscles reach the body of the tongue.

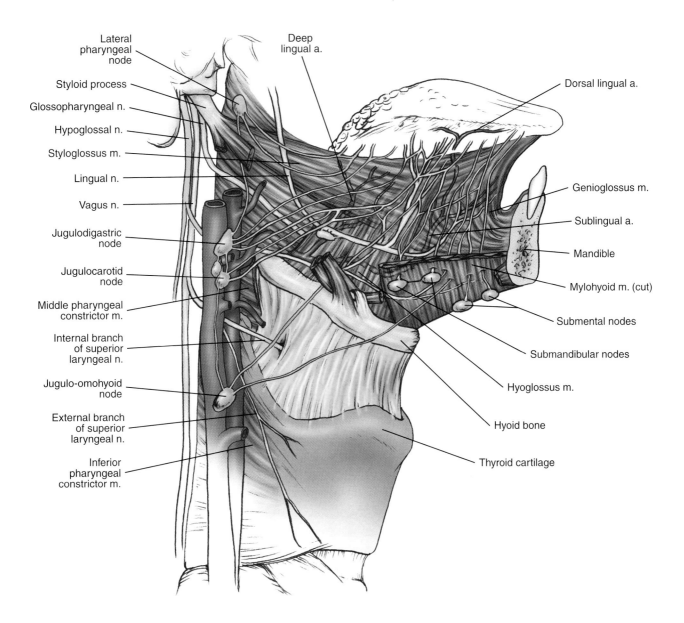

The tongue is a muscular structure composed of three sets of paired intrinsic muscles and three sets of paired extrinsic muscles. The intrinsic muscles are the longitudinal (superior and inferior), vertical, and transverse muscles. These muscles make up the body of the tongue and function to alter the shape of the tongue during speech and swallowing. The extrinsic muscles include the paired genioglossus, hyoglossus, and styloglossus muscles, which serve to move the tongue and change its shape.

The hyoglossus is a flat muscle that arises from the body and greater horn of the hyoid bone, partly above and partly behind the mylohyoid muscle, and extends superiorly and anteriorly into the tongue, interlacing with fibers of the other muscles. The styloglossus muscle originates from the styloid process and stylohyoid ligament, and runs anteroinferiorly and medially to insert into the side of the tongue. The genioglossus muscle originates from the mental spine on the inner surface of the mandible, immediately above the geniohyoid muscle, and fans out as it extends posteriorly. The lower fibers insert on the body of the hyoid bone, but the majority of fibers run superiorly and posteriorly to insert into the tongue, from the base to the tip. The palatoglossus muscles, which insert onto the posterolateral tongue, probably do not function in tongue movement (see section on soft palate). The area through which these muscles enter the tongue to attach to the body is the root. The midline of the tongue has a fibrous septum that attaches it to the hyoid bone posteriorly and provides an avascular plane that separates the two sides of the tongue. The septum is present through the entire tongue but does not reach the dorsum.

The connective tissue that separates the muscular bundles of the tongue provides a weak barrier to the spread of tumor. This results in deep invasion of the tongue by malignant tumors because significant symptoms do not occur until speech or swallowing are affected or the lingual nerve is invaded. Tumors of the tongue frequently are large before diagnosis. Also, the deeply invasive nature of carcinoma of the tongue results in greater difficulty in obtaining clear resection margins without resecting large portions of the tongue. It is recommended that approximately 2 cm of normal tissue be resected around tongue cancers and that frozen-section sampling of the margins be performed. This is especially true in tongue base tumors, which grow large before becoming symptomatic, frequently invading the root of the tongue. With invasion of the root of the tongue, surgical extirpation requires total glossectomy because all attachments of the tongue are transected with removal of the root.

The relationship of the oral tongue to the floor of mouth is important in maintaining tongue mobility. Squamous cell carcinoma of the oral tongue is most commonly located on the lateral surface of the middle third of the tongue, in proximity to or involving the floor of mouth. After resection of tumors of the tongue or floor of mouth, attempts should be made to reconstitute a sulcus between the tongue and the mandibular alveolus to prevent or minimize tethering of the tongue, allowing optimum postoperative rehabilitation of speech and swallowing. With resection of up to half of the tongue, primary closure, healing by secondary intention, skin grafting, or a thin pliable flap (i.e., platysma flap, free radial forearm) will accomplish this goal and allow better tongue function postoperatively. More extensive resection of the tongue presents more difficult problems and usually requires reconstructive techniques to restore bulk to the tongue (i.e., pectoralis major or other pedicled myocutaneous flap, or free tissue transfer). A bulky or sensate flap is necessary for reconstruction of the tongue base to prevent or minimize aspiration.

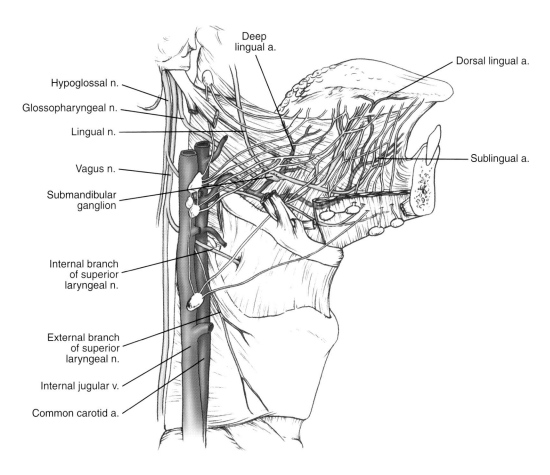

The arterial supply to the tongue is from the paired lingual arteries, which originate from the external carotid artery at the level of the greater horn of the hyoid bone. The lingual artery passes deep to the hyoglossus muscle and gives off one or two deep lingual branches that supply the tongue base. The sublingual artery originates near the anterior border of the hyoglossus muscle and continues forward between the mylohyoid and genioglossus muscles to supply these muscles, the geniohyoid muscle, and the sublingual gland. The remainder of the lingual artery proceeds forward as a dorsal lingual artery between the genioglossus and longitudinal muscles. It reaches the ventral surface of the tongue just deep to the mucosa, where it is accompanied by the deep lingual vein, which can be seen through the thin mucosa of the ventral tongue. The remainder of the venous drainage accompanies the arterial branches, ultimately joining the deep lingual vein to form the lingual vein, which empties into the internal jugular vein. Only at the tip of the tongue is there any anastomosis across the midline between the lingual arteries.

The hypoglossal nerve (cranial nerve XII) supplies motor innervation to the extrinsic and intrinsic muscles of the tongue. As is travels beneath the lateral fascia of the hyoglossus muscle, it innervates the extrinsic muscles, and as it reaches the anterior border of this muscle, it penetrates the tongue around the midportion of the oral tongue to supply the intrinsic muscles. Sensory innervation of the tongue is from the lingual nerve (a branch of V3) and the glossopharyngeal nerve (cranial nerve IX). The lingual nerve travels in the floor of the mouth above the hypoglossal nerve, between the mylohyoid and hyoglossus muscles, to innervate the anterior two thirds of the tongue and floor of mouth. The chorda tympani branch of the facial nerve travels with the lingual nerve and supplies taste to the anterior two thirds of the tongue. Sensation and taste are supplied to the base of the tongue by the glossopharyngeal nerve. This nerve enters the oropharynx laterally through the interspace between the superior and middle pharyngeal constrictor muscles and enters the base of the tongue posterior to the hyoglossus muscle.

During glossectomy, preservation of at least one hypoglossal nerve is necessary to maintain some tongue mobility and prevent severe oral dysfunction. Referred otalgia to the ipsilateral ear is a common symptom of carcinoma of the tongue because V3 (the mandibular division of the trigeminal nerve) also provides sensory branches to the external auditory canal, tympanic membrane, and temporomandibular joint through the auriculotemporal nerve. The glossopharyngeal nerve also provides sensation to the middle ear via Jacobsen's nerve.

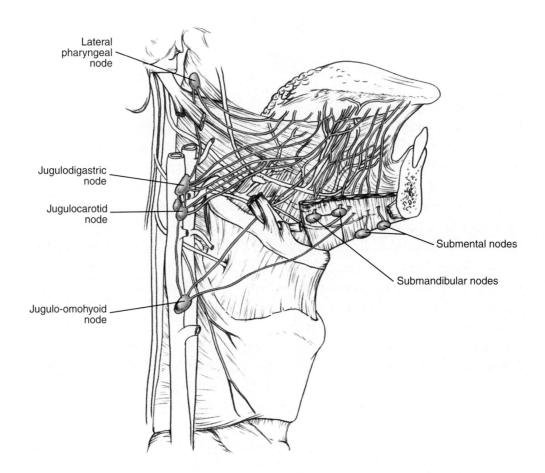

The tongue has an extensive submucosal lymphatic plexus that ultimately drains to the deep jugular lymph node chain. In general, the closer to the tip of the tongue the lymphatic vessels arise, the lower the first echelon node. The tip of the tongue drains to the submental nodes, the lateral tongue to the submandibular and lower jugular nodes (jugulo-omohyoid), and the tongue base to the jugulocarotid and jugulodigastric nodes. In addition, there is communication of lymphatic vessels across the midline of the tongue, which results in a high incidence of bilateral metastases of tumors of the tip of the tongue and the base of the tongue and tumors that approximate the midline of the tongue. The rich lymphatic network results in early metastases to cervical lymph nodes, even from small tumors (T1 or T2). Therefore consideration of treatment of one or both sides of the neck, either by neck dissection or radiation therapy, is advised in most tongue cancers.

Floor of Mouth

The floor of mouth is a crescent-shaped region of the oral cavity extending from the root of the tongue to the lower gingiva. Posteriorly it ends at the level where the anterior tonsillar pillar meets the tongue base. Anteriorly it is divided into two sides by the lingual frenulum. On either side of the lingual frenulum are the papillae of the submandibular ducts. Posterolateral to these papillae lie the sublingual folds, elevated areas of mucosa over the sublingual glands.

The floor of mouth is supported by a muscular sling composed of the mylohyoid, geniohyoid, and hyoglossus muscles. The paired mylohyoid muscles extend from the mylohyoid line on the inner surface of the mandible to insert on the hyoid bone, meeting in the midline as a median raphe. It is innervated by the mylohyoid branch of the lingual nerve. The hyoglossus muscle lies posterior and deep to the mylohyoid muscle, extending from the greater horn and body of the hyoid bone to insert into the body of the tongue. This muscle partly supports the posterior floor of mouth. The geniohyoid muscles, which are paired triangular muscles extending from the apex of the mental spine of the mandible to the body of the hyoid bone, are located in the midline floor of mouth superficial to the mylohyoid muscles but deep to the genioglossus muscles. Their lateral borders are in contact with the mylohyoid muscle. These muscles function in laryngeal elevation with speech and swallowing and are innervated by V3.

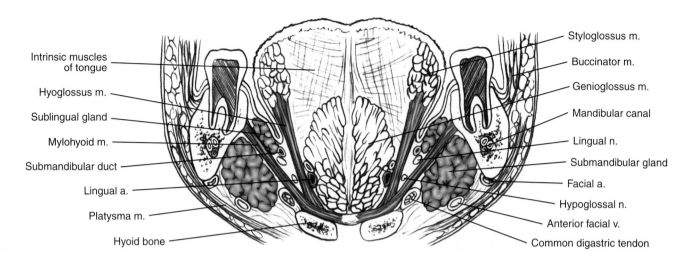

Intrinsic muscles of tongue

Hyoglossus m.

Sublingual gland

Mylohyoid m.

Submandibular duct

Lingual a.

Platysma m.

Hyoid bone

Styloglossus m.

Buccinator m.

Genioglossus m.

Mandibular canal

Lingual n.

Submandibular gland

Facial a.

Hypoglossal n.

Anterior facial v.

Common digastric tendon

The submandibular gland lies mostly superficial to the mylohyoid muscle. The space between the mylohyoid and hyoglossus muscles is an important surgical area. Posteriorly these muscles are separated by the tail of the submandibular gland, which wraps around the posterior border of the mylohyoid muscle before sending the submandibular duct anteriorly to open in the floor of mouth next to the lingual frenulum. The posterior part of the submandibular duct is surrounded by the sublingual gland. The lingual nerve, which gives sensory innervation to the floor of mouth, enters the floor of mouth superiorly to the submandibular duct and crosses it laterally before ascending on the medial surface of the duct adjacent to the hyoglossus muscle. The hypoglossal nerve always lies along the most inferior part of this plane deep to the fascia of the hyoglossus muscle.

Deep to the plane of the hyoglossus muscle lie three structures: the lingual artery, which supplies the floor of mouth, and more posteriorly the glossopharyngeal nerve and the stylohyoid ligament. The floor of mouth musculature, specifically the mylohyoid muscle, provides a fairly good barrier to the deep spread of tumor in the floor of mouth.

The lymphatic drainage in the floor of mouth arises from an extensive submucosal plexus. The anterior floor of mouth drains into the submental and preglandular submandibular nodes, with the medial anterior floor of mouth having cross-drainage to the contralateral side of the neck. The posterior floor of mouth drains directly to the ipsilateral jugulodigastric and jugulocarotid nodes.

Treatment of tumors of the floor of mouth greater than 2 cm should include treatment of the neck because of the approximately 40% risk for occult cervical metastases. For midline lesions, consideration should be given to bilateral prophylactic selective (supraomohyoid) neck dissection.

Tumors of the floor of mouth usually spread superficially to adjacent structures such as the root of tongue and the mandible prior to invading deeply into the floor of mouth. It is important to perform bimanual palpation to evaluate the depth of invasion and to determine whether the lesion is fixed to the mandible. This will allow adequate surgical planning, with resection, including a 1.5 to 2 cm margin of normal tissue around the tumor. This frequently includes resection of a portion of the tongue and may require cortical, rim, or segmental mandibular resection. The depth of invasion is important for planning reconstruction after tumor ablation, as reconstruction options are vastly different if the resection results in a full-thickness defect, connecting the oral cavity to the neck. Primary closure is sometimes possible for full-thickness defects, but more commonly pedicled flaps (i.e., platysma, sternocleidomastoid, nasolabial, pectoralis major) or free tissue transfers (radial forearm or lateral arm) are necessary to reconstitute the floor of mouth and prevent tethering of the tongue.

In resecting floor of mouth tumors attention must be given to the position of the submandibular duct. Tumors may spread along the submandibular duct to involve the submandibular triangle. In this instance, the submandibular duct and gland should be resected along with the primary tumor, usually as part of a neck dissection. If the submandibular duct is not involved but excision of floor of mouth tumor results in transecting the submandibular duct, the duct should be reimplanted into the remaining floor of mouth mucosa or the submandibular gland should be removed.

Buccal Mucosa

The buccal mucosa forms the lateral wall of the oral cavity. It consists of the mucous membranes lining the internal surface of the cheeks and lips, extending posteriorly to the pterygomandibular raphe and vertically to the mucosa of the alveolar ridges. Topographically, the only structure present is the papillae of the parotid gland duct (Stensen's duct), which opens into the buccal mucosa opposite the second maxillary molar. The buccinator muscle, which originates in the superior constrictor muscle posteriorly and inserts into the perioral musculature, forms the lateral muscular wall of the oral cavity. The buccinator muscle assists in providing oral competence. Lateral to this muscle lie the buccal fat pad and the buccal branches of the facial and trigeminal nerves.

The motor innervation of the buccinator muscle is through the buccal branch of the facial nerve. Sensory innervation to the buccal mucosa is from the buccal branch of the trigeminal nerve, with the infraorbital nerve and the mental branches of V3 supplying the anterior buccal mucosa. The vascular supply is from the facial vessels. Lymphatic drainage of the buccal mucosa is into the submental and submandibular nodes.

Deep invasion of the buccal mucosa by squamous cell carcinoma can result in invasion of the buccal fat pad. When this occurs, full-thickness resection of the cheek is necessary to obtain adequate surgical margins. Also, with deep cheek invasion consideration should be given to performing a parotidectomy to remove intraparotid lymph nodes, which may be at risk for metastases. Recontruction of full-thickness defects of the cheek may be accomplished with pedicled flaps, rotational flaps, or more pliable fasciocutaneous free flaps.

Lower Alveolar Ridge

The lower alveolar ridge is the mucosa and alveolar process of the mandible in the oral cavity. It is bounded by the junctions with the floor of mouth mucosa on the lingual surface and the buccal mucosa. It extends posteriorly to the retromolar trigone. The mucosa of the alveolar ridge, or gingiva, is tightly adherent to the underlying periosteum and bone. The periosteum provides the first line of defense against tumor spread into the mandible. The healthy dentulous mandible provides a barrier to tumor invasion into bone because of the tight periodontal ligaments. In the edentulous mandible, as is frequently the case with oral cavity cancer, cortical remodeling of the alveolus results in vertical loss of height of the mandible and areas of incomplete cortical bone that can be a site of tumor invasion.

The vascular supply of the lower alveolar ridge and teeth is by the inferior alveolar artery, a branch of the internal maxillary artery. Sensory innervation of the mandibular teeth is from the inferior alveolar nerve, a branch of V3. These structures enter the mandible on the medial aspect of the ramus through the mandibular foramen, travel through the inferior alveolar canal, and exit at the mental foramen, opposite the second bicuspid, as the mental nerve and artery. The gingiva of the lower alveolus receives sensory innervation from the lingual nerve on the lingual aspect and from the buccal and mental branches crowded on the buccal aspect. The lymphatic drainage for the lower alveolus is through the submental, submandibular, and upper jugular nodes.

The alveolar ridge is more often involved with tumor as a result of extension from adjacent structures than by primary tumor involvement. This is true of the underlying mandible also. Treatment of mandible and oral cavity cancers is an important consideration with respect to both oncologic resection and reconstruction, and oral rehabilitation. When oncologically safe, the best function and cosmesis are provided with mandible-sparing procedures, either completely sparing the mandible or resecting a partial thickness, thus preserving mandibular arch continuity. Tumors with radiologically demonstrable or gross invasion are best treated with segmental resection and sampling of the margin of the inferior alveolar nerve to ensure clear margins. If invasion is superficial and does not involve the medullary canal, a rim or cortical mandibular resection can be considered, although segmental resection is oncologically safer. Tumors that are fixed to the mandibular periosteum but are not invading bone can be safely treated with a rim or cortical mandibulectomy, in which the alveolar process and medullary cavity are removed, saving an inferior cortical rim. For tumors within 1 cm of the mandible but not involving the periosteum, stripping the periosteum and evaluating this as a surgical margin on frozen section may be adequate. If the periosteum is involved, partial bony resection is indicated. For patients who have had previous radiation therapy to the oral cavity, segmental resection of the mandible is the recommended treatment for tumors that invade the periosteum or bone. Partial-thickness resection brings with it the risk of osteoradionecrosis.

The need for mandibular reconstruction after segmental resection of the mandible is dependent on multiple factors. Lateral mandibular defects do not require reconstitution of the bony arch, in most circumstances, for adequate function and cosmesis. Patients with full dentition should undergo reconstruction of the lateral arch to restore postoperative dental occlusion. With anterior mandibular arch defects, reconstruction is necessary for adequate function and cosmetic results. This is best accomplished with free tissue transfer (fibular or iliac crest free flaps), although pedicled myocutaneous flaps and reconstruction plates may work in some cases.

Retromolar Trigone

The retromolar trigone is the portion of the alveolar gingiva overlying the ramus of the mandible. Its anterior base is posterior to the last molar. The superior apex lies at the maxillary tuberosity. It is laterally bounded by the oblique line of the mandible as it extends up to the coronoid process and is medially bounded by a line from the distal lingual cusp of the last molar to the coronoid process. This small triangular area blends laterally with the buccal mucosa and medially with the anterior tonsillar pillar. The mucosa of the retromolar trigone is tightly adherent to the underlying bone, which allows malignant tumors to infiltrate the mandible at an early stage. Also, the lingual nerve enters the mandible just posterior and medial to the retromolar trigone and may become involved with tumor relatively early. By the time of diagnosis, tumors of the retromolar trigone commonly invade surrounding structures, including the tonsil, soft palate, buccal mucosa, floor of mouth, and tongue. Conversely, the retromolar trigone is frequently involved with tumors extending from these adjacent areas. This makes it difficult to determine where the tumor originated.

Sensory innervation of the retromolar trigone is through the branches of the glossopharyngeal and lesser palatine nerves (V2). The blood supply is similar to that of the nearby tonsil, predominantly from the tonsillar and ascending palatine branches of the facial artery, with contributions from the dorsal lingual, ascending pharyngeal, and lesser palatine arteries. Venous drainage is to the pharyngeal plexus and common facial vein. Lymphatic drainage is to the upper deep jugular chain.

Hard Palate and Upper Alveolar Ridge

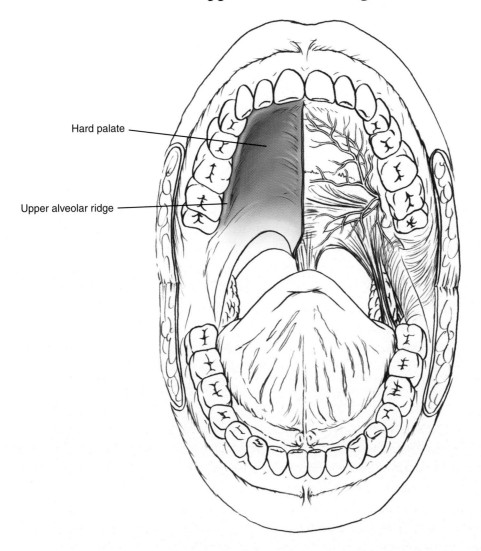

Hard palate

Upper alveolar ridge

The upper alveolar ridge is the mucosa and alveolar process of the maxilla. It is bounded laterally by the gingivobuccal sulcus and medially is continuous with the hard palate. The hard palate is the roof of the oral cavity, extending from the alveolar ridge to its junction with the soft palate posteriorly. The hard palate is composed of mucosa covering the bony hard palate. The bony palate consists of the premaxilla, which is that part anterior to the incisive foramen and includes the incisor teeth. The secondary palate is posterior to the incisive foramen and is formed by the paired palatine processes of the maxilla and the horizontal plates of the palatine bones.

Multiple foramina are present in the hard palate and transmit the neurovascular bundles. The incisive foramen transmits the nasopalatine nerve and the posterior septal artery from the anterior nasal cavity to supply the premaxilla and lingual surface of the premaxillary gingiva.

Posterolaterally, near the junction of the hard and soft palates, are the greater and lesser palatine foramina, which transmit the greater and lesser palatine nerves and blood vessels from the pterygopalatine fossa. The greater palatine nerve and vessels supply the hard palate and lingual surface of the upper alveolus, excluding the premaxilla. Different neurovascular bundles supply the teeth and the buccolabial surfaces of the upper alveolus. The posterosuperior alveolar vessels, which descend on the infratemporal surface of the maxilla, supply the upper alveolar teeth and the buccolabial gingiva. Sensory innervation to the maxillary teeth and the buccolabial gingiva posterior to the premaxilla is from the posterosuperior alveolar nerves. The labial gingiva of the premaxilla is supplied by the branches of the infraorbital nerve. All of these nerves and vessels are terminal branches of the maxillary nerve (V2) and the sphenopalatine branch of the internal maxillary artery, respectively.

Lymphatic vessels of these structures, especially the hard palate, are sparse compared with other sites in the oral cavity. Lymphatic drainage from the hard palate and lingual surface of the upper alveolus is to the upper jugular or lateral retropharyngeal nodes. The premaxilla also drains to the submandibular nodes. The buccolabial surface of the upper alveolus drains to the submandibular nodes. The sparse lymphatics draining the hard palate result in infrequent cervical metastases from malignancies of the hard palate (10% to 25%). For this reason, neck dissection is reserved for clinically positive lymph nodes.

The foramina of the hard palate provide pathways of extension of malignancy to the nasal cavity through the incisive foramen, and the pterygopalatine fossa through the palatine foramina. Evaluation of tumors of the hard palate and upper alveolus requires radiologic evaluation for possible perineural spread to the skull base. Magnetic resonance imaging (MRI) with gadolinium is useful for this purpose.

Although squamous cell carcinoma is the most common malignancy found in the hard palate, minor salivary gland tumors are nearly as frequent. Adenoid cystic carcinomas are the most common lesions, followed by mucoepidermoid carcinomas. These tumors have a higher likelihood of neural spread.

Treatment of hard palate and upper alveolar ridge malignancies, except in small tumors or those superficial tumors limited to the mucosa, may require partial or total maxillectomy. This results in communication of the oral and sinonasal cavities. Unlike other areas of the oral cavity where flap reconstruction is usually performed, palatal rehabilitation is best achieved with use of a palatal obturator or modified denture to restore oral competence.

OROPHARYNX

Along with being continuous with the oral cavity anteriorly, the oropharynx forms a tube continuous with the nasopharynx superiorly and the hypopharynx inferiorly. The oropharynx is first considered as part of the larger structure, the pharynx, and then separately. The pharynx is constructed of a myofascial framework that encloses the pharyngeal lumen and its contents. The external surfaces of the pharynx make up portions of the borders of important deep neck spaces involved in various disease processes, such as the parapharyngeal space.

The pharyngeal wall is composed of stratified squamous epithelium that covers the internal surface of the myofascial layer, which extends from the skull base superiorly to the level of the inferior border of the cricoid cartilage inferiorly. This myofascial layer is composed of three paired muscles, which are U-shaped with the opening anteriorly. These muscles form a telescoping structure, with the lower muscles overlapping the upper muscles at the inferior border. All three sets of muscles insert posteriorly on a midline posterior pharyngeal raphe, which is suspended superiorly from the pharyngeal tubercle of the basiocciput.

These paired pharyngeal constrictor muscles (superior, middle, and inferior) are covered internally and externally by fascial layers. Internally the constrictor muscles are covered by the pharyngobasilar fascia, which is thick superiorly and thin inferiorly and covers the constrictor muscles the length of the pharynx. Superiorly the pharyngobasilar fascia is attached to the pharyngeal tubercle of the occiput, extends along the petrous portion of the temporal bone, and attaches anteriorly to the medial pterygoid plate and the pterygomandibular raphe. This upper, thick portion of the fascia suspends the superior constrictor muscle from the skull base. The external surface of the pharyngeal constrictor muscle is covered by the buccopharyngeal fascia, which covers the pharynx at the level of the superior constrictor muscle and fuses below this level with the middle layer of deep cervical fascia, which forms the remainder of the external fascial covering of the pharynx.

The superior pharyngeal constrictor muscle originates from the medial pterygoid plate and pterygomandibular raphe anteriorly, its fibers extending posteriorly in a horizontal and slightly superior and inferior direction to insert on the posterior pharyngeal midline raphe. This muscle surrounds the oropharynx.

Between the overlapping layers of pharyngeal constrictor muscles are intervals through which structures enter the pharynx. The interval between the superior and middle constrictor muscles is traversed by the stylopharyngeus muscle, which extends from the styloid process and extends inferiorly and anteriorly in an oblique fashion to attach to the medial aspect of the middle constrictor muscle. The glossopharyngeal nerve, which supplies sensory innervation to the base of tongue and the pharynx, also traverses this interspace and, along with the lingual artery, runs deep to the hyoglossus muscle. The stylohyoid ligament, which attaches to the lesser cornu of the hyoid bone, also traverses this interval. This interval between the superior and middle pharyngeal constrictor muscles lies at the inferior pole of the tonsil and provides a pathway of extension of tumor to the parapharyngeal space, which lies lateral to the superior constrictor muscle.

The motor innervation of the pharyngeal muscles is from the pharyngeal plexus, which is composed of the pharyngeal branches of the glossopharyngeal and vagus nerves. The glossopharyngeal nerve supplies only the stylopharyngeus muscle and the vagal contribution supplies all the other muscles, including the muscles of the soft palate (with the exception of the tensor palatini muscle, which is supplied by the mandibular branch of the trigeminal nerve).

The vascular supply of the oropharyngeal mucosa is from the ascending pharyngeal artery, a branch of the external carotid artery. The venous drainage of the pharynx is through the pharyngeal plexus on the posterior surface of the pharynx, which drains into the pterygoid plexus, the superior and inferior thyroid veins, and the facial vein, and directly into the internal jugular vein. The lymphatic drainage of the oropharyngeal mucosa varies depending on the anatomic level. The posterior drainage is through the retropharyngeal lymph nodes (nodes of Rouvier), located behind the pharynx at the level of the carotid bifurcation. Drainage of the lateral pharyngeal structures is to the jugulodigastric and midjugular lymph nodes in the deep jugular chain.

The oropharynx is located at approximately the level of the second and third cervical vertebrae. Its boundaries extend superiorly from the junction of the hard and soft palates to the inferior margin at the level of the plane of the hyoid bone. Anteriorly it extends to the junction of the anterior two thirds and posterior third of the tongue, at the level of the circumvallate papillae. The oropharynx contains the soft palate and uvula, palatine tonsils and tonsillar fossae, base of tongue, valleculae, and lateral and posterior oropharyngeal walls.

Soft Palate

The soft palate is a dynamic muscular structure that extends from the level of the hard palate anteriorly and ends posteriorly in a midline protuberance, the uvula. Laterally the soft palate blends with the tonsillar area. The soft palate closes off the oropharynx from the nasopharynx during speech and swallowing to prevent nasopharyngeal reflux of air and food.

The soft palate is composed of stratified squamous mucosa covering a muscular framework composed of five muscles. All of these muscles, with the exception of the tensor vili palatini muscles, are innervated by the vagus nerve contribution to the pharyngeal plexus.

The levator veli palatini muscle forms most of the bulk of the soft palate. It arises from the floor of the petrous portion of the temporal bone and the medial portion of the cartilaginous eustachian tube, medial to the pharyngobasilar fascia. It travels inferomedially in an oblique fashion to fuse with the contralateral muscle in the posterior portion of the soft palate. Its function is to elevate the soft palate.

The tensor veli palatini muscle is the only soft palate muscle innervated by the mandibular branch of the trigeminal nerve and not the vagus nerve. It arises from the medial pterygoid plate, spine of the sphenoid bone and lateral portion of the cartilaginous eustachian tube, lateral to the pharyngobasilar fascia. It descends inferiorly to hook around the hamulus on the pterygoid bone and extends medially as a narrow tendon to insert on the posterior hard palate as the palatine aponeurosis. This muscle functions to laterally tense the palate and to open the eustachian tube orifice. Resection of the soft palate therefore frequently results in eustachian tube dysfunction and serous otitis media.

The musculus uvulae arise from the posterior hard palate and palatine aponeurosis on each side of the midline, extend posteriorly, and fuse as they form the uvula. Their function is to draw the uvula upward and forward.

The palatoglossus muscle forms the anterior tonsillar pillar, which is the anterior border of the tonsillar fossa, and demarcates the anterior margin of the lateral oropharynx. This thin muscle arises from the inferior portion of the soft palate, where it is fused to the contralateral palatoglossus muscle, and it projects inferiorly to attach to the lateral and dorsal tongue. Its function is to draw the palate down and narrow the pharynx.

The palatopharyngeus muscle forms the posterior tonsillar pillar and part of the posterior portion of the tonsillar fossa. It arises as two heads, from the hard palate and palatine aponeurosis and more posteriorly from the contralateral palatopharyngeus muscle. The muscle inserts on the fascia of the lower constrictor muscles. The palatopharyngeus muscle draws the palate down and narrows the pharynx, in addition to elevating the pharynx.

Sensory innervation of the soft palate is through the lesser palatine branches of the maxillary division of the trigeminal nerve. Blood supply is from the lesser palatine arteries, which are branches of the internal maxillary artery and travel with the nerve through the lesser palatine foramen.

As with the hard palate, resection of tumor involving the soft palate creates a defect that allows communication of the upper respiratory tract (i.e., the nasopharynx) and the oral cavity. These defects are best addressed with use of a palatal obturator or modified denture to close the soft palate defect.

Tonsil (Palatine Tonsil)

The palatine tonsil, commonly referred to as the tonsil, is a lymphatic structure containing indentations called crypts. It resides in the tonsilar fossa. This fossa is bound anteriorly by the palatoglossal arch and posteriorly by the palatopharyngeal arch, containing the muscles of the corresponding name and referred to as the anterior and posterior tonsillar pillars, respectively. The tonsillar fossa is bound superiorly by the soft palate and inferiorly by the base of tongue mucosa. Tonsillar tissue frequently extends superiorly and inferiorly into these structures. Laterally the tonsil has a capsule formed by the pharyngobasilar fascia. A layer of loose connective tissue separates the capsule from the superior constrictor muscle. Lateral to the superior constrictor muscle is the parapharyngeal space, of which the lateral border consists of the medial pterygoid muscle and angle of the mandible. Extension of a tumor through the buccopharyngeal fascia results in parapharyngeal space involvement. This may result in trismus because of the direct irritation or invasion of the medial pterygoid muscle.

The inferior pole of the tonsil lies at the level of the interspace between the superior and middle constrictor muscles. The glossopharyngeal nerve traverses this interspace between the superior and middle constrictor muscles at the inferior pole of the tonsil and is at risk in deep dissection during tonsillectomy.

The blood supply of the tonsil consists of five sources, all branches of the external carotid artery system. The main supply is inferiorly from the tonsillar branch of the facial artery. The ascending pharyngeal, dorsal lingual, ascending palatine branch of the facial artery, and descending palatine artery also supply the tonsil. Sensory innervation of the tonsil is through the glossopharyngeal nerve and from the greater and lesser palatine branches of the maxillary division of the trigeminal nerve. The phenomenon of referred otalgia in tumors of the tonsil is mediated through common projections of the oropharyngeal fibers of the glossopharyngeal nerve and Jacobsen's nerve (the tympanic branch of the glossopharyngeal nerve), which innervates the middle ear mucosa. Lymphatic drainage of the tonsils is primarily to the jugulodigastric lymph nodes.

Base of Tongue

The base of tongue is the posterior portion of the tongue, posterior to the circumvallate papillae and sulcus terminalis. It extends posteriorly to the level of the valleculae and is laterally continuous with the inferior pole of the tonsils. The base of tongue contains submucosal lymphatic collections referred to as lingual tonsils, which together with the palatine tonsils and adenoids (pharyngeal and tubal tonsils) form Waldeyer's ring, a first line of immunologic defense. This is an uncommon area of primary lymphoma presentation.

The sensory innervation of the base of tongue is through the glossopharyngeal nerve, which supplies general and special visceral afferent fibers for taste. The base of tongue musculature is innervated by the hypoglossal nerve. The arterial supply of the base of tongue is through the lingual arteries. The base of tongue has a rich submucosal lymphatic drainage system primarily to the jugulodigastric lymph nodes. Lymphatic drainage to both sides of the neck is common. This necessitates addressing both the ipsilateral and contralateral neck when treating tumors of the base of tongue because of the likelihood of bilateral metastases, even with small tumors.

The base of tongue extends posteriorly into paired concavities called the valleculae along the base of the lingual surface of the epiglottis. The valleculae are separated in the midline by a median glossoepiglottic fold and are bounded laterally by lateral glossoepiglottic folds, which attach the epiglottis to the base of tongue.

The remainder of the oropharynx consists of the posterior pharyngeal wall and the lateral pharyngeal wall posterior to the posterior tonsillar pillar.

Pharyngeal Relationship to Deep Neck Spaces

The oropharynx has important relationships to surrounding potential deep neck spaces, including the retrovisceral spaces and the parapharyngeal space (lateral pharyngeal space). Although not part of the pharynx, these spaces may be involved with disease that originates in the pharynx or encroaches on the pharynx. Knowledge of the anatomy of these spaces and their relationship to the pharynx is integral to understanding the surgical approaches to these spaces and the perils and pitfalls of these approaches.

Parapharyngeal Space (Lateral Pharyngeal Space)

The parapharyngeal space is typically described as an inverted pyramid–shaped space located lateral to the pharynx. Its superior extent is at the skull base, including a small portion of the temporal bone and a fascial connection from the medial pterygoid plate to the spine of the sphenoid medially. It extends inferiorly to the level of the greater cornu of the hyoid bone at its junction with the posterior belly of the digastric muscle. The superior medial border is formed by the fascia of the tensor veli palatini and medial pterygoid muscles and the pharyngobasilar fascia. Inferiorly the medial border is formed by the superior constrictor muscle. The anterior border is formed by the pterygomandibular raphe. The lateral boundaries are the medial pterygoid muscle, the mandible, the portion of the deep lobe of the parotid gland, and a small portion of the digastric muscle posteriorly. The posterior border is the prevertebral fascia.

The parapharyngeal space is divided into a prestyloid and a poststyloid compartment by fascia extending from the styloid process to the tensor veli palatini muscle. The prestyloid compartment contains lymphatic tissue, the internal maxillary artery, and branches of the mandibular division of the trigeminal nerve. The poststyloid compartment contains the carotid artery, the internal jugular vein, cranial nerves IX, X, XI, and XII, and the cervical sympathetic chain.

Masses in the parapharyngeal space are seen as fullness or bulging in the lateral pharyngeal wall, displacing the tonsil medially or the soft palate medially and inferiorly, with contralateral deviation of the uvula. Trismus is a frequent finding, especially with parapharyngeal space abscesses or large tumors, and is due to irritation or involvement of the medial pterygoid muscle, which forms the lateral extent of the parapharyngeal space. Removal of tumors in the parapharyngeal space should be performed by external approaches to ensure control of the great vessels and major nerves in the retrostyloid compartment, especially in the case of tumors that may be displacing the neurovascular structures.

SURGICAL APPLICATIONS

The most important aspects of surgical resection of oral cavity and oropharynx tumors are adequate preoperative assessment of tumor extent and reconstructive needs and good intraoperative exposure. Adequate tumor resection with a 1 to 2 cm margin of normal tissue and frozen-section control of margins requires appropriate exposure. Many approaches to the oral cavity and oropharynx are available and the choice depends on the location, size, and invasiveness of the tumor, along with the reconstructive considerations. The possible need for mandibular resection is an important consideration in choosing a surgical approach. The following sections will discuss surgical approaches to the oral cavity and oropharynx, indications for use of each approach, and specific procedures for tumor resection.

The range of approaches includes peroral, translabial, transmandibular, and transpharyngeal routes. Each has its merits and drawbacks. The head and neck oncologic surgeon should be familiar with all of these approaches and capable of utilizing the best approach for each individual case.

PERORAL RESECTION

Resection using the peroral route is limited to those tumors that can be adequately exposed, removed with adequate margins, and reconstructed through the mouth without additional incisions. This mainly includes small anterior tongue tumors (T1 or T2), small floor of mouth tumors, small hard and soft palate lesions, and tonsil tumors. Limited anterior mandibular alveolar ridge resection in conjunction with floor of mouth resection may be performed perorally, although better exposure is afforded by translabial approaches. Peroral resection may be combined with neck dissections as indicated. Deeply invasive or advanced tumors, the need for mandibular resection, and posterior oral cavity and most oropharyngeal tumors are contraindications to peroral resection.

Anterior Partial Glossectomy

To optimize exposure of anterior oral cavity tumors, nasotracheal intubation is preferred. As with all head and neck tumors, prior to tumor resection a direct laryngoscopy and esophagoscopy are performed to rule out the possibility of a second primary tumor and to completely assess the extent of the primary lesion.

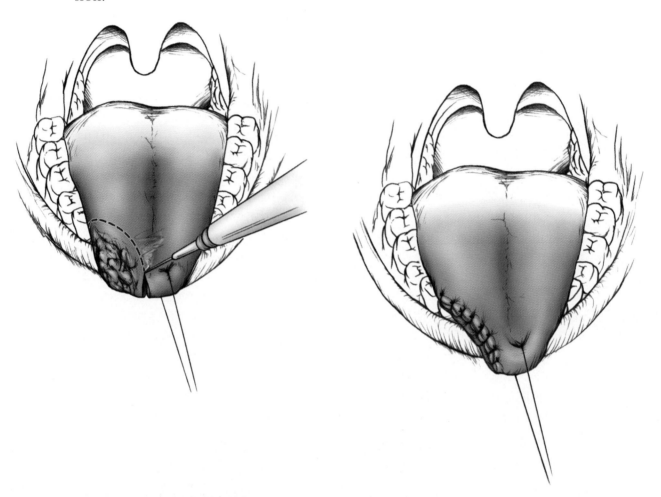

The jaws are opened using a side-biting oral retractor or an oral bite-block on the side opposite the lesion. The cheeks are retracted with army-navy or cheek retractors. The tongue is grasped with a towel clip or a silk suture placed through the tip of the tongue for anterior traction. When possible, palpation of the margins of the tumor with the thumb and forefinger of one hand is performed while the tumor is resected with an electrocautery. Care is taken not to bevel the cut toward the tumor to provide an adequate margin. For all but very superficial tumors or carcinoma in situ, obtaining a 1 to 2 cm cuff of normal tissue is preferred. Frozen-section margins are checked circumferentially and at the deep surface to ensure complete tumor removal. Hemostasis is obtained with the electrocautery. Primary closure is accomplished with 3-0 chromic or Vicryl sutures in one or two layers for lateral tongue defects and two layers for midline tip of tongue defects.

Anterior Floor of Mouth Resection

Peroral resection of anterior floor of mouth tumors is generally reserved for T1 and T2 tumors and some T3 tumors that are not deeply invasive. Mandibular invasion must not be present to use this approach, although anterior rim mandibulectomy can be performed to resect tumors approximating or adherent to the periosteum.

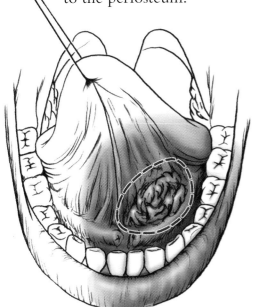

The patient is under general anesthesia and nasotracheally intubated. Tracheotomy can be performed but is not usually necessary for transoral resection or early floor of mouth lesions. For all but superficial T1 tumors, unilateral or bilateral selective neck dissections are performed prior to addressing the floor of mouth primary tumor. The alveolar ridges are retracted apart using a posteriorly placed bite-block or side-biting oral retractor. The cheeks are retracted with cheek retractors. The tongue is retracted superiorly.

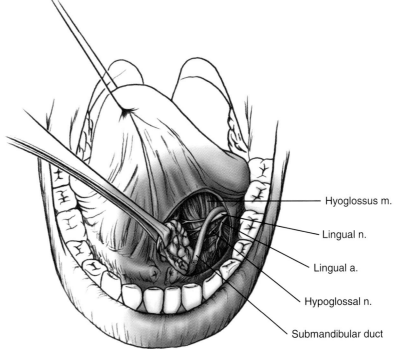

Hyoglossus m.

Lingual n.

Lingual a.

Hypoglossal n.

Submandibular duct

The electrocautery is used to make mucosal cuts circumferentially around the tumor with a 1 to 2 cm cuff of uninvolved mucosa. This frequently requires resection of a portion of the ventral tongue mucosa and musculature and possibly the lingual gingiva of the lower alveolar ridge. Submucosal dissection is carried through the sublingual glands down to the floor of mouth muscular sling (geniohyoid and mylohyoid muscles). These muscles usually provide a good barrier to deep spread of early tumors. One or both of the submandibular ducts may be transected during the deep resection. In most cases, unilateral or bilateral neck dissection will be performed; therefore these ducts do not require repair. If neck dissection is not performed, the ducts should be reimplanted into the floor of mouth mucosa with fine (5-0 or 6-0) absorbable sutures.

Attempts to perserve the lingual and hypoglossal nerves should be made, identifying them in the neck deep to the mylohyoid muscle and following them into the floor of mouth.

Prior to removal, the specimen should be marked with sutures to alert the pathologist to the appropriate orientation of the tissue. Margins then are obtained for frozen-section analysis. A scalpel or sharp scissors is used to obtain circumferential mucosal margins and deep margins from the remaining defect, not from the specimen. Hemostasis is obtained.

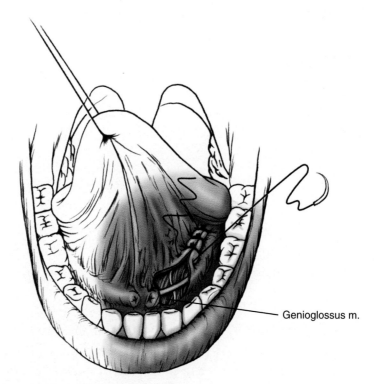

Genioglossus m.

For defects that are not through the floor of mouth muscular sling (i.e., communicating to the neck), several reconstructive options are available. When possible, primary closure of the mucosa is preferred, and this is performed with 3-0 chromic or Vicryl sutures. When primary closure is not possible or results in excess tethering of the tongue, healing by secondary intention is preferred. Split-thickness skin grafting may also be performed.

Floor of Mouth Resection With Marginal Mandibulectomy

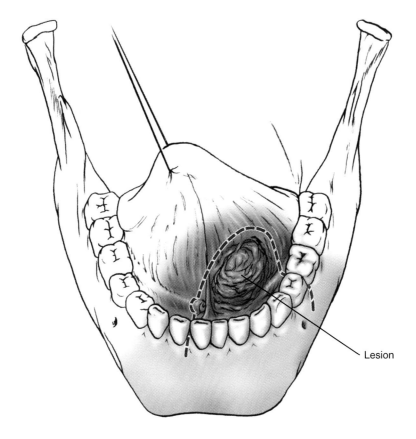

Lesion

For anterior floor of mouth tumors approaching or involving the periosteum of the anterior mandibular arch without gross bony involvement, a marginal mandibulectomy can be performed perorally, removing the alveolar process of the mandible, after exposure is obtained as previously described. The portion of alveolar ridge to be resected is demarcated by making mucosal cuts through the buccolabial gingiva down to the mandibular bone. In the dentulous patient, the teeth in the line of the osteotomy sites are extracted so that the osteotomy can be made through the tooth socket. After the teeth are extracted, the mucosal cuts are made in the floor of mouth and ventral tongue mucosa. The mucoperiosteum of the mandible is elevated on either side of the osteotomy sites, taking care not to elevate the mucosa in the proximity of the tumor.

An oscillating saw is then used to make the bony cuts, with the inferior cut angled posteroinferiorly to remove more of the inner cortex of the mandible to increase the margin of safety of the resection. The bony cuts are made completely through the bone with the saw so that the resected segment is completely free. A rim of mandible of at least 1 cm should be preserved to retain adequate strength of the residual mandibular arch. Also, performing the inner cortical mandibular cut above the level of the mylohyoid line retains integrity of the floor of mouth muscular sling.

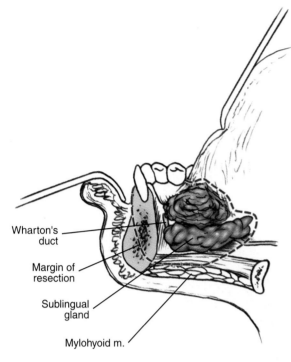

Wharton's duct

Margin of resection

Sublingual gland

Mylohyoid m.

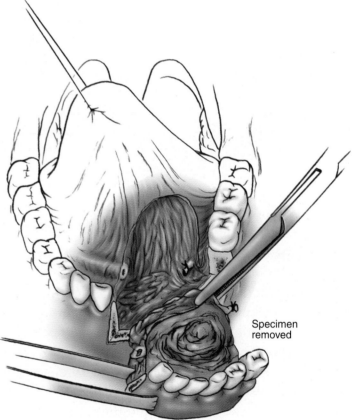

Specimen removed

After the osteotomies are made, access to the floor of mouth mucosal cuts is improved and the resection proceeds as above. When possible, the lingual nerve is preserved.

Closure of this defect frequently requires use of a split-thickness skin graft, as primary closure may result in significant tethering of the tongue. A Zimmer dermatome is used to harvest a graft approximately 0.016-inch thick, from the upper lateral thigh. The graft should be large enough to cover all exposed floor of mouth and mandible surfaces without tenting the graft, allowing re-creation of the gingivolabial and gingivobuccal sulci. The split-thickness skin graft is sutured in place circumferentially with a 4-0 chromic running suture and deep quilting sutures are used to help immobilize the graft centrally. Piecrusting of the graft is performed to allow drainage areas for serum and blood.

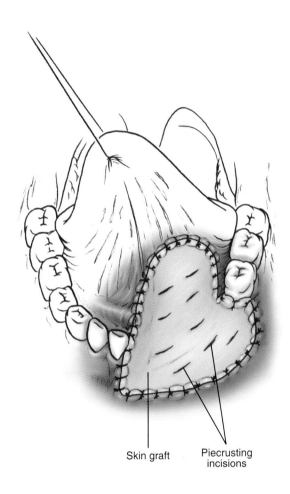

Skin graft   Piecrusting incisions

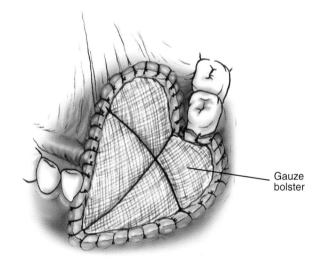

Gauze bolster

A bolster of Xeroform gauze is placed over the graft and sutured with 3-0 silk tieover sutures. This places pressure on the graft to increase the chances of graft take. The bolster should be left in place for 5 days, then removed.

Healing of the defect by secondary intention is possible, but attempts should be made to cover the exposed mandible with advancement of mucosa. Full-thickness defects that communicate with the neck may require flap closure with a platysma flap, sternocleidomastoid flap, or free tissue transfer.

Tracheotomy generally is not required unless a large amount of ventral tongue is removed, resulting in tongue edema, or a large bolster is necessary, resulting in posterior displacement of the tongue. The use of a temporarily placed nasopharyngeal trumpet to stent the oropharyngeal airway is an alternative to tracheotomy in managing the possibly narrowed upper airway after anterior floor of mouth resection. If there is any concern for possible airway compromise, tracheotomy should be performed.

Soft Palate Resection

Small (T1 and T2) posterior midline soft palate and uvula tumors can be resected easily through a peroral approach. Orotracheal intubation is performed, and the patient is placed supine with the head extended. A McIvor mouth gag is placed and opened as wide as possible. The soft palate is palpated to get an idea of the depth of invasion of the tumor. Local anesthetic consisting of 1% lidocaine with 1:100,000 epinephrine is injected into the soft palate at the proposed line of resection.

The uvula is grasped with a forceps and retracted inferiorly. The electrocautery is used to resect the soft palate, leaving a 1.5 cm margin of normal tissue. Care is taken to make the mucosal and muscular cuts through the soft palate perpendicular to the plane of the soft palate to avoid beveling, which can result in a closer margin than planned. Frozen-section control is performed, as with all head and neck tumors. If necessary, the resection can extend laterally to include one or both tonsils and tonsillar fossae. Hemostasis is obtained with cautery.

The mucosa is closed in a single layer with 3-0 Vicryl or chromic sutures when possible, or the wound can be left to granulate.

For limited resections, velopharyngeal insufficiency is not usually a permanent problem. Larger soft palate tumors that require more anterior soft palate resection result in permanent velopharyngeal insufficiency, which can be treated with the use of a palatal prosthesis to obturate the defect.

Tonsil Resection

Peroral resection of tonsil cancers is indicated for T1 and some T2 tumors that are not deeply invasive and do not involve the tongue. After direct laryngoscopy and esophagoscopy and, in the case of T2 tumors, selective neck dissection are performed, the patient is positioned supine with the neck extended. A McIvor mouth gag is placed and opened. Digital palpation is performed to determine the depth of invasion of the tumor. Local anesthetic is injected around the lesion for mucosal vasoconstriction.

The mucosal incisions are made with an electrocautery, while the tonsil is retracted medially with an Allis clamp, leaving a 1.5 cm margin around the tumor.

The superior pole of the tonsil or the superior mucosal resection edge is grasped with an Allis clamp and retracted medially. The dissection is then carried through the submucosa. At this point it is important to find the plane between the capsule of the tonsil and the musculature of the tonsil bed (superior constrictor muscle, palatoglossus and palatopharyngeus muscles), which allows a more bloodless dissection.

A Hurd elevator can be used to help bluntly find and dissect this plane by putting pressure on the tonsil from a lateral to medial direction. When this plane is identified, blood vessels are cauterized or ligated as they are encountered.

Dissection is carried out in a superior to inferior and anterior to posterior direction. For peroral resections, dissection is kept superficial to the superior constrictor muscle. If this muscle is involved with tumor, it should be resected. Since this muscle constitutes the medial border of the parapharyngeal space, which contains the great vessels and lower cranial nerves, resection of this area should be performed in combination with a neck approach for lateral exposure.

After the surgical specimen is removed, it is oriented with sutures for the pathologist. Meticulous homeostasis is obtained with the electrocautery and suture ligation with chromic sutures. Deep cautery in the tonsil bed is avoided because of proximity of the internal carotid artery. These wounds can be left to granulate, or smaller wounds may allow primary mucosal closure with 3-0 Vicryl or chromic sutures.

EXTERNAL APPROACHES

Tumors in the posterior oral cavity or oropharynx and larger tumors of the anterior oral cavity require additional surgical exposure than can be provided with peroral approaches. This requires mobilization of the soft tissue alone, or may also involve mandibular division or resection.

Lip-Splitting Incision

Surgical access to larger oral cavity and oropharyngeal tumors is limited by the size of the oral cavity opening. A lip-splitting incision frequently is used and allows excellent exposure. This may be performed with elevation of the cheek flap to expose the lateroposterior oral cavity, body and angle of the mandible, and oropharynx, or combined with an anterior mandibulotomy without elevation of a cheek flap (see p. 47).

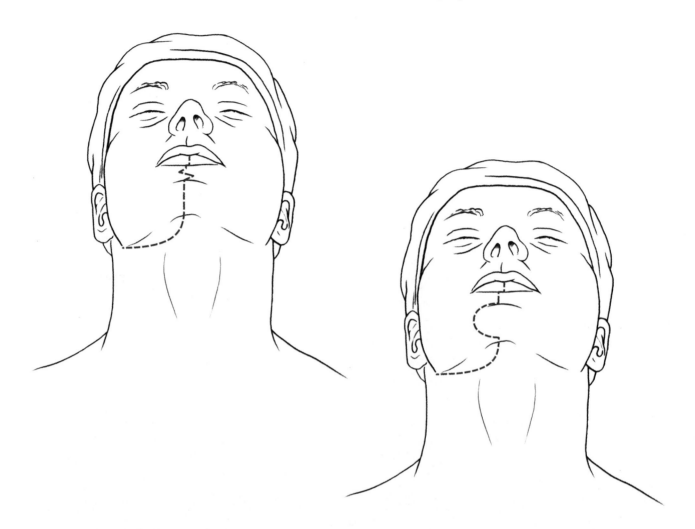

Since this type of access is nearly always performed in conjunction with neck dissection, the procedure begins with extension of the neck excision superiorly through the mental skin. The design of the translabial incision can be varied, either extending vertically through the midline of the mentum or curving around the mentum to follow the natural mental crease. I prefer to make a vertical excision through the mentum, incorporating a Z-plasty in the skin between the mental crease and the vermilion border, and a stair-step incision through the vermilion. This prevents vertical scar contraction and helps camouflage the incision. Reapproximation of the vermilion border at the time of closure is aided by incorporation of a small horizontal incision at the vermilion border. The incision through the mental skin is made down to the mandibular periosteum. The incision through the lip is performed with a fresh No. 11 blade. A stab incision is first carried through the full thickness of the lip at the horizontal limb of the vermilion border incision, followed by sharp vertical division of the lip. This transects the inferior labial artery, which runs deep to the mucosa, which can be cauterized or ligated. The limbs of the Z-plasty incision are then made with sharp stabs through the full thickness of the skin and mucosa. A mucosal incision is then made in the gingivobuccal sulcus, down to the mandible.

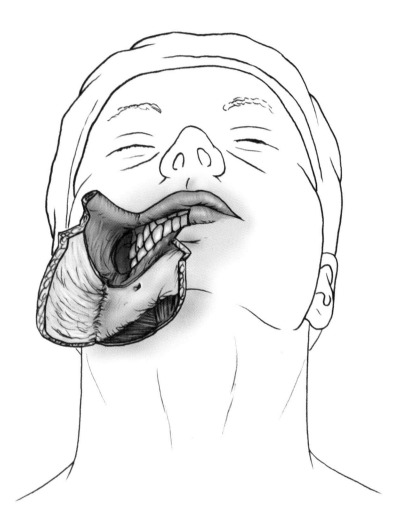

The gingivobuccal incision is carried posteriorly to the level of the mandibular ramus, transecting the mental nerve during flap elevation. The cheek flap will be continuous with the previously elevated neck flap.

This approach provides access for resection of posterolateral oral cavity and oropharyngeal tumors and can be combined with rim mandibulectomy or segmental mandibular resection. After resection and reconstruction are complete, closure first involves reapproximation of the gingival and buccal mucosa with 3-0 Vicryl or chromic sutures. The lip is closed in three layers, with approximation of the lip musculature with 4-0 Vicryl sutures, mucosal closure with 4-0 chromic sutures, and meticulous approximation of the skin, particularly the vermilion border, with 5-0 fast-absorbing gut or Prolene sutures. The mental skin is closed with deep 4-0 Vicryl sutures. The Z-plasty incision is closed with interrupted 5-0 fast-absorbing gut sutures and the mentum with a running suture. Accurate approximation of the vermilion border and Z-plasty are of the utmost importance to prevent notching and contraction of the lower lip, respectively.

Visor Flap

The visor flap provides much more limited exposure than the lip-splitting incision, allowing access only to the anterior oral cavity. Its advantage is that facial incisions are not necessary. The major disadvantage, aside from limited exposure, is the need to transect both mental nerves, resulting in lower lip and chin anesthesia.

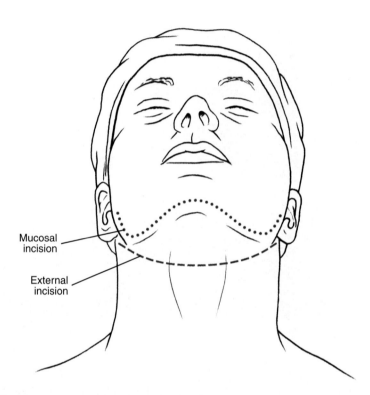

Mucosal incision

External incision

The visor flap procedure involves an external incision that extends between the angles of the mandibles, usually performed in conjunction with unilateral or bilateral neck dissection. The flap is elevated in a subplatysmal plane to the inferior rim of the mandible. An intraoral incision is then made with the electrocautery in the gingivobuccal sulcus from one angle of the mandible to the other. This mucosal incision is carried down to the mandible, transecting the mental nerves. This allows connection of the intraoral and external incisions.

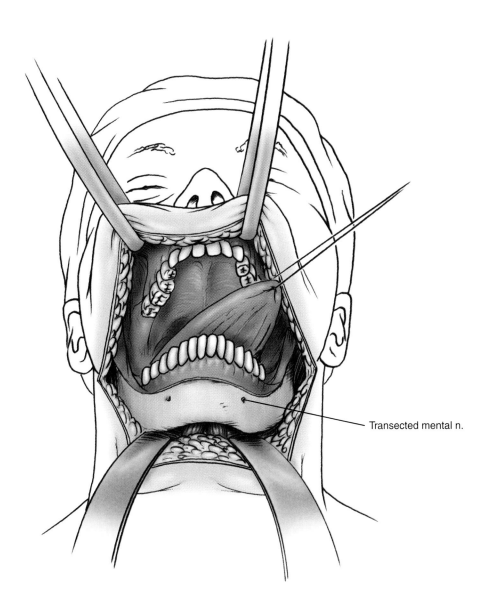

Transected mental n.

Large Penrose drains are placed around each side of the lip for superior retraction. This allows exposure of the anterior oral cavity. This is especially useful for larger floor of mouth cancers requiring segmental resection of the anterior mandibular arch. Unilateral visor flaps can be used for lateral mandible exposure for mandibulotomy, but exposure is more limited.

Closure is with 3-0 Vicryl sutures in the gingivobuccal sulcus to provide a watertight seal. The neck is closed as usual in two layers, including reapproximation of the platysma muscle and subcutaneous tissue and closure of the skin. Drainage is through the neck with suction drains through separate stab incisions.

MANDIBULAR OSTEOTOMIES

Further exposure of the posterior oral cavity, oropharynx, parapharyngeal space, and skull base is obtained with transmandibular approaches, involving transection or segmental resection of the mandible.

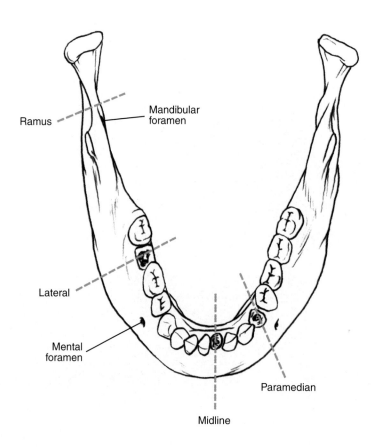

Mandibular osteotomies can be performed in the midline, paramedian (anterior to the mental foramen), or lateral (on the body or angle of the mandible) portions of the mandible or on the ascending ramus (posterior to the mandibular foramen). All but the ramus osteotomy require exposure through a lip-splitting incision or visor flap. Mandibular osteotomies also require a tracheotomy because of postoperative edema.

Mandibulotomies, whether lateral or medial, follow the same general principles. A midline mandibulotomy is depicted here. The mandible is exposed, usually by a lip-splitting incision. The mandibular periosteum on either side of the proposed incision is elevated with a periosteal elevator. In dentulous patients, the tooth in the line of the proposed osteotomy site is extracted (i.e., a molar for lateral osteotomies, canine or premolar for paramedian osteotomies, and a central incisor for midline osteotomies). Osteotomies between adjacent teeth are not performed because of the risk of devitalizing both teeth. The bony cut is marked on the mandible, designed to extend through the extraction socket. A stair-step pattern affords a greater surface contact area for osteosynthesis.

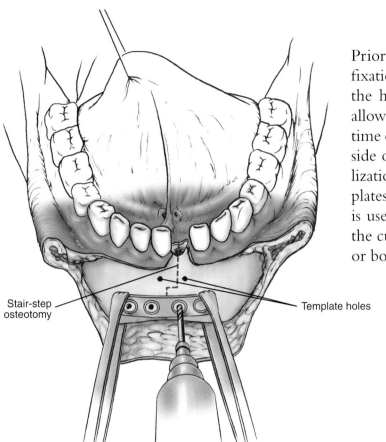

Stair-step
osteotomy

Template holes

Prior to making the bony cuts, mandibular fixation plates are fitted to the mandible and the holes are drilled and screws placed to allow better reapproximation of bone at the time of closure. At least two screws on either side of the osteotomy are needed for stabilization of the mandible. The screws and plates are then removed. An oscillating saw is used to make the bone cuts. Bleeding at the cut ends can be controlled with cautery or bone wax.

When the bone cuts are complete, the edges of the bone can be distracted away from each other. The lingual gingiva is then incised with an electrocautery, allowing exposure of the floor of mouth mucosa. Tumor excision is then performed as indicated.

After the resection and closure of the surgical defect the mandible is reapproximated using the previously fashioned fixation plates. The plates and screws are replaced, allowing reapproximation of the mandible and restoration of dental occlusion. The remainder of the closure is performed as previously described.

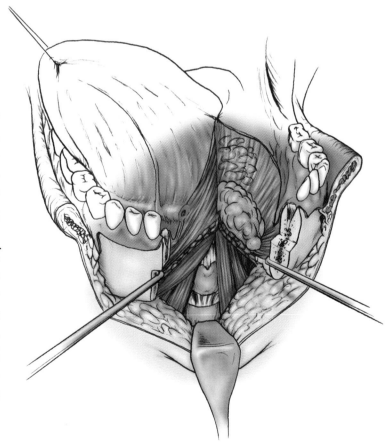

Lateral Mandibulotomy Approach to Tonsil Resection

Lateral mandibulotomy provides direct access to the posterior oral cavity and oropharynx, including the tonsil, retromolar trigone, base of tongue, soft palate, and posterior pharyngeal wall. It is particularly useful when the tumor approaches the mandible and the possibility exists for the need to perform a segmental mandibulectomy. The disadvantage is that it results in transection of the inferior alveolar nerve, with resultant lower alveolar and chin anesthesia. Here it is discussed in the context of resection of a tonsil cancer.

A tracheotomy and neck dissection are performed prior to addressing the oral cavity primary tumor. The best access for this approach is obtained with a lip-splitting incision and a lateral cheek flap, as previously described. The lateral mandibular approach can also be performed through a visor flap.

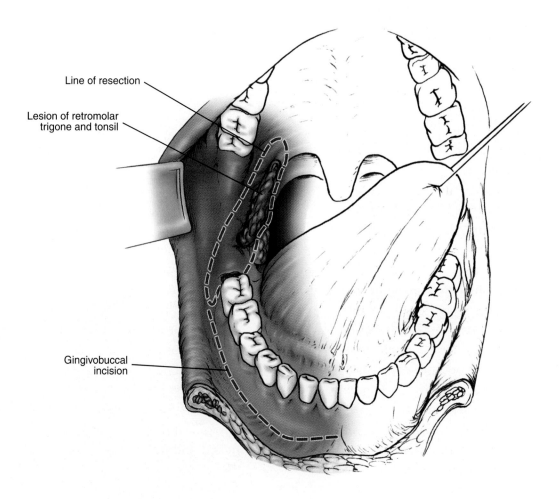

Line of resection

Lesion of retromolar trigone and tonsil

Gingivobuccal incision

If tumor approaches or involves the periosteum of the mandible, marginal resection should be performed, leaving an intact inferior rim of mandible. If this is to be performed, care should be taken in elevating the cheek flap so that the mucosal incision does not approach within 2 cm of the lateral extent of the gingival or retromolar trigone tumor margin. A mucosal incision is made with an electrocautery, leaving a 1.5 to 2 cm margin of normal tissue around the tumor.

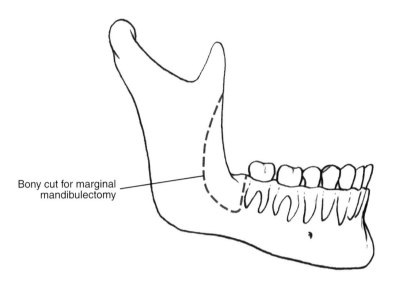

Bony cut for marginal mandibulectomy

The portion of bone to be removed is determined and the appropriate teeth extracted so that the vertical limbs of the osteotomy can proceed through the extraction sockets. The periosteum is elevated along the lateral aspect of the osteotomy site inferiorly, only so as not to elevate the periosteum over the upper alveolus, which will be resected. An oscillating saw is used to perform the osteotomies, first performing the vertical limbs and then the horizontal osteotomies. The horizontal limb of the osteotomy is angled slightly inferiorly as needed to remove more of the medial cortex of the mandible. In dentulous patients, the osteotomy site is made below the tooth roots. Care should be taken to ensure that the osteotomies are completely through the bone and that undue force is not placed on the bone to complete the osteotomies to avert possible fracture of the residual inferior cortex. At least 1 cm of inferior cortical bone should be preserved to maintain strength of the mandibular arch.

After the alveolar ridge osteotomies are performed and the bone is mobile, the soft tissue resection can proceed in an anterior to posterior and superficial to deep direction, maintaining a 1.5 to 2 cm margin of normal tissue. After the tumor is removed, it is oriented for the pathologist and frozen-section margins are obtained.

Closure of this type of defect usually can be performed with a combination of primary closure and skin grafting. Care is taken not to produce excess tethering of the tongue when approximating tongue mucosa to buccal mucosa, if it can be avoided.

Skin grafting over the alveolar ridge is frequently possible if radiation therapy has not been administered to the mandible and prevents tethering of the tongue. If greater exposure is needed, the rim mandibulectomy can be performed in conjunction with a lateral mandibulotomy.

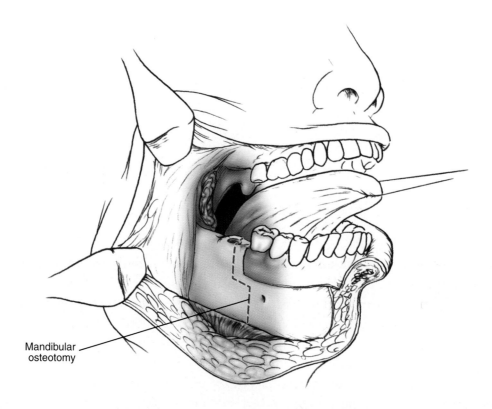

Mandibular
osteotomy

For tumors requiring more exposure but not requiring segmental mandibular resection, a lateral mandibular osteotomy can be performed. The site of the proposed osteotomy is usually approximately at the level of the anterior mucosal margin of the resection. Prior to performing the osteotomy, the mandibular fixation plates are fitted, the holes drilled, and the screws placed. The screws and plate are then removed. The osteotomy is performed in a stair-step fashion as previously described (see pp. 36 and 37).

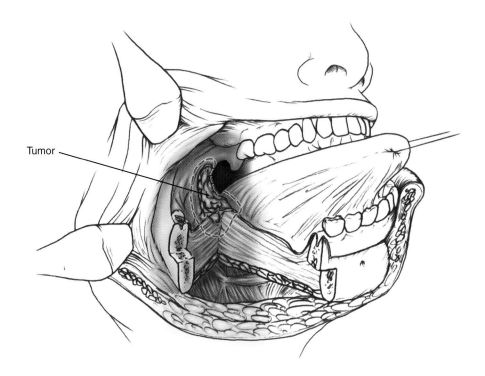

Tumor

Lateral distraction of the anterior and posterior mandibular segments allows exposure to the lingual gingiva, which is transected and the soft tissue resection performed as needed. This approach allows good access to the lateral posterior floor of mouth, posterior tongue and tongue base, tonsil, and soft palate. It also provides good access to the parapharyngeal space.

After soft tissue resection is completed, the defect is closed with either primary closure, split-thickness skin grafting, or a flap. Closure of the mandibulotomy involves replacement of the plates and screws. The lip-splitting excision is closed as previously described. The patient is given a soft diet for approximately 6 weeks postoperatively to allow for appropriate healing of the mandibulotomy.

For tonsil and other oropharyngeal tumors with mandibular invasion, a segmental mandibular resection should be performed. This is referred to as a composite resection. A lip-splitting incision is performed and a cheek flap elevation carried out as previously described.

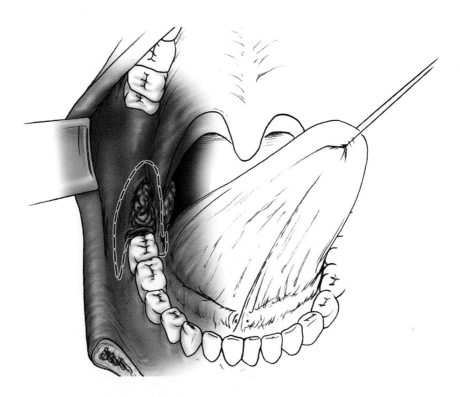

Care should be taken in elevating the cheek flap so as not to make any mucosal incisions within 2 cm of the tumor. The degree of mandibular resection is determined based on the extent of bony invasion.

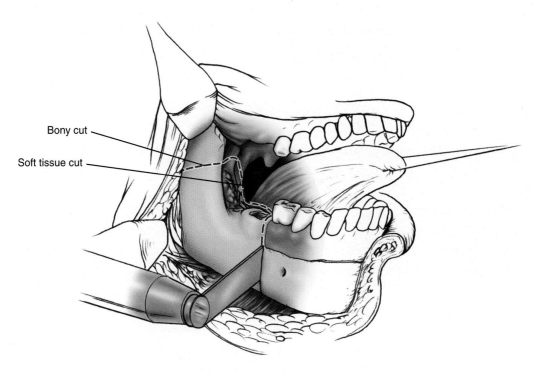

At least a 2 cm margin of noninvaded normal bone is resected on either side of the tumor. For tumors with deep bony invasion into the medullary space, the entire medullary canal from the mandibular foramen to the mental foramen should be resected, as the tumor may have spread through the medullary canal. The appropriate teeth are extracted to allow the osteotomy site to be performed through an extraction socket in the dentulous patient. Mucosal incisions are performed through the gingiva at the proposed osteotomy site. Elevation of the mucoperiosteum is performed only on the distal side of the proposed osteotomy site (on the mandible to remain). Mucoperiosteum should be minimally elevated on the portion of the mandible to be resected. An oscillating saw is used to perform the osteotomies. In segmental resections of the mandible, a stair-step incision is not necessary and a cut that is perpendicular to the long axis of that particular portion of the mandible is preferred. This usually involves a vertical cut through the body of the mandible and a horizontal cut thorough the ascending ramus. To prevent injury to the underlying soft tissues, a malleable retractor is placed on the underside of the mandible during the osteotomies to prevent the saw from penetrating the mucosa of the tongue or floor of mouth. This is especially important when performing the ascending ramus osteotomy, since deep penetration of the saw could cause inadvertent injury to the branches of the internal maxillary artery or the internal carotid artery.

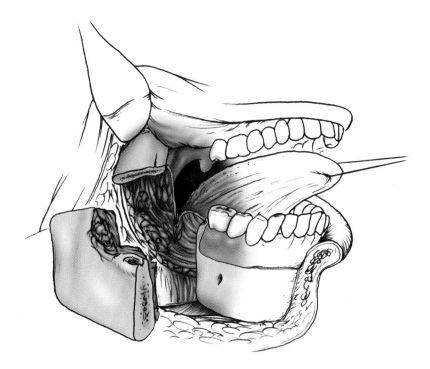

After the osteotomies are completed, the anterior aspect of the transected mandible is distracted laterally to allow exposure to the medial soft tissues. The electrocautery is used to perform the deep tissue resections in an anterior to posterior direction. The final soft tissue cuts will involve resection of the medial pterygoid muscle from the medial aspect of the mandible. For patients who have trismus secondary to medial pterygoid muscle involvement, the pterygoid muscle should be resected as high as possible from the pterygoid plates.

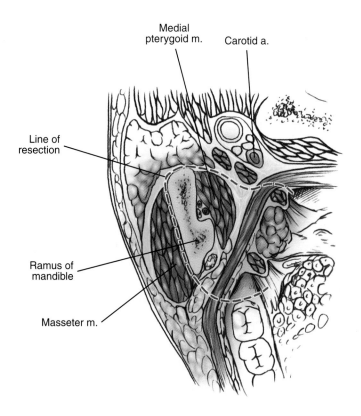

Medial pterygoid m.

Carotid a.

Line of resection

Ramus of mandible

Masseter m.

Because of the close proximity of the carotid artery to the deep tissues of the tonsil, exposure of the carotid artery and protection with a malleable retractor is necessary to prevent injury, especially during the posterior mandibular cuts and transection of the pterygoid musculature. After the tumor resection is completed, the tissues are oriented for the pathologist and frozen-section margins are obtained. Good hemostasis, especially in the area of the pterygoid muscles, is then obtained with cautery and suture ligation. Occasionally, dissolvable hemostatic packing is necessary to control persistent oozing from the pterygoid venous plexus.

Reconstruction of the defect, if mandibular reconstruction is not planned, can sometimes be performed by primary closure of the deep tissue and mucosa. Closure with a distant flap is usually necessary, especially if excessive tethering of the tongue occurs with primary closure.

A pectoralis major myocutaneous flap is the most frequently used form of closure. It provides bulk and epidermal closure, restoring contour to the lateral oral cavity and reducing tongue tethering. In most patients reconstitution of continuity of the mandibular arch is not necessary in lateral defects.

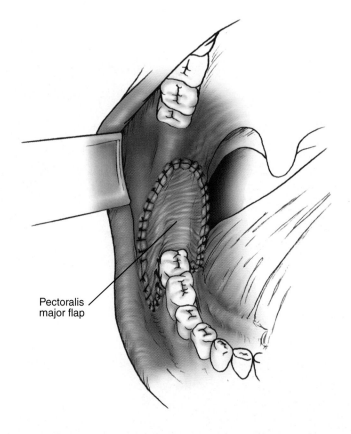

Pectoralis major flap

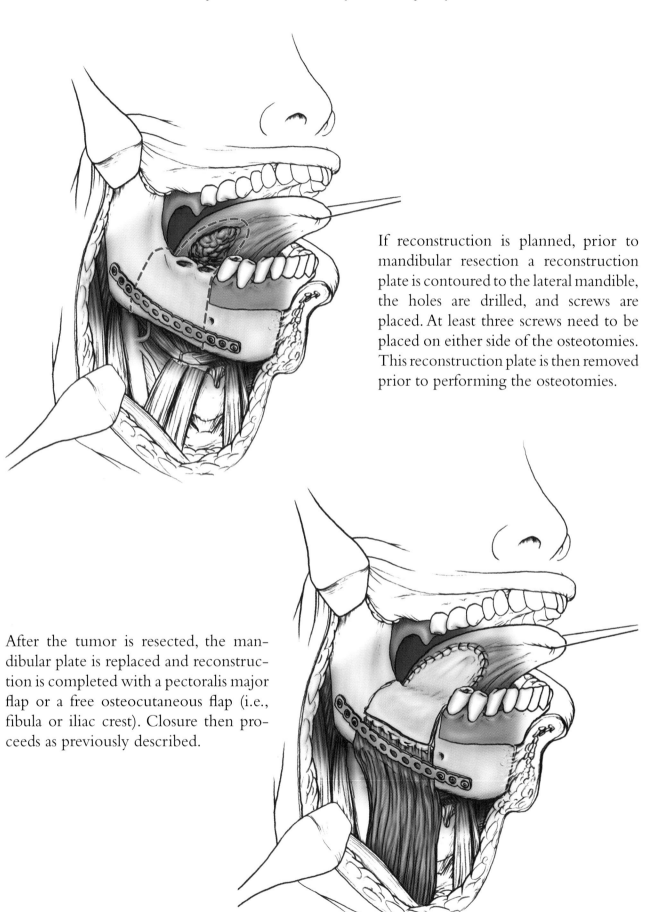

If reconstruction is planned, prior to mandibular resection a reconstruction plate is contoured to the lateral mandible, the holes are drilled, and screws are placed. At least three screws need to be placed on either side of the osteotomies. This reconstruction plate is then removed prior to performing the osteotomies.

After the tumor is resected, the mandibular plate is replaced and reconstruction is completed with a pectoralis major flap or a free osteocutaneous flap (i.e., fibula or iliac crest). Closure then proceeds as previously described.

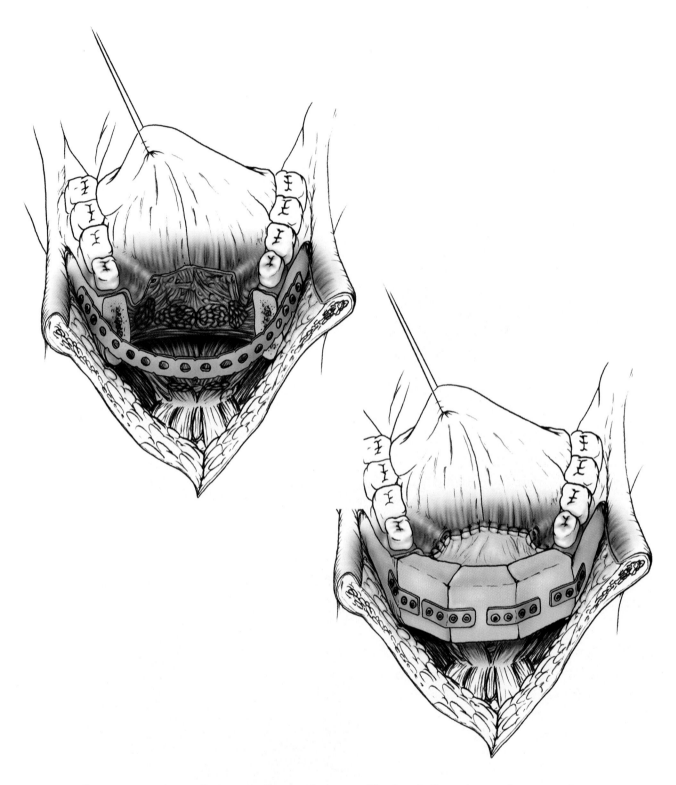

Reconstruction of segmental anterior mandibular defects (e.g., after resection of advanced lip or anterior floor of mouth tumors) is always necessary to restore oral function and cosmesis. This is best accomplished with a free osteocutaneous flap, usually the fibula free flap, but the iliac crest is suitable when more soft tissue is needed. The skin is used to reconstruct the floor of mouth, the chin skin, or both.

Mandibular Swing Approach to Resection of Oropharyngeal Tumors

The mandibular swing procedure provides excellent exposure of the oral cavity and entire oropharynx along with the parapharyngeal space. It is indicated for posterior oral cavity and oropharyngeal tumors that do not require segmental mandibular resection. If segmental mandibular resection may be necessary, this approach is not used because subsequent segmental resection would be committed to include the entire hemimandible. A lateral mandibulotomy approach is best in this situation. The mandibular swing procedure also has the advantage of sparing the mental nerve.

The procedure begins with a tracheotomy and neck dissection (if necessary). The neck incision is continued superiorly into a lip-splitting incision. If a midline mandibulotomy is to be performed, no cheek flap elevation is performed. If a paramedian osteotomy is to be used, a cheek flap is elevated only to the level of the mental foramen, preserving the mental nerve (a midline mandibulotomy is depicted).

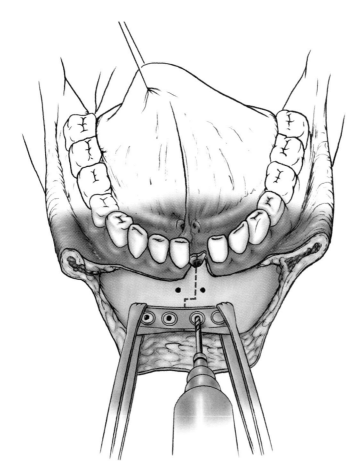

A mandibular fixation plate is fitted to the osteotomy site, the holes are drilled and screws placed, and the plate is removed. The mandibulotomy is performed through an extraction socket in dentulous patients, usually through a central incisor. After the mandibulotomy is performed, the ends of the mandible are distracted laterally, exposing the floor of mouth mucosa. An incision is made in the floor of mouth mucosa with the electrocautery from anterior to posterior, just medial to the lingual gingiva. A 1 cm cuff of floor of mouth mucosa should be preserved laterally for ease of closure at the end of the procedure. The submandibular duct orifice should be included with the mandibular segment. The deep incision is carried through the floor of mouth musculature, separating the muscular sling from the mandible. This allows significant distraction of the mandibular segments.

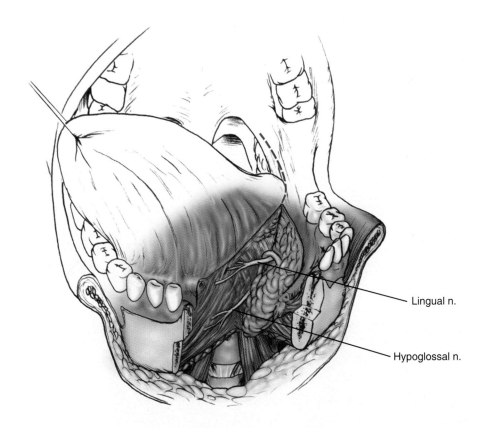

The lingual and hypoglossal nerves should be identified and preserved if possible. The mucosal incision can be carried superiorly along the anterior tonsillar pillar to include the tonsil or extended up onto the soft palate to access the superior parapharyngeal space.

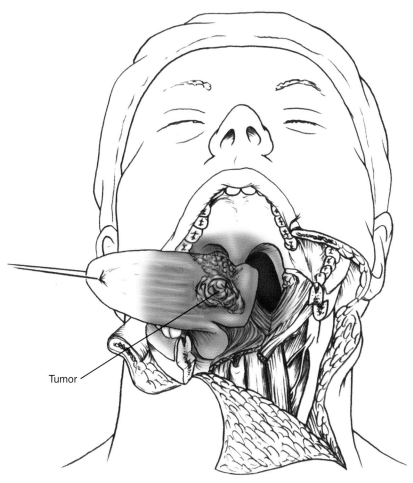

Tumor

The mucosal incision can also be carried posteriorly through the palatoglossal fold and down the lateral pharyngeal wall at its junction with the base of tongue to the level of the hyoid bone. This provides excellent exposure of the base of tongue and valleculae. The tumor is visualized and the Bovie used to resect it with a 2 cm margin of normal tissue. Frozen-section control of margins is performed.

If possible, primary closure of the tongue with interrupted 3-0 chromic or Vicryl sutures is preferred. Other options include a tongue setback procedure to move the oral tongue posteriorly or a pedicled myocutaneous flap or free flap.

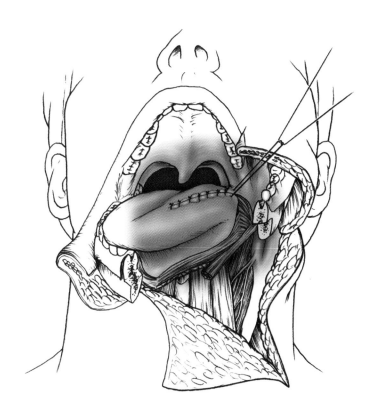

Total Glossectomy

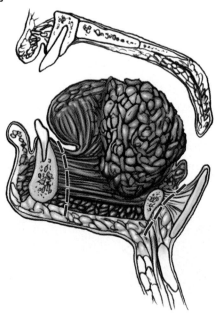

For tumors involving the entire tongue or root of tongue, total glossectomy is indicated. Total glossectomy can be performed with the mandibular swing approach by making bilateral floor of mouth incisions extending all the way back to the hyoid bone. The infrahyoid musculature is then transected from the inferior surface of the hyoid bone to release the tongue from the supraglottic larynx.

Reconstruction of total glossectomy defects requires large bulky flaps such as a pectoralis major myocutaneous flap, latissimus dorsi flap (pedicled or free), or rectus abdominis free flap to restore bulk. Other alternatives include a large sensate radial forearm or lateral arm free flap to restore sensation. The ultimate goal is to try to prevent aspiration while maintaining the larynx. Frequently after total glossectomy, prolonged or permanent gastrostomy tube feedings are required. In patients who have recurrent aspiration after total glossectomy, a laryngeal closure procedure or total laryngectomy is indicated.

An alternative to total glossectomy with a lip-splitting incision is the combined intraoral and cervical approach. Bilateral floor of mouth incisions are performed and the tongue is pulled through the floor of mouth and the posterior resection performed transcervically. The exposure for this procedure is much more limited than with a midline mandibulotomy, and reconstruction is much more difficult.

The wound is closed with interrupted 3-0 Vicryl sutures to reapproximate the floor of mouth musculature and to close the mucosa with a watertight seal. The mandibulotomy and lip-splitting incisions are closed as previously described. The neck wounds are drained with closed suction drains.

It is important in resecting large tongue tumors (i.e., hemiglossectomy or subtotal glossectomy) to try to preserve the contralateral lingual artery and hypoglossal nerve to prevent complete loss of tongue function.

LATERAL PHARYNGOTOMY FOR RESECTION OF OROPHARYNGEAL TUMORS

The lateral pharyngotomy approach is indicated for small (T1 or T2) tumors of the oropharynx, including the base of tongue, tonsil, and posterior pharyngeal wall. It averts the need for facial incisions and can be combined with a lateral mandibulotomy for further superior exposure. Inferior exposure can be extended to the level of the pyriform sinuses. The incision can also be extended anteriorly to allow complete oral tongue exposure.

Tracheotomy and selective or modified neck dissection are performed through standard incisions. After this, the lateral pharyngotomy is initiated.

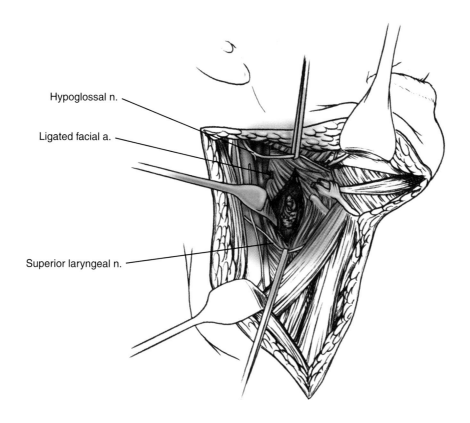

The hypoglossal nerve is identified and followed anteriorly to its entrance into the floor of mouth lateral to the hyoglossus muscle. The hypoglossal nerve is freed circumferentially from its surrounding venous structures. The overlying posterior belly of the digastric and stylohyoid muscles is transected. The ansa hypoglossi branch of the hypoglossal nerve is transected. This allows the hypoglossal nerve to be retracted superiorly out of the field. The facial and lingual arteries are ligated at their origin from the external carotid artery. The superior laryngeal nerve is identified at the level of the greater horn of the hyoid bone and mobilized along its course from the carotid sheath to its entrance through the thyrohyoid membrane. The hyoid bone may be freed from its attachments to the middle constrictor muscle and the greater horn or half of the hyoid bone removed.

A vertical incision is made through the middle constrictor muscle, exposing the mucosa. The mucosa is then incised in an area at least 1.5 cm from the tumor. Intraoral palpation with a finger in the oropharynx may assist in determining a safe area for the mucosal incision.

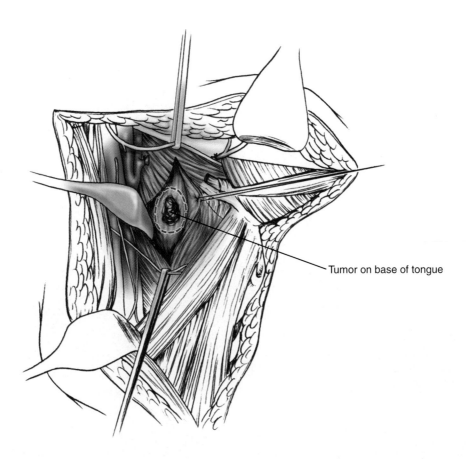

Tumor on base of tongue

After the mucosa is opened, the tumor can be visualized with good headlight illumination through the pharyngotomy. Mucosal incisions are then carried out, leaving a margin of normal mucosa at least 1.5 to 2 cm around the tumor. In the case of a tongue base tumor, a vertical pharyngotomy is performed, exposing the base of tongue. The tumor is then excised under direct visualization. As mentioned, more anterior exposure can be obtained by incising the floor of mouth musculature and the mucosa along the gingivolingual sulcus or by performing a lateral mandibulotomy.

After the tumor is resected, frozen-section margins are evaluated. Good hemostasis is obtained. Closure of the defect depends on the extent of tissue loss.

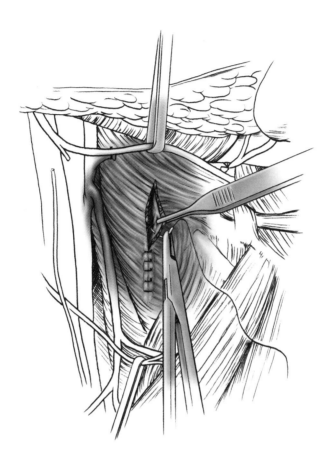

When possible, primary closure is preferred, but for large defects flap closure is necessary.

When primary closure is performed, the lateral pharyngeal wall mucosa is closed with interrupted 3-0 Vicryl sutures, with an attempt to evert the mucosal edges toward the pharyngeal lumen. The middle and superior constrictor muscles and the digastric and stylohyoid muscles are reapproximated with 3-0 Vicryl sutures. This reinforces the mucosal closure. The neck is drained with suction drains, which are kept away from the site of mucosal closure to prevent formation of a fistula. The neck is then closed as previously described.

Care is taken during the lateral pharyngotomy approach to avoid injury to the hypoglossal and superior laryngeal nerves, as injury to these structures can result in significant swallowing problems and aspiration postoperatively.

Anatomic Basis of Complications

- Because of the proximity of the carotid artery system and the internal jugular vein and its branches, there is the risk of significant bleeding. Repair or ligation of these vessels should be performed when necessary, and the internal carotid artery may require stenting or grafting. Airway obstruction can be the result of dislodgement of the endotracheal tube. Most major procedures on the oral cavity and oropharynx should include a tracheotomy. This allows bypassing the upper aerodigestive tract and minimizes the chance of airway obstruction.

- Airway obstruction can result secondary to soft tissue edema of the oral cavity or laryngeal or pharyngeal structures postoperatively, or as a result of compression of these structures due to hematoma or fluid collection. The likelihood of airway obstruction is essentially eliminated when a tracheotomy is performed as part of the surgical procedure. In those patients who do not undergo tracheotomy, oral cavity and oropharyngeal edema can sometimes be bypassed using a nasal or nasopharyngeal trumpet.

- Oral and pharyngeal dysfunction can result in significant postoperative problems in patients who have undergone upper aerodigestive tract surgery. This can be the result of cranial nerve injuries such as injury to the hypoglossal nerves, causing tongue weakness or paralysis; the glossopharyngeal nerve, causing pharyngeal hypesthesia; or the vagus nerve, causing poor pharyngeal phase of swallowing and vocal cord paralysis. In addition oral and pharyngeal tissue volume loss can significantly affect swallowing. Tethering of the tongue as a result of tight mucosal closure or tissue loss can also reduce swallowing efficiency. All of these factors can result in dysphagia, dysarthria, and possibly aspiration and subsequent aspiration pneumonia. Avoidance of postoperative oral feedings and use of a nasogastric or gastrostomy tube should be considered until the patient is able to safely swallow and protect the airway.

- Orocutaneous or pharyngocutaneous fistulas are tracts that extend from the mucosal surface to the skin. Multiple factors, including malnutrition and underlying microvascular disease, in the head and neck cancer patient may predispose to the development of this problem. Other factors that may lead to fistula include mucosal closure under tension, incomplete mucosal closure, infection, and the presence of a foreign body or residual tumor. Also hypothyroidism increases the likelihood of fistula formation. Initial treatment for a fistula includes conservative treatments such as external and/or internal packing of the wound to allow granulation or placement of a compression dressing to prevent further drainage. The patient should not have anything by mouth until the fistula is healed.

Anatomic Basis of Complications—cont'd

- Mandibular complications may occur as a result of osteotomies or poor wound healing. Malocclusion can occur when a mandibular osteotomy site is not appropriately realigned. This can be minimized by accurate placement of mandibular fixation plates prior to performing an osteotomy to allow accurate reapproximation after the procedure has been completed. Nonunion or malunion of the mandible may occur as a result of inadequate bone contact or mobility at the reapproximated bone edges. Again, accurate realignment and fixation of the osteotomized bone will prevent this complication. Also full mucosal closure over the osteotomy site will minimize the chances of this complication. The patient should be maintained on a soft diet for approximately 6 weeks after mandibular osteotomies. Mandibular fracture may result if a partial rim or cortical mandibulectomy has been performed but an inadequate amount of bone remains to support the mandibular arch.

- Loss of a pedicled myocutaneous flap or free tissue flap can result. Avoiding compression of the vascular pedicle is extremely important in the postoperative period. Surveillance of the capillary refill and venous drainage of the flap is necessary to ensure early detection of flap complications.

KEY REFERENCES

Baker SR. Malignant neoplasms of the oral cavity. In Cummings CW, Fredrickson JM, Harker LA, eds. Otolaryngology—Head and Neck Surgery, 2nd ed. St Louis: Mosby–Year Book, 1993, pp 1248-1305.

This extensive chapter provides a thorough presentation of the anatomy of the oral cavity, incidence and presentation of oral cavity tumors, and treatment options, including reconstructive considerations.

Hughes CJ, Gallo O, Spiro RH, et al. Management of occult neck metastases in oral cavity squamous carcinoma. Am J Surg 166:380-383, 1993.

The authors report on the risk for recurrence of squamous cell carcinoma in the neck after neck dissection because of oral cavity primaries. The neck failure rate was twice as high (26%) in patients who did not have a neck dissection at the time of treatment of the primary tumor but at the subsequent appearance of neck metastases. Those patients who underwent elective neck dissection (N0 disease) or therapeutic neck dissection (N+ disease) at the time of initial treatment had neck failure rates of 16% and 15%, respectively. The authors advocate that elective neck dissection (even with T1 oral cavity tumors, especially of the tongue) enhances regional control and improves the patient's quality of survival. No survival advantage was noted in this study.

Spiro RH, Gerold FP, Strong EW. Mandibular "swing" approach for oral and oropharyngeal tumors. Head Neck Surg 3:371-378, 1981.
The versatile median mandibulotomy with paralingual extension, or mandibular "swing"
procedure, is described for the resection of oral cavity and oropharyngeal tumors. A review of
65 patients is presented. The procedure is indicated for tumors not involving the mandible
that are not suitable for transoral resection. Morbidity is reduced compared with that with
segmental mandibulotomy and exposure is equivalent.

Thawley SE, O'Leary M. Malignant neoplasms of the oropharynx. In Cummings CW,
Fredrickson JM, Harker LA, eds. Otolaryngology—Head and Neck Surgery, 2nd
ed. St. Louis: Mosby–Year Book, 1993, pp 1306-1354.
This chapter thoroughly describes the anatomic and functional considerations of oropharyn-
geal cancer, with emphasis on surgical treatment and reconstruction. Additional surgical ap-
proaches, including the midline labiomandibular glossotomy and transhyoid pharyngotomy,
are described.

Urken ML. Composite free flaps in oromandibular reconstruction: Review of the literature. Arch Otolaryngol Head Neck Surg 117:724-732, 1991.
This article provides an overview of the options in oral cavity and oropharynx reconstruc-
tion, with emphasis on microvascular free tissue transfer.

SUGGESTED READINGS

American Joint Commission on Cancer. Manual for Staging of Cancer, 4th ed.
Philadelphia: JB Lippincott, 1992, p 27.

Ariyan S. Pectoralis major, sternomastoid, and other musculocutaneous flaps for head
and neck reconstruction. Clin Plast Surg 7(1):89-109, 1980.

Brennan CT, Sessions DG, Spitznagel EL, et al. Surgical pathology of the oral cavity
and oropharynx. Laryngoscope 101:1175-1197, 1991.

Byers RM. Anatomic correlates in head and neck surgery. The lateral pharyngotomy.
Head Neck 16(5):460-462, 1994.

Cunningham NJ, Johnson JT, Myers EN, et al. Cervical lymph node metastasis after
local excision of early squamous carcinoma of the oral cavity. Am J Surg 152:361-
366, 1986.

Day GL. Oral cavity and pharynx. In Cancer—Rates and Risks, 4th ed. Bethesda,
Md.: 1996, pp 175-178.

Day GL, Blot WJ. Second primary tumors in patients with oral cancer. Cancer 70:14-
19, 1992.

Derrick AJ, Haughey BH. Carcinoma of the base of the tongue. In Gates GA, ed.
Current Therapy in Otolaryngology—Head and Neck Surgery, 5th ed. St. Louis:
Mosby–Year Book, 1994, pp 277-283.

Esclamado RM, Burkey BB, Carroll WR, et al. The plastysma myocutaneous flap: Indications and caveats. Arch Otolaryngol Head Neck Surg 120(1):32-35, 1994.

Graney DO, Petruzzelli GJ, Myers EN. In Cummings CW, Fredrickson JM, Harker
LA, eds. Otolaryngology—Head and Neck Surgery, 2nd ed. St. Louis: Mosby–Year
Book, 1993, pp 1101-1112.

Hollinshead WH, Rosse C. Textbook of Anatomy, 4th ed. New York: Harper & Row,
1985, pp 906-909.

Johnson JT, Leipzig B, Cummings CW. Management of T1 carcinoma of the anterior aspect of the tongue. Arch Otolaryngol 106:249-251, 1980.

Koch WM, Lee DJ, Eisele DW, et al. Chemoradiotherapy for organ preservation in oral and pharyngeal carcinoma. Arch Otolaryngol Head Neck Surg 121(9):974-980, 1995.

Komisar A. The functional result of mandibular reconstruction. Laryngoscope 100:364-374, 1990.

McGregor IA, MacDonald DG. Spread of squamous cell carcinoma to the nonirradiated edentulous mandible—A preliminary report. Head Neck Surg 9:157-161, 1987.

Moore DM, Calcaterra T. Cancer of the tongue base treated by a transpharyngeal approach. Ann Otol Rhino Laryngol 99(4 Pt 1):300-303.

Olsen KD. Tumors and surgery of the parapharyngeal space. Laryngoscope 104(5 Pt 2 Suppl 63):1-28.

Urken ML, Buchbinder D, Weinberg H, et al. Functional evaluation following microvascular oromandibular reconstruction of the oral cancer patient: A comparison study of reconstructed and nonreconstructed patients. Laryngoscope 101:935-950, 1991.

Weber RS, Ohlms L. Functional results after total or near total glossectomy with laryngeal preservation. Arch Otolaryngol Head Neck Surg 117:512-515, 1991.

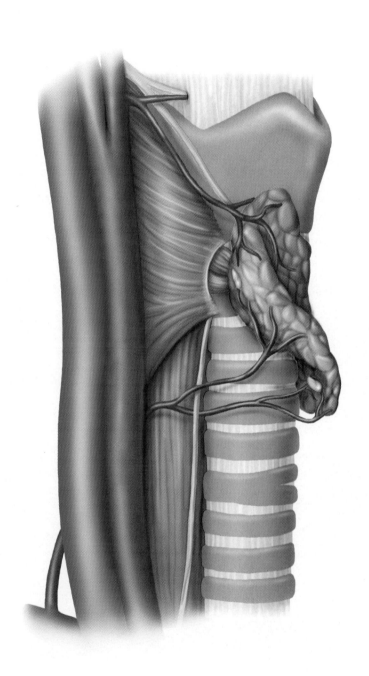

Neck

Anterior Neck

Collin J. Weber, M.D., and †William C. McGarity, M.D.

Lateral Neck

Grant W. Carlson, M.D.

Surgical Applications

Anterior Neck

Thyroidectomy

Subtotal Thyroidectomy

Modified Neck Dissection

Resection of Substernal
  Goiter

Parathyroidectomy

Lateral Neck

Radical Neck Dissection

Modified Neck Dissection

Parotidectomy

Submandibular Gland
  Resection

Carotid Body Tumor
  Resection

Tracheostomy

†Deceased.

B ecause of the nature of the tumors involved, the neck is discussed in two sections. The section on the anterior neck describes primarily tumors of the thyroid and parathyroid glands. The section on the lateral neck describes anatomy and procedures related to tumors of the salivary glands and metastatic neoplasms involving the lymphatic vessels, the nerves, and vascular structures of the neck.

Anterior Neck

Collin J. Weber, M.D., and †William C. McGarity, M.D.

Surgical resection remains the treatment of choice for most thyroid and parathyroid tumors. Goiters and thyroid nodules are problems of enormous magnitude, present in more than 7% of the world's population. Tracheal compression from goiter may respond only to thyroidectomy, and thyroid nodules may harbor carcinoma, occurring in approximately 20% of solitary thyroid nodules and 5% of multinodular goiters. Thyroid nodules have an annual incidence of 40 per million (approximately 12,000 new cases occur each year in the United States). The overall mortality is low, four per million per year (approximately 1000 deaths per year in the United States). However, this is a disease that most often affects women in the prime of life, frequently before age 40 years, and the average 10-year mortality for follicular thyroid carcinoma is 29%.

Total or subtotal thyroidectomy is the mainstay of therapy for thyroid carcinoma. Patient survival is statistically better following bilateral thyroidectomy than after unilateral thyroidectomy. Application of total thyroidectomy for this disease requires that the surgeon have detailed knowledge of the anatomy of the thyroid and parathyroid glands and the recurrent and superior laryngeal nerves.

For the most part, goiter is a benign process, responsive to iodine repletion therapy. However, subtotal or total thyroidectomy is conventional therapy for hyperthyroidism and symptomatic goiter, particularly when airway compromise is present. Thyroid lobectomy is reserved for benign thyroid nodules.

Hyperparathyroidism (due to solitary adenomas or hyperplasia involving multiple parathyroid glands) occurs in about one patient per 1000 (4:1 female predominance). Symptoms are multiple (renal stones and bone disease), and parathyroidectomy is the treatment of choice. More than 95% of patients can be cured with a single well-planned neck exploration. However, success depends on the surgeon's knowledge of anatomic variations in location and number of parathyroid glands and locations of the laryngeal nerves.

†Deceased.

EMBRYOLOGY OF THE THYROID AND PARATHYROID GLANDS

It is essential that the surgeon treating thyroid and parathyroid diseases be familiar with their embryology. The thyroid gland originates from the midline of the pharyngeal anlage, the foramen cecum. A process of evagination takes place, and the thyroid divides into two lobes, connected by an isthmus, that migrate caudad to the normal paratracheal location.

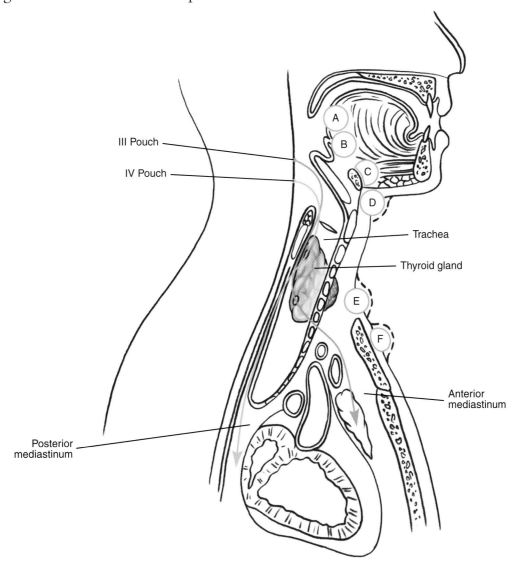

The migratory tract of the thyroid, the thyroglossal duct, begins at the base of tongue and runs adjacent to or through the hyoid bone. Normally the epithelium of the thyroglossal duct disappears. Occasionally it remains, and at any site along the duct, cysts, fistulas, or ectopic thyroid tissue may develop. Thyroglossal cysts may be located in front of the foramen cecum, at the foramen cecum, in the suprahyoid area, in the infrahyoid area, in the area of the thyroid gland, and in the suprasternal area.

Embryologically the superior glands migrate from the fourth branchial pouches with the lateral lobes of the thyroid, and the inferior glands migrate from the third branchial pouches with the thymus. Because of their embryonal motility, the inferior parathyroid glands have a more variable location than the superior glands. As illustrated, abnormal migration of the inferior parathyroids may cause them to descend into the anterior mediastinum, frequently within the thymus, and superior parathyroids often descend into the paraesophageal posterior mediastinum. The inferior gland may not descend completely and reside near the upper pole of the thyroid, often with a remnant of undescended thymic tissue. Rarely a parathyroid gland may be intrathyroidal (1%).

SURGICAL ANATOMY

The skin of the anterior neck is innervated by the cervical plexus and has transverse skinfolds, which may be used as sites for an inconspicuous skin incision. Since there is little tension in the longitudinal axis of the neck, horizontal incisions are preferable in thyroid surgery.

The blood supply to the skin of the neck is abundant, and loss of skin from compromise of the circulation is rare. The amount of subcutaneous fat is variable and tends to be more prominent in the mid-region, between the platysma muscles. Unless the cervical plexus is damaged, there is rarely loss of sensation in the upper flap following thyroidectomy.

The platysma muscle lies in the superficial fascia anterolateral in the neck and is innervated by the descending branch of the seventh nerve, which exits at the lower pole of the parotid gland, near the posterior facial vein. There it is associated with the mandibular branch of the facial nerve. If this descending branch is surgically sacrificed, skin tone of the neck is impaired. If the mandibular branch is injured, the depressor muscle of the corner of the mouth cannot function, and the lateral lower lip will elevate with smiling. If the platysma is transected in the submandibular region, slight weakness of the lower lip may result because the platysma muscle fibers blend with the depressor muscle.

The so-called strap muscles include the sternohyoid, sternothyroid, and omohyoid muscles, all of which are innervated by the ansa hypoglossi nerve. The thyrohyoid muscle is innervated by the hypoglossi nerve.

The sternohyoid muscles are on either side of the midline and arise from the clavicle and posterior manubrium. They run superiorly to insert on the lower border of the hyoid. The two bellies usually separate slightly at the sternal notch. The raphae may be displaced with one-sided thyroid enlargement, and the midline may be difficult to locate. The raphae are thus more easily identified at the hyoid or at the level of the thyroid notch. This muscle acts to depress the hyoid bone.

The sternothyroid muscles also arise from the posterior aspect of the manubrium and run superiorly over the lobes of the thyroid, deep to the sternohyoid, to insert on the lower border of the thyroid cartilage. Their action is to depress the larynx after deglutition.

The omohyoid muscle has an inferior and a superior belly and a common tendon on each side of the larynx and thyroid. The inferior belly arises from the upper border of the scapula and suprascapular ligament and crosses obliquely the lower posterior triangle of the neck deep to the sternomastoid. It ends in a common tendon with the superior belly. At this point, it crosses the carotid sheath attached to the deep cervical fascia. It continues superiorly as the superior belly, alongside the sternohyoid, and inserts on the lateral aspect of the body of the hyoid bone. It stabilizes the hyoid bone in deglutition.

The thyrohyoid muscles arise just above the insertion of the sternothyroid on the thyroid cartilage and cover the ala and the thyrohyoid membrane to insert on the hyoid bone. These muscles may elevate the larynx or depress the hyoid, depending on the extent of fixation of the suprahyoid muscles.

All strap muscles may be removed, divided, or denervated without serious changes in respiration, deglutition, or voice. Some surgeons routinely divide the strap muscles in all thyroidectomies to obtain adequate exposure of the gland and the superior pole vessels. This step is rarely necessary, except with extremely large, diffusely toxic glands or huge nodular goiters with large substernal components.

Adequate exposure of the superior pole vessels can be readily obtained by dividing the medial aspect of the insertion of the sternothyroid muscle. In the event of direct involvement of strap muscles with invasive cancer or thyroiditis, the sternothyroid muscle can be sacrificed. If total thyroidectomy follows an earlier partial thyroidectomy during which seeding by cancer cells occurred, both sternohyoid and sternothyroid muscles can be sacrificed.

THYROID

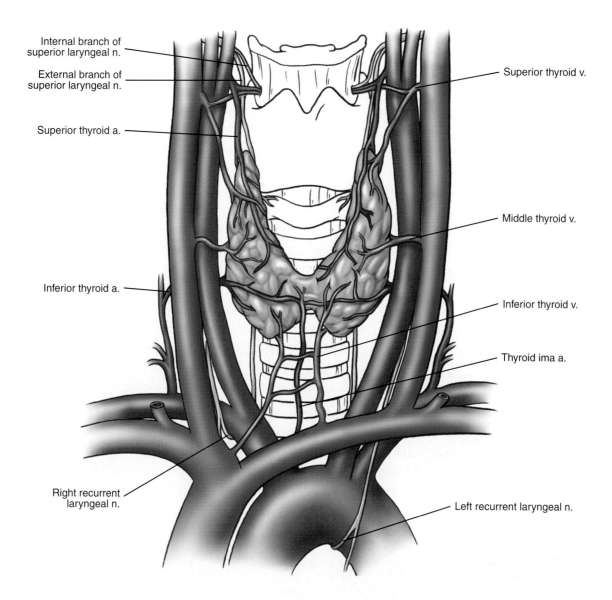

Internal branch of
superior laryngeal n.

External branch of
superior laryngeal n.

Superior thyroid a.

Inferior thyroid a.

Right recurrent
laryngeal n.

Superior thyroid v.

Middle thyroid v.

Inferior thyroid v.

Thyroid ima a.

Left recurrent laryngeal n.

The normal thyroid gland usually appears as a small, flat, reddish tan, bilobed structure lying on either side of the larynx and trachea, with a flat band of similar tissue, the isthmus, crossing the first three tracheal rings just below the cricoid cartilage.

One lobe, usually the right, may be smaller than the other (7%) or even be completely absent (1.7%). The isthmus is absent in about 10% of thyroid glands.

The thyroid gland normally extends from the level of the fifth cervical vertebra to that of the first thoracic vertebra. It may lie higher (lingual thyroid), but rarely lower.

Projecting superiorly from the isthmus may be a slender strip of thyroid tissue, the pyramidal lobe, to either side of or at the midline. This structure ascends toward the hyoid bone. In 50% of cases it is merely a residual fibrous tract. In pathologic conditions, such as Graves' disease or chronic thyroiditis, however, this lobe may become quite prominent. Cancer and benign nodules may develop in this or any other part of the thyroid.

Like many other organs, the thyroid gland has a connective tissue capsule continuous with the septa that makes up the stroma of the organ. This is the true capsule of the thyroid.

External to the true capsule is a more or less well-developed layer of fascia derived from the pretracheal fascia. This is the false capsule, the parathyroid sheath, or surgical capsule. Anteriorly and laterally this fascia is well developed; posteriorly it is thin and loose, permitting enlargement of the thyroid gland posteriorly. Thickenings of the fascia fix the posterior aspect of each lobe to the cricoid cartilage. These thickenings are the ligaments of Berry.

The thyroid is intimately related to the trachea and larynx. Each lobe is pear shaped, and the anterolateral aspect is covered by the sternothyroid muscle. The posterolateral aspect is related to the carotid sheath and its contents. Its superior deep surface abuts the inferior constrictor muscle. The recurrent laryngeal nerve is intimately adjacent to the middle third of the gland. The cricothyroid and thyrohyoid muscles separate the gland from the thyroid and cricoid cartilages. At the anterolateral aspect of the cricoid cartilage is an intimate union with the gland through the suspensory ligament.

As normal variants, one lobe of the thyroid may be larger than the other, and the blood supply may vary accordingly. Also, the gland may vary in size with age or with demand such as pregnancy. In healthy infants, the thyroid may weigh 1.5 to 2 gm; in the normal adult, it weighs between 15 and 25 gm.

Blood Supply
Arterial Supply

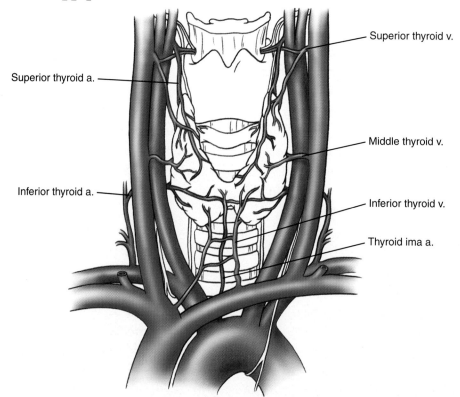

The thyroid gland receives more blood per gram of tissue (5.5 ml/gm/min) than do most other organs. One consequence is that hemostasis may be a major problem of thyroid surgery, especially in patients with toxic goiter. Two paired arteries, the superior and inferior thyroid arteries, and an inconstant midline vessel, the thyroid ima artery, supply the thyroid.

The superior thyroid artery arises from the external carotid artery just above, at, or just below the bifurcation of the common carotid artery, and it passes downward and anteriorly to reach the superior pole of the thyroid gland. In part of its course, the artery parallels the superior laryngeal nerve. The six superior thyroid branches are the infrahyoid, the sternocleidomastoid, the superior laryngeal, the cricothyroid, the inferior pharyngeal constrictor branch, and finally the terminal branches of the superior thyroid artery, which supply the thyroid and occasionally the parathyroid glands. Usually the terminal branches further divide into two, an anterior and a posterior branch, and occasionally a so-called lateral branch. The anterior branch anastomoses with the contralateral artery; the posterior branch anastomoses with branches of the inferior thyroid artery. From the posterior branch, a small parathyroid artery may pass to the superior parathyroid gland.

The inferior thyroid artery usually arises from the thyrocervical trunk, but in about 15% of individuals it arises from the subclavian artery. The inferior thyroid artery ascends behind the carotid artery and the jugular vein, passing medially and posteriorly on the anterior surface of the longus coli muscle. After piercing the prevertebral fascia, the artery divides into two or more branches as it crosses the ascending recurrent laryngeal nerve. The nerve may pass anterior or posterior to the artery or between its branches. The lowest branch of the artery sends a twig to the inferior and superior parathyroid glands and supplies the posterior surface of the thyroid gland. During thyroidectomy, ligation of the inferior thyroid artery should be distal to the terminal branches to the parathyroids to avoid ischemia of the parathyroid glands. Careful dissection of this artery and its branches is most important in total thyroidectomy or lobectomy, so that preservation of both the parathyroids and the recurrent nerves is assured. The upper branch supplies the posterior surface of the gland, usually anastomosing with a descending branch of the superior thyroid artery. On the right, the inferior thyroid artery is absent in about 2% of individuals; on the left, it is absent in about 5%. The artery is occasionally double.

The thyroid ima artery is unpaired and inconstant. It arises from the brachiocephalic artery, the right common carotid artery, or the aortic arch. Its frequency has been reported at 1.5% to 12.2%. It may be as large as an inferior thyroid artery or be a mere twig. Its position anterior to the trachea makes its recognition important in tracheostomy.

Venous Drainage

Veins of the thyroid gland form a plexus of vessels lying in the substance and on the surface of the thyroid. The plexus is drained by three pairs of veins.

The superior thyroid vein accompanies the superior thyroid artery. Emerging from the superior pole of the thyroid, the vein passes superiorly and laterally across the omohyoid muscle and the common carotid artery to enter the internal jugular vein alone or with the common facial vein.

The middle thyroid vein arises on the lateral surface of the gland. It crosses the common carotid artery to enter the internal jugular vein. This vein may be absent, and occasionally is double. The extra vein is inferior to the normal vein and has been called the "fourth" thyroid vein. The importance of these middle thyroid veins is their vulnerability to injury during thyroidectomy.

The inferior thyroid vein is the largest and the most variable of the thyroid veins; the right and left sides are usually asymmetric. The right vein leaves the lower border of the thyroid gland, passes anterior to the brachiocephalic artery, and enters the right brachiocephalic vein. The left vein crosses the trachea to enter the left brachiocephalic vein. In rare instances, the right vein crosses the trachea to enter the left brachiocephalic vein, sometimes forming a common trunk with the left vein. The common trunk is called the thyroid ima vein.

The thyroid veins may be found considerably engorged and dilated in the presence of intrathoracic goiter and may pose a difficult problem for the surgeon. Delivery of the goiter from the substernal area and thoracic inlet is required to relieve venous stasis and to prevent excessive bleeding. However, care must be taken to ensure that they are not untied, open, or torn veins, which may later result in hemorrhage or cause air embolus. This is best discovered by means of a Valsalva maneuver, performed by the anesthesiologist.

Inadvertent division of a large vein in the anterior neck may lead to fatal air embolism, since the neck is higher than the right atrium and there is negative venous pressure. Venous obstruction secondary to substernal goiter may make control of hemorrhage difficult until the goiter is delivered out of the neck and the venous obstruction is relieved.

Transverse communicating veins may be seen between the inferior branches. There is great variation in the pattern found. This can be a significant problem, since it interferes with the accuracy of parathyroid tumor localization with selective venous sampling of parathyroid hormone.

Lymphatic Drainage

The thyroid is rich in intraglandular lymphatic capillaries, which encircle the thyroid follicles and are adjacent to parafollicular cells that secrete calcitonin. Tagged thyroglobulin can be identified in both the lymphatic and venous collecting vessels. This rich intraglandular lymphatic capillary network makes its way to a position below the capsule of the gland, where it gives rise to collecting trunks within the capsule. The collecting trunks are in close association with the capsular veins and follow them to the major sources of venous drainage.

The number of collecting trunks depends on the configuration and blood supply of the gland. The chief efferent pathways are superior, lateral, and inferior and follow the superior blood vessels, the inferior thyroid artery, middle vein, and the inferior venous plexus.

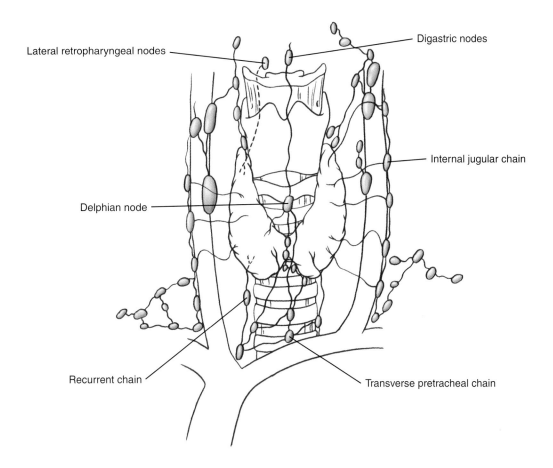

The primary zone of lymphatic drainage is to the midline Delphian, tracheoesophageal, and superior mediastinal nodes. The nodes of the lateral neck (internal jugular, posterior triangle) constitute a zone of secondary drainage.

Several broad patterns of lymphatic drainage of the thyroid gland have been proposed. Three to six vessels arise from the superior margin of the isthmus and from the median margins of the lateral lobes. These vessels pass upward anterior to the larynx and end in the digastric lymph nodes. Some vessels may enter one or more prelaryngeal (Delphian) nodes just above the isthmus. Secondary drainage may be to upper jugular nodes on either side or to pretracheal nodes below the thyroid by a vessel passing from the Delphian nodes downward over the front of the thyroid. Several lymph vessels drain the lower part of the isthmus and the lower medial portions of the lateral lobe. They follow the inferior thyroid veins to end in the pretracheal and brachiocephalic nodes.

Lymphatic trunks arise from the lateral border of each lobe. Superiorly they pass upward with the superior thyroid artery and vein; inferiorly they follow the inferior thyroid artery. Between these two groups, some vessels pass laterally, anteriorly, or posteriorly to the carotid sheath to reach lymph nodes of the internal jugular chain. Occasionally such vessels drain into the right subclavian vein, jugular vein, or thoracic duct without passing through a lymph node. Posterior lymphatic vessels arise from the inferior and medial surfaces of the lateral lobes to drain into nodes along the recurrent laryngeal nerve. Occasionally a posterior ascending trunk from the upper part of the lobe reaches the retropharyngeal nodes.

The superior route of lymphatic flow drains the anterior and posterior portions of the upper third or more of each lobe as well as the medial portion adjacent to the isthmus. The collecting trunks cross in front of the cricoid cartilage and encompass and drain the pyramidal lobe when it is present. These superior collecting trunks follow the superior thyroid veins behind the insertion of the sternnothyroid muscle and may pierce it in some instances. They continue to the subdigastric internal jugular nodes (middle jugular nodes). The posterior portion of the upper third of the lobe may also drain to the lower retropharyngeal nodes as well as to the midjugular nodes.

The inferior pathway drains the medial and posterior lower half of the lobe, the inferior pole, and the lower portion of the isthmus. The collecting trunks are numerous and go into the pretracheal, paratracheal, and recurrent laryngeal chain of nodes. The lymphatics may continue retrograde to the vicinity of the thymus, following the course of the innominate veins. The anterosuperior mediastinal nodes are in communication with the lower thyroid lymphatic pathways and nodes.

Lymphatic Spread of Thyroid Carcinoma

The regional lymph nodes most likely to be involved with thyroid carcinoma (papillary or medullary) are the most immediate paraglandular nodes. When total thyroidectomy is done, these nodes should also be removed, namely those in the pretracheal and paratracheal and recurrent laryngeal nerve chains.

Feind reported metastatic involvement of middle jugular lymph nodes in 85 of 111 specimens from patients with thyroid carcinoma. In 67 of these, lower jugular nodes were positive for disease. Submandibular and mediastinal nodes were rarely affected.

On the side of the obvious primary lesion, the middle internal jugular nodes should be inspected and biopsied to check for lateral cervical spread. If these nodes are obviously involved, neck dissection is done. If the lateral nodes prove positive in the final pathology report, neck dissection may be indicated. In Feind's series, in which only random sections or levels were taken of the specimens studied, about 40% had multifocal disease or intraglandular metastatic disease.

Based on these data, it has been recommended that when grade I papillary or follicular cancer is diagnosed, total thyroidectomy is warranted. Some authorities disagree with this approach and favor thyroid lobectomy, especially in the case of small primary thyroid tumors. However, the recent large summary reports by Mazzaferri and Hay et al. document enhanced long-term survival following bilateral, as opposed to unilateral, thyroidectomy for thyroid carcinoma.

Nerve Supply
Recurrent Laryngeal Nerves

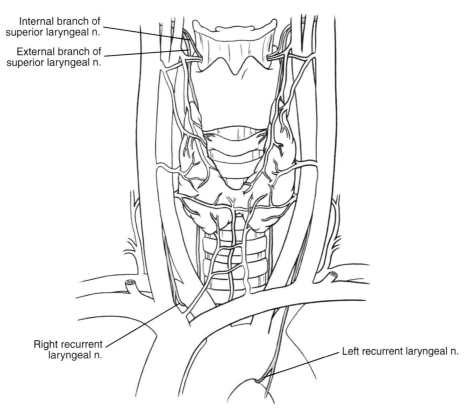

Internal branch of superior laryngeal n.
External branch of superior laryngeal n.
Right recurrent laryngeal n.
Left recurrent laryngeal n.

In intimate relation to the thyroid gland are the two recurrent laryngeal nerves. The right nerve branches from the vagus nerve as it crosses anterior to the right subclavian artery. The recurrent nerve loops around the artery from posterior to anterior and ascends in or near the tracheoesophageal groove, passing posterior to the right lobe of the thyroid gland to enter the larynx behind the cricothyroid articulation and the inferior corner of the thyroid cartilage. The left recurrent nerve arises where the aorta crosses the vagus nerve. It loops under the aorta and ascends in the same manner as the right nerve.

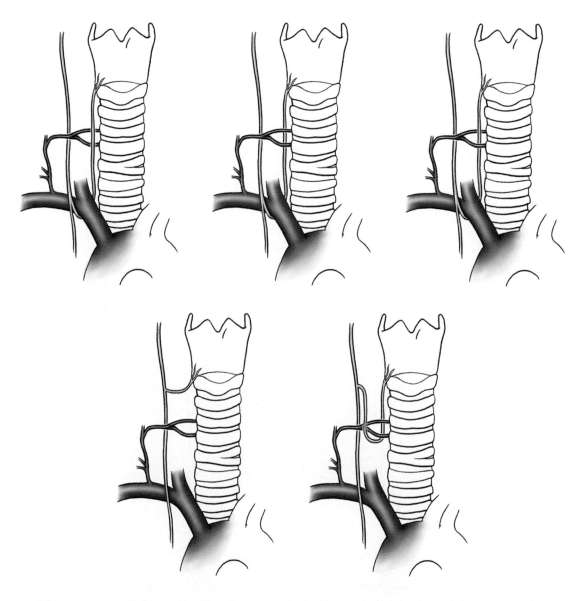

The course of the recurrent laryngeal nerve relative to the inferior thyroid artery may vary, increasing the likelihood of injury to the nerve during thyroid surgery. The recurrent laryngeal nerve crosses the inferior thyroid artery at the middle third of the gland. For practical purposes, there are three major types of crossing. The nerve may cross anterior to, posterior to, or between the branches of the artery. Alternatively, it may branch above the inferior thyroid artery (nonrecurrent nerve), or it may loop beneath the artery. No one pattern can be considered "normal"; the surgeon must be prepared for any configuration of artery and nerve.

Most laryngeal nerves, approximately 80%, are located either posterior to or between the branches of the inferior thyroid artery. In Skandalakis' series, the right nerve was most frequently between arterial branches (48%); the left nerve was usually behind the artery (64%). Henry et al. found that the nonrecurrent nerve may pass directly to the larynx with no relation to the inferior thyroid artery or may loop around the artery (0.63% of patients). In these cases the right subclavian artery arises from the descending aorta and passes to the right behind the esophagus. This anomaly is asymptomatic, and the thyroid surgeon will rarely be aware of it prior to operation. Less common (0.04%) is a nonrecurrent left nerve in the presence of a right aortic arch and a retroesophageal left subclavian artery.

In the lower third of its course, the recurrent laryngeal nerve ascends behind the pretracheal fascia at a slight angle to the tracheoesophageal groove. In the middle third of its course, the nerve may lie in the groove, medial to the suspensory ligament of the thyroid gland (ligament of Berry), within the ligament, or within the substance of the thyroid gland.

Skandalakis examined the course of the recurrent laryngeal nerve in 102 cadavers (204 sides). In about half of the specimens the nerve lay in the tracheoesophageal groove; in the other half the nerve was usually anterior to the groove (paratracheal), with a few situated more posterior (paraesophageal). Eight of 204 nerves lay within the thyroid gland. The nerve is safest and least visible when it lies in the tracheoesophageal groove. It is the most vulnerable when it transverses the thyroid parenchyma or runs within the suspensory ligament of the thyroid. It must be identified and protected before the ligament is divided.

The recurrent laryngeal nerve fibers are both sensory and motor. They supply sensation to the trachea and subglottic region of the larynx. The motor branches innervate the abductor and adductor muscles of the larynx. The nerve ascends into the neck adjacent to the trachea, in the tracheoesophageal groove. Each recurrent nerve gives off sensory branches to the trachea, continues deep to the respective thyroid lobe, and passes either in front of or behind the inferior thyroid artery or its branches. Just above this, the nerve assumes a position very close to the thyroid and bifurcates. The bifurcation is motor and sensory. The sensory branch joins the sensory branch of the superior laryngeal nerve to form the loop of Galen. At the position close to the thyroid, a projection of thyroid tissue overhangs the nerve. This lobulation may be very large in Graves' disease and, in some instances, actually projects behind the cricopharyngeus muscle. The nerve, in close association with the thyroid, pierces just below the inferior constrictor muscle to gain access to the muscles of the larynx.

Superior Laryngeal and Other Nerves

The superior laryngeal nerve arises from the inferior ganglion (nodosum) of the vagus nerve just outside the jugular foramen of the skull. The nerve passes inferiorly, medial to the carotid artery. At the level of the superior corner of the hyoid bone it divides into a large sensory internal laryngeal branch (to the mucous membrane of the pyriform fossa and the larynx above the cords) and a smaller (external laryngeal) branch, supplying motor function to the cricothyroid muscle.

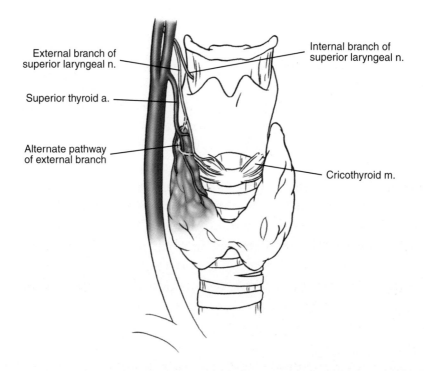

The superior laryngeal nerve branches with the carotid arteries. Injury to the external branch of the superior laryngeal nerve ("opera singer's nerve") causes early fatigue of the voice. The internal laryngeal branch is rarely identified by the surgeon, except where there is a greatly enlarged upper pole of the thyroid gland rising above the superior border of the thyroid cartilage. There is also a relationship between the internal and external branches of the superior laryngeal nerve with the superior thyroid artery and the upper pole of the thyroid gland.

The cervical sympathetic chain lies deep to the common carotid artery between the prevertebral fascia and the carotid sheath. In the upper neck it continues deep to the internal carotid artery. The retropharyngeal lymphatic vessels are in communication with those of the anterior cervical chain and cross this trunk. These lymphatics and their lymph nodes may be involved in metastatic thyroid cancer. In advanced disease, the sympathetic chain may be directly invaded from these involved nodes, and eradication may result in a Horner's syndrome. Rarely Horner's syndrome may result from compression by a large goiter or Grave's disease.

The hypoglossal (twelfth cranial) nerve, a motor nerve to the tongue, emerges from the hypoglossal canal on the occipital base of the skull. It is in close contact with the ninth, tenth, and eleventh cranial nerves. It lies between the internal jugular vein and the internal carotid artery and descends to the lower border of the posterior belly of the digastric muscle, where it crosses both the internal and external carotid arteries. It then crosses anteriorly just deep to the anterior facial vein, follows the stylohyoid muscle to gain the submandibular triangle, and innervates the tongue muscles. The nerve is likely to be injured as it crosses the carotid arteries and must be identified before the internal jugular vein is transected during neck dissection.

The descending branch of the hypoglossal nerve leaves the parent nerve at the crossing of the carotid arteries and descends on the surface of the internal and common carotid arteries. There it is joined by the descending cervical nerve (C2 and C3), which arises from the cervical plexus. This joining or nerve loop is termed the ansa hypoglossi, whose branches innervate the thyrohyoid muscle. Sacrifice of either the ansa hypoglossi or descending cervical nerve has no serious consequence.

In neck dissection, injury to the brachial plexus and phrenic nerve must be avoided. However, the cervical plexus may be sacrificed distal to the takeoff of the phrenic nerve at roots C3 and C4. The brachial plexus occupies the anteroinferior angle of the posterior triangle of the neck. In the neck, the plexus lies behind the inferior belly of the omohyoid muscle. It emerges posterior to the scalenus anticus and anterior to the scalenus medius. The upper trunk of the plexus is visible, and the nerve to the rhomboids is often easily seen. It is important that the prevertebral fascia not be violated. All the motor nerves given off lie in this fascia.

The phrenic nerve in the neck is also in the prevertebral fascia and descends from roots of C3 and C4 of the cervical plexus. The part of the cervical plexus arising from C1, C2, C3, and C4 may be sacrificed distal to the motor takeoffs or distal to prevertebral fascia, without serious consequences. The phrenic nerve remains in the prevertebral fascia of the scalenus anticus as it crosses from the lateral to the medial border of this muscle in its descent. On the left side, the nerve is in close association with the thoracic duct.

The spinal accessory (eleventh cranial) nerve emerges from the jugular foramen of the skull and gives off a branch to the inferior ganglion of the vagus, thereby providing motor branches to the pharynx and larynx. The spinal accessory nerve crosses the internal jugular vein immediately to descend deep to the occipital artery and posterior belly of the digastric muscle, where it reaches the deep surface of the sternocleidomastoid muscle. The nerve pierces the muscle, giving off a branch to the muscle, and emerges between the muscle's posterior border and the trapezius muscle, running inferiorly in the lateral aspect of the posterior triangle of the neck. The nerve finally enters and innervates the trapezius muscle.

Lymphatic collecting trunks accompany the nerve from the base of the skull. However, they are rarely involved by metastatic thyroid cancer. It is thus reasonable to save this nerve in a neck dissection. When the nerve is sacrificed during radical neck dissection for aggressive head and neck cancers, disability from the resultant shoulder drop is disfiguring and presents a physical and emotional handicap for the patient to overcome.

The descending branch of the seventh cranial nerve supplies the platysma muscle, but also gives off a mandibular branch as it leaves the lower pole of the parotid salivary gland. This branch goes to the depressor muscles of the lower lip. This small branch courses deep to the platysma muscle, usually close to the angle of the mandible at the lower border of the masseter muscle, and joins the facial vessels as they cross the mandible.

Exposure of Laryngeal Nerves

Exposure of the recurrent nerve during any procedure on the thyroid is a sound surgical principle and should be done wherever possible. If the nerve cannot be found readily, the surgeon must avoid the areas in which it may be hidden.

Visual identification, with avoidance of traction, compression, or stripping of the connective tissue, is wise. Complete anatomic dissection is not required. The recurrent laryngeal nerve forms the medial border of a triangle bounded superiorly by the inferior thyroid artery and laterally by the carotid artery. The nerve may be identified where it enters the larynx just posterior to the inferior cornu of the thyroid cartilage. If the nerve is not found, a nonrecurrent nerve should be suspected, especially on the right. In the lower portion of its course the nerve may be palpated as a tight strand over the tracheal surface. There is more connective tissue between the nerve and the trachea on the right than on the left.

The external laryngeal branch, together with the superior thyroid vein and artery, passes under the sternothyroid muscles. The nerve then passes beneath the blood vessels into the lower part of the thyropharyngeal muscle to continue inferiorly and innervate the cricothyroid muscle. In most patients, there is a plane of dissection between the vessels and the nerve. In about 25% of individuals the nerve lies beneath the fascia together with the vessels and may pass between branches of the superior thyroid artery.

PARATHYROID
Topography

The parathyroid glands are spherical or ovoid, somewhat flattened bodies varying in size from 4 to 6 mm in length and 3 to 4 mm in width and thickness. Each gland weighs approximately 40 mg. The two inferior glands usually are slightly heavier than the superior glands. The consistency is slightly softer than normal thyroid tissue. The normal parathyroid gland is yellowish brown, but may be more tan if the fat content is increased. When the tissue becomes adenomatous, it becomes more reddish, almost the color of liver.

Parathyroid Number and Location

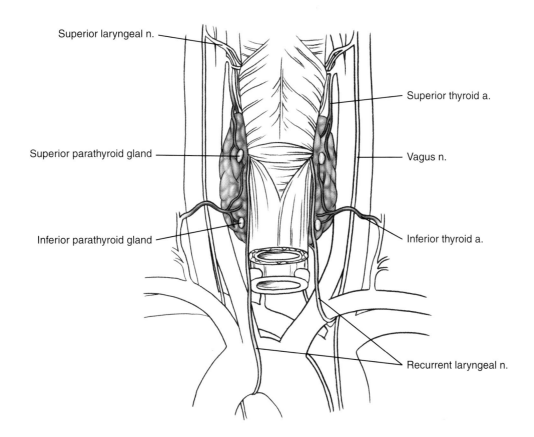

The parathyroid glands usually are found on the dorsal surface of the thyroid gland. This posterior view of the neck demonstrates the relationship of the inferior thyroid arteries and recurrent laryngeal nerve to the parathyroid glands on the dorsal aspect of the thyroid. Superior parathyroid glands most commonly are located above the inferior thyroid artery at the junction of the middle and upper thirds of the posterior surface of the thyroid. Inferior parathyroid glands lie below the inferior thyroid artery on the posterolateral aspect of the inferior pole of the thyroid gland. The normal parathyroid gland usually is underneath a thin film of opaque fascia, surrounded by fat globules that are lighter in color. Typically there are four parathyroid glands, but the number may vary from two to seven. Approximately 6% of all individuals have five parathyroid glands. These accessory parathyroids occupy somewhat unusual locations; for example, they may lie within the mediastinum. They are occasionally found within the substance of the thyroid, in 1% of cases.

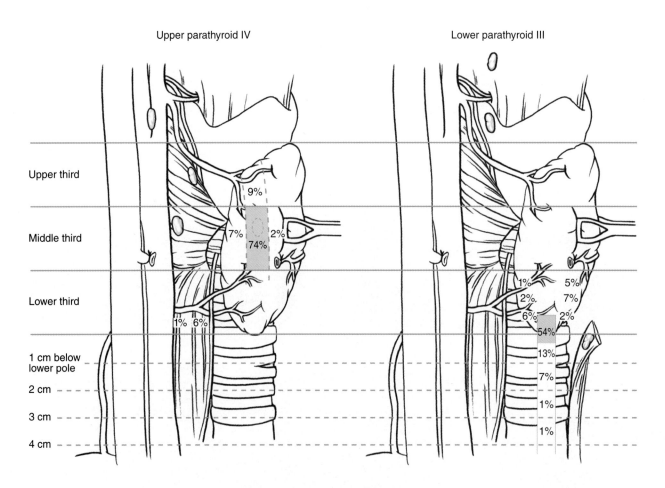

Lateral views of the anatomic locations of upper and lower parathyroids, as dissected by Gilmour, are illustrated. Extreme locations are very rare, although glands have been found as high as the bifurcation of the carotid artery and as low as the mediastinum.

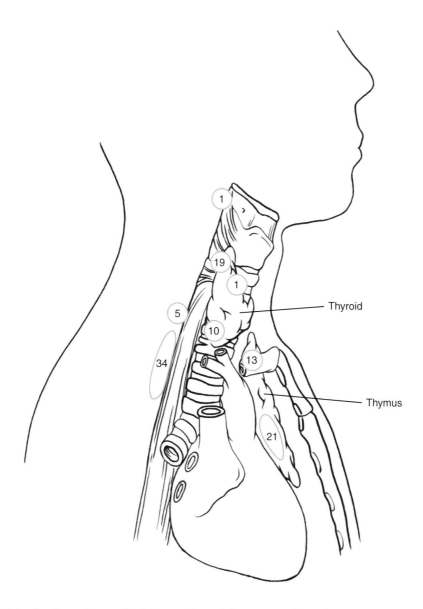

Illustrated is the location of 104 parathyroid tumors found at reoperation after failure to cure hyperparathyroidism at initial surgery, as described by Wang.

More than four or fewer than four parathyroid glands are not uncommon. For example, Gimour reported that 6.1% of patients had only three parathyroids. Where fewer than four glands are found, the possibility of ectopic glands is hard to rule out. Two parathyroid glands may appear fused to one another. Such a pair can be differentiated from a bilobed gland by the presence of a cleavage plane between them.

Blood Supply

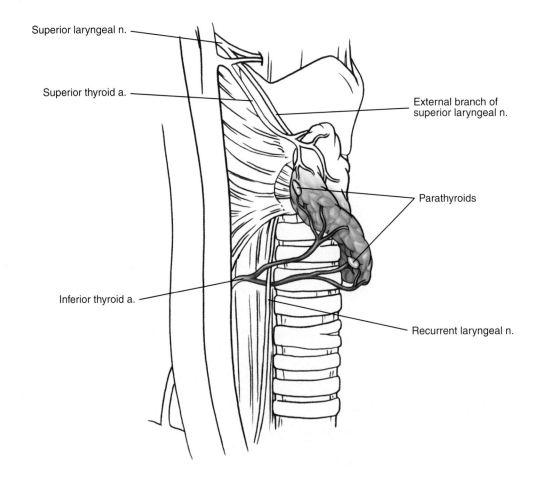

Superior laryngeal n.

Superior thyroid a.

External branch of superior laryngeal n.

Parathyroids

Inferior thyroid a.

Recurrent laryngeal n.

The inferior thyroid artery is the major blood supply to all four parathyroid glands. Each gland receives an artery, which enters the hilus at a slight depression in the capsule. Occasionally the superior thyroid artery supplies or adds additional blood vessels to the superior parathyroid glands.

The largest series (354 postmortem subjects) analyzing the parathyroid vascular supply is that of Aleryd, who found that both the superior and inferior parathyroids were usually supplied by the inferior thyroid artery, 86.1% on the right side and 76.8% on the left. In the majority of cases in which the inferior thyroid artery was absent, both the upper and lower parathyroids were supplied by the superior thyroid artery. When the glands are enlarged, a large vascular pedicle may be very helpful in locating them. Rarely an inferior parathyroid adenoma may be intrathymic and receive its blood supply from a branch of the internal mammary artery.

SURGICAL APPLICATIONS
Thyroidectomy

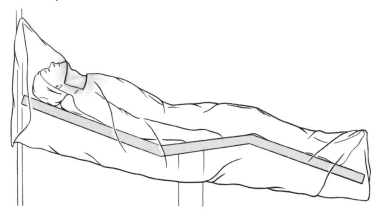

The patient is placed in a semisitting ("lounge chair") position. The head of the table is tilted upward approximately 30 degrees to increase exposure and decrease venous engorgement. A rolled sheet is placed longitudinally between the shoulders to allow maximum hyperflexion of the neck. Surgical drapes should allow access so that the entire anterior aspect of the neck from the chin to the suprasternal notch is exposed.

Incision

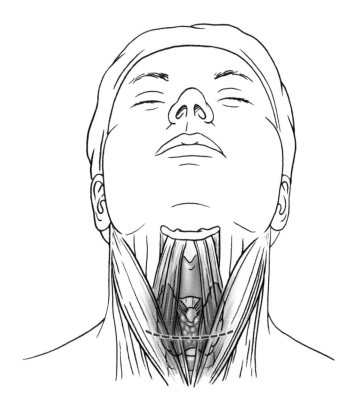

The optimal incision for thyroidectomy must be long enough that the skin flap can be elevated for adequate exposure of the thyroid gland, yet cosmetically placed within a transverse skin crease, curving gently upward on both ends.

The incision is made about 3 cm above the clavicles, and the scar will be about 1.5 cm above the clavicle in the upright position. It should not be straight, but curved upward slightly. It should be symmetric, extending the same distance on each side from the midline, and should be curved equally on both sides so as not to be askew.

Elevation of the Skin Flap

The skin, subcutaneous fat, and platysma are elevated as one layer. The fascial plane between the posterior sheath of the platysma and the sternohyoid muscle is relatively avascular. After the skin incision has been completed, the platysma muscle is identified laterally and its fibers divided, exposing the fascia of the prethyroid muscles (the sternohyoid and the sternothyroid) underlying deep investing. The superficial veins are not elevated with the flap. Avoiding injury to the superficial veins prevents unnecessary bleeding.

By applying upward traction, the flap is raised above the thyroid notch by combined sharp and blunt dissection in a relatively avascular plane. This plane is identified by firm upward traction on the skin and countertraction below on the midline tissues of the neck. One of the most important technical steps in the thyroidectomy is high elevation of the upper flap, which allows adequate anatomic exposure. Next the inferior flap is developed to the level of the sternal notch, taking care to avoid injury to anterior jugular veins. A self-retaining retractor is placed in the wound.

Prethyroid Muscles (Sternohyoid and Sternothyroid)

Although rarely necessary, the prethyroid muscles may be divided in difficult cases (e.g., huge goiters) to obtain adequate exposure to perform thyroidectomy safely. If the muscles are severed high, preserving their innervation from the ascending branch of the ansa hypoglossi nerve, no disability results. Disfiguring atrophy of the prethyroid muscles, with sunken neck and prominent trachea, may result from dividing the prethyroid muscles and their innervation too low in the neck.

The medial borders of the sternohyoid and sternothyroid muscles are best identified in the midline low in the neck. The midline of the trachea above the suprasternal notch should be determined by palpation, and this area explored. The investing fascia is incised vertically. Often a small amount of free fatty tissue is a clue to the midline. It may be necessary to divide communicating anterior jugular veins crossing the midline. Both the sternohyoid and deeper sternothyroid muscles are freed from the anterolateral surfaces of the thyroid, using blunt and sharp dissection and electrocautery to avoid bleeding from small vessels present in this plane.

Middle Thyroid Vein, Recurrent Nerve, and Parathyroid Identification

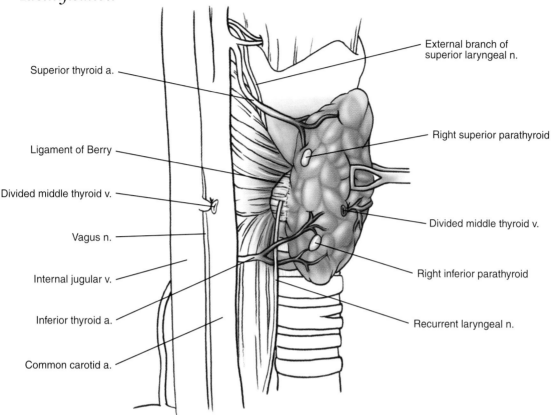

The strap muscles are retracted laterally, and the thyroid lobe is retracted medially with a gauze-covered index finger, a "peanut" dissector, or a Babcock clamp. This allows identification, ligature, and division of the middle thyroid vein. With the middle thyroid vein divided, the right thyroid lobe may be retracted further toward the left. Areolar planes adjacent to the thyroid, trachea, and esophagus are dissected gently, allowing visualization of the inferior thyroid artery, the inferior and superior parathyroids, and the fascial attachments of the thyroid to the trachea (ligament of Berry). There may be two or more veins draining (and tethering) the lateral and inferior aspects of the thyroid lobe. It is important to dissect and divide these veins meticulously to avoid injury to the internal jugular vein or hemorrhage and discoloration of the operative field, which can make identification of the parathyroids and recurrent laryngeal nerve more difficult.

In cases involving large goiters, the internal jugular vein may be adherent to the capsule of the thyroid. Patience and careful retraction of the lobe are necessary to identify the location of the middle thyroid vein, and it may be necessary to divide multiple branches of the vein close to the capsule of the thyroid.

It is essential to identify the location and course of the recurrent laryngeal nerve. It should be sought and found prior to division of any major structures except the obviously blood-filled middle thyroid vein(s). The recurrent laryngeal nerve is a glistening, white, string-like structure emerging from the para-esophageal mediastinum and coursing cephalad in the tracheoesophageal groove, crossing either beneath or anterior to the transversely oriented inferior thyroid artery.

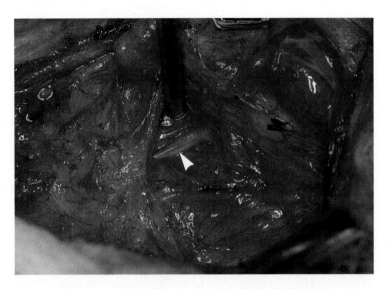

The left lobe of the thyroid is retracted anteriorly by surgical clamp; the patient's head is to the right. The left recurrent laryngeal nerve (arrow) courses from mediastinum (left side of photo) cephalad to disappear beneath the cricothyroid membrane.

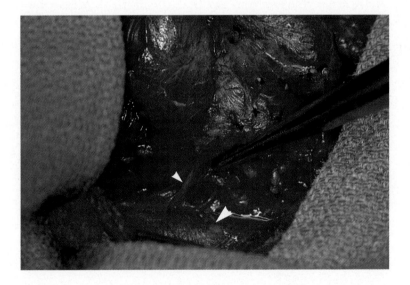

It is essential for the surgeon to be cognizant of the variations in anatomic location of the recurrent laryngeal nerve, especially its "nonrecurrence" (small arrow) when it exits directly from the carotid sheath (large arrow) and courses from lateral to medial to pierce the cricothyroid membrane. The right thyroid lobe is retracted anteriorly, surgical forceps points toward the trachea, and the patient's head is to the left.

In most cases the recurrent laryngeal nerve is reliably and quickly identified as it crosses the inferior thyroid artery. Great care must be taken to avoid traction or cautery injuries to the nerve throughout the remainder of the procedure. Before clamping and cutting any structure, it is wise to ascertain its proximity to the nerve. It is best to keep the nerve in view at all times, since traction on the thyroid can distort its location markedly. A meticulous, bloodless dissection is advisable.

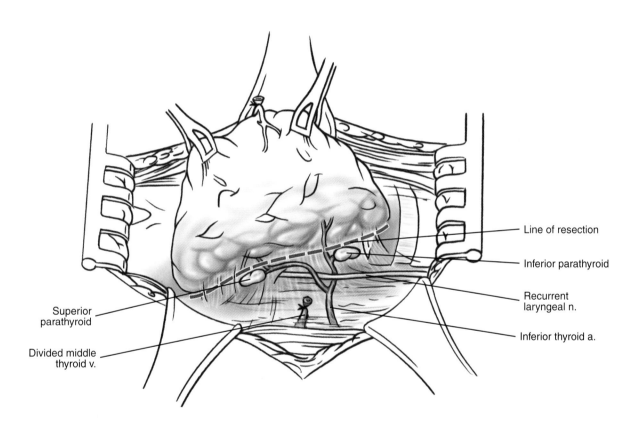

At this point in the procedure both parathyroids should be visualized, noting their blood supply and relationship to the thyroid capsule. It is usually possible to separate them from the surface of the thyroid and to divide branches of the inferior thyroid artery distal to the origin of its branches to the parathyroids, thus preserving them in situ in the neck.

Division of Superior Vessels and Identification of External Branch of Superior Laryngeal Nerve

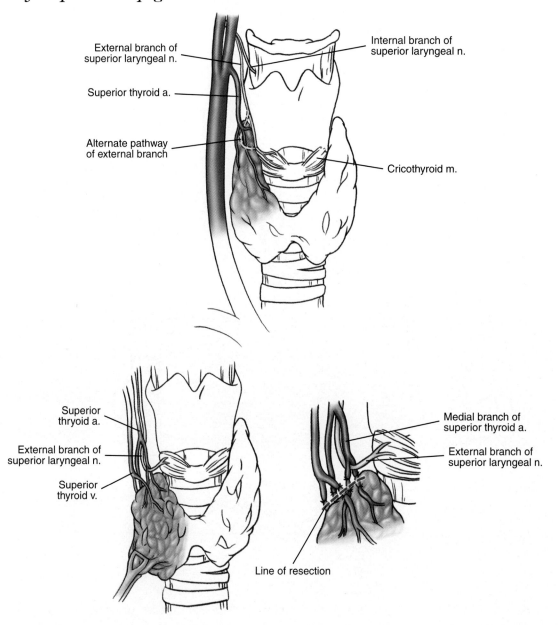

Once these vital structures are identified, it is usually advantageous to dissect and divide the branches of the superior thyroid artery and vein. This allows much better mobilization of the lobe for the final pretracheal dissection. It is important to identify the external branch of the superior laryngeal nerve. Although it is usually higher and medial to the main trunk of the superior thyroid artery, considerable variation in its location has been documented. It may intertwine itself with branches of the artery. It is wise to divide the distal

branches of the artery and vein individually to avoid nerve injury. Double ligatures of silk are advisable on this artery, tied in continuity prior to division,
since it can retract caphalad if control is lost, causing hemorrhage and placing
the nerve in jeopardy.

After the superior pole vessels are divided, the thyroid lobe may be retracted
toward the opposite side, fully exposing the recurrent laryngeal nerve and
parathyroid (see p. 85).

Division of the Ligament of Berry and Isthmus and Parathyroid Sparing

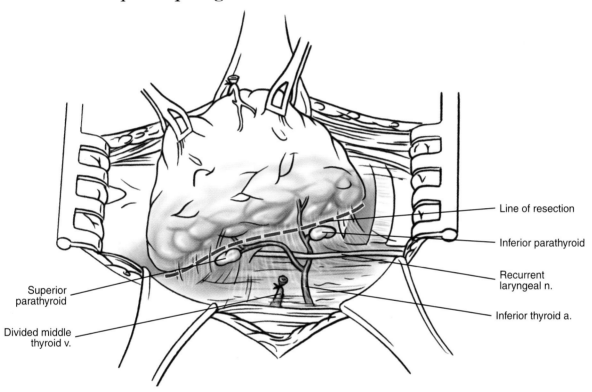

The lobe is mobilized forward and medially, putting its posterior adventitial attachments on slight traction. Keeping the recurrent laryngeal nerve in view at
all times to ensure that it is not being stretched, the thyroid is progressively mobilized upward by dividing its fascial attachments to the trachea and by dividing
the distal secondary branches of the inferior thyroid artery near the surface of
the thyroid. The parathyroid glands are gently dissected from the thyroid capsule, taking care to preserve their blood supply wherever possible. If a parathyroid gland is devascularized, it may be removed, minced finely into small
(1 mm × 1 mm) pieces in saline solution, and autotransplanted into a small intramuscular pocket in the sternocleidomastoid muscle with the aid of a 16-
gauge angiocatheter and a 1 ml syringe.

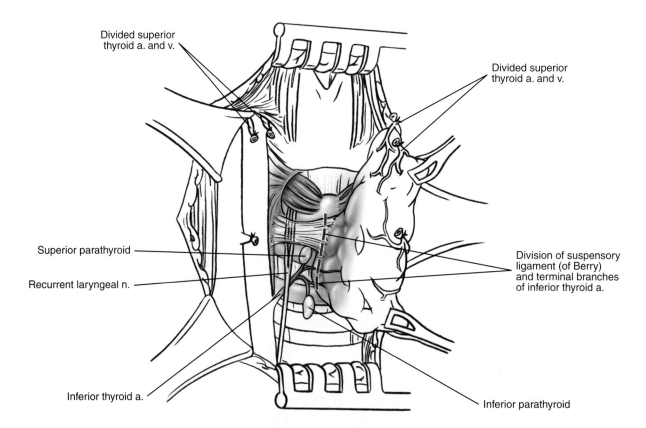

As dissection progresses cephalad, portions of the tough ligament of Berry are dissected free from the tracheal surface, anteromedial to the path of the recurrent laryngeal nerve, and divided in continuity, keeping the nerve in view at all times. It is important to ligate this ligamentous tissue, because it contains multiple small arterial and venous twigs that can retract beneath the path of the nerve, endangering the nerve as they are subsequently clamped and ligatured. Freeing of the ligament of Berry allows complete mobilization of the lobe toward the isthmus.

The isthmus is freed from its attachments to the trachea in the midline and divided after placement of circumferential suture-ligatures for hemostasis. Care must be exercised in separating the isthmus from the underlying pretracheal fascia to avoid injuring the trachea. At the upper aspect of the isthmus, the suspensory ligament is divided to complete the mobilization of the gland, and any pyramidal tissue is resected.

At this moment in thyroidectomy it is necessary to decide the amount of gland to resect. This is determined by the pathologic condition for which the thyroidectomy is being performed. In hyperthyroidism, usually about 90% to 95% of the gland is removed, leaving approximately 2 to 5 gm. Concerns regarding persistence of hyperthyroidism or ophthalmopathy have led many surgeons to perform total thyroidectomy for this condition. With a diffuse hyperplastic gland, such as that found in Graves' disease, it is better to err on the side of more complete removal, because surgically produced hypothyroidism is more easily controlled than persistent or recurrent hyperthyroidism. In toxic nodular and nontoxic nodular goiters, the risk for late recurrence (10 to 20 years) of the goiter has prompted total thyroidectomy in younger patients. In benign tumors, lobectomy to remove the tumor completely will suffice. In malignant tumors, total thyroidectomy is indicated in most cases.

In most cases it is wise to pass off the initial lobe for frozen section, since occult carcinoma may be identified. If completion of a total thyroidectomy is indicated, the contralateral lobectomy is done precisely as described for the first lobectomy.

Subtotal Thyroidectomy

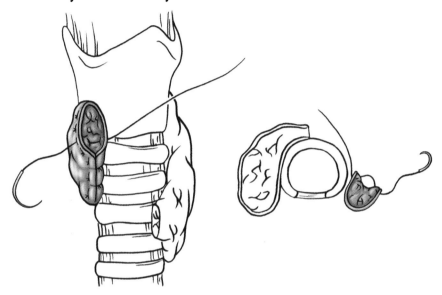

In some instances it is desirable to leave a thyroid remnant in situ. Subtotal thyroidectomy may be done as follows. After the thyroid lobe has been dissected in the usual manner and the recurrent laryngeal nerves and parathyroid glands have been identified, the resection margin is selected. Using a No. 2-0 or 3-0 silk suture on an atraumatic detachable needle, sutures are placed around the resection margin through the capsule and including 1 to 2 mm of underlying parenchyma. The suture is tied down onto the gland, occluding any capsular vessels. This is performed around the entire circumference of the lobe, with each suture spanning approximately a 3 to 5 mm length of capsule; normally 15 to 20 such sutures are required per lobe. Once all of the sutures have been placed, the capsule is sharply incised with a new blade, 1 to 2 mm above the suture line. The incision in the parenchyma is angled posteriorly to wedge out the thyroid tissue, leaving the capsule protruding 1 to 2 mm above the parenchyma. The cut ends of the capsule are then approximated using interrupted No. 3-0 silk to facilitate hemostasis and reestablish capsular continuity.

For closure of the thyroidectomy wound, the patient's head is slightly flexed to remove tension on the prethyroid muscles. The prethyroid muscles are approximated with mattress sutures. The platysma is reapproximated with absorbable sutures. This is important in that the platysmal closure takes tension off the subsequent finely sutured skin closure. Drains, if used, should be of the closed type (e.g., Hemovac) and are brought beyond the ends of the incision. Skin sutures of fine monofilament may be removed on the second postoperative day. Absorbable skin sutures are convenient, but may cause hypertrophic scars in some patients.

Modified Neck Dissection

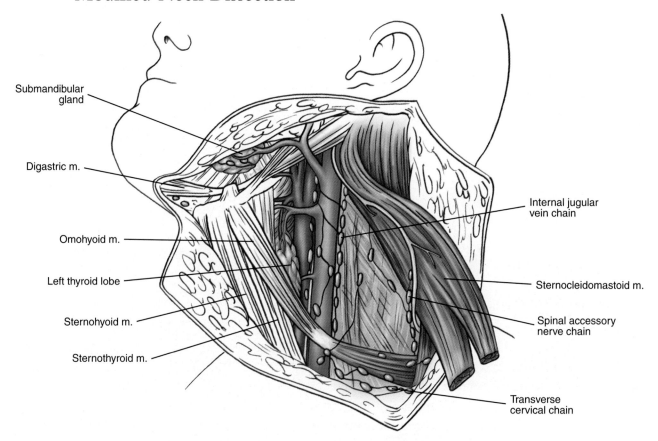

Submandibular gland

Digastric m.

Omohyoid m.

Left thyroid lobe

Sternohyoid m.

Sternothyroid m.

Internal jugular vein chain

Sternocleidomastoid m.

Spinal accessory nerve chain

Transverse cervical chain

When the paraglandular lymph nodes are clinically involved with thyroid carcinoma, a modified neck dissection is indicated. Because residual microscopic disease can be eradicated with subsequent radioactive iodine therapy, the disfigurement of a classic radical neck dissection is rarely warranted. The standard collar incision is extended laterally and upward along the posterior border of the sternocleidomastoid muscle. The space between the sternocleidomastoid and strap muscles is dissected. The sternal head of the sternocleidomastoid may be divided for exposure. The regional nodes of the thyroid are most likely to be involved. The paraglandular, paratracheal, internal jugular, scalene, and posterior triangle nodes are easily accessible by reflecting the transected sternocleidomastoid muscle. The spinal accessory nerve and the submandibular salivary gland should be preserved. Modified radical neck dissection can be performed through an extended transverse lower neck incision.

The internal jugular nodes are dissected from the vein and removed along with surrounding fat. Node-bearing tissue from the posterior triangle is dissected in continuity with the jugular nodal specimen. It is rare to have either spinal accessory nerve or submandibular nodes involved with thyroid carcinoma. This nerve and the submandibular compartment can thus be spared. The sternocleidomastoid muscle also is spared unless grossly involved or seeded with tumor from a previous neck node biopsy.

The spinal accessory nerve is preserved in all instances, because major disability from neck dissection relates to shoulder dysfunction resulting from its sacrifice. No increased incidence of recurrence within the neck area results from preservation of this all-important structure. When modifying standard radical neck dissection in patients with differentiated thyroid carcinoma, the structures preserved are, in order of descending cosmetic importance, the spinal accessory nerve, the submaxillary area, the jugular vein, and the sternocleidomastoid muscle. More complete neck dissection may be necessary in the case of medullary and undifferentiated carcinomas, however, since patients are generally older and have a greater tendency for local recurrence (for more information on this topic, see discussion of the lateral neck, p. 104).

Resection of Substernal Goiter

Most substernal goiters may be removed through the neck. Venous hemorrhage is more troublesome than arterial hemorrhage. Venous hemorrhage before delivery of a substernal goiter into the neck may be serious. The superficial and deep thyroid veins may be greatly enlarged and dilated secondary to the tourniquet effect of the goiter pressing on the superior thoracic strait. Extreme care must be exercised to avoid tearing these veins. The arterial supply to the substernal goiter arises in the neck, and it may be ligated before attempting mobilization of the goiter. After ligation of the inferior and superior thyroid arteries, a cleavage plane is sought between the capsule of the thyroid and the surrounding tissue. The trachea may be compressed and pushed to one side. The best cleavage plane is usually laterally and posteriorly. By finger dissection the goiter is freed from the pleura and the cellular tissue in the mediastinum and is delivered into the neck.

The thyroid surgeon should be familiar with a method of exposing the anterosuperior mediastinum. This may be necessary to remove a large substernal goiter or to perform anterosuperior mediastinal dissection in malignant disease. In some cases the assistance of a thoracic surgeon may be wise. A vertical incision is made from the midportion of the collar incision at the substernal notch in the midline downward to the level of the border of the fourth costal cartilage. The sternum is bared down to the periosteum. The undersurface of the sternum is freed by blunt dissection, and the sternum is divided using a sternal saw. Mediastinal tissues are further dissected from the undersurface of the sternum and the attached cartilages. The divided sternum is retracted laterally, and wide exposure to the anterior surface of the mediastinum is obtained. Beginning at the pericardium, the fascia with the lymph nodes, the fibroareolar tissue, the thymus, and the remaining thyroid remnants are dissected from the great vessels and the trachea. The recurrent laryngeal nerves must be constantly in view. In this fashion the transsternal dissection can be combined with thyroidectomy and neck dissection.

Parathyroidectomy
Indications and Pathology

In 97% of patients hyperparathyroidism can be cured with a single well-planned neck exploration. However, surgical treatment sometimes is difficult because of the minute size of the parathyroid glands, their varied location, and the various types of disease. Comprehensive knowledge of parathyroid embryology, pathology, and surgical anatomy is essential if the treatment is to be successful. The surgeon's goal should be to identify all parathyroid glands in the neck and remove only the enlarged glands responsible for parathyroid hyperfunction. Confirmation of the location and histology of normal parathyroids by frozen-section biopsy is optional but provides invaluable information in patients with multiglandular disease and helps enormously in guiding repeat operations in those patients in whom initial neck exploration does not result in cure.

In approximately 70% to 80% of the cases reported, primary hyperparathyroidism is caused by a solitary parathyroid adenoma. About 2% of patients have multiple nodular hyperplasia, and approximately 20% to 30% of patients with primary hyperparathyroidism have diffuse or nodular hyperplasia. Occasionally a patient may have both an adenoma and hyperplasia. About 1% of patients with primary hyperparathyroidism have parathyroid carcinoma.

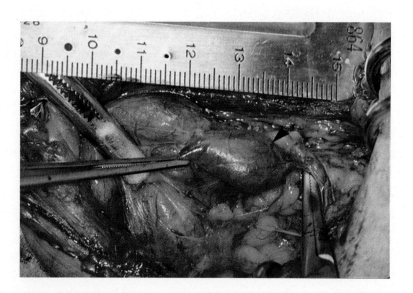

The average adenoma is 1 to 3 cm in diameter; however, they can be much larger. Adenomas are encapsulated and are slightly firmer than the surrounding tissue. Their capsule is reddish brown and their cut surface is yellowish brown. Illustrated is a right lower parathyroid adenoma (arrow). Surgical clamps are on vascular pedicles of the adenoma, sponge forceps retract the right thyroid lobe anteriorly and cephalad, and the patient's head is to the left.

The hyperplastic gland is usually irregular, but can simulate an adenoma, and the size varies from slightly larger than normal to 3 to 4 cm in diameter.

All four glands may be the same size or they may vary in size, and one gland may be enlarged while the other three glands are near normal in size, making it difficult to distinguish grossly between an adenoma and hyperplasia, because uninvolved parathyroids are seldom atrophic in the presence of an adenoma.

Histologically, the normal parathyroid gland is made up of sheets of epithelial cells separated by sinusoids and fat. There are three cell types: chief cells, which show scanty cytoplasm and large deeply staining nuclei; water-clear cells, distinguished by their vacuolated cytoplasm and small eccentric nuclei; and oxyphil cells, which have granules in their cytoplasm that stain deep red with acid dyes. A normal parathyroid gland is composed predominately of chief cells with scattered water-clear and oxyphil cells throughout the glands. There are fat cells between sheets of parathyroid cells. The percentage of fat cells vs. chief cells increases with age, from 10% in childhood to approximately 50% in adulthood.

Adenomas and hyperplastic glands are usually composed predominately of chief cells. Water-clear cell hyperplasia and adenomas rarely occur. Even more rare is the occasional oxyphil adenoma. Histologically, chief cell adenomas are composed of closely packed small cells that resemble the cells of a normal parathyroid except they are more tightly packed and there is little or no fat seen. To confirm the diagnosis of adenoma, the pathologist must find a capsule and an associated fragment of normal parathyroid tissue that is being compressed by the adenoma. Hyperplastic parathyroids are composed of chief cells plus varying amounts (5% to 30%) of fat.

Carcinoma of the parathyroid is usually larger than an adenoma, with firm to hard consistency. Histologically, it is usually made up of closely packed chief cells. The diagnosis of a malignancy cannot be made on the histologic features of the cells; there must be evidence of invasion of adjacent structures or distant metastasis.

Operative Techniques

The initial steps in parathyroidectomy are identical to those for thyroidectomy. The patient's neck is comfortably hyperextended by placing a folded sheet longitudinally between the shoulders to give good exposure of the operative field. The head of the table is tilted upward approximately 30 degrees to increase exposure and decrease venous engorgement.

A transverse incision is made 3 cm above the clavicles in or parallel to a crease in the neck. The scar will be 1.5 cm above the clavicles when the neck is in normal position. Lower incisions over the clavicle and sternum are more likely to develop hypertrophic scars and keloids, since the skin is somewhat tethered to these structures, and therefore the incision is put under transverse tension with motion of the neck. The incision is extended through the skin, subcutaneous tissue, and platysma muscle and is continued to the lateral border of the sternocleidomastoid muscle on each side. The skin flaps are dissected along the avascular plane between the platysma and the investing layer of deep cervical fascia, as described for thyroidectomy. The upper flap is dissected to the level of the superior thyroid notch and the lower flap to the manubrium, exposing the suprasternal notch. The wound edges are draped, and a self-retaining retractor is applied to facilitate good exposure. The strap muscles and sternohyoid and sternothyroid muscles are separated in the midline in the avascular plane, up to the superior thyroid notch of the thyroid cartilage and extending inferiorly to the jugular notch of the manubrium. It is unnecessary to divide the anterior jugular veins unless they communicate across the midline.

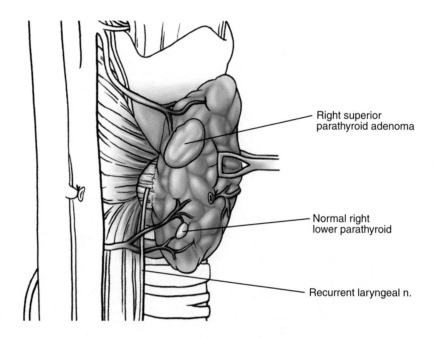

Right superior
parathyroid adenoma

Normal right
lower parathyroid

Recurrent laryngeal n.

The sternothyroid muscle is then dissected free from the thyroid lobe to expose the thyroid and the superior mediastinal tissue. It is rarely necessary to divide the strap muscles during parathyroid exploration. The middle thyroid vein is identified, divided, and ligated. The thyroid lobe can then be retracted medially and anteriorly.

The area bordered medially by the lateral surface of the thyroid gland and laterally by the carotid sheath is now dissected. Gentle anteromedial traction on the thyroid lobe with the use of a "peanut" dissector or Babcock clamp tends to tense up the structures, making their identification easier. This gives a clear view of the posterior aspect of the thyroid gland. It is seldom necessary to ligate the superior pole vessels of the thyroid gland; however, when it is required for good exposure, mobilization should be done carefully to prevent injury to the external branch of the superior laryngeal nerve.

After adequate exposure has been obtained, the inferior thyroid artery and recurrent laryngeal nerve are first identified in the lower portion of the neck, usually in the groove between the trachea and the esophagus. In about two thirds of cases, the nerve runs posterior to the inferior thyroid artery, but it may be anterior to or between branches of the artery. The nerve enters the larynx under cover of the anterior constrictor muscle of the pharynx. The superior parathyroid glands are normally above the inferior thyroid artery, and the inferior parathyroid glands are below the inferior thyroid artery.

The superior parathyroid gland is in its normal position in approximately 75% of cases, posterior to the thyroid lobe at the level of the upper and middle thirds of the thyroid gland. It usually hangs from the thyroid gland or lies near or is closely attached to the dorsal surface of the thyroid gland. The superior parathyroid gland usually is found lateral and dorsal to the recurrent laryngeal nerve as it enters the larynx under cover of the inferior constrictor of the pharynx.

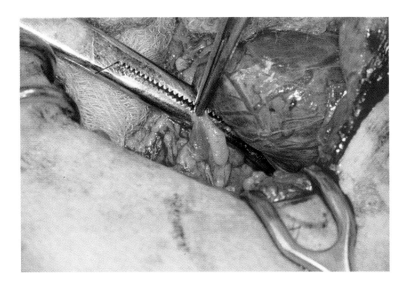

The normal parathyroid gland has a yellow-brown color slightly darker than fat and is rarely larger than 6 × 3 × 3 mm. Surgical forceps holds fat near this left lower parathyroid (arrow), and a surgical clamp retracts the left thyroid lobe anteriorly; the patient's head is to the right. Parathyroid tissue can be confused with fat, lymph nodes, and thyroid and thymus glands.

The superior parathyroid gland is usually covered or surrounded by fat and a thin capsule or opaque fascia. On gentle palpation of the suspected gland, one can see a small "body" moving beneath the fat capsule. The entire parathyroid gland should not be dissected free from the surrounding fat and capsule because of the danger of interfering with its blood supply. A tiny biopsy may be done to confirm diagnosis, using microsurgical technique, opposite its feeding artery. Two gross findings are helpful in identifying parathyroid tissue at the time of biopsy. Parathyroid tissue is quite vascular, and on biopsy a "blush" or diffuse bleeding is seen from the cut surface; fat does not exhibit such a blush. The gland holds its shape or body following biopsy; this does not occur if the tissue is fat.

The lower parathyroid gland is more difficult to identify than the superior gland. It is in its normal position in approximately 50% of individuals. The lower parathyroid gland is normally located on the posterolateral aspect of the inferior pole of the thyroid gland, below the inferior thyroid artery (see p. 85).

It sometimes may be in a fatty appendage of the distal thyroid pole. The inferior parathyroid gland is usually surrounded by fat and a thin capsule. On gentle palpation of the suspect gland, it may be seen moving within the fat and capsule. A small area of the parathyroid tissue is exposed by gentle dissection of the fat and capsule distal to its blood supply. The surgeon should expose only enough of the gland for identification and determination of size and for biopsy. The mass of parathyroid may be estimated in situ by taking its measurements in three dimensions and multiplying the volume by 0.6, which yields the volume of a prolate ellipsoid. The volume in cubic millimeters is approximately equal to the mass ring.

All four parathyroid glands should be identified before removing any parathyroid tissue. Generally the parathyroid glands can be identified by gross appearance. However, many surgeons prefer to biopsy each gland to confirm identification of the four parathyroid glands and to establish the histologic picture of each gland.

Extent of Parathyroidectomy

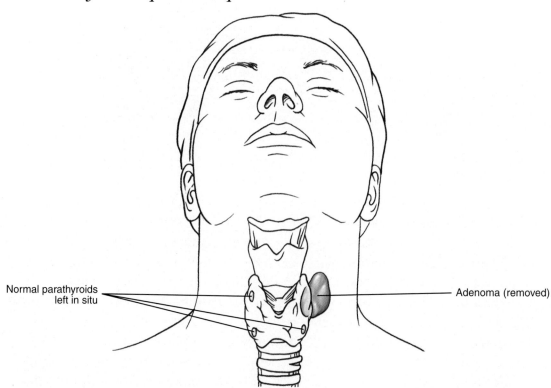

Normal parathyroids left in situ — Adenoma (removed)

If an adenoma is found and the other glands are histologically normal, the adenoma is removed (resected gland hatched). The adenoma is frequently tucked down under the lateral lobe of the thyroid in a space beside the esophagus. It may be just slightly posterior, in the groove between the esophagus and the trachea or thyroid cartilage. With careful dissection, a normal rim of parathyroid tissue can often be identified grossly inside the capsule of the adenoma. This may be labeled with a suture and brought to the attention of the pathologist so that it can be identified histologically. When an adenoma is removed, a frozen section is done to confirm the diagnosis of hyperfunctioning parathyroid tissue.

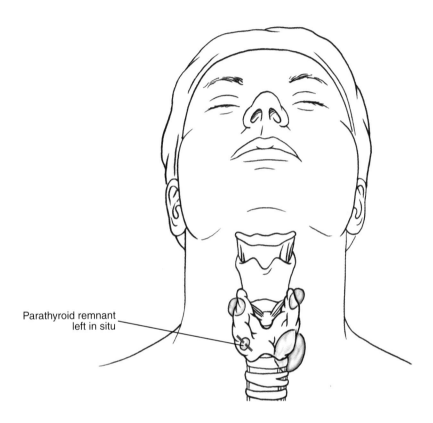

Parathyroid remnant
left in situ

If the parathyroid glands are hyperplastic, three and one half to three and three fourths are removed, and the equivalent of two normal glands is cryopreserved (resected tissue hatched). The gland remnant may be marked with a permanent suture for future identification. Alternately, all parathyroids may be removed from the neck, and the equivalent of one to two normal parathyroids may be minced into 1 mm^3 fragments and autografted into either the sternocleidomastoid or forearm muscle. In this instance, additional fragments may be cryopreserved as a safeguard in case the autografted tissue is insufficient. Total parathyroidectomy and autotransplantation have the advantage that recurrent parathyroid hyperfunction may be treated by partial autograft excision under local anesthesia. However, some autografts fail to function, particularly in marginally nourished patients receiving dialysis. In these patients a vascularized parathyroid remnant often functions better, and patients may be discharged sooner. Furthermore, in our experience, vascularized remnant regrowth is distinctly uncommon if the size of the remnant is small (the equivalent of one to two normal parathyroids in mass, less than 80 mg).

If there is carcinoma of the parathyroid, en bloc excision of the primary tumor and metastasis with definitive resection at the initial operation is the treatment of choice. An ipsilateral modified radical neck dissection should be done because of early local lymphatic involvement.

After hemostasis has been accomplished, a small closed suction drain is left on each side of the neck and brought out through a separate site. The strap muscles are approximated in the midline with interrupted 4-0 silk sutures. The platysma is sutured with interrupted 4-0 white absorbable suture and the skin edges approximated with interrupted mattress sutures. The drains are removed in 24 hours. The skin sutures are removed on the second day.

Abnormal Parathyroid Tumor Locations

The location of the inferior glands varies because of their embryologic motility. Abnormally located parathyroid glands may be found from the level of the angle of the jaw to the carina. Frequently missing superior parathyroid adenomas are found in the tracheoesophageal groove and the area posterior to the esophagus. The abnormal gland may be found lying below or lateral to the cervical vertebral bodies. The area along the carotid sheath should also be palpated and exposed. The capsule on the dorsal aspect of the thyroid gland should be inspected carefully. A branch of the inferior thyroid artery may lead the surgeon to the missing parathyroid gland. If the gland still is not found, transcervical thymectomy should be attempted. By gentle traction with clamps, the thymus can be withdrawn from the mediastinum into the cervical incision. Possible complications include bleeding and pneumothorax. Parathymic glands should be searched for above the thyroid to a level at the angle of the jaw near the submaxillary gland. If the missing parathyroid gland is still not found after an extensive search such as described, the thyroid lobe on the appropriate side should be removed because an intrathyroidal parathyroid adenoma may be present.

If a hyperfunctioning parathyroid cannot be found during initial surgery, exploration of the mediastinum should be delayed A careful operative record should be made for future reference. The hyperfunctioning parathyroid tissue may have been removed in the tissue or thyroid submitted for histologic study, or the blood supply to the hyperfunctioning parathyroid tissue may have been interrupted during the course of dissection. If significant hypercalcemia persists, the patient should be reevaluated. High-resolution, real-time sonography and computed tomography (CT) may be helpful. However, the single most reliable localization test currently is technetium-sestamibi scanning. Approximately 2% of parathyroid tumors are found within the mediastinum or the thymus or in the aortopulmonary window or precarinal spaces. The aortopulmonary window can be dissected via sternotomy. The precarinal space is best approached via right thoracotomy.

Anatomic Basis of Complications

NERVE INJURIES

- Nerves at risk during thyroidectomy and parathyroidectomy include the recurrent laryngeal nerves, the external branches of the superior laryngeal nerves, and the cervical sympathetic nerve trunks. In a series of 217 thyroid operations, Holt et al. found nine laryngeal nerve injuries, four of them permanent. In the same series there were three injuries to superior laryngeal nerves; one was permanent.

- Most recurrent laryngeal nerve injuries occur "just below that point to where the nerve passed under the lower fibers of the inferior constrictor muscle to become intralaryngeal." The usual cause is a hemostatic stitch. Another source of injury is mass ligation of the vessels of the lower pole of the thyroid. Such ligation may include a recurrent nerve more anterior than usual. The nerve should be identified before ligating the inferior thyroid vein.

- Sites of possible nerve injury in thyroidectomy are as follows:

  1. External branch of the superior laryngeal nerve during ligation of the superior thyroid vascular pedicle.

  2. Recurrent laryngeal nerve as it traverses the ligament of Berry during total lobectomy. The recurrent nerve usually courses posterior to the "adherent zone" (ligament of Berry); however, in 25% of cases it passes through it. The nerve traverses the thyroid itself at this level in 10% of patients. By retraction on the lobe, the recurrent nerve can be pulled forward into the operative field and be injured inadvertently.

  3. Recurrent laryngeal nerve during ligation of the inferior thyroid artery. It is important to ligate branches of the artery while keeping the nerve under direct vision lateral to the nerve.

  4. Recurrent laryngeal nerve during ligation of the inferior thyroid veins. The nerve is anterolateral to the trachea in about 10% of cases and may be caught and divided during ligation of the veins.

  5. Nonrecurrent nerve during ligation of the inferior thyroid artery. A nonrecurrent nerve may be mistaken for the inferior thyroid artery and ligated, because it takes a parallel horizontal course from the cervical vagus to the larynx. Fortunately, this anatomic variant is rare.

  6. Cervical sympathetic trunk during ligation of the inferior thyroid artery. If the inferior thyroid artery is ligated too far lateral, the cervical sympathetic trunk may be caught in the tie.

Continued.

Anatomic Basis of Complications—cont'd

- Specific causes of recurrent nerve injury have been detailed by Chang. Separation of the inferior thyroid artery from the recurrent laryngeal nerve requires care. Where the nerve passes between branches of the artery, the individual branches must be ligated and divided separately.
- Injury to the recurrent laryngeal nerve usually is complete. The vocal cord then takes up a paramedian or cadaveric position. When only one side is involved, the airway is adequate. However, the voice may be hoarse until one cord compensates by adducting over to the opposite cord. If the external branch of the superior laryngeal nerve is also injured, the cord becomes flaccid as well as paralyzed. This may cause noisy breathing on both inspiration and expiration.
- The recurrent laryngeal nerve carries both adductor and abductor fibers. The adductor fibers are more vulnerable to injury and may be preferentially damaged by traction, cautery, and other procedures. Such incomplete bilateral damage to the recurrent laryngeal nerves is more dangerous and more potentially life-threatening than is bilateral complete injury, since damage to abductor fibers results in unopposed function of adductor fibers, which draw the cords toward the midline, narrowing the glottic opening to a slit and resulting in severe respiratory distress.
- Injury to the external branch of the superior laryngeal nerve results in dysfunction of the cricothyroid muscle, with ensuing hoarseness that usually improves with time. The voice is usually "breathy" and aspiration of liquids is a frequent complication. Bilateral damage to both external branches results in flaccid vocal cords and extreme weakness of the voice on phonation. The superior thyroid artery should not be clamped above the upper pole of the thyroid because the external laryngeal nerve may be injured. Individual branches of the artery should be divided individually.
- Postoperative hoarseness is not always the result of operative injury to laryngeal nerves. One percent to 2% of patients have a paralyzed vocal cord prior to thyroid resection. Based on several large series, it is recommended that the patient be informed that, despite all precautions, there is a possibility (1% to 2%) of some vocal disability following thyroidectomy or parathyroidectomy.
- A sympathetic ganglion may be confused with a lymph node and removed when the surgeon operates for metastatic papillary carcinoma of the thyroid. Injury to the cervical sympathetic nerve results in Horner's syndrome (constriction of the pupil, ptosis of the upper eyelid, apparent enophthalmus, and dilation of retinal vessels).

Anatomic Basis of Complications—cont'd

HYPOPARATHYROIDISM

- With total thyroidectomy, transient hypocalcemia may occur in 5% to 10% of patients. The incidence of permanent hypoparathyroidism is less than 1% in patients operated on by experienced surgeons, especially with preservation or autotransplantation of resected tissue from a normal parathyroid gland.

VASCULAR INJURIES AND HEMORRHAGE

- Thyroid arteries must be ligated carefully. The superior thyroid artery tends to retract. The middle thyroid vein is short and easily torn and, if divided accidentally, will retract, making hemostasis difficult. With too much traction of the thyroid gland, the vein becomes flattened and bloodless, making it difficult to recognize. The tear is often at the junction of the vein with the jugular vein. The thoracic duct is rarely injured in thyroidectomy, although it may be injured during neck dissection. The duct may be ligated with impunity.

ORGAN INJURIES

- The pleurae are rarely injured, except in cases of huge goiter extending into the mediastinum. Both anteriorly and posteriorly, the two pleurae approach the midline and hence each other. Intrathoracic goiter may descend into the anterior or posterior medastinum, bringing the thyroid gland close to the pleurae.
- The trachea and esophagus may be injured in the presence of thyroiditis, calcified adenoma, or malignancy. The true capsule of the thyroid, the pretracheal fascia, the trachea, and the esophagus may be fixed to one another, and vigorous attempts at separation may perforate the trachea. Tracheal perforation may require immediate tracheostomy.

KEY REFERENCES

Edis A, Ayala L, Edgahl R. Manual of Endocrine Surgery. New York: Springer-Verlag, 1975, p 122.

The authors provide detailed accounts of the techniques of thyroidectomy and parathy-roidectomy as performed at the Mayo Clinic. They also outline the potential risks and complications of these procedures, including injury to the recurrent laryngeal nerve.

Feind CR. The head and neck. In Haagensen CD, Feind CR, Herter FP et al., eds. The Lymphatics in Cancer. Philadelphia: WB Saunders, 1972.

The author provides a comprehensive analysis of the lymphatic and vascular anatomy of the neck, particularly as it pertains to the thyroid and parathyroid glands.

Gilmour JR. The embryology of the parathyroid glands, the thymus and certain associated rudiments. J Pathol 45:507, 1937.

This is the largest and most authoritative study of the locations of the human parathyroids in the literature. The author has carefully mapped the most frequent locations, as well as aberrant sites, for both upper and lower parathyroids.

McGarity WC, Bostwick J. Technique of parathyroidectomy. Am Surg 42:657, 1976.

The authors provide a detailed report of the technique of parathyroidectomy, with careful attention to the pitfalls, risks, and potential complications, particularly those related to injury of the recurrent laryngeal nerve.

Sedgwick CE. Surgery of the thyroid gland. In Sedgwick C, Cady B, eds. Surgery of the Thyroid and Parathyroid Glands: Major Problems in Clinical Surgery. Philadelphia: WB Saunders, 1980, pp 159-187.

The author summarizes in great detail the Lahey Clinic technique for thyroidectomy, with sequential, step-by-step, detailed descriptions of safe approaches to the recurrent laryngeal nerve and parathyroid sparing.

SUGGESTED READINGS

Aleryd A. Parathyroid gland in thyroid surgery. Acta Chir Scand (Suppl) 389:1-120, 1968.

Boerner T, Ramanathan S. Functional anatomy of the airway. In Benumof J, ed. Airway Management: Principles and Practice. St Louis: Mosby, 1996, pp 3-21.

Caldarelli DD, Holinger LD. Complications and sequalae of thyroid surgery. Otolaryngol Clin North Am 13:85-97, 1990.

Chang-Chien Y. Surgical anatomy and vulnerability of the recurrent laryngeal nerve. Int Surg 65:23, 1980.

Hay ID, Bergstralh EJ, Goellner JR, et al. Predicting outcome in papillary thyroid carcinoma: Development of a reliable prognostic scoring system in a cohort of 1779 patients surgically treated at one institution during 1940 through 1989. Surgery 114:1050-1058, 1993.

Henry JF, Audiffret J, Denizot A, et al. The nonrecurrent inferior laryngeal nerve: Review of 33 cases, including two on the left side. Surgery 104:977-984, 1988.

Holt GR, McMurry GT, Joseph DJ. Recurrent laryngeal nerve injury following thyroid operations. Surg Gynecol Obstet 144:567, 1977.

Kaplan EL, Yashiro T, Salti G. Primary hyperparathyroidism in the 1990s. Ann Surg 215:300-301, 1992.

Lahey FH, Hoover WB. Injuries to the recurrent laryngeal nerve in thyroid operations. Ann Surg 108:545, 1938.

Leight GS. Nodular goiter and benign and malignant neoplasms. In Sabiston D Jr, ed. Textbook of Surgery, 14th ed. Philadelphia: WB Saunders, 1991, pp 579-590.

Lumsden AB, McGarity WC. A technique for subtotal thyroidectomy. Surg Gynecol Obstet 168:177-179, 1989.

Mazzaferri EL. Thyroid carcinoma: Papillary and follicular. In Mazzaferri E, Samaan N, eds. Endocrine Tumors. Boston: Blackwell, 1993, pp 278-333.

Riddell V. Thyroidectomy: Prevention of bilateral recurrent nerve palsy. Br J Surg 57:1, 1970.

Skandalakis JE, Droulias C, Harlaftis N, et al. Recurrent laryngeal nerves. Am Surg 42:620, 1976.

Thompson NW. Complications of parathyroid surgery. In Greenfield LJ, ed. Complications in Surgery and Trauma. Philadelphia: JB Lippincott, 1990, pp 660-673.

Wang C. The anatomic basis of parathyroid surgery. Ann Surg 183:271, 1976.

Weber CJ, Sewell CW, McGarity WC. Persistent recurrent sporadic primary hyperparathyroidism: Histology, complications, and results of reoperation. Surgery 116:991-998, 1994.

Lateral Neck

Grant W. Carlson, M.D.

The vast majority of solitary, nonthyroidal neck masses in adults represent metastatic cancer from a primary lesion located above the clavicle. Squamous cell carcinoma accounts for the vast majority of these neoplasms. Benign tumors and infectious causes comprise the majority of neck masses seen in children.

Tumors of the salivary glands and carotid body are infrequent causes of neck masses. Lymphoma commonly presents in the head and neck and is the most common tumor of childhood.

A complete head and neck examination can locate the primary cancer in over 90% of cases presenting as a neck mass. The diagnosis can usually be made by fine-needle aspiration cytology. Equivocal results or insufficient tissue may necessitate open biopsy. Computed tomography (CT) or magnetic resonance imaging (MRI) can improve the sensitivity of physical examination of the neck and parotid glands and guides treatment planning.

SURGICAL ANATOMY
Fasciae of Neck

Knowledge of the fascial layers of the neck is mandatory to extirpate cancer and treat infections of the head and neck. The fascia surrounds muscles, vessels, and viscera to form defined surgical planes and fascial envelopes. Metastatic squamous cell cancer of the head and neck follows predictable patterns, and the fascial planes enable resection with preservation of many vital structures.

The superficial fascia of the neck is composed of the platysma muscle, loose connective tissue, fat, and small unnamed nerves and blood vessels. The platysma is a voluntary muscle and is innervated by the cervical branch of the facial nerve. The muscle may be included in elevating skin flaps to improve vascularity. Superficial lymphatic channels lie above the muscle, and removal would require skin excision.

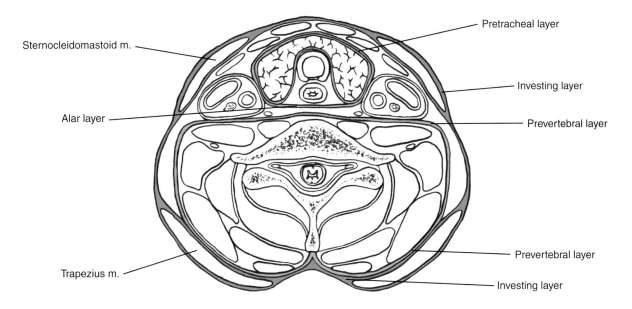

Sternocleidomastoid m.

Alar layer

Trapezius m.

Pretracheal layer

Investing layer

Prevertebral layer

Prevertebral layer

Investing layer

The cutaneous nerves of the neck and the external and anterior jugular veins lie between the platysma and the deep cervical fascia. The deep cervical fascia consists of areolar tissue that supports the muscles, vessels, and viscera of the neck. In certain areas it forms well-defined fibrous sheets called the investing layer, the pretracheal layer, and the prevertebral layer. The investing layer of the deep cervical fascia arises from the ligament nuchae and the spines of the cervical vertebrae and courses forward to completely surround the neck. It is attached to the external occipital protuberance, mastoid process, and zygoma. The investing layer envelops the trapezius and sternocleidomastoid muscles and the parotid and submaxillary glands. At the anterior border of the sternocleidomastoid muscle it contributes to the anterolateral wall of the carotid sheath and continues as a single layer to the midline. The pretracheal layer splits into an anterior portion that envelops the sternohyoid and sternothyroid muscles and a posterior layer that envelops the thyroid gland, forming the false capsule of the gland. Below, it extends into the thorax and blends with the fibrous pericardium. Laterally it blends with the carotid sheath and with the investing layer beneath the sternocleidomastoid muscle. The carotid sheath contains the common and internal carotid arteries, internal jugular vein, and vagus nerve. The nerve lies between and beneath the vessels. The deep cervical group of lymph nodes are found along the internal jugular vein, within the sheath. Removal of the nodes can be facilitated by removal of the internal jugular vein, as described in a classic radical neck dissection. With careful fascial dissection the nodes can be removed without vein sacrifice in a modified neck dissection. The prevertebral or deep layer encircles the muscles attached to the vertebral column: splenius capitis, levator scapulae, and the anterior, middle, and posterior scalene muscles. The deep cervical lymphatic channels are embedded in the loose connective tissue between investing and deep layers of the deep cervical fascia.

Triangles of the Neck

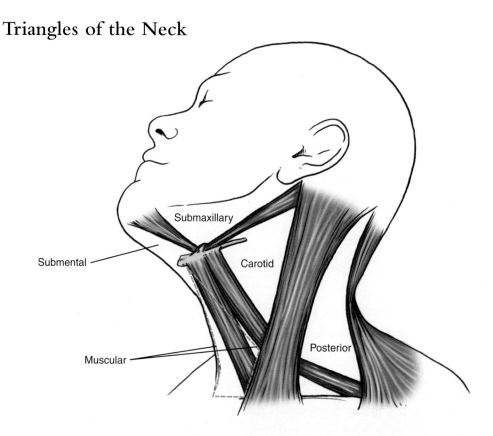

The sternocleidomastoid muscle divides the neck into two large triangles: anterior and posterior. It is attached to the lateral surface of the mastoid and the superior nuchal line of the occipital bone. Inferiorly it divides into two heads inserting on the clavicle and the sternum. At the anterior margin of the sternocleidomastoid muscle, thickened fascia attaches to the angle of the mandible, forming an angular band called Charpy's band. This band must be released to expose the tail of the parotid and carotid vessels. The anterior triangle is formed by the anterior edge of the sternocleidomastoid muscle, the midline of the neck from the manubrium to the symphysis of the mandible, and the inferior margin of the mandible. It is composed of four smaller triangles: submental, submaxillary, carotid, and muscular. The submental triangle is bounded laterally by the anterior belly of the digastric muscle, inferiorly by the hyoid bone, and medially by the midline of the neck. The floor is composed of the mylohyoid muscle. Within the triangle is the terminal portion of the submental artery and a few submental lymph nodes. These nodes drain the anterior part of the tongue, floor of mouth, and gingiva.

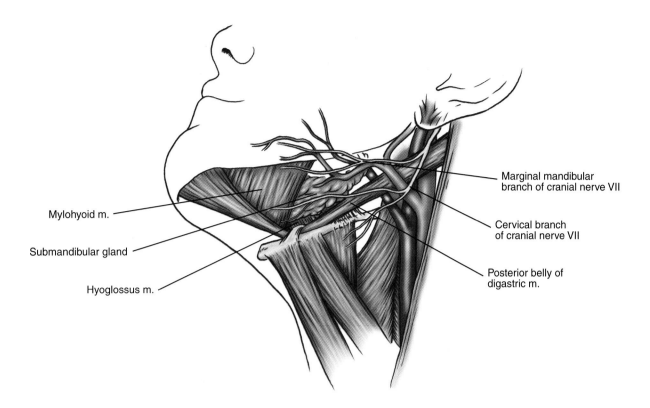

Mylohyoid m.

Submandibular gland

Hyoglossus m.

Marginal mandibular
branch of cranial nerve VII

Cervical branch
of cranial nerve VII

Posterior belly of
digastric m.

The submaxillary triangle is formed by the anterior and posterior bellies of the digastric muscles and the inferior border of the mandible. This area includes the most complicated anatomy in the neck and has clinical importance in the treatment of tumors of the submandibular gland as well as metastatic disease from the anterior tongue and floor of mouth. The roof is formed by the skin and the platysma muscle. The floor is composed largely of the mylohyoid muscle and a small amount by the hyoglossus muscle and the middle constrictor of the pharynx.

The carotid triangle is formed by the anterior border of the sternocleidomastoid muscle, inferiorly by the superior belly of the omohyoid muscle, and superiorly by the greater cornu of the hyoid bone and the posterior belly of the digastric muscle. The floor is formed anteriorly by the thyrohyoid muscle and posteriorly by the middle and inferior constrictors of the pharynx. Passing superficial within the triangle are tributaries of the common facial vein, the greater auricular nerve, and the cervical branch of the facial nerve. The superior thyroid, occipital, and ascending pharyngeal branches of the external carotid artery arise within the triangle.

The muscular triangle lies below the hyoid bone. It is formed anteriorly by the midline of the neck, superiorly by the superior belly of the omohyoid muscle, and inferiorly by the anterior border of the sternocleidomastoid muscle. The floor is composed of the sternohyoid and the sternothyroid muscles. Beneath the floor lies the thyroid gland, larynx, trachea, and esophagus. The anterior jugular veins course beneath the platysma muscle on either side of the midline. Just above the suprasternal notch the veins unite, then pass laterally beneath the sternocleidomastoid muscle to drain into the external jugular vein.

The sternocleidomastoid and trapezius muscles attach on a continuous line, extending from the external occipital protuberance along the superior nuchal line to the mastoid process. The proximity of the attachments forms the apex of the posterior triangle. The anterior and posterior boundaries are these two muscles, and the base is the middle third of the clavicle. The floor is formed by the splenius capitis, levator scapulae, and scalenus medius muscles, covered by prevertebral fascia. The roof is formed by the overlying skin; the platysma muscle is present only in the anterior part. Its absence makes it difficult to develop skin flaps in the posterior neck. The triangle contains the third part of the subclavian artery and the transverse cervical, suprascapular, and occipital arteries. The external jugular vein courses obliquely through the triangle to drain into the subclavian vein. Difficulty arises in dissection of the most inferior portion of the triangle, where troublesome bleeding may be encountered. The inferior belly of the omohyoid muscle serves as an important landmark. No important structure other than the external jugular vein is found until the muscle is divided. The spinal accessory nerve is the most important structure in the posterior triangle. It exits the jugular foramen, crossing ventral to the internal jugular vein and deep to the posterior belly of the digastric muscle. It lies deep to the sternocleidomastoid muscle and divides within the muscle to supply it, then continues through the lateral neck on the levator scapulae muscle to innervate the trapezius muscle.

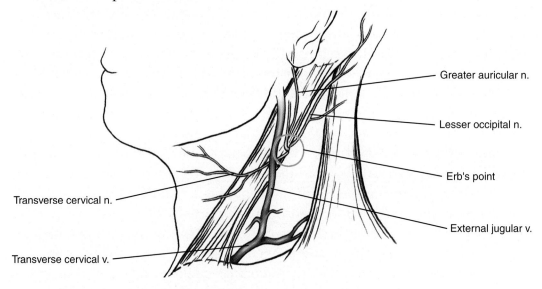

The nerve can be identified as it enters the deep surface of the sternocleidomastoid muscle approximately 4 cm below the mastoid. It can also be found at Erb's point just superior to where the greater auricular nerve surfaces from behind the sternocleidomastoid muscle. The nerve enters the deep surface of the trapezius approximately two fingerbreadths superior to the clavicle.

Submaxillary Gland

The submaxillary gland and associated lymph nodes fill the triangle overlapping the digastric muscles and extending upward deep to the mandible. Differentiating gland from lymph nodes can be difficult. The gland sends a prolongation of tissue with the submaxillary duct of Wharton under the mylohyoid muscle. The duct opens into the mouth on the side of the frenulum of the tongue. Superficial to the gland, the facial vein crosses the submaxillary triangle to reach the anterior border of the mandible. The facial artery enters the triangle under the posterior belly of the digastric and stylohyoid muscles. It ascends to emerge above or through the upper border of the gland. The marginal mandibular branch of the facial nerve courses through the triangle beneath the platysma muscle. It is the only important structure above the digastric muscle in a submaxillary dissection. The course of the nerve is variable and frequently has multiple branches. Dingman and Grabb found the nerve to be above the anterior ramus of the mandible in 81% of their cadaver dissections. In my experience, the nerve loops below the mandible to a varying degree in most patients. Skandalakis et al. reported that in 50% of cases the mandibular branch was above the mandibular border and therefore outside the submaxillary triangle. It courses over the facial vessels as it travels upward to supply the depressor anguli oris and the depressor labii inferioris muscles. To prevent injury during neck dissection, the facial vessels are divided below the nerve and used to retract the nerve above the mandible. Lymph nodes are present about the vessels, and the nerve may need to be sacrificed to facilitate removal. Injury to the nerve can result in facial asymmetry, occasionally with drooling. The hypoglossal nerve descends between the internal jugular vein and the internal carotid artery, giving branches to the thyrohyoid and geniohyoid muscles, and supplies the superior limb of the ansa cervicalis, which supplies the infrahyoid strap muscles. It enters the triangle deep to the posterior belly of the digastric muscles. It lies on the surface of the hyoglossus muscle and courses deep to the mylohyoid muscle to supply motor function to the tongue. The lingual nerve, a branch of the mandibular nerve, is found under the border of the mandible on the hyoglossus muscle above the hypoglossal nerve. It is attached to the submaxillary gland by the submaxillary ganglion and courses deep to the mylohyoid muscle to provide sensation to the anterior tongue and floor of mouth (see p. 107).

Cervical Lymph Nodes

One third of the lymph nodes in the body are concentrated in the head and neck region. Detailed knowledge of the cervical lymphatic channels is necessary to diagnose and treat cancer of the head and neck. The superficial lymphatics course in the subcutaneous tissue intimately associated with the skin and superficial fascia. They perforate the superficial layer of the deep cervical fascia to communicate with the deep cervical nodes. These superficial nodes are frequently involved in cervical metastases, especially during the late stages, but are of little significance from the surgical standpoint. Superficial lymphatic nodes involved with cancer cannot be removed without resection of large areas of skin, and their involvement implies a dismal prognosis.

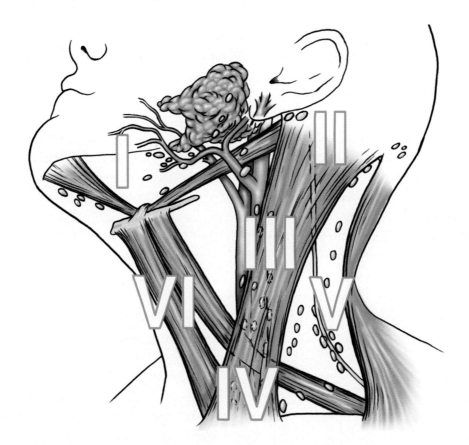

At the junction of the head and neck are groups of nodes named for their location: occipital, retroauricular, parotid, submandibular, submental, and retropharyngeal nodes. These groups of nodes form a cervical ring and are the first-echelon drainage for the scalp, the face, and the mucous membrane of the upper aerodigestive tract. Involvement of a particular nodal group provides a clue to the location of the primary lesion.

The lymph nodes in the posterior cervical triangle course along the spinal accessory nerve. The upper nodes in this group are in the anterior neck, where there is a coalescence of nodes from both the upper jugular and spinal accessory groups. These nodes drain the nose and upper extent of the aerodigestive tract. The spinal accessory nodes are infrequently involved in metastases from the oral cavity, but preservation may be impossible because of proximity to the anterior jugular chain. Small nodes course along the transverse cervical vessels, communicating with both the spinal accessory and jugular chains. They receive drainage from the skin of the lateral neck and chest. The nodes in this group are more frequently involved by metastatic carcinoma from below the clavicle (breast, lung, kidney, stomach, lower gastrointestinal tract) than from the neck itself.

The lymphatics of the anterior triangle course along the internal jugular vein. They are embedded in the fascia of the carotid sheath, and the majority lie on the anterolateral aspect of the vein. The jugulodigastric nodes are in the upper neck, below the posterior belly of the digastric muscle and behind the angle of the mandible. This is an important surgical area and is a frequent site of cervical metastases. The spinal accessory nerve must frequently be sacrificed to adequately remove metastatic nodes in this area. The middle jugular nodes are found where the omohyoid muscle crosses the carotid sheath. These drain the middle part of the aerodigestive tract and thyroid. The inferior nodes are below the omohyoid and drain the thyroid, esophagus, and trachea.

A system of levels for describing the location of lymph nodes in the neck was developed by the Memorial Sloan-Kettering group and provides standardization that is useful to accurately compare studies of cervical nodal disease.

Level I *Submental Group.* Nodal tissue between the anterior belly of the digastric muscles and above the hyoid bone.
Submandibular Group. Nodal tissue in the triangular area bounded by the anterior and posterior bellies of the digastric muscle and the inferior border of the mandible.

Level II *Upper Jugular Group.* Nodal tissue around upper portion of the internal jugular vein and the upper spinal accessory nerve. It extends from the skull base to the bifurcation of the carotid artery or the hyoid bone. The posterior limit is the posterior border of the sternocleidomastoid muscle and the anterior border is the lateral border of the sternohyoid muscle.

Level III *Middle Jugular Group.* Nodal tissue around the middle third of the internal jugular vein, from the inferior border of level II to the omohyoid muscle. The anterior and posterior borders are the same as for level II.

Level IV *Lower Jugular Group.* Nodal tissue around the inferior third of the internal jugular vein, from the inferior border of level III to the clavicle. The anterior and posterior borders are the same as for levels II and III.

Level V *Posterior Triangle Group.* Nodal tissue around the lower portion of the spinal accessory nerve and along the transverse cervical vessels. It is bounded by the triangle formed by the clavicle, posterior border of the sternocleidomastoid muscle, and anterior border of the trapezius muscle.

Level VI *Anterior Compartment Group.* Lymph nodes around the midline visceral structures of the neck, extending from the level of the hyoid bone superiorly to the surprasternal notch inferiorly. The lateral border is the medial border of the carotid sheath. Included are the perithyroidal and paratracheal lymph nodes, and nodes along the recurrent laryngeal nerves.

Blood Supply

The carotid sheath is a filmy fascial covering surrounding the carotid artery and internal jugular vein. The vast majority of the venous outflow from the head and neck courses through the internal jugular vein, the external jugular vein, and the anterior jugular vein. The internal jugular vein empties and fills during the inspiratory-expiratory cycle. Once divided at its lower end, it becomes distended with blood, which can make further dissection difficult. For this reason, some surgeons prefer to ligate the upper portion of the vein first. The internal jugular vein has no posterior branches. Dissection carried out from behind the sternocleidomastoid muscle moving forward can effectively exploit this.

The internal jugular vein begins at the jugular foramen in the skull as a continuation of the sigmoid sinus. It descends through the neck to unite with the subclavian vein behind the medial head of the clavicle to form the brachiocephalic vein. The facial vein is a main tributary of the internal jugular vein. It courses over the submandibular gland to drain the face. It must be divided to expose the carotid bifurcation. The external jugular vein begins behind the angle of the mandible by the union of the posterior auricular and retromandibular veins. It descends obliquely across the sternocleidomastoid muscle parallel to the greater auricular nerve. It enters the subclavian vein just above the clavicle in the posterior triangle.

The arterial supply to the extracranial head and neck is derived predominantly from the external carotid artery. The level of carotid bifurcation is variable but is most commonly at the angle of the mandible.

Nerve Supply

The anterior and lateral neck areas are innervated by the anterior rami of cervical nerves C2 to C4. The greater auricular nerve runs obliquely with the external jugular vein, across the sternocleidomastoid muscle to supply sensation to the skin of the external ear. The transverse cutaneous nerve passes across the midportion of the sternocleidomastoid muscle to provide sensation to the anterior and lateral portions of the neck.

The vagus nerve exits the jugular foramen at the skull base. It lies between the carotid artery and the internal jugular vein in the carotid sheath. The spinal accessory nerve also exits the jugular foramen. It usually courses over the internal jugular vein to enter the sternocleidomastoid muscle, which it innervates. It exits posteriorly behind the sternocleidomastoid muscle at Erb's point to innervate the trapezius muscle. The hypoglossal nerve exits the skull at the hypoglossal foramen. It descends between the internal carotid artery and the internal jugular vein beneath the digastric muscles. It enters the oral cavity after passing under the mylohyoid muscle.

SURGICAL APPLICATIONS

The primary role of lymph node dissection in head and neck cancer is to achieve locoregional control. Radical neck dissection, systematic removal of the cervical lymph nodes, was first described by Crile in 1906. The procedure removes all the lymph node–bearing tissue from the midline of the neck to the anterior border of the trapezius muscle and from the horizontal ramus of the mandible to the clavicle (levels I to V). The classic operation, popularized by Martin, includes removal of the sternocleidomastoid muscle, internal jugular vein, and spinal accessory nerve. The upper portion of the nerve exits the jugular foramen in close proximity to the internal jugular vein. Dissection of the nerve in this portion violates the anterior fascial compartment. The nerve then passes through the fascial envelope of the posterior triangle to innervate the trapezius muscle. Martin stressed that the nerve must be sacrificed to adequately extirpate the cervical lymphatics. Metastases to the posterior triangle are relatively infrequent unless levels I to IV nodes are involved.

Sacrifice of the spinal accessory nerve is extremely debilitating. Nahum described in 1961 the shoulder syndrome of pain, scapular displacement, and shoulder droop. Trapezius muscle paralysis limits abduction and support of the shoulder. Several studies have demonstrated successful grafting of the resected nerve with a portion of greater auricular nerve. Modifications of the radical neck dissection have been developed to preserve the spinal accessory nerve in early stage neck disease when level V metastases are infrequent.

The recurrence rate for tumor in the neck after radical neck dissection has been reported at 10% to 70%. Historically, the lack of control attributed to radical neck dissection was related to lack of control of the tumor primary site.

One has to look at the older data regarding recurrence after radical neck dissection to avoid the effect of combined treatment with radiation therapy. Strong found that tumor recurrence in the neck was 71% if multiple levels of nodes were involved initially. The problem with the study was that in 25% of cases the primary tumor was not controlled.

Schneider et al. found recurrence rates of 11% for N1 disease and 19% for N2 disease when the primary tumor was controlled. As reported by DeSanto et al., recurrence rates in dissected necks at 2 years after radical neck dissection were 7.5% for N0 disease, 20.2% for N1 disease, and 37.4% for N2 disease. These results indicate that the efficacy of radical neck dissection decreases as the severity of disease in the neck increases.

Modified neck dissection, or functional neck dissection, preserves one or more of the nonlymphatic structures sacrificed in radical neck dissection. Removal of levels I to V nodes with preservation of the spinal accessory nerve, sternocleidomastoid muscle, and internal jugular vein was suggested by Bocca et al. The theoretical advantages of modified neck dissection are as follows:

- Preservation of neck and shoulder girdle function
- Better cosmetic contour of the neck
- Protection of the internal carotid artery
- Ability to perform bilateral procedures
- Use as an elective operation in clinical N0 disease

Preservation of the spinal accessory nerve is an attempt to reduce the shoulder morbidity seen with a radical neck dissection. It is usually followed by a temporary, reversible phase of dysfunction resulting from traction or devascularization of the nerve. Preservation of the sternocleidomastoid muscle may improve the cosmetic contour of the neck and protect the carotid artery.

Bilateral cervical lymph node metastases are not an infrequent occurrence. Bilateral radical neck dissection usually is performed as a staged procedure over several weeks. Loss of both internal jugular veins may alter cerebral and facial circulation, although Crile thought the vertebral venous system would provide adequate collateral circulation. The perceived risks of bilateral jugular vein loss include death, brain damage, blindness, and permanent facial distortion. Beahrs reported a series of bilateral radical neck dissections and found a low complication rate.

Radical Neck Dissection
Sequence of Dissection

The classic description of the radical neck dissection begins with the division of the sternocleidomastoid muscle and internal jugular vein at the base of the neck. The operation then proceeds in a cephalad direction. This is technically easy, but involves sacrifice of the spinal accessory nerve without assessment of the upper neck; it can be difficult to ligate the upper end of the internal jugular vein. It also fails to take advantage of the fact that the major vessels of the neck have no posterior branches except the occipital artery arising under the posterior belly of the digastric muscle. Resectability of the nodal metastases cannot be assessed until the neck dissection is almost completed.

Beginning in the submandibular triangle and proceeding laterally and inferiorly has several advantages. The majority of nodal metastases are in the upper part of the neck, which allows early assessment of operability. This sequence allows assessment of the spinal accessory nerve's relationship to nodal metastases for possible nerve preservation. This operation is an attack on the tumor and not on the neck.

Surgical Exposure and Incisions

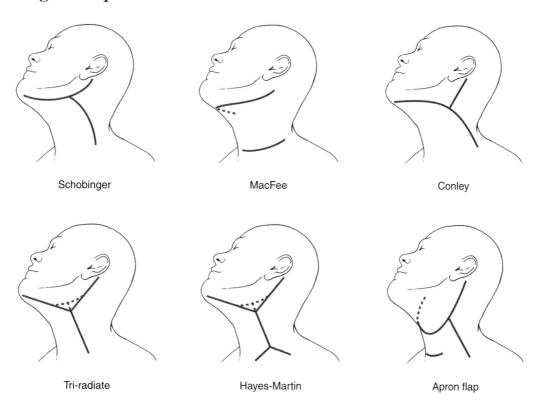

Schobinger   MacFee   Conley

Tri-radiate   Hayes-Martin   Apron flap

Many incisions have been described for use during a neck dissection. Each represents a compromise between exposure of the operative field and the need to provide soft tissue coverage for vital structures left in the neck. A superiorly based subplatysmal apron flap provides good surgical exposure and adequate soft tissue coverage of the major vessels. A vertical extension along the anterior border of the trapezius muscle can provide additional exposure to the posterior triangle. The incision can be incorporated into a lip-splitting incision.

The skin flap is elevated over the inferior edge of the mandible and fixed with sutures. The greater auricular nerve and the external jugular vein are preserved for possible nerve grafting or as recipient vessels for microvascular transfer.

Submental and Submandibular Dissection: Level I

First, the marginal mandibular nerve is identified. It usually has multiple branches that run in areolar tissue between the platysma and the fascia surrounding the submandibular gland. The facial vessels are identified crossing the inferior border of the mandible at the anterior border of the masseter muscle. The nerve branches course above these vessels. The vessels are ligated below the nerve and retracted superiorly to get the marginal nerve branches out of the operative field.

The submental dissection begins by incising the deep cervical fascia off the contralateral anterior digastric muscle and along the inferior border of the mandible. The fascia is grasped with mosquito clamps and is carefully dissected off the mylohyoid muscle, which forms the floor of the submental triangle. The dissection is continued laterally to the ipsilateral digastric muscle, where the submental vessels branching from the facial vessels are encountered. These are ligated and divided. Then the submandibular dissection is begun.

The digastric muscles provide a safe plane in which to operate. The submandibular gland is retracted laterally to expose the mylohyoid muscle. The free posterior margin of the mylohyoid muscle is key to the submandibular dissection. It is retracted medially to reveal the deep portion of the submandibular gland lying on the hyoglossus muscle. The lingual nerve is located superiorly under the mandible and attached to the gland via the submandibular ganglion. It must be carefully ligated to prevent troublesome bleeding. Wharton's duct is deep to the lingual nerve and is ligated carefully to prevent nerve injury. The hypoglossal nerve is located inferiorly below the digastric muscle (see p. 107) and is accompanied by a plexus of veins. The fascia and gland are retracted laterally with mosquito clamps. The facial artery is again ligated as it courses around the posterior surface of the gland.

Upper Neck Dissection: Level II

The posterior belly of the digastric muscle is key to the dissection in the upper neck. It is superficial to the vessels of the carotid sheath and hypoglossal nerve.

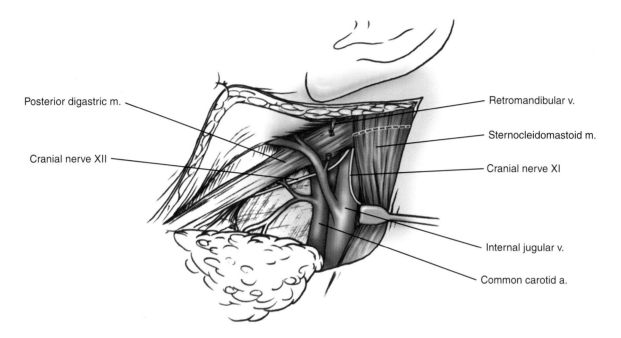

Posterior digastric m.

Cranial nerve XII

Retromandibular v.

Sternocleidomastoid m.

Cranial nerve XI

Internal jugular v.

Common carotid a.

The tail of the parotid gland is carefully divided to expose the retromandibular vein, which is then ligated and divided. The insertion of the sternocleidomastoid muscle is divided with the electrocautery and retracted inferiorly to expose the posterior digastric muscle. The occipital artery runs parallel and deep to the muscle, which is retracted with a vein retractor to expose the internal jugular vein and splenius capitis muscle. Cranial nerve XII crosses over the bifurcation of the carotid vessels at a variable distance above the bifurcation. The ansa cervicalis, which provides motor innervation to the strap muscles, branches from the hypoglossal nerve and is divided. The vagus nerve can be identified between the internal jugular vein and the carotid artery. Exposure of the carotid bifurcation may result in bradycardia and hypotension; 1% lidocaine solution can be injected into the carotid sinus if this becomes problematic. The spinal accessory nerve is usually identified exiting the jugular foramen anterior to the internal jugular vein. In as many as 30% of cases it travels posterior to the vein. Clinical assessment is made to determine whether nerve preservation is possible. If a short segment of nerve is adherent to tumor, it can be resected and a greater auricular nerve graft interposed using 9-0 nylon interrupted epineural sutures. The internal jugular vein is divided after placing two right-angle clamps proximally and one distally. The proximal stump is suture ligated, and a second tie is placed behind the second clamp. The contents of the submandibular triangle and upper neck dissection are now reflected inferiorly.

Posterior Neck Dissection

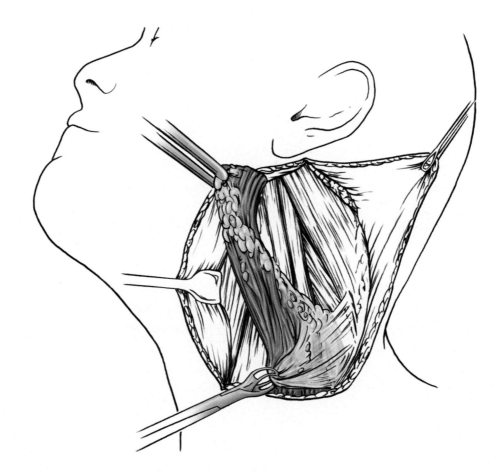

The posterior neck is dissected in continuity with the midneck dissection. The sternocleidomastoid muscle, nodal contents, and internal jugular vein have been reflected inferiorly and anteriorly, baring the splenius capitis muscle, which forms the floor. The prevertebral fascia is identified and removed with the specimen, thus transecting the cervical plexus branches of nerves C2 to C4 as they emerge from the fascia. Dissection continues along the anterior border of the trapezius muscle, exposing the levator scapulae muscle until the omohyoid muscle is identified. The spinal accessory nerve emerges from under the sternocleidomastoid muscle at the midpoint of the muscle. This posterior plane is relatively avascular.

Lower Neck Dissection

The omohyoid muscle is key to the inferior neck dissection. It is superficial to the carotid sheath and is used as a guide to divide the sternocleidomastoid muscle. The brachial plexus and the phrenic nerve are behind and on top of the anterior scalene muscle and are carefully preserved. The subclavian vein can sometimes be seen behind the clavicle and in front of the scalene muscle. The thoracic duct is located behind the junction of the internal jugular vein and subclavian vein.

The sternal and clavicular heads of the sternocleidomastoid muscle are divided, exposing the omohyoid muscle, which is also divided. The proximal portion of the internal jugular vein is dissected in a manner similar to that previously described. The supraclavicular fat surrounding the omohyoid muscle contains the transverse cervical vessels. The vein is more superficial than the artery and courses parallel to the omohyoid muscle, which may be superficial or deep to it. The vein enters the external jugular vein laterally and can be sacrificed without difficulty. Care is taken to not pull the fatty tissue from behind the clavicle. The entire specimen is removed en bloc.

Wound Closure

Two flat, closed suction drains are placed through separate inferior stab incisions. The platysma muscle is reapproximated with interrupted absorbable sutures. Interrupted absorbable dermal sutures are placed and the skin edges reapproximated with a running nylon suture. Neck dressings are not used, and a light film of antibiotic ointment is applied for 48 hours.

Modified Neck Dissection
Surgical Approach

The cervical lymphatics are removed by careful dissection of the investing and prevertebral layers of the deep cervical fascia (see p. 105). The sternocleidomastoid muscle, internal jugular vein, and spinal accessory nerve are preserved if possible. The entire dissection is performed through an anterior approach by retracting the sternocleidomastoid muscle laterally. The posterior triangle is dissected from underneath the muscle, with preservation of the cervical plexus. The exposure and submandibular dissection are identical for that described for the radical neck dissection.

Fascial Dissection

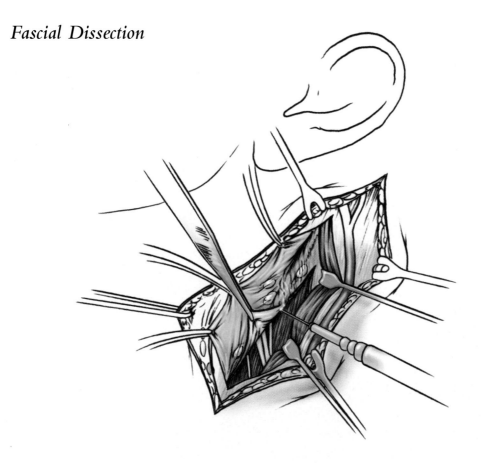

The investing layer of the deep cervical fascia is incised along the anterior border of the sternocleidomastoid muscle. When possible, the greater auricular nerve is preserved by carefully dissecting it out of the parotid tail. The investing fascia is grasped and retracted medially. The sternocleidomastoid muscle is retracted laterally, and the small perforating vessels entering the muscle from the fascia are cauterized. The fascial dissection is carried to the posterior edge of the sternocleidomastoid muscle where the investing fascia joins the prevertebral fascia. This fascia is reflected medially off the deep cervical muscles (splenius capitis, levator scapulae, and scalene muscles), preserving the cervical plexus and phrenic nerve branches.

Posterior Neck Dissection

The spinal accessory nerve exits behind the sternocleidomastoid muscle at approximately its midpoint (Erb's point). The greater auricular nerve courses obliquely over the sternocleidomastoid muscle at this point. Working from underneath the sternocleidomastoid muscle, the contents of the posterior triangle are reflected medially. The posterior margin of dissection is several centimeters from the edge of the trapezius muscle. The inferior limit of the dissection is the transverse cervical artery and the omohyoid muscle, usually several centimeters above the clavicle.

Central Neck Dissection

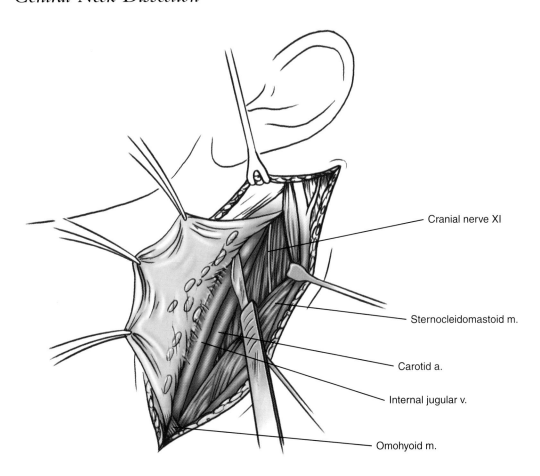

Normally the jugular vein is lateral, but traction of the investing fascia pulls it medial to the carotid artery. Thus the carotid artery is encountered first in dissection of the central neck. Sharp scalpel dissection directly against the vessel releases the fascia and adventitia. The vagus nerve is identified between the vessels, and the hypoglossal nerve is seen crossing the carotid artery at approximately its bifurcation. The fascial and nodal contents are then reflected over the internal jugular vein. The facial vein is ligated proximally to release the contents of the submandibular contents.

Upper Neck Dissection

Dissection of the upper neck is the most important and difficult portion of a modified neck dissection. Clinical judgment is necessary to determine whether the spinal accessory nerve can be preserved while adequately extirpating the cervical lymphatics.

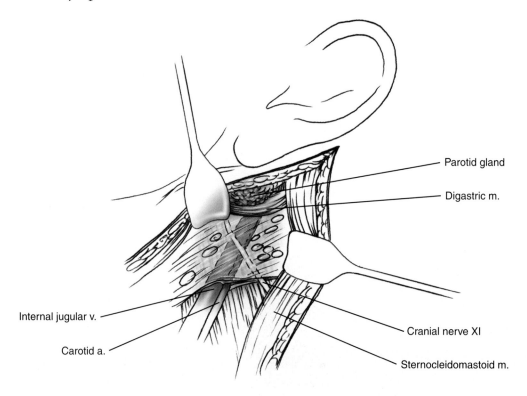

The upper third of the spinal accessory nerve must be identified prior to its entrance into the sternocleidomastoid muscle. The tail of the parotid gland is divided with the electrocautery, and the posterior facial vein is divided to expose the posterior belly of the digastric muscle. The spinal accessory nerve is identified exiting the jugular foramen underneath the digastric muscle. The nerve is carefully dissected out of the surrounding tissue until it enters the sternocleidomastoid muscle. The nerve is retracted medially with a vein retractor, and the sternocleidomastoid muscle is retracted laterally to expose the upper spinal accessory nodal tissue lateral to the nerve. The fascia overlying the splenius capitis muscle is incised and grasped with mosquito clamps. This tissue is reflected under the nerve and over the internal jugular vein and carotid artery to join the contents of the central neck dissection.

PAROTID GLAND

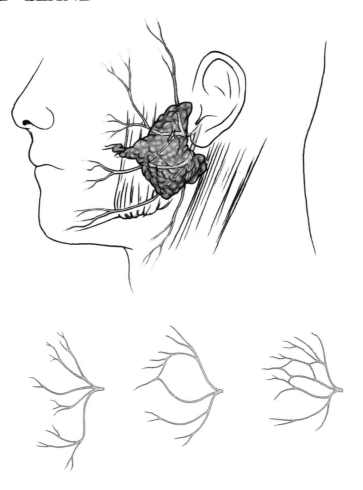

The parotid gland is the most common site of salivary neoplasms, accounting for 80% of the total. The majority of these tumors are benign, but precise knowledge of the anatomy is necessary to avoid facial nerve injury during parotidectomy. The parotid gland is an irregular, wedge-shaped organ that envelops the posterior border of the ascending ramus of the mandible. On its superficial surface it extends medially to cover a portion of the masseter muscle. The body of the gland fills the space between the mandible and the surface bounded by the external auditory meatus and the mastoid process. Deep to the ascending ramus the gland extends forward to a variable degree, lying in contact with the medial pterygoid muscle. Just below the condylar neck, above the attachment of the medial pterygoid to the bone, the gland extends between the two. In the region of the condyle, the gland lies between the capsule of the temporomandibular joint and external acoustic meatus. Laterally, at the junction of the mastoid process and sternocleidomastoid muscle, the gland lies directly on the posterior belly of the digastric muscle, the styloid process, and stylohyoid muscle. These structures separate the gland from the internal carotid artery, internal jugular vein, and cranial nerves IX to XII. Practically, these anatomic entities form the parotid bed, which is related to the so-called deep lobe of the parotid gland. Several important anatomic entities may be remembered with the mnemonic *VANS* where:

V = Internal jugular vein (one vein)
A = External and internal carotid arteries (two arteries)
N = Last four cranial nerves (IX, X, XI, XII)
    Glossopharyngeal nerve
    Vagus nerve
    Spinal accessory nerve
    Hypoglossal nerve
S = Styloid process plus three muscles
    Styloglossus
    Styloglossus pharyngeus
    Styloglossus hyoid

As to the topographic anatomy of these structures, remember:

Vein = Deep in the floor of the parotid bed
Artery = Anterior to the vein
Nerves
    Glossopharyngeal = Related to the S muscles
    Vagus = Between internal carotid artery and jugular vein
    Spinal accessory = Superficial to the carotid sheath but proceeding downward behind the posterior belly of the digastric muscle
    Hypoglossal = Same course as the spinal accessory

Remember also that the posterior belly of the digastric muscle is an excellent anatomic landmark because behind it are the carotid arteries, jugular vein, cranial nerves X, XI, and XII, and the sympathetic chain.

Stenson's duct passes from the anterolateral edge of the gland, over the masseter muscle. At the anterior margin of the muscle it turns medially to pierce the buccinator muscle and enters the oral cavity at the level of the upper second molar tooth. Accessory gland is occasionally found along the course of the duct and follows a line drawn from the floor of the external auditory meatus to just above the commissure of the lips. These are important landmarks in evaluating facial lacerations with possible duct injury.

There is no natural plane between the gland and the overlying skin. Surgical exposure requires raising the cheek flap in the subcutaneous plane just beneath the hair follicles. The gland is fixed by fibrous attachments to the external acoustic meatus, mastoid process, and fibrous sheath of the sternocleidomastoid muscle. These must be released to mobilize the gland, facilitating exposure of the facial nerve. One of the fascial attachments, the stylomandibular ligament, passes deep to the gland from the styloid process to the posterior border of the ascending ramus just above the angle, separating the parotid gland from the submandibular gland.

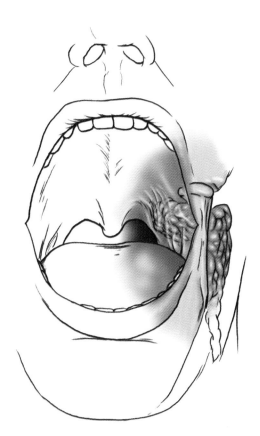

Together with the mandibular ramus, it forms a tunnel through which a process of the gland can extend into the parapharyngeal space. Occasionally tumors can develop in the process, resulting in swelling in the facial and lateral pharyngeal area rather than externally.

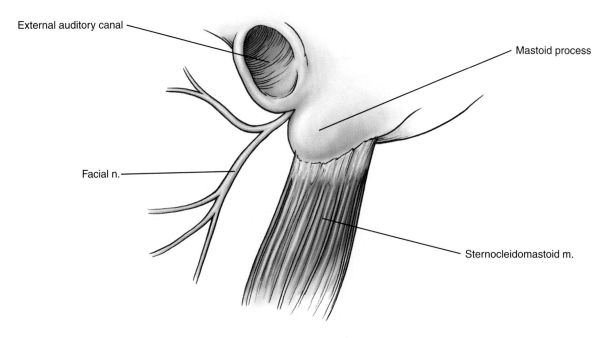

External auditory canal

Facial n.

Mastoid process

Sternocleidomastoid m.

The facial nerve is intimately associated with the parotid gland. It emerges from the skull through the stylomastoid foramen, immediately posterior to the base of the styloid process and anterior to the attachment of the digastric muscle. The main trunk of the facial nerve is always located in the triangle formed by the mastoid, the angle of the mandible, and the cartilaginous ear canal, medial to the mastoid. The trunk of the nerve bisects the angle between the mastoid and the cartilaginous ear canal 1.5 cm deep to the surface of the parotid gland. Before entering the gland the nerve has three branches: to the posterior auricular muscle, to the posterior belly of the digastric muscle, and to the stylohyoid muscle. The nerve enters the posterior surface of the gland about 1 cm after exiting the skull. It is superficial to the external carotid artery and the posterior facial vein. The nerve branches into an upper temporofacial division, which takes a vertical course, and a lower cervicofacial division, which is a transverse continuation of the main trunk. The point of branching is called the pes anserinus. From the pes the nerve divides into five branches: temporal, zygomatic, buccal, mandibular, and cervical. The temporal and zygomatic branches share the motor supply of the orbicularis oculi, and the temporal branch alone supplies the forehead musculature. The cervical branch supplies the platysma, and the remaining buccal and mandibular branches share in supplying the remaining facial muscles. The primary division is constant, but there is considerable variation in the origins, interrelations, and specific distribution of the peripheral branches. The pattern of branching is particularly variable, and rami often communicate between branches, sometimes within the gland but more often in front of its anterior border. The presence of these communicating rami explains the occurrence of unexpectantly mild paralysis following division of a branch.

The facial nerve runs within the substance of the gland, but within the gland the facial nerve is superficial, the veins are deeper, and the arterial branches are deepest. Traditionally the path of the nerve has been used to separate the parotid gland into superficial and deep lobes, but no true facial planes separate the two. Tumors generally develop superficial or deep to the plane of the nerve; thus the distinction of superficial and deep lobe tumors. Occasionally a tumor will arise in the plane of the nerve, separating the branches.

The external carotid artery enters the inferior surface of the gland and divides into the maxillary and superficial temporal arteries at the junction between the middle and upper third of the gland. The superficial temporal artery gives off the transverse facial artery to supply the face before continuing upward to emerge from the upper border of the gland. The maxillary artery passes forward and slightly upward behind the condylar neck in the part of the gland lying deep to it. The artery emerges from the gland and passes into the infratemporal fossa.

The venous drainage of the area is variable, but the superficial temporal vein generally enters the superior surface and receives the internal maxillary vein to become the posterior facial vein. Within the gland, it divides into a posterior branch, which joins the posterior auricular vein to form the external jugular vein. The anterior branch emerges from the gland to join the common facial vein. The facial nerve is superficial to the vessels, the artery is deep, and the veins lie between them.

Knowledge of the lymphatic channels of the parotid gland is important in evaluating skin cancers of head. Preauricular lymph nodes in the superficial fascia drain the temporal scalp, upper face, and anterior pinna. Lymph nodes within the parotid substance drain the gland, nasopharynx, palate, middle ear, and external auditory meatus. These lymphatics drain into the internal jugular and spinal accessory nodes.

The greater auricular nerve emerges from the posterior border of the sternocleidomastoid muscle at Erb's point (see p. 108). It crosses the midportion of the muscle approximately 6.5 cm beneath the external auditory meatus and travels parallel and superior to the external jugular vein to supply sensation to the ear and preauricular region. It passes on the surface of the parotid gland and can be preserved unless invaded by tumor by retracting it posteriorly. If the nerve must be sacrificed, it is preserved in saline solution for use as a possible nerve graft. Loss of the branches to the ear can cause disturbing numbness of the lobule, making it difficult to wear earrings, and sometimes causing frostbite in the winter.

The auriculotemporal nerve is a branch of the mandibular division of the trigeminal nerve. It traverses the upper part of the parotid gland and emerges from the superior surface with the superficial temporal vessels. It carries sensory fibers from the trigeminal nerve and secretory fibers from the glossopharyngeal nerve via the otic ganglion.

Parotidectomy
Preoperative Preparation

The history and physical examination are often diagnostic of parotid masses. A slow growing mass that has been present for many years is most likely a pleomorphic adenoma. Facial nerve paralysis usually indicates a malignant process. Computed tomography (CT) can be useful in equivocal cases, when a deep lobe tumor is suspected, and when malignancy is suspected.

Fine-needle apiration cytology is useful if malignancy is suspected. It aids in preoperative counseling about the risk for nerve injury, but should not determine operability.

Surgical Exposure and Incisions

Parotidectomy is performed under loupe magnification and headlight illumination. A bipolar cautery is used to protect the facial nerve from conducted electricity. Meticulous hemostasis is necessary to permit safe exposure of the nerve. No muscle relaxation is used, and a nerve stimulator is sometimes helpful to identify nerve branches.

The patient is positioned supine with the head extended and rotated to the opposite side. Draping allows exposure of the entire external ear, facial skin, and neck. A petroleum gauze plug is placed in the ear to prevent blood accumulation.

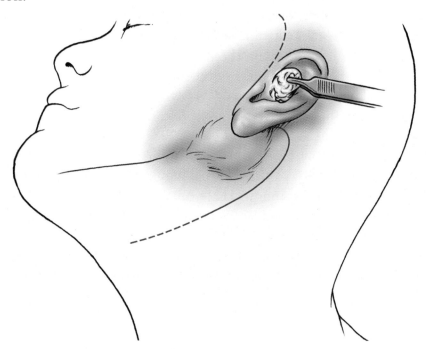

A preauricular incision is made, which may extend up to the zygoma depending on the location of the tumor. The incision curves around the ear and proceeds down the neck in a transverse skin crease. The anterior skin flap is developed in the subcutaneous plane just below the hair follicles. This is not a natural surgical plane and is usually made with a scalpel. Dissection continues medially onto the surface of the masseter muscle.

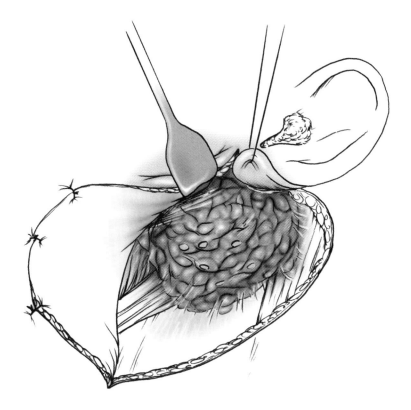

The posterior flap is developed in the subplatysmal plane over the anterior border of the sternocleidomastoid muscle. The skin flaps are secured with sutures.

After surgical exposure is obtained, the dissection begins at the inferior portion of the gland. The posterior facial vein is divided between clamps. The greater auricular nerve is identified crossing the sternocleidomastoid muscle. The nerve may have to be divided if it crosses the superficial aspect of the gland. If the nerve is sacrificed, it is placed in saline solution–moistened gauze to be used later as a possible nerve graft.

The tail of the parotid gland is grasped with mosquito clamps and carefully dissected off the sternocleidomastoid muscle. The anterior muscle border is identified from the mastoid process to the inferior end of the incision. Careful dissection is performed anterior and deep to the sternocleidomastoid muscle. The posterior belly of the digastric muscle is identified coursing in an oblique direction from the sternocleidomastoid muscle. The internal jugular vein and internal carotid artery are deep to this muscle. All of the salivary tissue is retracted anteriorly and superiorly to the digastric muscle. The ear lobe is retracted, and the dense fibrous attachments between the parotid gland, mastoid tip, and cartilaginous auditory canal are divided. This exposes the tragal pointer. The facial nerve lies 1 cm deep and slightly inferior to the pointer. During separation from the ear canal, bleeding from the superficial temporal vessels is controlled with the bipolar cautery.

Identification of Facial Nerve

Parotidectomy requires precise identification of the facial nerve. The main trunk is constantly found between the base of the styloid process and the mastoid process. The tail of the parotid gland must be separated from the sternocleidomastoid muscle. Lateral traction of the muscle exposes the digastric muscle, which is followed to its insertion on the mastoid tip. The nerve lies between the insertion of the muscle and the styloid process. In difficult cases, the nerve can be found by removing the mastoid tip with an osteotome. This exposes the nerve in the descending portion of the facial canal as it exits through the stylomastoid foramen. If the tumor mass overlies the main nerve trunk, an optional approach is to identify the posterior facial vein as it enters the gland. The marginal mandibular nerve can be seen crossing superficial to it and can be followed to the main trunk.

Between 1.0 and 1.5 cm from the stylomastoid foramen the nerve divides into the upper zygomaticofacial and lower cervicofacial divisions at the pes anserinus.

Tumor Resection

Resection of a parotid mass should be considered an attack on the tumor and not the gland itself. The majority of tumors of the parotid gland arise in the superficial portion. Removal of tumors in this portion is usually limited by the underlying nerve unless it is sacrificed. A pleomorphic adenoma has a well-defined capsule, but enucleation results in an unacceptable recurrence rate. When nerve branches disappear into the tumor, malignancy should be suspected. Nerve resection is indicated when clinically involved. The greater auricular nerve can be used as a nerve graft. Total parotidectomy is usually performed in the case of malignant neoplasms.

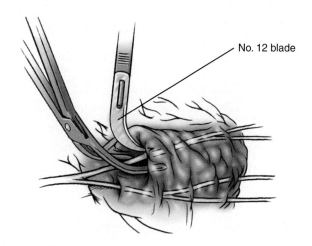

No. 12 blade

The individual nerve branches are dissected with a fine mosquito clamp. The overlying parotid mass is divided with a No. 12 knife blade. Hemostasis is con-

Anatomic Basis of Complications

- Facial nerve injury is related to tumor location and the experience of the operator. Temporary nerve paresis, especially of the marginal mandibular and temporal branches, is not uncommon. When removing the gland, care must be taken to not apply too much traction on the specimen. Hematoma and infection are extremely rare if proper surgical technique is used.
- Frey's syndrome is localized sweating and flushing during the mastication of food. This common disorder occurs in 35% to 60% of patients after parotidectomy with facial nerve dissection. The syndrome usually is noted several months after surgery, with varying degrees of severity. It may result from abberant regeneration of nerve fibers from postganglionic secreto-motor parasympathetic innervation to the parotid gland occurring through the severed axon sheaths of the postganglionic sympathetic fibers that supply the sweat glands of the skin. The majority of affected patients do not seek treatment.

trolled with the bipolar cautery. Lesions deep to the facial nerve necessitate removal of the superficial parotid tissue first. The remaining tissue can then be carefully dissected out between nerve branches.

Postoperative Care

A 7 mm flat closed suction drain is brought out through the inferior edge of the wound. Several interrupted deep dermal sutures are placed, followed by a running intracuticular stitch. The drain is removed after 2 to 3 days if the drainage is less than 30 ml per 24 hours.

SUBMANDIBULAR GLAND

The submandibular salivary gland is the site of approximately 10% to 15% of salivary neoplasms. Thirty percent to 55% of tumors will be malignant, and adenoid cystic carcinoma is the most common cancer. Most neoplasms are asymptomatic, but if a patient has evidence of neural involvement, such as marginal mandibular or hypoglossal paresis or loss of sensation, an aggressive malignant neoplasm is probable. Bimanual examination through the mouth allows assessment of possible extension under the mylohyoid muscle.

Submandibular Gland Resection

Tumors involving the submandibular gland are usually contained within the gland, and resection is confined to the gland and surrounding fat or lymph nodes. A curvilinear incision extending from the midline of the jaw to the mastoid, following the course of the digastric muscles, provides good exposure. The dissection is similar to that described for a level I radical neck dissection.

CAROTID BODY TUMOR

Chemodectomas or nonchromaffin paragangliomas usually arise from the carotid body or the adventitia of the carotid bulb at the carotid bifurcation and infrequently from the vagus nerve or glomus vagale. They are slow-growing tumors that if untreated will eventually cause symptoms in the majority of patients. Preoperative cranial nerve defects are seen in 10% of patients.

The diagnosis is suggested by the presence of a firm, slow-growing, nontender pulsatile mass in the region of the carotid bifurcation. The diagnosis is confirmed with an angiogram, which often reveals widening of the carotid bifurcation with prominent tumor vascularization. Rarely a carotid body tumor can produce vasoactive amines and mimic a pheochromocytoma.

Preoperative Assessment

Because a small carotid body tumor is easily removed, surgery is indicated in all but selected cases. Radiation therapy can control tumor growth in the majority of patients who are not surgical candidates. Preoperative embolization may ease the dissection and reduce blood loss. Vascular surgery consultation is indicated for large tumors, which may require resection and reconstruction of the internal carotid artery.

Carotid Body Tumor Resection

Surgical exposure can be obtained through an oblique horizontal incision in the upper neck or a vertical incision along the anterior border of the sternocleidomastoid muscle. Early proximal and distal control is obtained with vascular tapes. Transection of the mandibular ramus just posterior to the second molar is sometimes necessary to provide additional exposure of the extracranial internal carotid artery. This can be performed with entrance through the oral cavity.

The majority of carotid body tumors can be safely dissected from the carotid vessels. Only approximately 10% of carotid body tumors will necessitate resection of the internal carotid artery. A posterolateral approach is used to resect that portion of the tumor involving the internal carotid artery. Meticulous dissection is performed in a plane between the adventitia and the media of the vessel wall. The external carotid artery is sacrificed if patency of the internal carotid artery has been verified at preoperative angiography. Great care is taken to prevent injury to the vagus, hypoglossal, and superior laryngeal nerves, and the sympathetic chain.

Complications

Despite meticulous dissection, cranial nerve deficits (IX, X, XII) are noted post-operatively in approximately 40% of patients.

TRACHEA
Tracheostomy

The trachea, together with the esophagus and the thyroid gland, lies in the visceral compartment of the neck. The anterior compartment comprises the sternothyroid and sternohyoid muscles, covered anteriorly by the investing layer of the deep cervical fascia and posteriorly by the prevertebral fascia. The trachea begins at the level of the sixth cervical vertebra, and its bifurcation is at the level of the sixth thoracic vertebra in the erect position or the fourth to fifth thoracic vertebrae when supine.

The chief arterial blood supply to the trachea is the inferior thyroid arteries. At the tracheal bifurcation, these descending branches anastomose with the ascending branches of the bronchial arteries. The tracheal veins join the laryngeal vein or empty directly into the left inferior thyroid vein. The pretracheal and paratracheal lymph nodes receive the lymphatic vessels from the trachea.

Surgical Exposure and Incisions

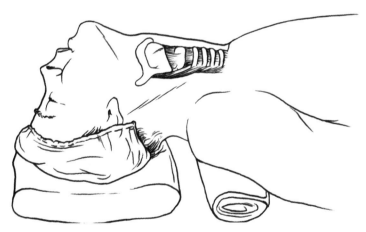

The patient is positioned with the head and neck hyperextended. Excessive neck extension can result in exposure of an excessive length of trachea, with the potential for placing the tracheostomy too low. A 4 cm transverse skin incision is made midway between the cricoid cartilage and the sternal notch. Skin flaps are developed in the subplatysmal plane superiorly to the thyroid notch and inferiorly to the sternum.

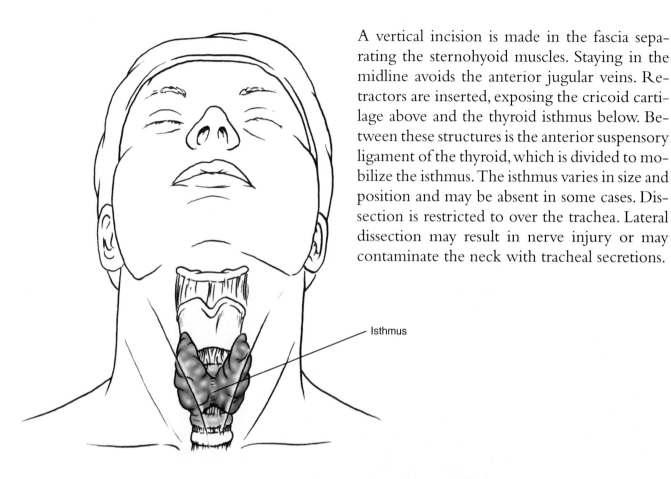

A vertical incision is made in the fascia separating the sternohyoid muscles. Staying in the midline avoids the anterior jugular veins. Retractors are inserted, exposing the cricoid cartilage above and the thyroid isthmus below. Between these structures is the anterior suspensory ligament of the thyroid, which is divided to mobilize the isthmus. The isthmus varies in size and position and may be absent in some cases. Dissection is restricted to over the trachea. Lateral dissection may result in nerve injury or may contaminate the neck with tracheal secretions.

Isthmus

The isthmus can usually be retracted superiorly with a vein retractor to expose the tracheal rings. Occasionally the isthmus must be divided between clamps and the ends suture ligated. Dividing the isthmus with the cautery may result in perioperative hemorrhage.

With the trachea exposed, lidocaine is injected into the tracheal lumen. Air within the syringe confirms the location within the lumen. A small portion of the second or third tracheal ring is removed to minimize the danger of fragmented cartilage being pushed into the tracheal lumen, reduce the risk of narrowing the lumen from inverted portions of trachea, and allow greater ease of reestablishing an airway if the tracheostomy tube inadvertently becomes dislodged during the first 48 to 72 hours after surgery. A No. 11 blade is used to first make a 5 mm horizontal incision directly above the tracheal ring of choice. The cut edge is grasped with an Allis clamp, and vertical cuts are then made through the tracheal ring. A window is removed after the inferior cut is made.

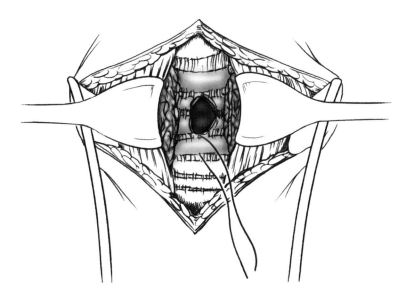

A midline suture is placed through the tracheal ring inferior to the window. This provides a traction suture to expose the trachea in the event of inadvertent decannulation.

The tracheostomy tube is inserted, the obturator removed, and the cuff inflated. The flanges of the tube are sutured to the skin of the neck. The skin incision is left open to prevent development of mediastinal emphysema. Proper position of the tube is confirmed with a chest radiograph.

Anatomic Basis of Complications

- Bleeding from the thyroid or great vessels may occur. The innominate artery or right common carotid artery may cross the trachea above the sternal notch, so care must be taken during an emergency tracheostomy. Midline dissection prevents injury to the esophagus and recurrent laryngeal nerves.
- False passage of the tracheostomy tube may result in a pneumothorax or pneumomediastinum. Improper tube placement may result in perforation of the lateral or posterior tracheal wall. Postoperative complications include erosion into a major vessel or the esophagus. Long-term tracheal intubation may result in tracheal stenosis.

KEY REFERENCES

Carlson GW. Surgical anatomy of the neck. Surg Clin North Am 73:837-852, 1993.
  This article reviews the surgical anatomy of the neck.
Carlson GW. Cervical lymphatics and squamous cell carcinoma of the head and neck. Surg Oncol Clin North Am 5:65-77, 1996.
  This article is a good review of the treatment of metastatic squamous cell carcinoma of the neck.
Sloan D, Goepfert H. Conventional therapy of head and neck cancer. Hematol Oncol Clin North Am 5:601-625, 1991.
  This is a good review of the treatment of head and neck cancer.
Vokes EE, Weichselbaum RR, Lippman SM, et al. Head and neck cancer. N Engl J Med 328:184-194, 1993.
  This article is an outstanding overview of the epidemiology, etiology, pathogenesis, diagnosis, and treatment of head and neck cancer.

SUGGESTED READINGS

Beahrs O. Surgical anatomy and technique of radical neck dissection. Surg Clin North Am 57:663, 1977.

Bocca E, Pignataro O, Oldini C, et al. Functional neck dissection: An evaluation and review of 843 cases. Laryngoscope 94:942-945, 1984.

Byers RM, Wolf PF, Ballantyne AJ. Rationale for elective modified neck dissection. Head Neck Surg 10:160-167, 1988.

Crile G. Excision of cancer of the head and neck: With special reference to the plan of dissection based upon 132 operations. JAMA 47:1780-1785, 1906.

DeSanto L, Beahrs O. Modified and complete neck dissection in the treatment of squamous cell carcinoma of the head and neck. Surg Gynecol Obstet 167:259, 1988.

Dingman RO, Grabb WC. Surgical anatomy of the mandibular ramus of the facial nerve based on dissection of 100 facial halves. Plas Reconstr Surg 29:266, 1962.

Lindberg RD. Sites of first failure in head and neck cancer. Cancer Treat Symp 2(21), 1983.

Mackay GJ, Carlson GW, Wood RJ, et al. Plastic and maxillofacial surgery. In Sabiston DC, ed. Textbook of Surgery: The Biological Basis of Modern Surgical Practice. Philadelphia: WB Saunders, 1996, pp 1298-1329.

Martin H. The case for prophylactic neck dissection. Cancer 4:92, 1951.

Mendenhall WM, Million RR, Cassisi NJ. Squamous cell carcinoma of the head and neck treated with radiation therapy: The role of neck dissection for clinically positive neck nodes. Int J Radiat Oncol Biol Phys 12:733-740, 1986.

Myers EN, Johnson JT. The significance of extracapsular extension of squamous cancer in lymph nodes. In Larson DL, Ballantyne AJ, Guillamondegui OM, eds. Cancer in the Neck: Evaluation and Treatment. New York: Macmillan, 1986, pp 65-71.

Nahum AM, Mullaly W, Marmor L. A syndrome resulting from radical neck dissection. Arch Otol 74:82-86, 1961.

Schneider JJ. Control by irradiation alone of nonfixed clinically positive lymph nodes from squamous cell carcinoma of the oral cavity, oropharynx, supraglottic larynx, and hypopharynx. AJR 123:42, 1975.

Schuller DE, Reiches NA, Hamaker RC, et al. Analysis of disability resulting from treatment including radical neck dissection or modified neck dissection. Head Neck Surg 6:551-558, 1983.

Shah JP. Patterns of cervical lymph node metastasis from squamous carcinomas of the upper aerodigestive tract. Am J Surg 160:405-409, 1990.

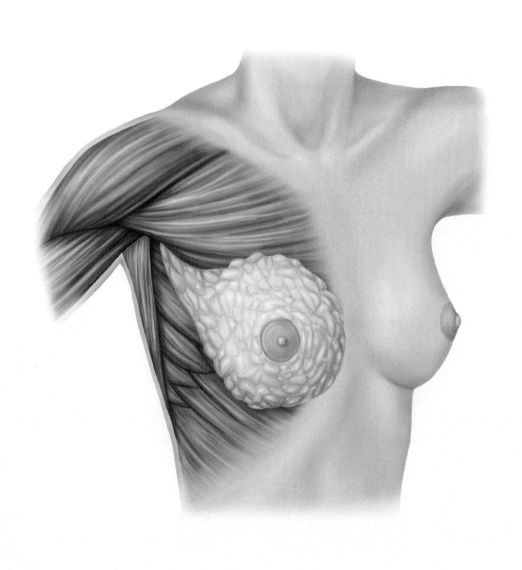

Chapter 3

Breast and Axilla

William C. Wood, M.D., and John Bostwick III, M.D.

Surgical Applications

Fine-Needle Aspiration and Core Needle Biopsy

Excisional Biopsy

Nipple Duct Excision

Lumpectomy, Segmental Resection, and Partial Mastectomy

Modified Radical Mastectomy (Total Mastectomy With Levels I and II Axillary Dissection)

Patey's Modified Radical Mastectomy

Radical Mastectomy

Total Mastectomy

Sentinel Node Biopsy

Axillary Dissection

Axillary Dissection With Lumpectomy

Breast Reconstruction

Implants and Expanders

Latissimus Dorsi Flap

Endoscopic Latissimus Dorsi Flap for Partial Mastectomy Deformity

TRAM Flap

Skin-Sparing Mastectomy With Immediate TRAM Flap Breast Reconstruction

*B*reast diseases are among the most common seen in any surgeon's practice. In the United States 180,000 new breast cancers are identified each year, with an additional 600,000 estimated biopsies. The techniques of breast surgery have a clear relationship to outcome, not only in local control of tumors but in the cosmetic results that the patient will enjoy or suffer throughout the remainder of her life. Both benign and malignant diseases of the breast require surgery, and the emotional responses evoked by the breast heighten the stakes for both patient and surgical team.

SURGICAL ANATOMY
Topography

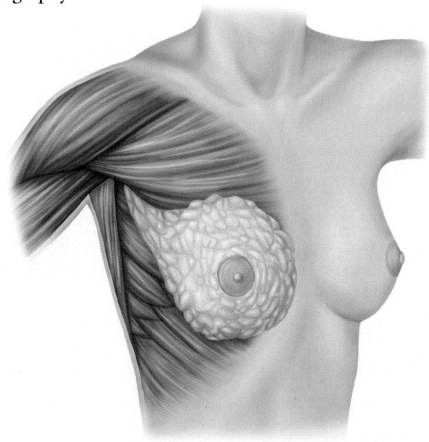

The adult female breast is located on the anterior chest wall. It extends from the second rib above to the sixth or seventh rib below, and from the sternal border medially to the midaxillary line laterally. The majority of the breast lies anterior to the pectoralis major muscle; the remainder lies anterior to the serratus anterior muscle; and the inferior margin is situated over the aponeurosis of the external oblique muscle. In 95% of women the upper outer quadrant of the breast extends through a hiatus in the deep fascia (hiatus of Langer) into the axilla proper. This, the axillary tail of Spence, is the only portion of the breast parenchyma beneath the deep fascia. In about 5% of women a distinct upper pole of palpable breast parenchyma extends directly superiorly. A retromammary space lies between the superficial fascia enveloping the breast and the deep fascia investing the pectoralis muscle. This space contributes significantly to the mobility of the breast on the chest wall.

Deep Fascia

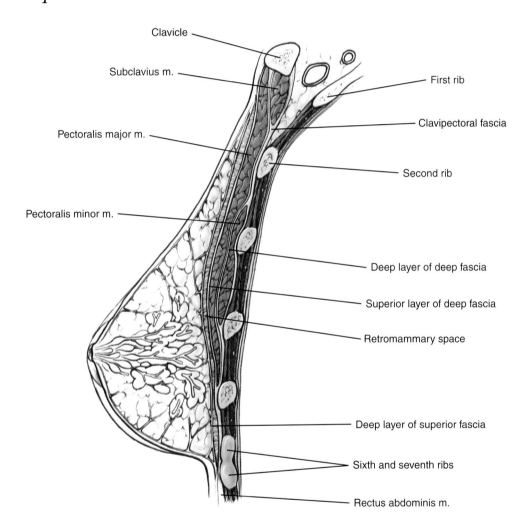

The breast is contained within layers of superficial fascia. The superficial layer of this superficial fascia is located near the dermis and is not distinct from it. The deep pectoral fascia envelops the pectoralis major muscle. The clavipectoral fascia surrounds the pectoralis minor muscle and a portion of the subclavius muscle.

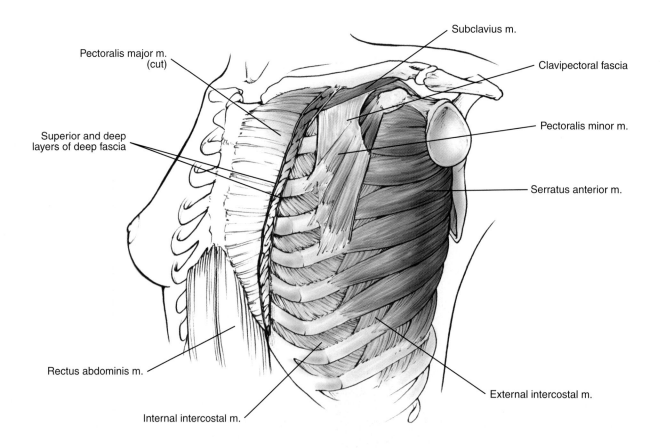

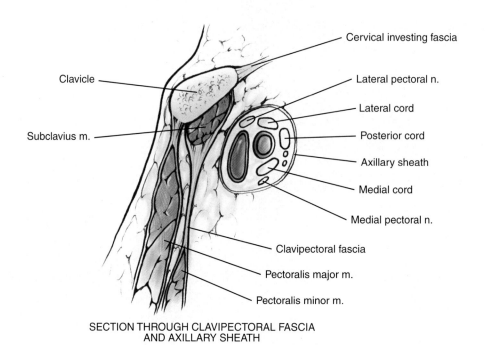

SECTION THROUGH CLAVIPECTORAL FASCIA
AND AXILLARY SHEATH

The axillary vessels and nerves to the arm are enclosed in a flimsy tubular fascial sleeve, the axillary sheath.

Nipple and Areola

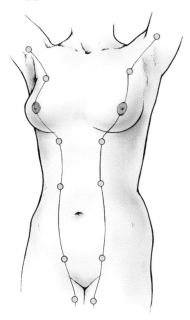

The nipple develops as a budding of the epidermis and the duct system, and potential glandular tissue arises from the epidermis in fetal life, forming a nipple bud at birth. Absence of the breast (amastia) or areola (aphelia) is rare; in these instances the underlying pectoralis muscles are often absent as well. When the nipple is present but no breast forms, the condition is termed amazia. Supernumerary nipples or breasts are termed accessory if they are along the embryonic milk line or ectopic if they lie elsewhere. Ectopic nipples or breasts are extremely rare. Breast cancer may arise in any of these areas of extramammary breast tissue.

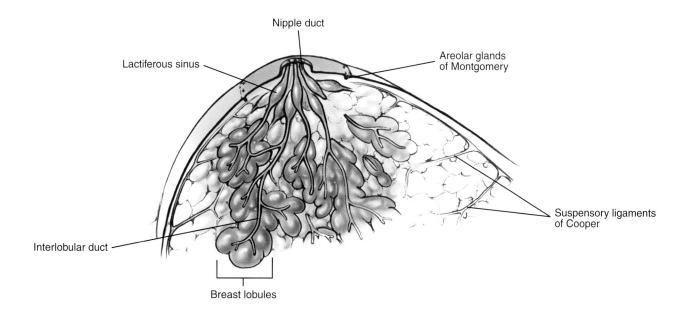

The nipple is pink in the nulliparous Caucasian breast but becomes pigmented to brown in early pregnancy. The pigmentation is correspondingly darker in women of darker complexion. The nipple is covered in keratinized stratified squamous epithelium. Its stroma contains dense connective tissue, with smooth muscle surrounding the lactiferous ducts.

The skin surrounding the nipple is the areola, which undergoes the same pigment changes as the nipple during pregnancy. Beneath the areola the large areolar glands of Montgomery may be seen by the naked eye. Beneath the nipple and areola is the erector areola muscle, bundles of smooth muscle fibers arranged circumferentially and radially that produce erection of the nipple when stimulated.

Parenchyma

The breast parenchyma consists of 12 to 20 lactiferous ducts branching and terminating in lobules of breast glandular tissue. Just beneath the nipple the lactiferous ducts converge into expanded lactiferous sinuses lined by stratified squamous epithelium. These constrict onto a terminal duct that runs vertically upward to end in the papilla of the nipple in the narrow orifice. Each of these ducts serves a segment of breast tissue. Although these ducts are sometimes represented as anatomically separate and distinct areas, that is an infrequent finding.

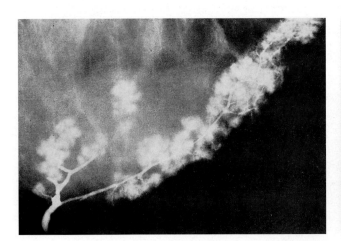 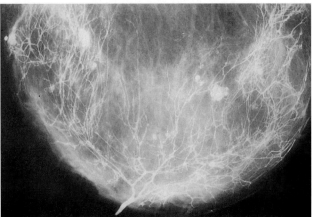

Radiographic imaging of the ductal system demonstrates the diffuse nature and interconnectedness of the breast lactiferous duct systems, precluding dissection of true segments of the breast.

The breast parenchyma is arranged in lobules suspended by fibrous bands that connect with the overlying dermis and the underlying superficial fascia. These are called the suspensory ligaments of Cooper and provide internal support to the breast. Interlaced throughout the breast is abundant adipose tissue between the lobules.

Axilla

The axilla is a pyramidal space with an apex, base, and four walls. The apex is the junction of the clavicle, scapula, and first rib. The base is the axillary fascia beneath the skin of the axillary fossa. The anterior wall is composed of the pectoralis major, pectoralis minor, and subclavius muscles and the clavipectoral fascia enveloping the muscles and conjoining them. The posterior wall is formed by the scapula and its overlying muscles: the subscapularis, latissimus dorsi, and anterius major. The medial wall consists of the lateral chest wall containing the second to sixth ribs and the serratus anterior muscle. The lateral wall is the narrowest, formed by the bicipital groove of the humerus. Within the axilla are lymph nodes and fatty tissue, the axillary sheath covering blood vessels and nerves, and the tendons of the long and short heads of the biceps and the coracobrachialis muscles. Surgery of the breast and axilla, particularly in patients with tumors that have distorted the normal anatomy or in those in whom the anatomy has been disrupted by prior surgery, requires a precise knowledge of the blood supply and nerves traversing these tissues, as well as the location of the breast parenchyma and the draining lymphatic vessels and lymph nodes.

Nerve Supply

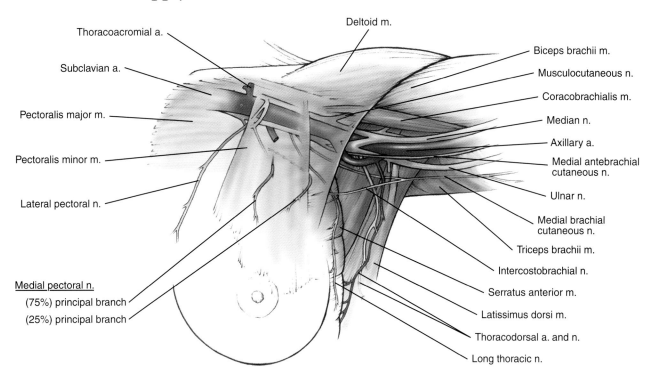

The major nerves of the breast and axilla are the brachial plexus, the lateral and medial pectoral nerves, the thoracodorsal nerve, the long thoracic nerve, the intercostobrachial nerve, and the anterolateral intercostal sensory nerves.

The brachial plexus lies within the axillary sheath. If dissection in the axilla is kept caudad to the inferior border of the axillary vein, the brachial plexus will neither be seen nor injured. The lateral pectoral nerve, named for its origin from the lateral cord of the brachial plexus, passes medially around the medial border of the pectoralis minor muscle together with the thoracoacromial vessels. It is the medial of the two pectoral nerves in its anatomic position. In the surgical anatomic literature some authors describe these nerves in terms of their origin and others by their location, creating needless confusion. We will follow the traditional terminology based on the cord of origin. The lateral nerve often divides with one or more branches penetrating the fibers of the pectoralis minor muscle to enter and innervate the pectoralis major muscle. Dividing these branches produces atrophic areas in the upper half of the pectoralis major muscle.

The medial pectoral nerve, named for its origin from the medial cord of the brachial plexus, passes laterally around the pectoralis minor muscle to innervate the lower half of the pectoralis major muscle. It sometimes has a branch that perforates the pectoralis minor muscle belly to supply the pectoralis major muscle. Injury to the medial pectoral nerve causes atrophy of the lateral and/or middle portion of the pectoralis major muscle, resulting in an aesthetic defect. The thoracodorsal nerve emerges from beneath the axillary vein and approximately 1 cm medial to the thoracodorsal vein. As it courses caudad it joins the thoracodorsal vein and runs together with it onto the latissimus dorsi muscle, where it crosses over or beneath the thoracodorsal vein to innervate the latissimus dorsi muscle.

The long thoracic nerve emerges from behind the axillary vein and runs along the chest wall in the fascia of the serratus anterior muscle in exactly the same anteroposterior plane as the thoracodorsal nerve. Once the thoracodorsal nerve is identified in the axilla, proceeding 2 to 3 cm directly medially to the chest wall leads to the long thoracic nerve and aids in its identification in difficult axillary dissections. It lies beneath the investing fascial plane of the serratus anterior muscle, but with traction may be drawn away from the chest wall into the axillary soft tissues. Injury to the long thoracic nerve is the most troubling of the axillary dissection. The serratus muscle fixes the shoulder to allow its motion and lifting. The defect of a paretic serratus is known as wing scapula. The intercostobrachial nerve, the highest of the anterolateral intercostal sensory nerves, supplies the upper axilla and medial posterior skin of the upper arm. It is usually easy to identify by palpation in the midplane of the axilla 1 to 2 cm beneath the axillary vein and anteriorly 1 to 2 cm to the plane of the thoracodorsal and long thoracic nerves. If the intercostobrachial nerve is cleared of its surrounding tissue and spared, there is less numbness associated with dissection of the axilla. The more inferior anterolateral intercostal sensory nerves are usually sacrificed during axillary dissection.

Lymphatic Drainage

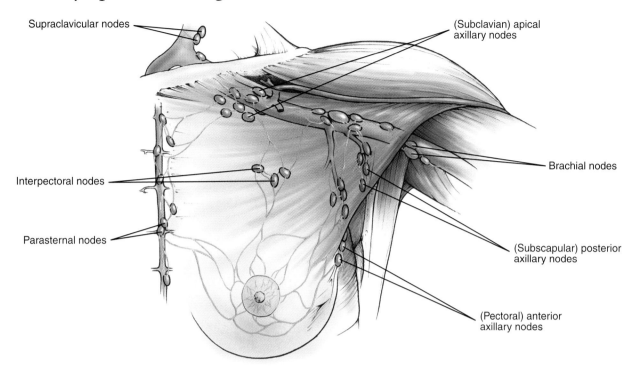

Supraclavicular nodes

(Subclavian) apical axillary nodes

Brachial nodes

Interpectoral nodes

Parasternal nodes

(Subscapular) posterior axillary nodes

(Pectoral) anterior axillary nodes

The lymphatic vessels of the breast drain both medially to the internal mammary lymph nodes and laterally to the axillary lymph nodes. Even from the most medial aspect of the breast, both lymphoscintigraphy and analysis of lymph node metastases suggest that the majority of lymphatic flow is toward the axillary lymph nodes. Three levels are illustrated. Level I nodes are lateral to the pectoralis minor muscle, level II nodes lie behind it, and level III nodes are medial to it.

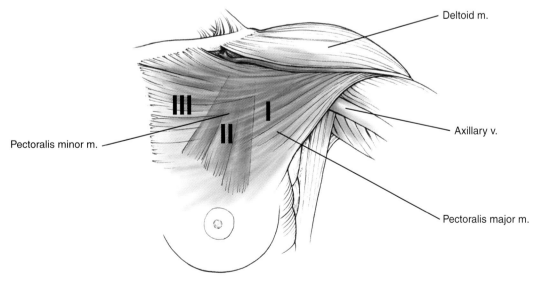

Deltoid m.

Pectoralis minor m.

Axillary v.

Pectoralis major m.

LEVELS OF AXILLARY LYMPH NODES

The lymphatic vessels draining the arm and those from the breast transverse the axilla. More radical axillary dissections (removing level III nodes or carrying the dissection anterior to the axillary vein) are associated with a higher incidence of arm and breast edema. A modified en bloc approach is used to clear the axillary nodal tissue. All the lymphatic vessels and nodes with interlacing fat and vessels are removed while carefully preserving the transversing essential structures.

Blood Supply

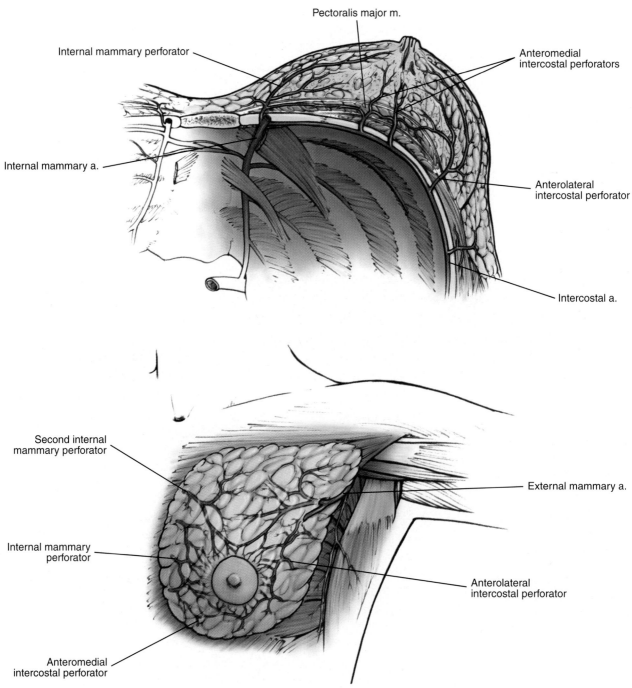

The blood supply to the breast is through the external mammary artery and perforating branches from the internal mammary artery. The venous drainage parallels this arrangement. These vessels may be divided as required, but may influence breast reconstructive options.

UNDERLYING MUSCULATURE

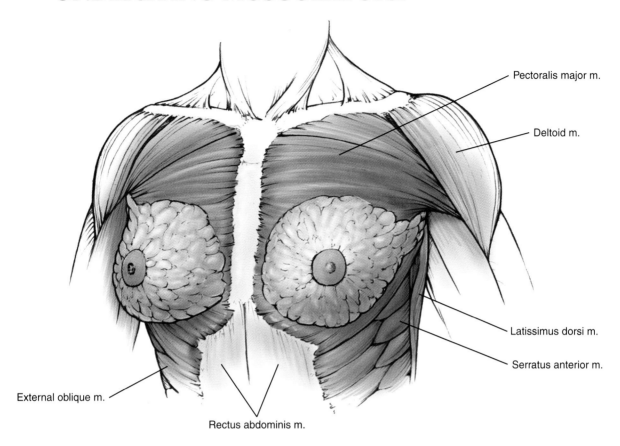

The breast overlies the deep fascia and underlying musculature. The upper medial portion of the breast is over the pectoralis major muscle. The lower portion of the breast covers the anterolateral serratus anterior muscle digitations, the upper external oblique muscle origins and its fascia, and the fascia over the upper origins of the rectus abdominis muscle. The breast parenchyma extends laterally to the lateral margin of the latissimus dorsi muscle, and the upper lateral breast parenchyma extends to the axilla. A substantial portion of the breast's blood supply, innervation, and lymphatic drainage passes up through these muscles. An intact muscular layer ensures maximal blood supply to the breast and can act as a biologic barrier between the breast parenchyma and a breast implant during reconstructive breast surgery. Current breast reconstruction techniques depend on an accurate knowledge of this musculature with its blood and nerve supplies.

Pectoralis Major Muscle

The pectoralis major muscle is a primary muscle of the upper chest wall. It extends from its broad origins over the anteromedial chest to insert onto the upper portion of the humerus. Located just beneath the upper medial breast area, it forms the anterior wall of the axilla, is the major component of the anterior axillary fold, and provides the primary fill for the infraclavicular area.

The pectoralis major muscle originates from the medial sternal half of the clavicle and from the outer anterior half of the sternum from the sternal notch down to the sixth or seventh costal cartilages. It also originates from the medial cartilages of the second through sixth or seventh ribs, and below from the external oblique and rectus abdominis fascia. The sternal and clavicular portions of the pectoralis major are usually distinct and separated by a fascial interval. The superficial layer of the deep fascia also extends from the external surface of the pectoralis major muscle across the sternum and joins the fascia above the opposite muscle.

The pectoralis major muscle fibers converge spirally toward the axillary region and form a broad origin for a double-laminated 5 cm tendon of insertion that attaches to the lateral lip of the intertubercular sulcus of the upper humerus.

Nerve Supply

The medial and lateral pectoral nerves innervate the pectoralis major muscle. C5-6 supply the clavicular portion of the muscle fibers, and C7-8 supply the sternal muscle fibers. These nerves are named for their respective cords of origin from the brachial plexus rather than for their position in relation to supply of the pectoralis major muscle. Two to five filaments of each pectoral nerve lead into the pectoralis major muscle. Some of these motor nerve filaments to the pectoralis major muscle course through the pectoralis minor muscle and are removed or can be damaged if this muscle is resected during an axillary dissection. Removal of the nerves innervating the pectoralis major muscle can cause muscle atrophy and infraclavicular flattening.

The medial pectoral nerve fibers provide motor innervation to the lateral and middle portion of the pectoralis major muscle. Selective interruption of these nerve fibers reduces the pectoralis major muscle pull over the upper portion of a subpectoral breast implant without producing significant functional compromise or noticeable atrophy of the upper breast area.

A modified radical mastectomy in which the pectoralis minor muscle is excised can also destroy these motor nerves to the pectoralis major muscle. During axillary dissection these nerves and the pectoralis minor muscle must be spared if pectoralis major function and bulk are to be preserved. It is difficult, however, to remove the lymph nodes at the apex of the axilla (level III) without sacrificing the medial pectoral nerve. Most oncologic surgeons believe that sufficient clearance of the lymph nodes can be obtained without taking the pectoralis minor muscle and the pectoral nerve.

Division of the pectoral nerves during a modified radical mastectomy results in muscle atrophy and decreased muscle thickness. At least 60% of the muscle bulk is generally lost 4 to 6 months after motor nerve division, simulating the appearance of a radical mastectomy in the infraclavicular area. This is especially noticeable when a significant thickness of the subcutaneous tissue is removed from the infraclavicular region. The anterior axillary fold, however, is preserved even when there is muscle atrophy, but it may be deficient because of muscle atrophy and removal of axillary breast tissue, which also contributes to the fullness of this fold. Pectoralis major muscle atrophy and infraclavicular hollowness are areas of concern that must be addressed during breast reconstruction.

Blood Supply

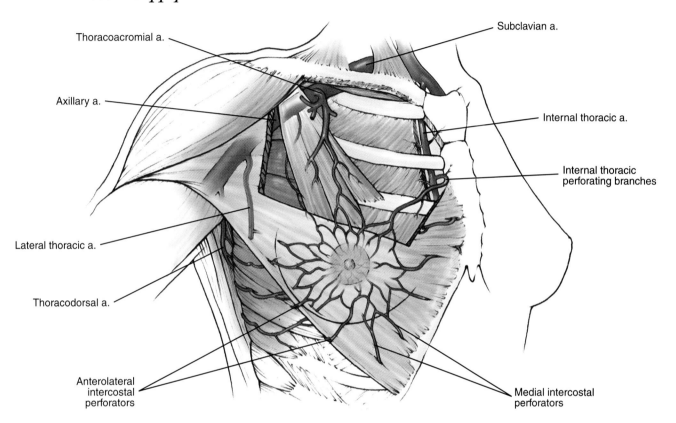

The blood supply to the pectoralis major muscle originates from a number of sources. The thoracoacromial artery, a major branch of the axillary artery, enters the deep surface of the pectoralis major muscle near its upper lateral portion and sends branches throughout the muscle. Perforating vessels from the thoracoacromial artery enter the deep surface of the breast. The thoracoacromial artery is a substantial vessel, 2 to 3 mm in diameter, and can nourish the entire pectoralis major muscle and the overlying skin and breast.

Another major group of vessels, branches of the internal thoracic artery, enter the pectoralis major muscle from the second to sixth intercostal spaces medially. Large direct perforating branches from the internal thoracic artery continue through the muscle and its fascia to enter the overlying medial breast. The entire pectoralis major muscle, skin, and breast can also be nourished by these internal mammary vessels from the internal thoracic artery.

The second intercostal arterial perforator is the longest of these perforating vessels. Located high and medial, this arterial branch provides the most direct flow to the upper inner quadrant of the breast. Because of the major collateralization within the breast, it can supply the entire breast parenchyma when there is normal microcirculation. The other three major perforating vessels of the internal mammary artery, the third, fourth, and fifth, are also major sources of inflow into the breast.

Another group, the medial intercostal perforating vessels, supply the lower portions of the pectoralis major muscle. They enter through the costal origins of the pectoralis major muscle through the fourth, fifth, and sixth intercostal spaces, then course superficially to supply the breast and overlying skin.

The anterolateral intercostal perforating vessels course anteriorly and enter at the junction of the lateral pectoralis major muscle through the intercostal spaces at the medial aspect of the serratus anterior muscle. Branches of these arteries supply the pectoralis major muscle; their primary flow enters the deep surface of the breast along with the accompanying veins and nerves. These intercostal perforators are from segmental vessels that communicate with the aorta posteriorly and the internal thoracic artery anteriorly.

Serratus Anterior Muscle

The serratus anterior muscle is a broad, flat shoulder girdle muscle that extends from the undersurface of the scapula to the lateral and anterolateral chest. It originates from extensive costal attachments of the anterolateral aspects of the first through the eighth or tenth ribs. These segmental muscular digitations are covered by a thick layer of deep fascia and are densely and broadly attached to the chest wall. The muscle passes backward posteriorly to insert beneath the tip as well as on the deep lateral surface of the scapula. The serratus anterior muscle holds and stabilizes the scapula to the chest wall, assists in rotating the scapula laterally, and draws the scapula forward around the chest. It is essential for reaching and pushing movements of the arm. It also functions and assists in respiration. The muscle and its fascia are beneath the lateral and inferior portions of the breast.

The fascia of the serratus anterior muscle is continuous with the pectoralis major fascia. It is dense and substantial in its lower portions and becomes thinned in its upper portions near the axilla, where it is associated with the pectoralis minor muscle. A musculofascial dissection that proceeds bluntly from the pectoralis major muscle laterally beneath the lower breast area goes below the lower serratus anterior fascia and elevates some of the serratus anterior muscle. Sharp dissection is necessary to elevate the full thickness of the serratus anterior muscle beneath the lateral breast. Blunt dissection laterally from the pectoralis major muscle in the upper breast often pushes out through the thin fascia over the pectoralis minor muscle and serratus anterior muscle, and the dissecting finger or instrument will go on top of this fascia to the subglandular breast position. Although the serratus anterior muscle and fascia form a distinct layer of coverage, it is not so substantial as the cover provided by the pectoralis major muscle and fascia.

Nerve Supply

The long thoracic nerve from the posterior roots of C5-7 supplies the serratus anterior muscle. This nerve is situated laterally and is covered by the external serratus fascia, but is superficial to the external surface of the serratus anterior muscle in the midaxillary line. The long thoracic nerve is carefully spared during mastectomy and axillary dissection. Its location must be kept in mind during breast reconstruction when the serratus anterior muscle and fascia are elevated for breast implant coverage and when elevating a latissimus dorsi flap.

External Oblique Muscle

The external oblique muscle is a primary muscle of support for the anterior abdominal wall and is an important consideration after a transverse rectus abdominis myocutaneous (TRAM) flap breast reconstruction procedure. It arises from the outer surfaces of the lower anterior and lateral ribs and curves around the lateral and anterior parts of the lower thorax and abdomen. These slips of origin are closely related to the origins of the serratus anterior muscle in the lower breast area and the origins of the lateral latissimus dorsi muscle farther down on the chest wall.

SURGICAL APPLICATIONS
Fine-Needle Aspiration and Core Needle Biopsy

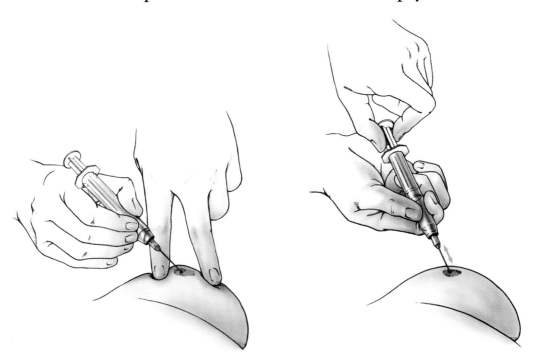

Simple cysts routinely encountered as palpable breast masses in clinical practice may be diagnosed and treated with fine-needle aspiration. If a solid lesion is encountered, the tip of the needle is passed up and down 10 to 15 times, in a traverse of only a few millimeters. Minimal pressure is applied on the plunger of the syringe to collect dishesive cells in the barrel of the needle. When the needle has been removed with no force of aspiration applied, the air-filled syringe may be replaced and the contents of the needle expressed onto a slide, smeared, and immediately placed in 95% alcohol. Even a few seconds of air drying is sufficient to greatly diminish the diagnostic value of such aspirate smears. Larger solid lesions suspected to be cancerous can also be assessed with fine-needle aspiration. Aspiration cytology is preferable to core biopsy for detecting dishesive cells associated with malignancies. Because there is a dense stromal response to cancer and this stroma tends to be captured with a Tru-cut needle, the Tru-cut needle biopsy is less effective for detection and diagnosis of cancer than fine-needle aspiration biopsy.

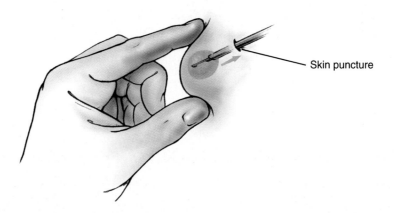

Skin puncture

Core needle biopsies are advantageous for histologic diagnosis of fixed tissue because they accurately distinguish between invasive and preinvasive lesions. A Tru-cut needle biopsy is illustrated. Whenever possible, the fine incision made with the tip of a No. 11 blade to allow a Tru-cut needle biopsy should be placed where it can be excised if a mastectomy can be performed. If the site is to be irradiated as part of breast-conserving therapy, it does not need to be reexcised.

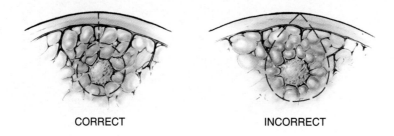

CORRECT   INCORRECT

Both fine-needle aspiration biopsy and core needle biopsy may be used to diagnose clinically occult, mammographically detected solid lesions. The accuracy of these techniques is under continuing investigation. Occult lesions requiring excision are localized by placement of a fine guiding wire hood (e.g., Kopans) or stiff tack (e.g., Wood–Kopans). These guidewires should be placed by a radiologist who understands the surgical approach to be used to remove the lesion. It is essential that the localizing wire pass directly through the clustered microcalcifications. What may appear to be tangential to or very near a cluster of calcifications on breast compression may actually be several centimeters away when compression is released.

Excisional Biopsy

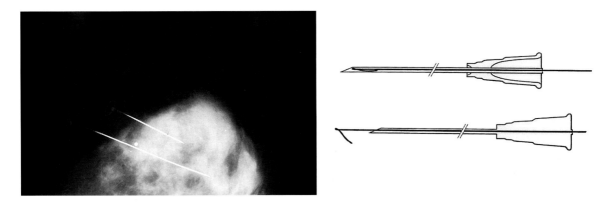

If a mass being excised without a diagnosis could potentially be benign, it is not advisable to remove a large margin of normal tissue surrounding the mass, possibly creating a cosmetic defect. Rather, a minimal margin of a few millimeters should be taken. Much has been written about the anatomic and cosmetic basis for orienting skin incisions for these procedures.

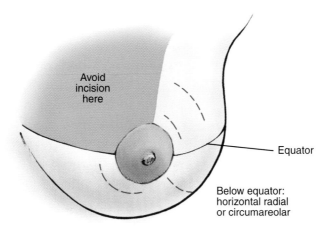

Incisions placed at the boundary between the areola and the surrounding breast skin tend by their location to heal with very inconspicuous scars. Circumareolar incisions should be used when possible in excising lesions.

Nipple Duct Excision

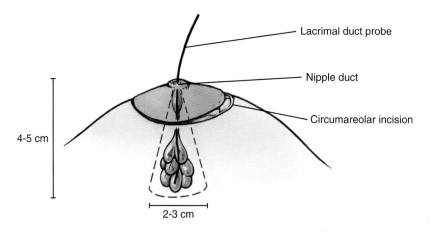

Both bloody discharge from the nipple and spontaneous clear discharge from a single nipple duct require biopsy. Each has approximately 20% likelihood of being caused by a neoplastic lesion. Excision of the involved nipple duct involves placement of a fine (4-0) lacrimal duct probe down the nipple duct, from which the discharge can be expressed. When the lacrimal probe is inserted into the breast, a trumpet-shaped piece of breast tissue is removed through a circumareolar incision that includes the terminal duct at the nipple skin, the lactiferous sinus beneath it, and the next 4 to 5 cm of enlarging breast tissue about that duct. The most common finding will be intraductal papilloma or ductal ectasia, with intraductal carcinoma or infiltrating duct carcinoma making up approximately 20%. This procedure is most comfortably performed with general anesthesia of short duration.

Lumpectomy, Segmental Resection, and Partial Mastectomy

Breast conservation therapy involves surgical removal of all gross tumor in the breast, removal of levels I and II axillary lymph nodes, and breast irradiation. A variety of terms are used to describe excision of a breast lesion with a margin of normal tissue enveloping it. These imply something about the margin of normal-appearing tissue removed, but are so imprecise that the generic term "lumpectomy" has become common parlance. Both retrospective analysis and prospective studies show that the greater the margin of normal-appearing breast tissue removed the lower the local recurrence rate. On the other hand, the greater the margin of tissue removed the poorer the resultant cosmetic appearance. The optimal balance of histologic tumor type and grade, nature of the tumor margin (infiltrative vs. pushing), size of the tumor, margin of surgical excision, and use of irradiation boost dose to the area closest to the resection cavity is only slowly being defined based on prospective data. Several principles are clear, however. Higher failure rates follow failure to establish a margin clear of invasive breast cancer. Tumors that have an extensive intraductal component (>25% of the tumor mass of intraductal tumor [ductal carcinoma in situ] in the adjacent tissue) have a more diffuse pattern of infiltration in the adjacent breast and appear to benefit from a slightly wider margin of excision designed to leave no residual tumor. A margin of a couple of millimeters is probably sufficient for a purely invasive tumor with a pushing margin, but a 1 cm margin will produce a lower failure rate in more diffuse tumor patterns. This may be performed as a secondary procedure at the time of the axillary clearance if the initial excisional biopsy is thought to provide an insufficient margin.

For breast carcinoma that will be treated with breast-sparing surgery followed by irradiation, there is no evidence that operating through a circumareolar incision located farther from the mass has any oncologic risk compared with a direct incision overlying the mass. Similarly, there is no oncologic justification for making a cosmetically less desirable incision; those lesions that can be easily approached through a circumareolar incision should be. When a mass is considered too large relative to the size of the breast to be amenable to initial breast conservation, core needle or incisional biopsy may be appropriate to provide sufficient tissue for accurate diagnosis. All small open biopsies can be performed with local anesthesia.

When lumpectomy of whatever extent has been accomplished, the cosmetic result is related to both the percentage of the breast that was resected as well as the manner of closure. The resection cavity should be addressed with fine snaps and the Bovie electrocautery until it is "bone dry." An external supportive dressing that shapes the breast tissue into ideal position and form should then be placed and supported by the patient's own brassiere. The dressing should not be removed for 5 days. No drains should ever be placed; the small hemoseroma that forms will be absorbed by natural retraction more evenly than can be achieved by surgical approximation of the breast tissue. Drains often lead to indentations.

Special Considerations for Specific Lesions
Fibroadenoma

If a fibroadenoma is to be excised in a young woman, there is no need to remove an additional surrounding margin of normal tissue. If the lesion is larger or the woman older and it may represent a phyllodes tumor, several millimeters of normal breast tissue should be removed in all directions to ensure total tumor excision. Invasive carcinoma should be removed with sufficient margin (usually 3 to 5 mm) to assure the pathologist that there is no cut-through or transgression of the tumor at its border. Tumors with an extensive intraductal component have a more diffuse pattern of infiltration at their margins. In excising or reexcising tumors with an extensive intraductal component, a margin of about 1 cm ensures confidence that no significant burden of tumor is left in the breast. Such lumpectomies or segmental mastectomies may be of no cosmetic consequence when the lesion is small or the breast large. For larger lesions in smaller breasts, treatment options for optimal cosmesis include (1) induction chemotherapy with excision of a considerably regressed primary lesion, (2) tailoring of the breast or insertion of a small subpectoral implant or flap, and (3) wrapping of the breast after resection so that it heals in the desired shape. Partial mastectomy or quadrantectomy is not an appealing option in these cases because of the resulting cosmetic defect in most women or change in breast size.

Paget's Disease of Nipple

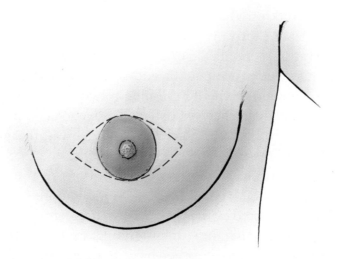

Intraductal carcinoma involving the skin of the nipple and areola can be treated with partial mastectomy with excision of the nipple–areolar complex and the underlying central ducts. If this is done in an elliptical fashion, the breast wrapped in such a way that the breast tissue is coapted, and the skin closed as a single layer, the result is a very normal breast mound with a transverse incision. Patients who desire may undergo nipple–areolar reconstruction and can expect a natural-appearing result. Orientation of the specimen is important to allow the pathologist to describe any close or positive margin in a way that can permit localized reexcision. The conserved breast can then be irradiated.

Mastectomy Procedures

Total mastectomy (simple mastectomy)

Extended total mastectomy, includes level I lymph nodes

Modified radical mastectomy, includes levels I and II lymph nodes

Patey's modified radical mastectomy, includes levels I to III lymph nodes and division or excision of pectoralis minor muscle for access to level III nodes

Radical mastectomy, includes both pectoralis muscles

Subcutaneous mastectomy

Total mastectomy sparing the nipple-areolar complex; a controversial technique that leaves residual breast tissue in the nipple and, as performed, often in the periphery of the breast

MASTECTOMY

From the near universality of radical mastectomy for all breast cancers in the first half of the twentieth century, a selective role for removal of the total breast has evolved. Earlier detection of breast cancer with mammography and randomized trials demonstrating equivalent survival with breast conservation therapy have contributed to the diminishing role of mastectomy. The diffuse nature of some in situ ductal carcinomas, the large size of some invasive carcinomas relative to the size of the breast, the presence of diffuse suspect breast microcalcifications rendering assessment of the extent of tumor impossible, the inability to use breast irradiation in some patients such as those with active collagen vascular disease, and the occurrence of multiple primary breast tumors continue to require removal of the entire breast in some women. Others, who are biologically good candidates for breast conservation therapy, have personal reasons for choosing mastectomy. A variety of mastectomy procedures have evolved that are directed toward the biology of the tumor being treated. Radical mastectomy is included, despite virtually no role in clinical practice, because it served as the basis for the proliferation of modifications.

Modified Radical Mastectomy (Total Mastectomy With Levels I and II Axillary Dissection)

Modified radical mastectomy is presented as the best for displaying the anatomy of the breast and axilla. Radical mastectomy and total mastectomy are described as variations of this procedure.

Incision

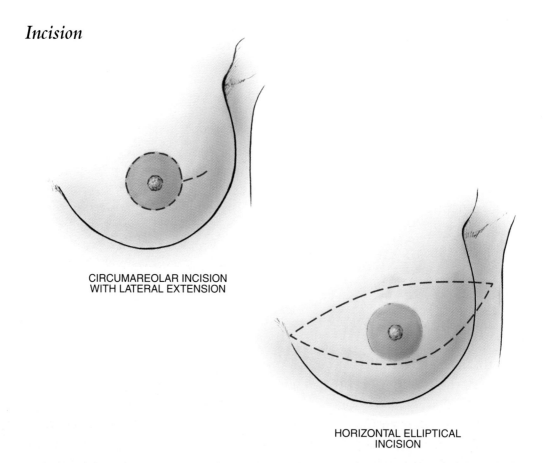

CIRCUMAREOLAR INCISION
WITH LATERAL EXTENSION

HORIZONTAL ELLIPTICAL
INCISION

The incision for a modified radical mastectomy is drawn to encompass the biopsy incision, the nipple, and the areola. If immediate reconstruction is to be done, the best cosmetic result is achieved by excising only the areolar skin (skin-sparing mastectomy) with a lateral incision several centimeters long if required to deliver the breast and axillary tissue. This incision generally gives sufficient access to allow modified radical mastectomy. It can be extended laterally to the anterior axillary line if required by the size and shape of the breast. There is no reason to extend the skin incision medially. If immediate reconstruction is not planned, an elliptical excision, usually oriented horizontally, is outlined. The extent of the ellipse medial to the nipple can be dropped downward to allow the maximum amount of anteromedial skin to be spared for later reconstruction without the scar being obvious in a bathing suit. The width of the ellipse is chosen to allow flaps long enough to touch without stretching for coaption at the conclusion of the procedure. If excess skin is left, it tends to form pachydermatous folding. Consequently, the tension on the closed flap should be similar to that of the remainder of the thoracic skin. The skin incision is carried down through the skin and subcutaneous tissue, stopping short of the parenchyma of the breast. In very slender patients the breast parenchyma may abut the skin. Typically there are several millimeters of adipose tissue that are clearly subcutaneous before any breast parenchyma is encountered.

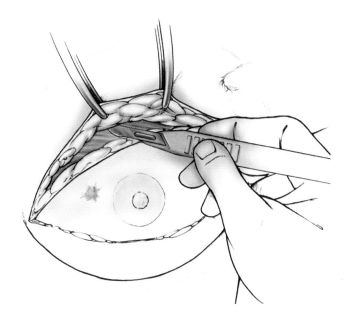

The skin flaps are elevated to just beneath the clavicle superiorly, onto the sternum medially, inferiorly along the inframammary fold down to the depth of the rectus aponeurosis, and centrally and laterally to the lateral border of the latissimus dorsi muscle. When flaps have been raised and the described margins outlined, the breast is lifted off the pectoralis major fascia, taking the investing fascia of that muscle.

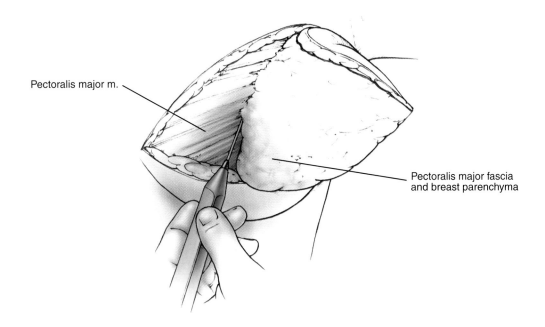

Pectoralis major m.

Pectoralis major fascia and breast parenchyma

This approach ensures removal of the entire breast parenchyma. As the pectoralis major fascia and the overlying breast are dropped off the lateral border of the pectoralis major muscle, it is possible to slip between the posterior fascia of the muscle and the muscle belly. A retractor in this plane raised superiorly extends nearly to the humerus. Dropping down 2 cm from the highest portion of the interpectoral fascia, a transverse incision is made through the pectoralis major fascia, then deeper so that the clavipectoral fascia is incised at the same level, from the pectoralis minor muscle that lies within the fascia laterally. Making the transverse incision at this level spares the axillary lymphatic vessels returning from the arm, minimizing the risk of later arm swelling. This approach reveals the inferior margin of the axillary vein immediately subadjacent to the clavipectoral fascia. Sweeping the fatty tissue inferiorly and away from the axillary vein will reveal some external thoracic and axillary vein branches entering the inferior margin of the axillary vein. These can be divided. Dorsal to this the thoracodorsal vein enters the more dorsal aspect of the axillary vein 2 to 2.5 cm from the chest wall.

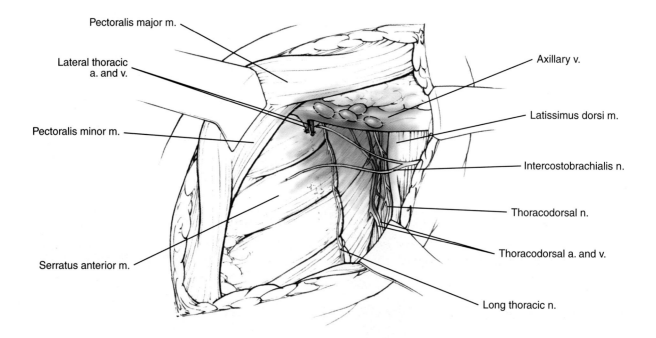

The subscapular vein and thoracodorsal vein may enter separately, adjacent to one another, or more commonly fuse as a common trunk. Some anatomists refer to this as the thoracodorsal vein with a subscapular branch, others to the subscapular vein with a thoracodorsal branch. Just medial to the thoracodorsal vein the thoracodorsal nerve emerges from beneath the axillary vein to join the thoracodorsal vein and the thoracodorsal artery. These pass inferiorly to enter the latissimus dorsi muscle. Just lateral to the thoracodorsal vessels the surgeon's finger can pass between the lateral aspect of the thoracodorsal vessels immediately beneath the axillary vein and the latissimus dorsi lateral border previously identified. The tissue encompassed between the surgeon's two fingers may now be completely divided, with one exception. The intercostobrachial nerve supplying sensation to the skin of the axilla and medial posterior arm is now palpated against the surgeon's finger. Drawing down on the axillary contents just described causes sufficient tension that the intercostobrachial nerve is easily identified. It may be dissected free of the surrounding axillary contents, and should be spared whenever possible. With that nerve spared, but the other lateral axillary contents divided, visual access into the medial axilla is excellent.

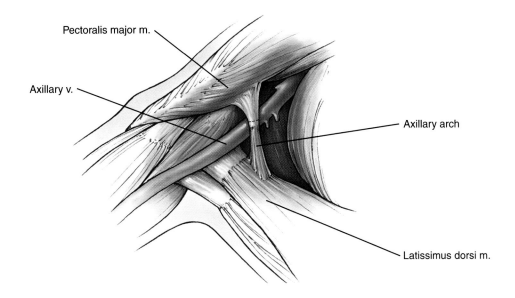

In approximately 5% of patients an axillary arch is present. Those fibers forming the arch may be divided to provide access to the axilla. The long thoracic nerve is identified on the chest wall beneath the fascia of the serratus anterior muscle, at exactly the same anteroposterior depth as the thoracodorsal nerve. In any axillary dissection identification of the thoracodorsal vein also serves to identify the thoracodorsal nerve, making it easy to locate the long thoracic nerve.

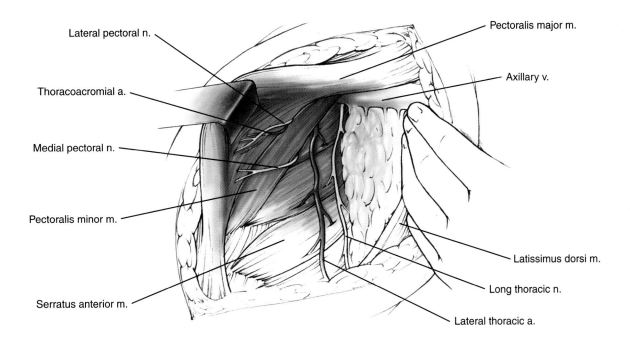

The axillary contents may be cleared away, sparing only the medial origins of the two intercostal contributions of the intercostobrachial nerve. The medial pectoral nerve is also visualized and carefully spared when removing the level

II lymph nodes. These are the lymph nodes that lie behind the pectoralis minor muscle. The medial pectoral nerves sweep around the border of the pectoralis minor muscle or may have an additional branch that penetrates the lateral fibers of the pectoralis minor muscle. They pass anteriorly to innervate the lateral half of the pectoralis major muscle. If these nerves are inadvertently removed, the lateral aspect of the pectoralis major muscle atrophies, producing thinning that is more important cosmetically than functionally. All the lymphatic tissue behind the pectoralis minor muscle is swept out inferiorly with the other axillary contents. These include breast tissue comprising the tail of Spence that has entered the axilla, as described above. Two suction drains are placed, one to drain the axilla and one in the anterior chest wall. The skin is then closed as a single layer or the reconstructive portion of the procedure is begun.

Patey's Modified Radical Mastectomy

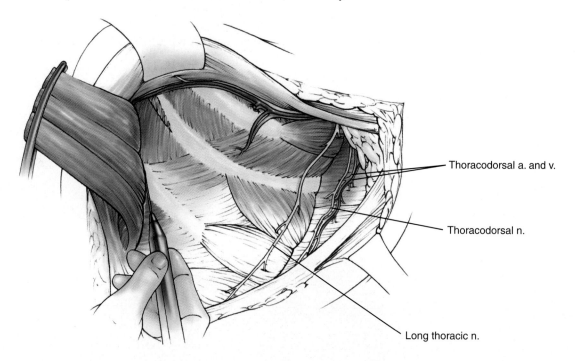

Thoracodorsal a. and v.

Thoracodorsal n.

Long thoracic n.

The operation described by Patey includes removal of the level III lymph nodes. This can be accomplished by preparing the arm into the operative field so that it may be brought across the chest, relaxing the pectoralis major muscle. With a retractor beneath the relaxed pectoralis major muscle, the pectoralis minor muscle may be encircled and divided. Its origin is removed together with the level III axillary lymph nodes after the muscle has been divided. When dividing the pectoralis minor muscle, it is important to identify the lateral pectoral nerves and thoracoacromial artery and vein entering the pectoralis major muscle medially so that they may be spared and to spare the medial pectoral nerves lying lateral to the pectoralis minor muscle. The level III nodes include Rotter's nodes, the eponym for the interpectoral nodes. In patients with bulky nodal

Possible Causes of Lymphedema Following Axillary Dissection

- Too radical excision of lymphatic vessels, including those draining the arm
- Obesity
- Infection with scarring of the lymphatic vessels draining the arm
- Node dissection coupled with irradiation of the axilla
- Tumor involving and blocking lymphatic vessels

disease, a full axillary dissection can be performed. Because the axillary lymph nodes are contiguous with the supraclavicular nodes above the clavicle and with the intrathoracic nodes through the thoracic inlet, it is apparent that the axillary lymph nodes are not a qualitatively different compartment but simply an arbitrary division of the lymphatic vessels of this region. Removing the level III nodes in addition to the levels I and II nodes increases the risk for arm edema from approximately 3% to approximately 10%.

Radical Mastectomy

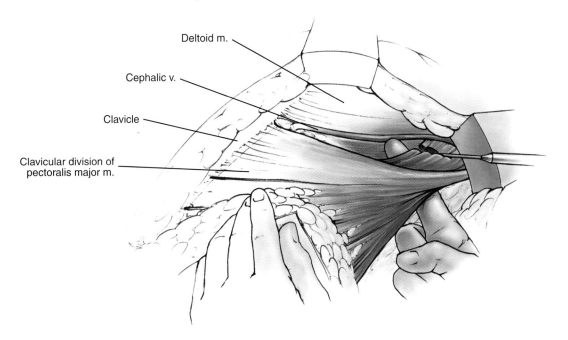

In an era of multimodality therapy, induction chemotherapy and radiation therapy have all but eliminated the indications for radical mastectomy. Although radical mastectomy is no longer of clinical utility, technically this is an easier procedure than modified radical mastectomy. After skin flaps are elevated as described for modified radical mastectomy, the pectoralis major muscle is divided just before it inserts on the humerus. The cephalic vein marks the level at which the pectoralis major muscle is separable from the deltoid muscle above.

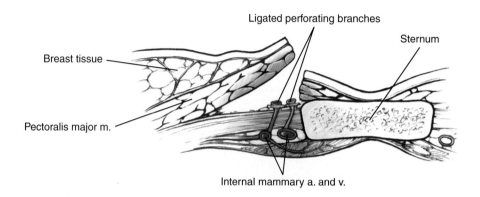

In taking the origin of the pectoralis major muscle medially, perforating branches from the internal mammary vessels are seen. These are grasped and ligated, clipped, or electrocoagulated. If allowed to retract beneath the intercostal muscles, they could cause considerable hemorrhage in the subpleural space between the chest wall and the pleural cavity.

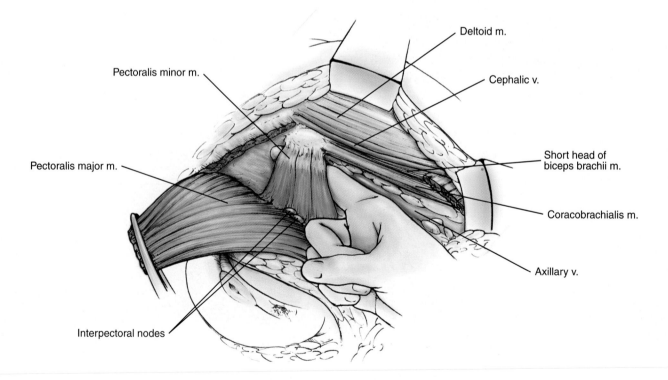

Beneath the pectoralis major muscle, the clavipectoral fascia and pectoralis minor muscle are divided. Removal of the pectoralis major and minor muscles in addition to those structures incorporated in a modified radical mastectomy completes the procedure. Tumor recurrences involving the pectoralis major muscle after breast-conserving therapy may require a radical mastectomy.

Total Mastectomy

Total mastectomy is performed as described for modified radical mastectomy, but without axillary dissection. It is essential to enter the lower axilla to remove the tail of Spence and the breast tissue lying within the first level of the axilla.

Sentinel Node Biopsy

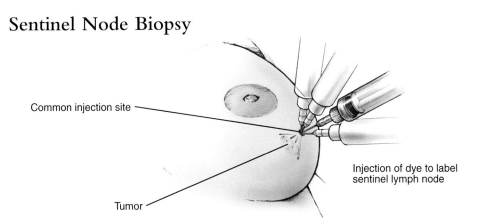

Common injection site

Injection of dye to label sentinel lymph node

Tumor

Dr. Donald Morton proposed that each area of skin probably drains through a lymphatic pathway to a specific lymph node. If the lymph node draining the area where a melanoma is located is removed, it should be more specific than the entire regional lymph node basin and, if free of metastatic cells, may mean that the other nodes in the region are also free. He and Dr. Guiliano applied the same reasoning to breast cancer, and subsequent trials appear to bear out their hypothesis. The sentinel lymph node can be identified by injection of lymphazurin blue dye or by use of radioactive technetium sulphur colloid and a nuclear medicine scanning instrument to provide an image or a hand-held Geiger counter probe to locate the node or nodes (it is not rare for two or more nodes to be identified).

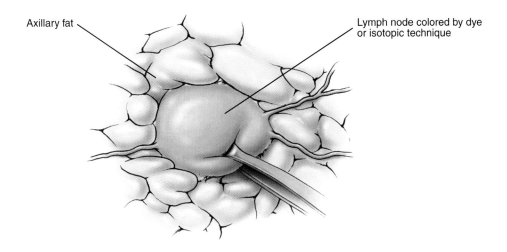

Axillary fat

Lymph node colored by dye or isotopic technique

The dye is injected at the edge of the tumor or at a small excision site. It must be placed into the breast parenchyma, not the subcutaneous tissue or the pectoral fascia deeply. Then 3 minutes after the injection of about 4 ml in the upper breast, 5 minutes for the central breast, and 7 minutes for the lower breast, a transverse axillary incision is made. The axillary contents at the junction of level I and level II nodes are divided in superficial cuts, each about 2 mm deeper, searching for the blue-dyed lymphatic vessel. When seen, it will be smaller than the veins, which will also be blue, usually 1 mm or 0.5 mm in diameter. It may be grasped with an Allis clamp and traced proximally to identify the most proximal lymph node along its course. This is the sentinel node and will usually be bright blue at this time, fading over the next 5 to 10 minutes. The region is searched for additional blue nodes or a second lymphatic vessel. Sometimes the tumor in a node prevents the node from turning blue even though it lies along the course of an identified sentinel lymphatic vessel. With the isotopic technique the incision and search for the lymph node are directed by the hand-held probe. The removed node is checked for activity with the probe. The axilla is checked again for additional "hot" nodes.

Axillary Dissection

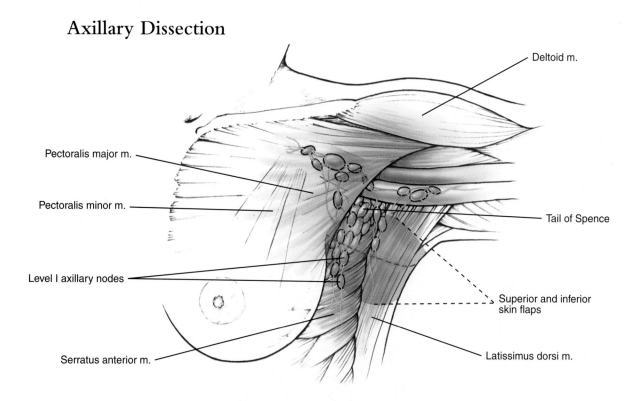

A transverse skin incision is made from the pectoralis major muscle anteriorly to the latissimus dorsi lateral border posteriorly 2 to 3 cm down from the junction of the axillary skin and the brachial skin. This incision may be oriented to lie in normal skin lines. It is carried through the skin and immediate subcutaneous tissue, but only a millimeter or two of subcutaneous tissue is spared. The lymphatic vessels are rich and approach the level of the skin. Consequently the skin flaps for an axillary dissection are relatively thin. The procedure was described earlier (see pp. 161 to 164). In patients with melanoma or squamous cell carcinoma lymph node metastases to all three levels of axillary lymph nodes should be removed (see p. 164). A single suction drain is placed through a separate stab wound.

Axillary Dissection With Lumpectomy

Axillary dissection is typically limited to levels I and II lymph nodes when performed with lumpectomy for breast conservation. When the two operations are combined, it is usually preferable to perform the axillary dissection first. Then with separate instruments the lumpectomy is performed and the breast wrapped. Wrapping the breast immediately after completion of the lumpectomy prevents development of a seroma or hematoma during the axillary dissection.

BREAST RECONSTRUCTION
John Bostwick III, M.D.

Breast reconstruction is an important component of the treatment and rehabilitation of the woman with breast cancer. Most patients seek proper management of breast cancer with breast preservation or restoration. This goal can often be accomplished with lumpectomy plus irradiation, with removal of limited portion of the breast. When a considerable portion of breast tissue is excised or mastectomy is necessary, the breast can be reconstructed with a number of reliable procedures that meet the patient's psychologic and aesthetic expectations for breast restoration. Breasts can be rebuilt with implants or tissue expanders placed beneath the musculofascial layer, with muscle or musculocutaneous flaps of the patient's own tissues obtained from the abdomen and back (less frequently from the buttocks and hip), or with a combination of these modalities. The choice of reconstructive method depends on the amount and quality of the tissue remaining after the mastectomy, patient preferences, and the surgeon's experience with each technique. If flap reconstruction is selected, familiarity with the surgical anatomy of the TRAM and latissimus dorsi flaps and the position of the vascular pedicles after transfer for breast reconstruction is a requirement. The source of the blood supply to the flaps is a major consideration because interventions that compromise it can result in even greater problems.

With the development and refinement of skin-sparing mastectomy techniques as well as new endoscopic procedures, tissue expansion advances, and autologous tissue refinements, the results of immediate reconstruction have improved considerably and are frequently better than those that can be expected after delayed reconstruction. Often immediate reconstruction can permit the oncologic surgeon to remove less breast skin than would ordinarily be removed for mastectomy alone, thus reducing or shortening the breast scar. The preserved skin used to cover the new breast reduces the need for skin expansion and requires less skin to be transferred from the abdomen or back if autologous breast reconstruction has been selected. The surgeon can also help preserve the natural anatomic landmarks of the breast, such as the inframammary fold, medial cleavage, and lateral limits of the breast. These boundaries can then be used to more accurately define breast shape, producing a reconstructed breast that often has optimal symmetry with the remaining breast. The reduced scar is made less conspicuous later when it is partially covered by the new nipple-areola reconstruction. Essentially the same techniques are used for immediate breast reconstruction as for delayed breast reconstruction. Immediate reconstruction is often preferred for breast restoration, provided it does not interfere with proper management of the breast cancer or unduly delay adjunctive treatment.

Implants and Expanders
Surgical Anatomy

For breast reconstruction with breast implants and expanders consideration must be given to the normal topographic position of the breast, and the devices must be positioned to give the most natural appearance. Shaped or anatomic implants and expanders are available that provide more versatile options for achieving breast symmetry and more natural contour. These devices may be textured as a means of reducing the incidence of capsular contracture. Textured implants do not perform as well when overlying skin cover is thin and may be unnaturally palpable or may exhibit visible wrinkling through the skin.

If an immediate reconstruction is being performed, the implant can be placed through the mastectomy incision. When the mastectomy scar is not in the best location, a small incision can be made near the new inframammary crease and the implant or expander placed through this new incision. When implant or expander reconstruction is used, the implants and expanders are usually placed beneath the chest wall musculature, that is, the pectoralis major muscle and serratus anterior muscle. Sometimes the lower portions of the breast implant are covered with the fascia of the external oblique muscle and the rectus abdominis muscle. When oncologic requirements permit, the external fascia of these muscles is maintained to provide an additional layer of cover for these devices. This muscle and fascia cover protects the breast implant from exposure through overlying thin skin, especially during immediate breast reconstruction. It also appears to protect the device from capsular contracture.

Surgical Applications

Breast reconstruction with placement of a breast implant or tissue expander beneath the musculofascial layer is a simple outpatient procedure. These operations do not rule out autologous tissue breast reconstruction later if needed. Patients who are ideal candidates for this type of breast reconstruction are thin and have relatively small, rounded breasts without ptosis. This breast contour is much easier to match than that seen in heavier women with large ptotic breasts. The operation is appropriate for a woman who has some ptosis or heaviness of the opposite breast if she is amenable to undergoing a procedure to modify the other breast.

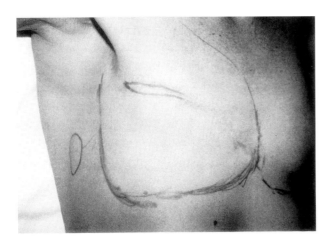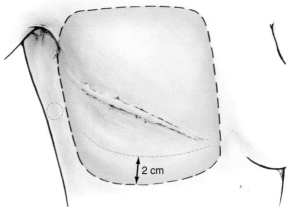

Preoperative markings are made for a left inframammary submusculofascial breast augmentation. The tissue expander selected should be of similar width as the proposed augmented breast. It will be placed through the lateral mastectomy scar. It is also positioned 2 cm below the opposite inframammary crease to recruit and expand skin from the upper abdomen for reconstruction of the lower breast. The position of the expander port is also noted.

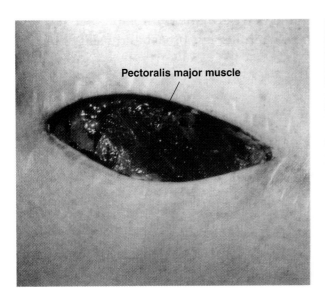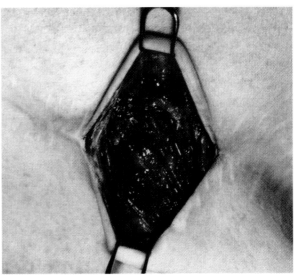

After an ellipse of the lateral mastectomy scar is excised, the dissection is made down to the lateral margin of the pectoralis major muscle. The skin is elevated superiorly and inferiorly to expose a 6 cm segment of the pectoralis major muscle.

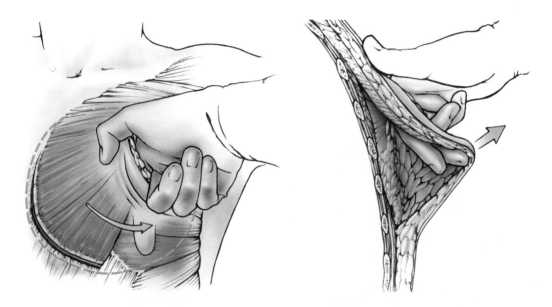

The pectoralis major muscle is lifted from its underlying attachments with blunt finger dissection. A lighted retractor is useful at this point for dividing the origins of the pectoralis major muscle from the second rib down to the new inframammary crease. The inferior dissection is most critical. It is essential to free any tight restricting cicatrix in the lower breast region so there is less resistance to expansion than encountered in the upper portion. Dissection then swings laterally to lift the mastectomy skin off the lateral fascia. The upper dissection is completed by elevating the upper fibers of the serratus anterior muscle and its attached fascia.

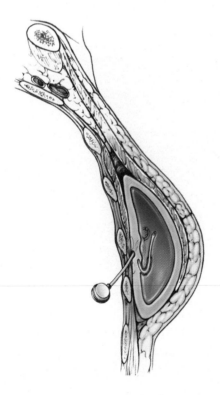

The device and valve are positioned, and a test inflation is done to ascertain whether the device is functioning properly. The muscular layer in the region of the mastectomy scar is completely closed, and the incision is aligned with skin staples and closed with two layers of buried absorbable sutures. After the initial procedure 200 ml of saline solution is left in the tissue expander. The final volume is adjusted in the postoperative period.

Results

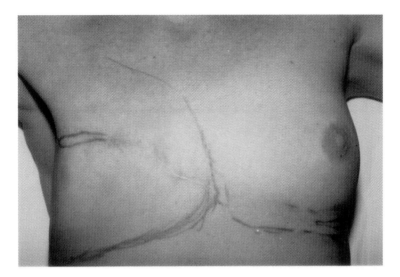

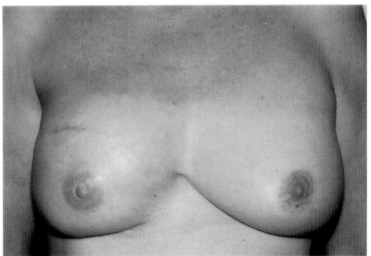

This patient is shown 2½ years after breast reconstruction with a temporary tissue expander, which was exchanged for permanent implants to give better projection and contour. Left breast augmentation was also performed to achieve breast symmetry.

Latissimus Dorsi Flap

The latissimus dorsi flap was the first major musculocutaneous flap used for breast reconstruction. The flap provides muscle, subcutaneous tissue, and skin. It is particularly useful for replacing tissue in the lateral and upper portions of the reconstructed breast, and the muscle provides a protective cover for breast implants. When the patient has excess back tissue and does not require a large breast reconstruction, additional subcutaneous tissue can be harvested from the back for autologous tissue breast reconstruction. In some patients undergoing lumpectomy plus radiation therapy the defect is large relative to the breast size or a large breast parenchyma resection is necessary to adequately remove the breast cancer. For these patients, after determination that the tumor is completely excised, endoscopic harvest of the latissimus dorsi muscle and its overlying subcutaneous tissue is also a possibility to provide fill for the breast defect through the axillary lymph node dissection incision. This living tissue is usually radiolucent on mammograms and does not present problems for patient follow-up.

Surgical Anatomy

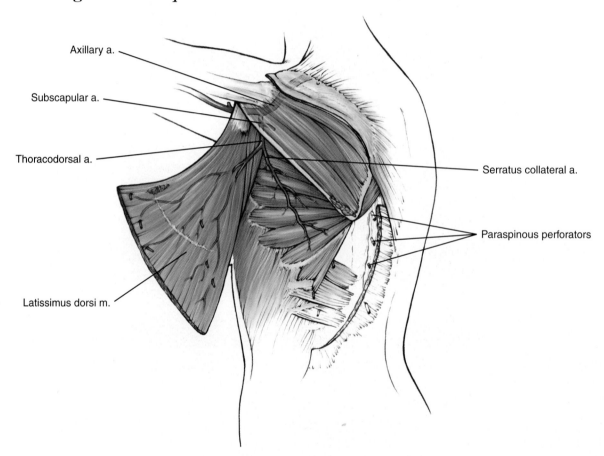

The vascularity and reliability of the latissimus dorsi musculocutaneous flap are more forgiving than that of the TRAM flap. The flap is based on the thoracodorsal pedicle, a branch of the subscapular artery arising from the axillary artery, which is usually spared with axillary lymph node dissection. This is not the case after radical mastectomy.

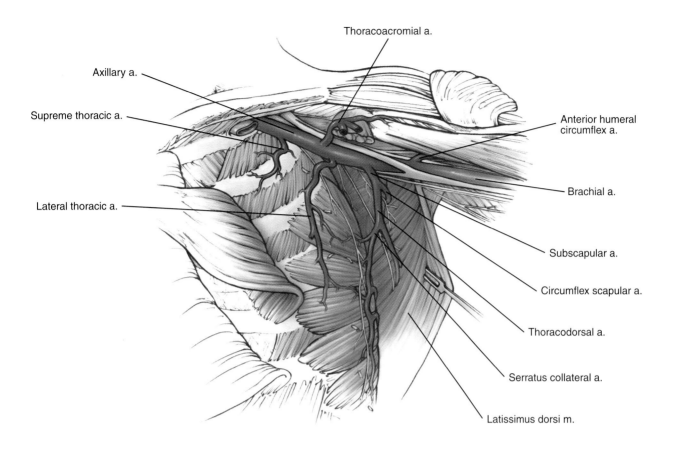

Thoracoacromial a.

Axillary a.

Supreme thoracic a.

Anterior humeral circumflex a.

Brachial a.

Lateral thoracic a.

Subscapular a.

Circumflex scapular a.

Thoracodorsal a.

Serratus collateral a.

Latissimus dorsi m.

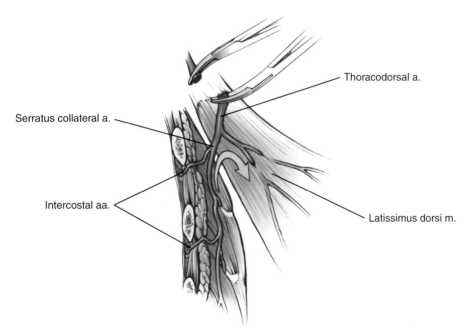

Thoracodorsal a.

Serratus collateral a.

Intercostal aa.

Latissimus dorsi m.

The thoracodorsal artery has a relatively large diameter, 1 to 2.5 mm. An intramuscular vascular pattern radiates from the thoracodorsal pedicle to nourish the latissimus dorsi flap. Successful latissimus dorsi flap reconstruction, both primary and secondary, depends on the reconstructive surgeon's knowledge of this intramuscular branching of the thoracodorsal artery. The primary intramuscular vessel courses vertically in the same direction as the pedicle, approximately 3 cm inside the lateral edge of the latissimus dorsi muscle. The intramuscular network, radiating from the entrance of the thoracodorsal pedicle into the latissimus dorsi muscle 10 cm below the axilla, permits splitting the latissimus dorsi into two or three muscle strips to support several skin islands if these are needed for specialized secondary procedures. The largest perforating vessels branch from this primary vessel; therefore verticolateral orientation of the latissimus dorsi flap provides the safest skin island. Several other major branches extend in a radial manner from the primary pedicle. The intramuscular branching pattern permits division of the latissimus dorsi muscle while preserving the proximal blood supply and the integrity of the musculocutaneous unit. A collateral pedicle from the serratus anterior fascia is also usually preserved and is a constant vessel in this region. The latissimus dorsi flap can survive on this vessel when the thoracodorsal pedicle has been injured or divided. The flap can be harvested either laterally or transversely for a variety of flaps that can be customized to replace the tissue needed for the reconstructed breast. When there has been previous axillary lymph node dissection, the reconstructive surgeon should always assume the thoracodorsal pedicle has been injured. Patient selection is important when using the latissimus dorsi flap. If there is severe radiation damage of the axilla there may be some concern about the patency of the thoracodorsal pedicle and the ultimate vascular nourishment of the flap.

The thoracodorsal nerve, arising from the C6–8 roots of the posterior cord of the brachial plexus, is the motor nerve to the latissimus dorsi muscle. This nerve along with the thoracodorsal vessels passes downward through the axilla and enters the muscle with the thoracodorsal vascular pedicle. The thoracodorsal nerve is responsible for muscular contraction of the latissimus dorsi muscle. If this muscle contraction is a problem to the patient after latissimus dorsi flap reconstruction, it can be divided during a secondary procedure. This division paralyzes the muscle and induces denervation atrophy of the latissimus dorsi muscle without compromising the blood flow to the flap through the muscle and skin island as long as the collateral vessels from the serratus anterior muscle are preserved.

The surgeon should also be familiar with the anatomy of the insertion of the latissimus dorsi muscle, which is through a 3 cm broad tendon attached to the bottom of the intertubercular groove of the humerus. The tendon and proximal latissimus dorsi muscle actually encircle the teres major muscle, which is the muscle that primarily contributes to the form of the posterior axillary fold.

Surgical Applications

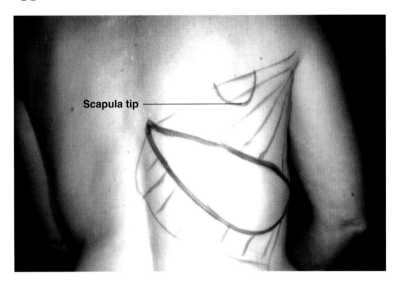

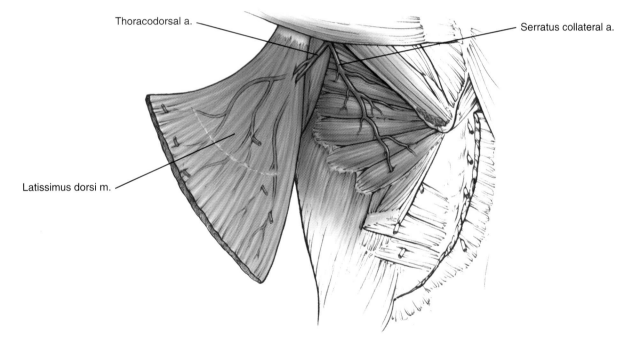

The limits of the entire latissimus dorsi muscle and the location of the skin island above the muscle to be transferred are noted and marked according to estimated requirements. The markings for the skin island are in the natural skin lines across and around the back. A transverse skin island is usually designed over the upper portion of the muscle.

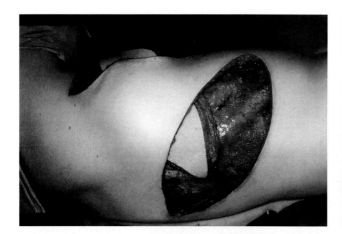
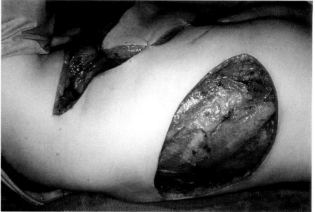

After the mastectomy incision is opened anteriorly, the flaps are elevated as out-lined by the preoperative markings. Dissection is delayed in the axilla near the axillary vein until the patient is in a supine position and the vessel is clearly vis-ible. After a subcutaneous tunnel is developed high in the axilla, the flap is trans-ferred first into the axillary incision and then into the anterior chest wall.

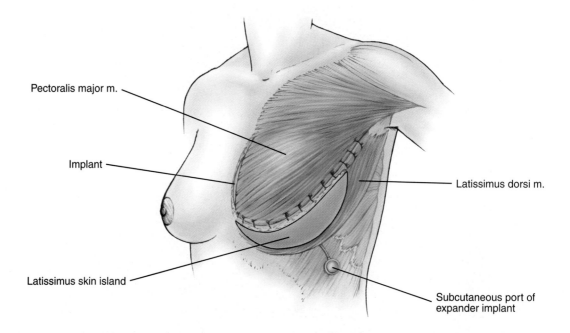

For completion of the operation the patient is placed in a supine position with the arms positioned symmetrically and abducted at a 60-degree angle.

The latissimus dorsi muscle is sutured to the elevated pectoralis major muscle and the skin just above the inframammary crease. When an axillary fold is needed, some of the outer layer of skin and a portion of the latissimus dorsi muscle are brought around and stitched out onto the upper arm to simulate a new anterior axillary fold. After the skin island is closed inferiorly, an opening is left laterally for placement of the tissue expander. The expander is inflated with saline solution in the postoperative period. For immediate breast reconstruction, the upper part of the expander is placed under the pectoralis major muscle above and the lower part is covered by the latissimus dorsi muscle. When skin is needed, it replaces the skin removed at the time of mastectomy.

Results

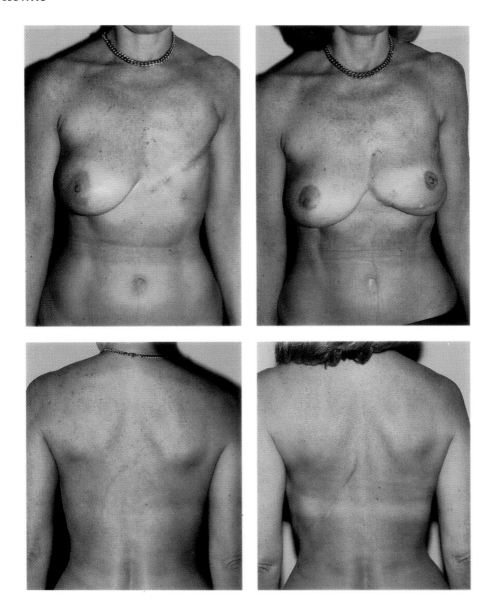

This 42-year-old woman underwent a modified radical mastectomy. After completing chemotherapy she requested breast reconstruction. She had significant breast asymmetry, but because her lower abdomen was attractive she did not want a scar in this area. Her breast was reconstructed with a latissimus dorsi musculocutaneous island flap taken from a natural crease in the direction of the natural skin lines of her back and a breast implant. The back scar has remained thin and does not concern this patient.

Endoscopic Latissimus Dorsi Flap for Partial Mastectomy Deformity

Large local excisions of breast parenchyma are sometimes necessary to obtain clear margins during breast-conserving surgery, and healing of the resulting defect can cause significant breast deformity. After radiation therapy the additional fibrosis and scarring further distort the treated breast. Combined endoscopic techniques and latissimus dorsi reconstruction can be performed to fill these partial mastectomy defects, obviating these significant deformities and restoring a natural breast contour. After wound healing and radiation therapy it is not possible to simply reopen the wound, recreate the defect, and fill the area with either autologous tissue or an implant. Rather, the deformity must be prevented or the defect filled with autologous tissue before the breast is irradiated.

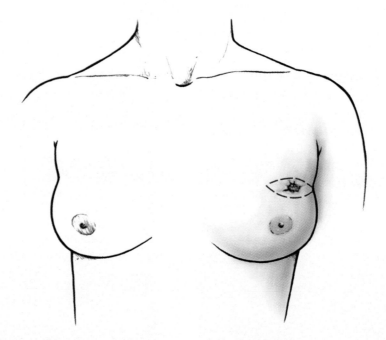

For partial breast reconstruction, such as after quadrantectomy, the latissimus dorsi muscle and its overlying fat and subcutaneous tissue can be harvested through the axillary incision used for the axillary node dissection and a separate, small lower lateral incision with the use of the endoscope. With this technique, postoperative breast appearance is enhanced, there is less fibrosis in the area, and mammography is not compromised.

Surgical Applications

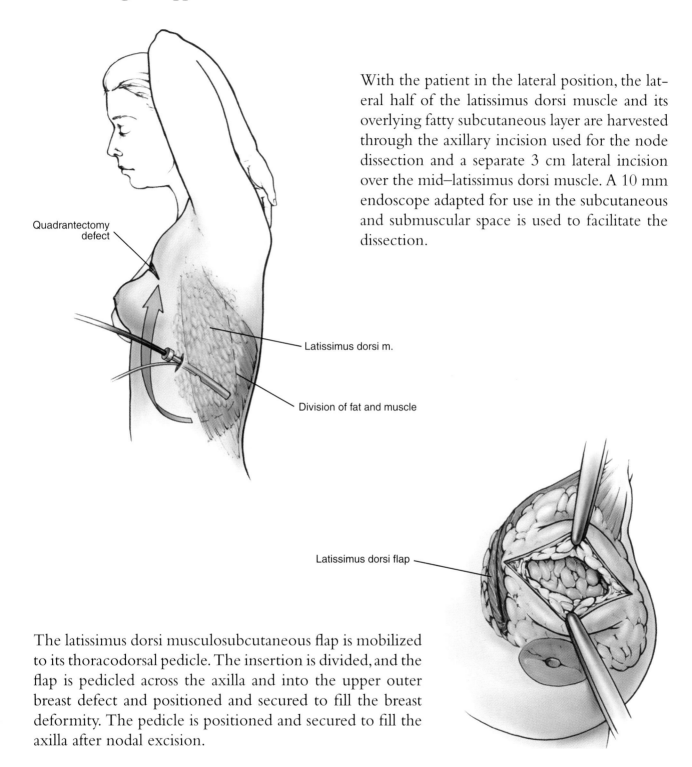

Quadrantectomy
defect

Latissimus dorsi m.

Division of fat and muscle

With the patient in the lateral position, the lateral half of the latissimus dorsi muscle and its overlying fatty subcutaneous layer are harvested through the axillary incision used for the node dissection and a separate 3 cm lateral incision over the mid–latissimus dorsi muscle. A 10 mm endoscope adapted for use in the subcutaneous and submuscular space is used to facilitate the dissection.

Latissimus dorsi flap

The latissimus dorsi musculosubcutaneous flap is mobilized to its thoracodorsal pedicle. The insertion is divided, and the flap is pedicled across the axilla and into the upper outer breast defect and positioned and secured to fill the breast deformity. The pedicle is positioned and secured to fill the axilla after nodal excision.

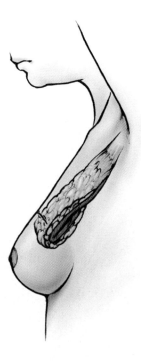

Closure of the wound gives a normally shaped breast that will be given radiation therapy several weeks later.

Results

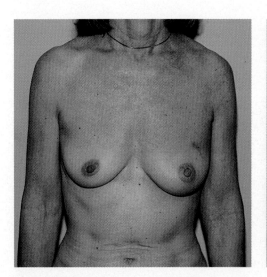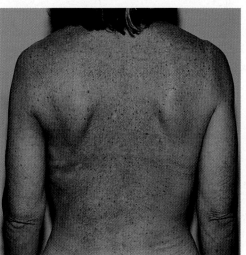

This woman underwent quadrantectomy and immediate breast reconstruction with an endoscopically harvested latissimus dorsi musculosubcutaneous flap. The photograph was taken 1 year after reconstruction and 6 months following radiation therapy to the left breast.

TRAM Flap

The transverse rectus abdominis musculocutaneous (TRAM) flap is the musculocutaneous flap most frequently used for breast reconstruction. Excess tissue in the lower abdominal wall is harvested based on the underlying rectus abdominis muscle and its contained epigastric system. The tissue is either pedicled on the superior epigastric system or transferred as a composite free tissue flap based on the inferior epigastric system.

Surgical Anatomy

The TRAM flap is unforgiving of technical shortfalls and requires detailed knowledge of the surgical anatomy of the breast and abdominal wall. Its blood supply is less reliable when patient selection, operative technique, and perioperative management are extended beyond recognized limits. For example, if the pedicle is divided while placing an implant to enlarge the reconstructed breast, the blood supply to the TRAM flap can be compromised and portions of the flap lost.

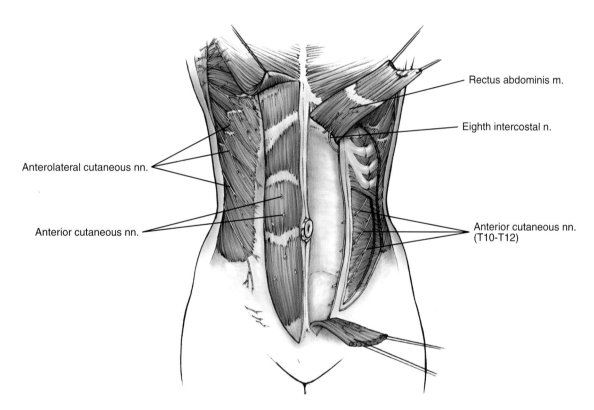

The vertical epigastric vascular system provides the major source of blood supply to the rectus abdominis muscle and the overlying musculocutaneous territories of the anterior abdominal wall. The superior epigastric artery, a terminal branch of the internal mammary artery, nourishes the superiorly based TRAM flap.

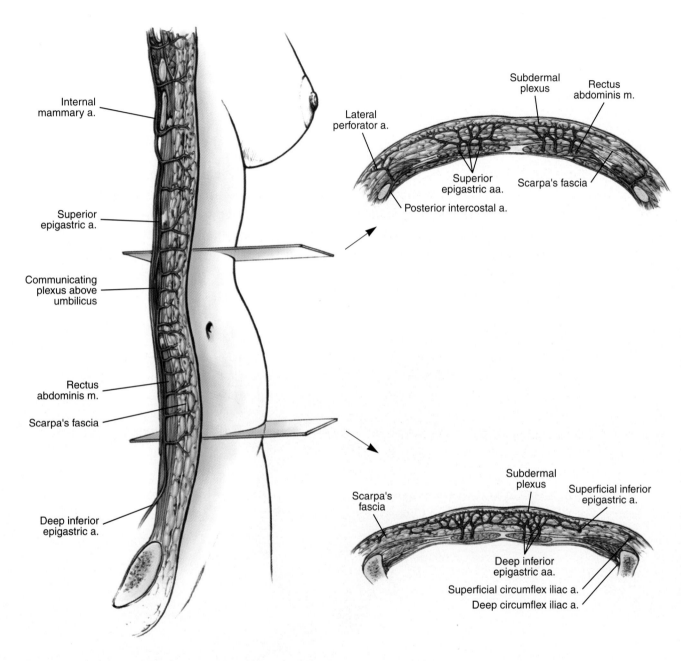

Internal
mammary a.

Lateral
perforator a.

Subdermal
plexus

Rectus
abdominis m.

Superior
epigastric aa.

Posterior intercostal a.

Scarpa's fascia

Superior
epigastric a.

Communicating
plexus above
umbilicus

Subdermal
plexus

Superficial inferior
epigastric a.

Scarpa's
fascia

Rectus
abdominis m.

Scarpa's fascia

Deep inferior
epigastric aa.

Superficial circumflex iliac a.

Deep circumflex iliac a.

Deep inferior
epigastric a.

Musculocutaneous perforating arteries extend from the vertical epigastric system within the rectus abdominis muscle and pass through the anterior rectus sheath, providing nourishment for the skin and subcutaneous tissue of the anterior abdominal wall. These perforating vessels branch into axially coursing vessels that are primarily located above the superficial layer of the abdominal wall fascia and are especially concentrated in the subdermal plexus. In the upper abdomen these vessels supply the primary flow into the thoracoepigastric flap, with the subdermal plexus providing significant collateral flow.

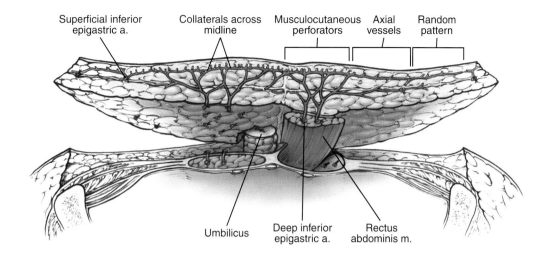

Axial vessels branching from the direct periumbilical rectus abdominis muscular perforators nourish the lateral extensions of the TRAM flap that are not directly over the rectus abdominis muscle. A rich vascular network and interconnected vessels branch in the subcutaneous tissues across the midline of the abdomen. The vascular network is present primarily at the level of the subdermal plexus and communicates with the axial vascular system and subdermal plexus of the contralateral anterior abdominal wall, providing flow to the skin on the contralateral side. TRAM flap elevation across the entire anterior abdominal wall laterally to the anterior axillary line is dependent on this collateral flow and that of the subdermal plexus across the midline into the opposite sides of the abdominal wall subcutaneous vascular network. Radiation, atherosclerosis, age-associated problems, anatomic variations, previous operations, and vasoconstrictors can affect normal flow in this vascular network. A midline incision effectively destroys this midline vascular connection. Decreased vascularity to the TRAM flap and a small skin island may be problems in patients who smoke. Division of the lower deep inferior epigastric artery and vein and the superficial inferior epigastric artery and vein 1 to 2 weeks before the flap elevation procedure (surgical delay) permits more flow into the system from the superior deep epigastric artery.

Surgical Applications

The TRAM flap procedure provides autologous tissue for breast reconstruction. With this procedure, a woman's breasts can be restored with her own, sometimes abundant abdominal tissues, with the added benefit of abdominoplasty. The lower abdominal wall skin replaces large portions of missing breast skin, and autogenous lower abdominal wall fat is used for the missing breast parenchyma, obviating the need for breast implants with their associated concerns. Many patients need autologous tissue breast reconstruction for a satisfactory result; others choose this approach to avoid breast implants. The TRAM flap is the most technically demanding of the commonly used techniques for breast reconstruction, with the exception of microvascular free tissue transfers. In addition to a thorough knowledge of the surgical anatomy of the TRAM flap and abdominal wall, this procedure takes an aesthetically experienced eye and judicious shaping of the flap to produce the expected result.

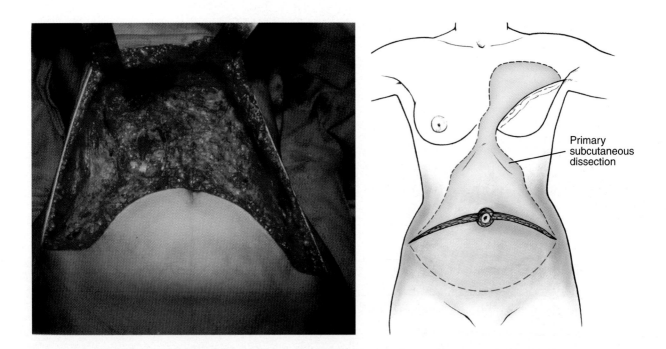

Primary
subcutaneous
dissection

The incision is made across the upper portion of the ellipse, and the abdominal flap is elevated over the costal margin toward the area of the tunnel. If flap closure is too tight, the lower incision can be moved upward on the abdominal wall.

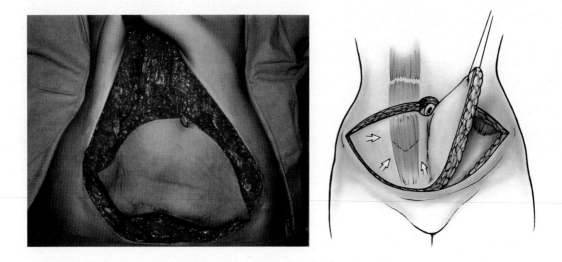

The dissection extends 3 to 4 cm above the costal margin and centrally up to the level of the inframammary crease to prepare the lower portions of the tunnel.

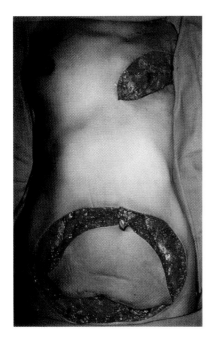 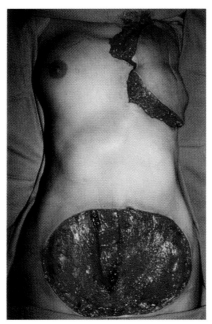 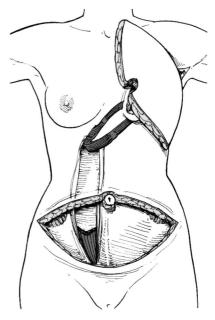

The mastectomy scar is excised elliptically, and the mastectomy wound is re-created above the muscle layer according to the preoperative markings. It is essential not to go too low with the inframammary crease dissection. The final crease position during flap and breast shaping is determined toward the end of the procedure and after abdominal closure with the patient sitting upright. The contralateral TRAM island flap is then transposed to the breast region in the vertical position.

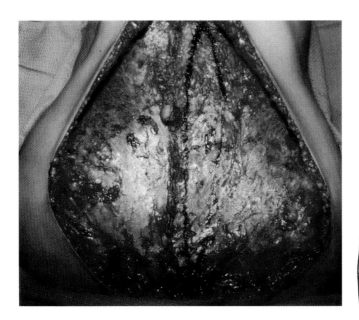 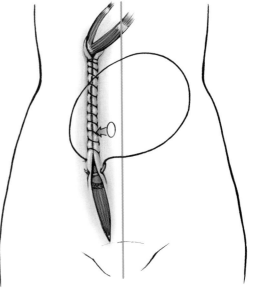

The lower portion of the incision is closed, first by suturing the anterior sheath to the posterior sheath at the level of the arcuate line. Next a large vertical non-absorbable running suture is used for repair, from just below the pedicle to the pubic area. Two layers of sutures are used to secure the closure. The plication should leave about 1 cm of laxity at the costal margin; more than this will create an upper abdominal bulge.

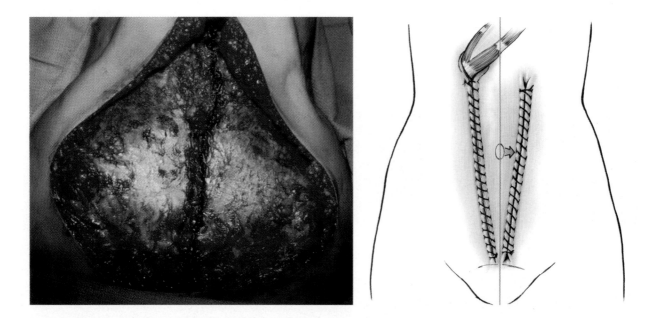

An opposite plication vertically over the rectus fascia further tightens the abdominal wall, flattens the umbilicus, and gives better abdominal symmetry. Without this plication for the unipedicle flap, the abdomen will have a bulge on the side of the retained muscle. The plication must go all the way to the pubis to prevent a later bulge.

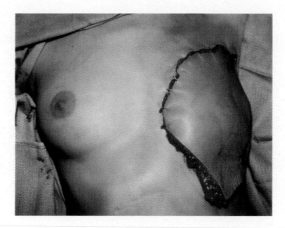

The breast is shaped with the vertical mound shaping technique, from above downward. The upper flap is buried and deepithelialized to give upper breast fill. A small portion of the flap is turned under and deepithelialized to give some lower projection and ptosis.

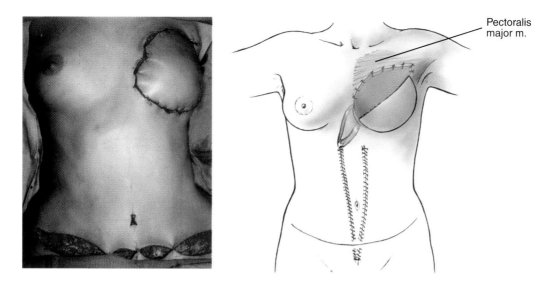

The position of the umbilicus and the final shaping of the breast are shown. Before abdominal closure the subscarpal fat is removed from the upper abdominal flap throughout the future lower abdominal area. This thins the abdominal wall flap, removes fat that may have become desiccated during the procedure and therefore is less viable, and removes the fat that is more likely to be poorly vascularized and thus prone to fat necrosis, postoperative firmness, delayed healing, poor tissue adherence, and seroma.

Results

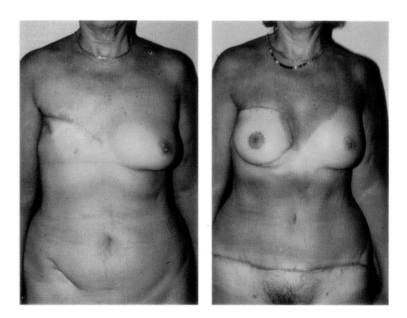

This 52-year-old woman requested breast reconstruction to match her opposite breast. She had an appendectomy scar on the right side. A contralateral unipedicle TRAM flap and the horizontal mound shaping technique were used for breast reconstruction. The nipple-areola was reconstructed with specialized tissues from the opposite nipple and the upper inner thigh. The photographs were taken 9 months after breast reconstruction.

Skin-Sparing Mastectomy With Immediate TRAM Flap Breast Reconstruction

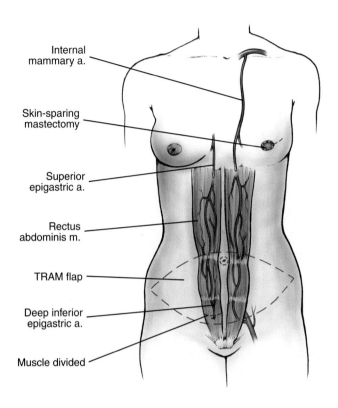

Internal
mammary a.

Skin-sparing
mastectomy

Superior
epigastric a.

Rectus
abdominis m.

TRAM flap

Deep inferior
epigastric a.

Muscle divided

The skin-sparing mastectomy is combined with immediate breast reconstruction with autologous tissue from the lower abdomen. The TRAM flap is pedicled on the contralateral muscle.

Surgical Applications

The TRAM flap is transferred to the breast through an upper abdominal tunnel. It remains attached to the rectus abdominis muscle. The flap is tailored and positioned to give symmetry with the opposite breast. It is deepithelialized except for the skin island, which will be used to replace the areola.

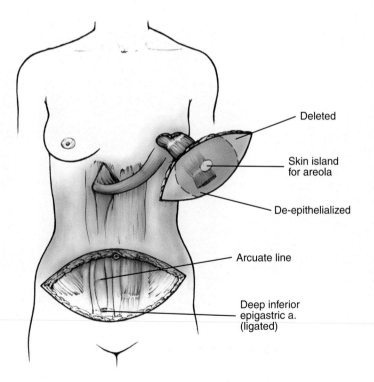

Deleted

Skin island
for areola

De-epithelialized

Arcuate line

Deep inferior
epigastric a.
(ligated)

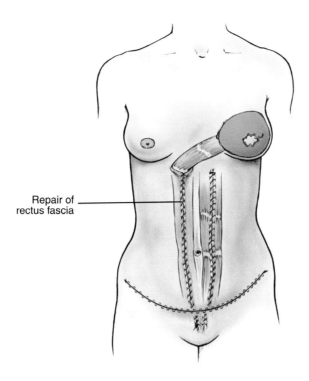

Repair of rectus fascia

The abdominal tissue is fashioned into a breast. After repair of the vertical rectus abdominis fascia from xiphoid to pubis and vertical plication of the opposite rectus abdominis fascia, the lower abdomen is closed as a transverse scar.

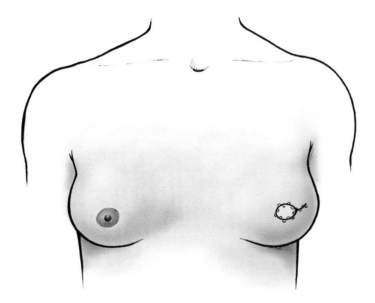

The reconstructed breast is shown with short periareolar incision with side excision closed. The reconstructed breast is allowed to heal for 3 to 6 months before the nipple is reconstructed.

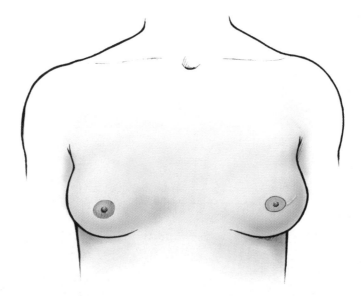

The nipple is reconstructed several months after breast reconstruction, with local flaps of skin and subcutaneous tissue. The areola is tattooed 2 months later.

Results

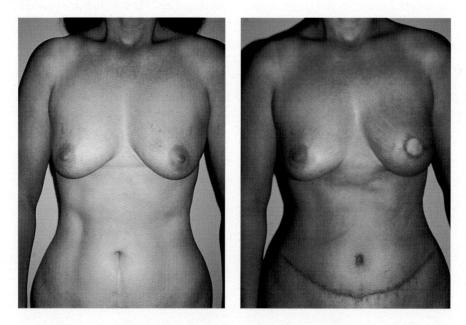

This patient underwent skin-sparing mastectomy and immediate breast reconstruction with a TRAM flap. The tissue from the abdomen was used to replace the breast tissue and a round piece of the abdominal wall skin was used to fill the defect left after the nipple-areola was removed. She is shown 6 months after breast reconstruction before her nipple-areola reconstruction was performed.

Anatomic Basis of Complications

MAJOR

- Injury to long thoracic nerve results in a winged scapula.
- Too extensive resection of brachial lymphatic vessels results in increased risk for arm lymphedema.

MINOR

- Injury to the thorocodorsal nerve weakens the latissimus dorsi muscle.
- Injury to the medial pectoral nerves results in partial atrophy of the pectoralis major muscle.
- Total division of the intercostobrachial nerve results in numbness and dysesthesia under the arm.

KEY REFERENCES

Berger K, Bostwick J III. A Woman's Decision: Breast Care, Treatment, and Reconstruction, 3rd ed. St. Louis: Quality Medical Publishing, 1998.
   This book gives broad coverage for the information concerning breast care, treatment of breast disease, including breast cancer, and options for breast reconstruction after mastectomy. It includes in-depth interviews with 14 women who have undergone treatment of breast cancer and tell the stories of their personal experiences with its management.

Bostwick J III, Eaves FE III, Nahai F. Endoscopic Plastic Surgery. St. Louis: Quality Medical Publishing, 1995.
   This book outlines the field of endoscopic plastic surgery and includes chapters on endoscopic axillary breast augmentation and endoscopic harvesting of the lattissimus dorsi flap.

Bostwick J III, Jurkiewicz MJ. Recent advances in breast reconstruction: Transposition of the latissimus dorsi muscle singly or with the overlying skin. Am Surg 46:537, 1980.
   This paper presents the range of possibilities of breast reconstruction using the latissimus dorsi flap after radical mastectomy and modified radical mastectomy.

Bostwick J III. Plastic and Reconstructive Breast Surgery. St. Louis: Quality Medical
Publishing, 1990.
*This comprehensive text outlines the approach to aesthetic and reconstructive breast surgery.
Detailed anatomy of the breast and the flaps necessary to carry out the full range of breast
reconstruction are included.*

Carlson GW, Bostwick J III, Styblo TM, Moore B, Bried JT, Murray DR, Wood WC.
Skin sparing mastectomy: Oncologic and reconstruction considerations. Ann Surg
255(5):570-578, 1997.
*This article incorporates the reference and studies of GW Carlson supporting the anatomic
background of this procedure.*

Fisher B, Lerner H, Margolese R, Pilch J, Poisson R, Shibata H. The technique of
segmental mastectomy (lumpectomy) and axillary dissection: A syllabus from the
National Surgical Adjuvant Breast Project workshops. Surgery 102:828-834,
1987.
*This is a very practical illustrated guide to technique. It is opinion, rather than evidence
based, but is still a useful reference.*

Guiliano AE, Guenther JM, Kirgafi DM, Morton DL. Lymphatic mapping and sentinel lymphadenectomy for breast cancer. Ann Surg 220:391-401, 1994.
*This article provides a description of sentinel lymph node excision by the group that intro-
duced the procedure.*

Hartrampf CR Jr, Scheflan M, Black PW. Breast reconstruction following mastectomy with a transverse abdominal island flap. Anatomical and clinical observa-
tions. Plast Reconstr Surg 69:216, 1982.
*Initial paper describing the TRAM flap includes relevant anatomy and description of pa-
tient selection and technique.*

Poulard B, Teicher I, Wise L. Preservation of the intercostobrachial nerve during axillary dissection for carcinoma of the breast. Surg Gynecol Obstet 155:891-892,
1982.
The technique of preservation of this clinically important sensory nerve is described.

Radovan C. Breast reconstruction after mastectomy using the temporary expander.
Plast Reconstr Surg 69:195, 1982.
*This initial paper outlines the use of the tissue expander for breast reconstruction. This tech-
nique is an important advance that extended and enhanced the possibilities of breast reconstruction using breast implants.*

Scanlon EF. The importance of the anterior thoracic nerves in modified radical mastectomy. Surg Gynecol Obstet 52:789-791, 1981.
This article demonstrates the importance of preservation of the pectoral nerves.

SELECTED READINGS

Carlson GW. Skin sparing mastectomy: Anatomic and technical considerations. Am Surg 62(2):151-155, 1996.

Cooper A. On the Anatomy of the Breast. London: Longmans, 1840.

Cunningham L. The anatomy of the arteries and veins of the breast. J Surg Oncol 9:71-85, 1977.

Haaaenson CD. Anatomy of the mammary glands. In Haaaensen CD, ed. Diseases of the Breast, 3rd ed. Philadelphia: WB Saunders, 1986, p 1.

Lappert P, Toth B. Modified skin incisions for mastectomy: The need for plastic surgical input in preoperative planning. Plast Reconstr Surg 87:1048-1053, 1991.

Skiles H. Contributions to the surgical anatomy of the breast. Edinburgh Med J 37:1099, 1892.

Spratt JS. Anatomy of the breast. Major Probl Clin Surg 5:1-13, 1979.

Turner-Warwick RT. The lymphatics of the breast. Br J Surg 46:574-582, 1953.

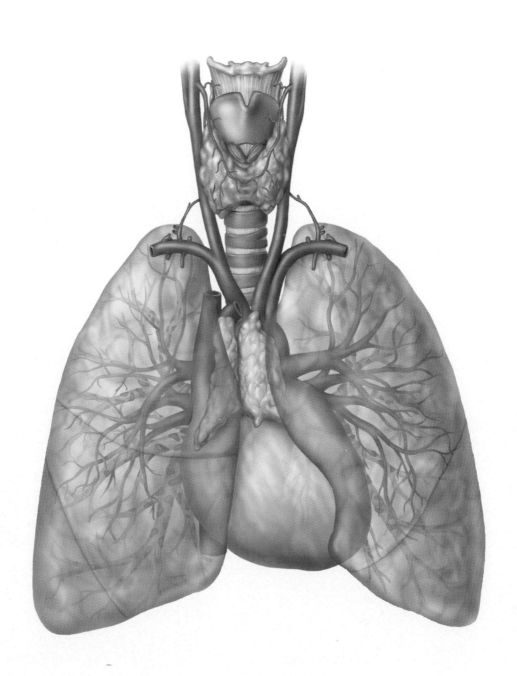

Chapter **4**

Mediastinum, Thymus, Cervical and Thoracic Trachea, and Lung

Robert B. Lee, M.D.

Surgical Applications

Mediastinum
  Diagnosis and Resection of
    Mediastinal Tumors

Thymus
  Resection of Thymic Gland
    Tumors

Cervical and Thoracic Trachea
  Bronchoscopy
  Incisions for Tracheal and Major
    Bronchial Resections
  Resection and Reconstruction of
    Cervical Trachea
  Resection and Reconstruction of
    Thoracic Trachea
  Reconstruction After Carinal
    Resection

Lung
  Posterolateral Thoracotomy
  Limited or Muscle-Sparing
    Thoracotomy
  Median Sternotomy Incision
  Pulmonary Resection
  Right Upper Lobectomy
  Right Middle Lobectomy
  Right Lower Lobectomy
  Left Upper Lobectomy
  Left Lower Lobectomy
  Right and Left Pneumonectomy
  Mediastinal Lymph Node
    Dissection

Mediastinum

The mediastinum exists by definition, not as a single organ. It is an area defined by arbitrary anatomic boundaries within which many intrathoracic organs reside. The mediastinum's existence by definition has led not only to confusion but to controversy regarding its anatomic subdivisions. This in turn has led to confusion in the radiologic, medical, and surgical literature reporting frequency of different tumors within the mediastinum. The organs and tumors within the mediastinum are many. This section defines the mediastinum and its compartments, the contents within, surgical procedures for diagnosis, and representative resection techniques within each compartment.

SURGICAL ANATOMY

The mediastinum is that anatomic space defined as the intrathoracic region, bounded laterally by the parietal pleura, superiorly by the thoracic inlet, inferiorly by the superior surface of the diaphragm, anteriorly by the sternum (jugular notch to xiphoid), and posteriorly by the anterior longitudinal spinal ligaments, which run along the first through the eleventh thoracic vertebrae. Although the costovertebral region (paravertebral sulci) are not by definition within the mediastinum, it has been commonly accepted that masses here are considered within the mediastinum. A mass lesion may arise and predominate within a given region; however, extension into another division as the mass enlarges is common. The site in which the greatest bulk of a given lesion resides defines its compartment of origin.

Division of Mediastinum

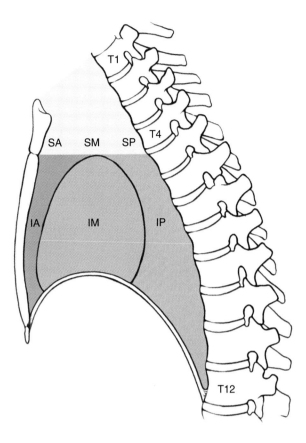

The arbitrary division of the mediastinum into compartments has led to confusion. Traditionally anatomists divided the mediastinum into a superior and an inferior section, with anterior, middle, and posterior sections within each. Shields suggested a simplified division in 1972.

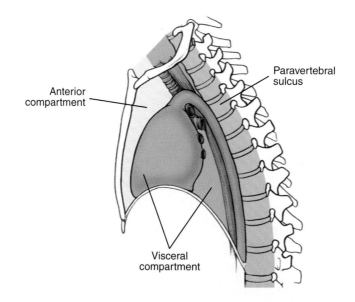

Using Shield's definition, the superior anterior, middle, and posterior sections are the anterior and visceral compartments and the bilateral paravertebral sulci.

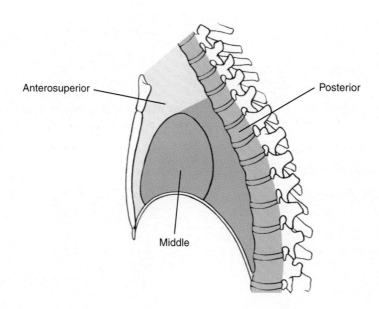

This schema closely corresponds to the division I have found most clinically useful, which combines the anterior and superior compartments into one anterosuperior mediastinal compartment.

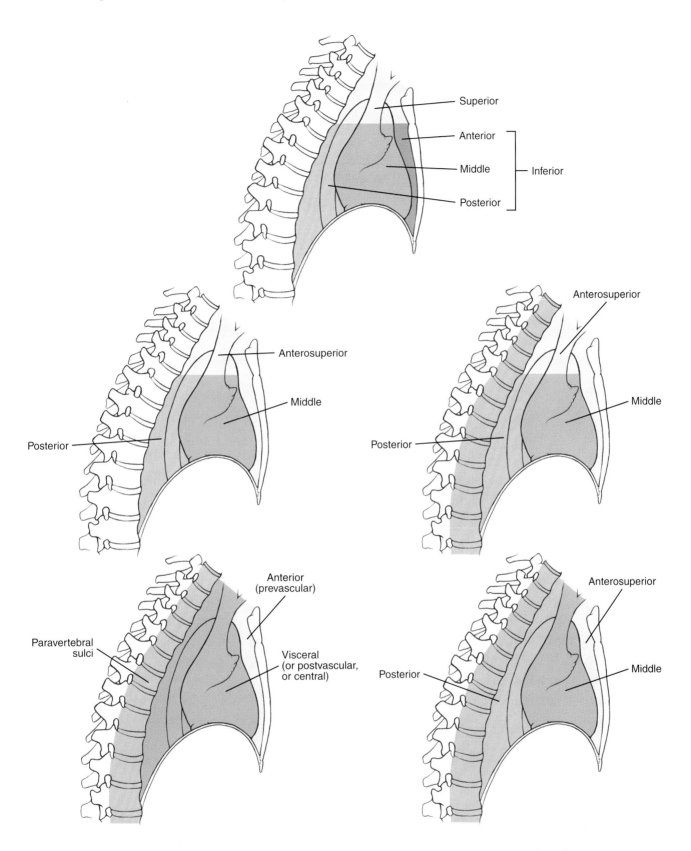

The other compartments are the middle and posterior. Walsh gives the clearest description of the different nomenclatures used to compartmentalize the mediastinum. His fourth diagram (in the lower left) is similar to that of Shields, and is used for the present discussion.

The anatomy of the mediastinum is the definition of the boundaries of its compartments and the organs within. An in-depth discussion of each structure is beyond the confines of this text. A more detailed anatomic description of the thymus, trachea, main stem bronchi, and esophagus follow.

The anterior, or prevascular, compartment is bounded posteriorly by an imaginary arbitrary plane along the anterior surface of the great vessels and the pericardium, anteriorly by the posterior aspect of the sternum, and laterally by the mediastinal parietal pleura. The superior extent is the thoracic inlet; the inferior extent is the diaphragm. The visceral or middle compartment originates anteriorly at the imaginary plane forming the posterior extent of the anterior compartment. The posterior extent is the anterior aspect of the vertebral bodies. The lateral and superoinferior boundaries are the same as for the anterior compartment. The posterior compartment, or costovertebral sulci, begins at the dorsal aspect of the vertebral bodies and extends posteriorly to the transverse vertebral processes. Superior and inferior boundaries are the same as for the previous vertically oriented compartments.

Structures and Lesions
Anterior Compartment

The anterior (prevascular) compartment may contain the thymus, retrosternal thyroid, and parathyroid glands, fat, germ cell rests, and lymph nodes. The only organs rightfully residing in the anterior compartment are the thymus and anterior mediastinal lymph nodes. When present, the thyroid and parathyroid glands and germ cell rests are ectopic. In adults 54% of mediastinal tumors develop in the anterior space, 20% in the visceral (central) space, and 26% in the posterior (paravertebral) space. In children 63% of mediastinal tumors develop in the posterior (paravertebral) space, compared with 11% in the visceral (middle) space and 26% in the anterior (anterosuperior) space.

The true incidence and prevalence of masses within each compartment will remain unclear and debatable as long as no single definition of the compartments is uniformly accepted as standard. At present it is accurate to say that, with a recognized increase in lymphoproliferative diseases and increased recognition of thymic tumors in the myasthenia gravis in patients screened with chest computed tomography (CT), the anterior (prevascular) compartment is the "hot zone" in which abnormal lesions are most frequently found.

Table 4-1   *Structure and Lesions in the Anterior Superior Mediastinum*

Structure	Tumor
Thymus	Thymoma
	Thymolipoma
	Thymic carcinoid
	Thymic cyst
	Thymic hyperplasia
	Thymic carcinoma
Thyroid	Substernal goiter
	Ectopic thyroid without connection to neck
Parathyroid	Ectopic parathyroid adenoma
	Parathyroid carcinoma
Fat	Lipoma
	Liposarcoma
Lymph nodes	Malignant diseases
	Hodgkin's lymphoma
	Non–Hodgkin's lymphoma
	Metastatic carcinoma
	Benign processes
	Castleman's disease (nodal hyperplasia)
	Infectious mononucleosis
	Granuloma
	Fungal diseases
	Histoplasmosis
	Coccidioidomycosis
	Tuberculosis
	Sarcoidosis
	Wegener's granulomatosis
Germ cell rests	Benign processes
	Teratoma (dermoid)
	Malignant lesions
	Seminoma
	Nonseminomatous germ cell tumors
	Embryonal carcinoma
	Choriocarcinoma
	Endodermal sinus tumor (yolk sac)
	Teratocarcinoma

From Walsh GC. General priniciples and surgical considerations in the management of mediastinal masses. In Roth JA, Ruckdeschel JC, Weisenburger TH, eds. Thoracic Oncology. Philadelphia: WB Saunders, 1995, p 448.

Because in adults the thymus is the site of most mediastinal masses, and specifically, anterior mediastinal masses, the thymus and thymic resection are discussed separately. Thyroid goiter extending into the mediastinum, with or without malignancy, and ectopic parathyroid glands are addressed in Chapter 2. Germ cell tumors, which constitute approximately 15% of masses in the adult anterior mediastinum, are discussed in detail by Allen et al.

The most frequent challenge for the thoracic surgical oncologist when masses are detected in the anterior mediastinum is the distinction between thymoma, a surgically treated disease, and lymphoma, a medically treated disease. Although thymomas usually predominate in this region, lymphoma occurs 22% of the time in adults and 45% of the time in children. Many of the lymphomas in this region are not primary lesions but part of a systemic lymphoproliferative disorder (non-Hodgkin's lymphoma, 43%; Hodgkin's lymphoma, 67%). Fever, night sweats, weight loss, anorexia, and the "B" symptoms of lymphoma are useful in distinguishing lymphoma from thymoma. Generalized weakness, easy fatigability with repetitive motion, and oculobulbar symptoms suggest the diagnosis of myasthenia gravis and associated thymoma. Contrast-enhanced CT evaluation of the chest is absolutely essential prior to any invasive diagnostic techniques. Lymphomas tend to be bilateral and more diffuse, whereas thymomas often predominate on one side, as seen on chest CT scans. Fine-needle aspiration biopsy has previously been discouraged in differentiating lymphoma from thymoma, for fear of disrupting the thymic capsule and disseminating thymic carcinoma. I routinely perform fine-needle aspiration biopsy when lymphoma is suspected to obtain tissue for flow cytometry and cytology. These techniques have a high rate of specificity in differentiating lymphoma from thymoma, thus averting a more invasive surgical procedure. The superior posterior mediastinum is the home of neurogenic tumors. The most common are neurolinomas, benign (70%) and malignant (30%).

Middle Compartment

The visceral (middle) compartment contains the trachea, proximal main stem bronchi, thoracic esophagus, pericardium, heart and great vessels, lymph nodes, phrenic, vagus, and sympathetic nerves, and thoracic duct. Tracheobronchial and esophageal tumors are discussed subsequently. Although containing the greatest number of "true organs," the visceral compartment contains the least number of tumors (20%) in the adult population if esophageal and tracheobronchial malignancies are excluded.

Cardiac tumors are rare. Metastases to the heart are 20 to 30 times more frequent than primary cardiac tumors. Benign tumors of cardiac origin account for 75% of cardiac tumors. Of the benign cardiac tumors, myxoma primarily of the atria constitute the vast majority. Malignant cardiac tumors are most often sarcomas (rhabdomyosarcoma and angiosarcoma), rapidly progressive to death within weeks, and most often (80% of the time) associated with systemic metastasis at the time of diagnosis. Both primary and metastatic cardiac tumors can be resected with cardiopulmonary bypass and reconstructive surgery. Cardiac transplantation has made right-sided endomyocardial biopsy safe and commonplace. Thus, in any patient with a known prior malignancy and newly found right chamber cardiac mass, biopsy should be attempted and diagnosis made prior to surgical resection. In most cases resection of a metastatic cardiac neoplasm without assured control of the original primary lesion is contraindicated. Bronchogenic carcinoma extending into the cardiac chamber without lymph node metastasis can be resected by the experienced cardiothoracic surgeon with acceptable morbidity and mortality and at least 30% 5-year survival. I have used transesophageal echocardiography to evaluate bronchogenic carcinoma for resection. It accurately allows exclusion of unresectable tumors and guides the approach in attempts at resection.

Pericardial tumors are uncommon. As with cardiac tumors, metastasis to the pericardium or direct involvement by nearby primary malignancies is more common than primary tumors arising from the pericardium. In fact, as patients with breast and lung primary tumors survive longer, malignant pericardial effusion associated with pericardial involvement is becoming more common. Bronchogenic carcinoma is the most frequent tumor metastatic to the pericardium (33%), followed by breast carcinoma (25%) and hematologic malignancies (15%). The most frequent primary pericardial malignant tumor is mesothelioma. Extremely rare, it was found in 0.0022% of 500,000 autopsies in one series. Angiosarcoma is another primary pericardial tumor. Teratomas of the pericardium occur most frequently in children, but are rare.

Within the visceral compartment are several lymph node groups. The paratracheal, tracheobronchial, subcarinal, and subaortic lymph nodes are well known to the thoracic surgeon as sites of metastasis of primary bronchogenic carcinoma. Most frequently enlargement of these lymph nodes is due to metastases; however, sarcoidosis may produce profound asymptomatic nodal enlargement and requires differentiation from primary lymphoma and metastasis before initiation of treatment. A less well-known group of mediastinal lymph nodes is described by Shields as located around the pericardial attachments to the diaphragm, draining the diaphragm and liver. They may on occasion be involved by lymphoma.

Table 4-2   *Structures and Lesions in the Middle (Visceral) Mediastinal Compartment*

Structure	Tumor
Trachea	Bronchogenic cyst
	Bronchial adenoma
	Adenocystic carcinoma
	Carcinoid tumor
	Mucoepidermoid
	Bronchial mucous gland adenoma
	Mixed salivary gland tumor
	Squamous cell carcinoma
Esophagus	Primary malignancies
	Adenocarcinoma or squamous cell carcinoma
	Small cell carcinoma
	Mesenchymal tumor
	Leiomyosarcoma
	Rhabdomyosarcoma
	Lymphoma
	Benign lesions
	Duplication cyst
	Leiomyoma
	Esophageal diverticulum (pulsion or traction)
Pericardium	Pericardial cyst
	Pericardial diverticulum
	Hemangiopericytoma
Heart	Fibroma
	Rhabdomyosarcoma
Aorta and arch vessels	Aneurysm (saccular or diffuse)
	Coarctation
	Arch anomalies
	Double aortic arch
	Right arch with left ligamentum
	Left arch with aberrant right subclavian artery
	Leiomyosarcoma, leiomyoma

From Walsh GC. General principles and surgical considerations in the management of mediastinal masses. In Roth JA, Ruckdeschel JC, Weisenburger TH, eds. Thoracic Oncology. Philadelphia: WB Saunders, 1995, p 448.

Table 4-2 *Structures and Lesions in the Middle (Visceral) Mediastinal Compartment—cont'd*

Structure	Tumor
Veins	Ectasia and aneurysm formation
	Venous anomalies
	Persistent left superior vena cava
	Anomalous pulmonary venous drainage
	Azygos continuation of the inferior vena cava
	Leiomyoma, leiomyosarcoma
Lymph nodes	Sarcoidosis
	Lymphoma
	Metastatic carcinoma
Phrenic and vagus nerves	Nerve sheath tumors
Sympathetic nerves	Paraganglioma (chemodectoma)
Thoracic duct	Cysts
Lymphatic vessels	Lymphangioma (cystic hygroma)
	Lymphangiopericytoma

Posterior Compartment

The posterior compartment (paravertebral or costovertebral sulci) contains peripheral intercostal nerves, sympathetic ganglia, and paraganglia. Owing to its contents this area is the most common site of mediastinal neurogenic tumors. The majority of posterior compartment tumors are benign; the incidence of malignancy is low in adults (<5%), but is slightly increased in children. Tumors in this compartment tend to enlarge, but generally remain asymptomatic and are identified on chest radiographs obtained for other purposes. Most authors recommend excision without prior tissue diagnosis, because these lesions are well characterized on CT and nuclear magnetic resonance imaging (MRI).

Mediastinal paragangliomas are highly vascular and frequently chemically active. Miller and I discuss the diagnosis and treatment of these uncommon mediastinal tumors in Wood and Thomas' text.

Table 4–3 *Structures and Lesions in the Posterior (Costovertebral Sulcus) Compartment*

Structure	Tumor
Peripheral intercostal nerve	Benign processes
	Neurofibroma
	Neurilemmoma (schwannoma)
	Malignant lesions
	Neurosarcoma
Sympathetic ganglia	Benign
	Ganglioneuroma
	Malignant
	Ganglioneuroblastoma
	Neuroblastoma
Paraganglia	Pheochromocytoma
	Chemodectoma (paraganglioma)

From Walsh GC. General principles and surgical considerations in the management of mediastinal masses. In Roth JA, Ruckdeschel JC, Weisenburger TH, eds. Thoracic Oncology. Philadelphia: WB Saunders, 1995, p 449.

SURGICAL APPLICATIONS

Diagnosis and Resection of Mediastinal Tumors

Anterior Compartment

Thymectomy is the most frequent resection performed in the anterior mediastinum and is detailed in length in the subsequent section.

Prior to embarking on resection of an anterior mediastinal mass, noninvasive diagnostic techniques (e.g., CT, nuclear MRI, ultrasonography, serum tumor markers) and clinical examination should be performed and the results scrutinized. Even after exhaustive investigation, differentiation between thymoma and lymphoma may be a challenge. I have resected one anterior mediastinal mass after such an exhaustive investigation, including two fine-needle aspiration biopsies and thoracoscopic excisional biopsy, only to find that the suspected thymoma was a lymphoma arising within the thymus gland proper.

Fine-needle aspiration biopsy with a 20-, 22-, or 25-gauge needle, with fluoroscopic or CT guidance, should be performed if the clinical history and imaging studies support the diagnosis of lymphoma. The use of flow cytometry has made subtyping of lymphoma increasingly accurate. Fine-needle aspiration biopsy is also sensitive (90%) in diagnosing metastatic carcinoma in the mediastinum.

Extended or substernal mediastinoscopy, as described by Ginsberg et al., can be used to access the anterior compartment. Through the same 2 cm cervical incision used for standard mediastinoscopy, the strap muscles are mobilized and retracted laterally. The scope is advanced anterior to the thymus and thus anterior to the innominate vein. Great care must be taken not to produce excessive traction on the innominate vein to prevent a tear. Further advancement of the scope permits entrance into the prevascular space anterior to the great vessels, allowing biopsy of anterior mediastinal masses and aortopulmonary lymph nodes. Because of the proximity of the great vascular structures, this procedure is somewhat more risky than standard mediastinoscopy and should be performed only by the seasoned thoracic surgeon.

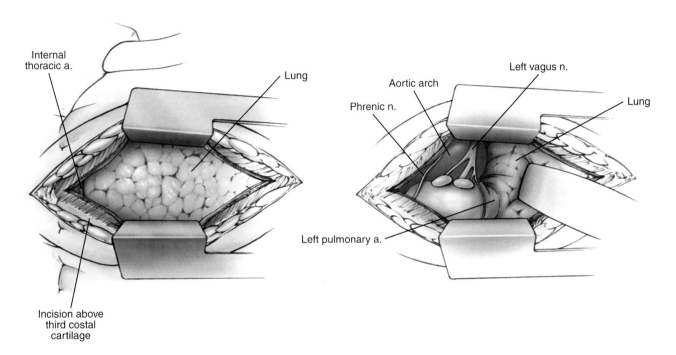

Anterior or parasternal mediastinotomy (Chamberlin procedure) is the more frequently performed procedure for access to the anterior compartment. A 5 to 8 cm incision is made from the lateral sternal border laterally over the third or fourth costal cartilage. The incision is deepened with the electrocautery through the overlying pectoralis muscle. The intercostal muscles are detached from a superior edge of the third or fourth rib as far laterally as practical and medially to the internal thoracic vessels. The internal thoracic vessels should be avoided and preserved. The pleura may be dissected and retracted laterally or entered. As originally described, the third cartilage was excised. I have not found this uniformly necessary. This approach allows access to hilar and aortopulmonary lymph nodes and anterior compartment masses. The surgeon should identify clearly the surrounding vascular structures prior to any incisional or excisional biopsy. This same approach can be used on the opposite side for anterior compartment masses predominating on the right.

Middle Compartment

Operations within the middle compartment mandate precise planning and diagnosis prior to embarkation. Contrast-enhanced chest CT is mandatory, and on occasion aortic arch aortography should be performed before any attempt at fine-needle aspiration or excisional biopsy to prevent any catastrophic biopsy of aneurysmal vascular structures. Surgery of the trachea and esophagus are detailed subsequently. With exclusion of vascular lesions, tracheal lesions, and esophageal lesions, surgery of the middle mediastinum is performed to resect pericardial and cardiac lesions.

The pericardium is approached most frequently through a full median sternotomy. This allows excision of pericardial cysts or tumors. On occasion a pericardial mass will involve the phrenic nerve or be posterior to the phrenic nerve. In this situation the approach should be transthoracic through a standard posterior lateral thoracotomy on the affected side. In cases of tumor, excision of the phrenic nerve is acceptable but usually unnecessary. The mass should be excised with sharp and electrocautery excision, and 2 cm margins verified as negative for tumor on frozen-section analysis. On the left side a wide excision should be performed to avert herniation or entrapment of the left ventricle. When wide excision is not indicated the defect may be closed with absorbable Vicryl mesh. When right-sided lesions are excised, the defect should be reconstructed with Vicryl mesh to prevent herniation of the right atrium or torsion and herniation of the entire heart through the defect. This unlikely occurrence is extraordinarily rare if a pneumonectomy has not been performed in conjunction with the pericardial resection. Excision of metastatic pericardial lesions may be performed for diagnosis. The anterior and lateral pericardium down to the phrenic nerve should be excised and the pleura entered to avert later constrictive processes or accumulation of malignant pericardial effusion.

The heart and cardiac chambers are approached through a full median sternotomy. This allows the best exposure and control of vascular structures. Cardiopulmonary bypass may be instituted through this incision. Resection of intracardiac tumors is most often performed through the right atrium and across the intra-atrial septum or through the tricuspid valve. Such resections are generally performed by cardiac surgeons or thoracic surgical oncologists who also perform cardiac surgery. Proper planning by the experienced cardiothoracic surgeon allows resection of primary and metastatic cardiac tumors not previously thought possible. I have excised 50% of the right ventricular free wall and reconstructed the defect with bovine pericardium. The patient recovered uneventfully and remains alive at 36 months without cardiovascular sequelae or limitation. Kirklin and Barratt-Boyes' text provides further in-depth discussion of the management and resection of intracardiac tumors.

Mediastinoscopy is frequently performed to diagnose masses and stage lymph node involvement in the middle (visceral) compartment. With the patient under general anesthesia, a 2 cm transverse incision is made 1.5 cm above the sternal notch. The underlying strap muscles are divided in the midline, the pretracheal fascia is bluntly or sharply dissected, and the pretracheal space entered. The pretracheal space is then gently examined with the surgeon's index finger. This permits not only detection of masses but gentle mobilization of the areolar tissue surrounding the trachea. The scope is then gently placed within the pretracheal space and advanced underneath the innominate vessels under direct vision. The right paratracheal space, precarinal, subcarinal, and left paratracheal space are then examined in that order. Areas of intended biopsy should be aspirated with a needle prior to biopsy to avert biopsy of a vascular structure. Great care should be exercised in the area of the azygos vein and pulmonary artery, the structures most frequently inadvertently injured during mediastinoscopy. Injury to the trachea and esophagus has also been described.

Posterior Compartment

Resection of tumors in the posterior mediastinum involves excision of tumors arising from peripheral intercostal nerves or sympathetic ganglia. Often a diagnosis cannot be confirmed by preoperative fine-needle aspiration biopsy. The surgeon is justified in proceeding with excision because these lesions will continue to enlarge at varying rates, ultimately producing pain or pressure due to compression of nearby structures. Neurofibromas, neurolemmomas (schwannoma), and ganglioneuromas are the most frequently seen posterior mediastinal neurogenic tumors. Both neurofibromas and neurolemmomas have a malignant potential (2% to 3%). They are often associated with von Recklinghausen's disease. Paragangliomas are frequently vascular and vasoactive. Resection is justified and should be aggressive. Complete resection is associated with alleviation of symptoms and cure, whereas other therapeutic modalities are ineffectual.

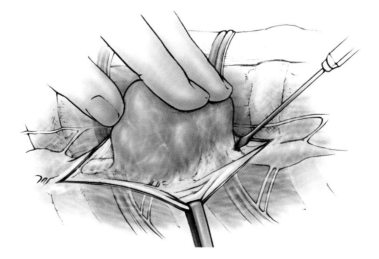

All neurogenic tumors should be approached through an ipsilateral posterolateral thoracotomy. The lung is retracted anteriorly and the parietal pleura incised circumferentially 2 cm around the mass. Those tumors not entering the

vertebral neural foramina may be easily excised with sharp scissors and electrocautery. As the dissection approaches closer to the vertebral column, the
electrocautery should be abandoned in favor of the scissors and ligating clips
to prevent possible transmission of electrical current into the spinal cord.

Neurogenic tumors of the posterior mediastinum with intravertebral
foraminal extension deserve additional planning and neurosurgical consultation. Extension into the vertebral column is suggested when widening of the
foramina or vertebral body erosion is suggested on plain chest radiographs.
Chest CT with fine (3 to 5 mm) sections through the tumor and adjacent vertebral column gives a more definitive image. When these neurogenic "dumbbell" tumors are suspected, nuclear MRI of the thorax with sagittal, coronal,
and cross-sectional images is highly desirable if not essential. Nuclear MRI has
all but replaced thoracic spinal column myelography. Once the tumor is confirmed to be a dumbbell tumor with extension into the vertebral column, inclusion of a neurosurgical oncologic surgeon on the surgical team is appropriate.

A posterior nonthoracotomy approach has been described by the Japanese,
but the standard approach is through an ipsilateral thoracotomy. This approach
allows excellent visualization for excision and control of the vascular structures
feeding the tumor, as well as laminectomy if indicated.

The inner space entered is dependent on the level of the lesion, but generally is within the fourth, fifth, or sixth inner space. The parietal pleura is incised and the previously collapsed lung retracted anteriorly. A nasogastric tube
should be in place to aid in identifying the esophagus. The extent of rib, vertebral body, and nerve involvement is assessed. With scissors and the electrocautery, the dissection is begun inferiorly and proceeds laterally and superiorly,
leaving the medial aspect attached. This allows the area of the intervertebral
foramina to be approached last. Traction should be avoided and the electrocautery abandoned to avert inadvertent injury to the spinal cord. At this point
the neurosurgeon is involved to perform a laminectomy and intradural excision of the tumor. This allows en bloc removal of tumor while minimizing possible injury to the spinal cord. The aorta and lung are rarely invaded unless the
tumor is a malignant infiltrative type. The tumor blood supply is from segmental intercostal vessels, which can be ligated. The neurosurgeon will assist
in confirming absence of a cerebrospinal fluid leak. If a cerebrospinal fluid leak
is identified, a pedicled intercostal muscle flap may be used to seal the leak. A
single-tube thoracostomy drain is usually all that is required. Closure of the
thoracotomy is standard.

Anatomic Basis of Complications

- Poor preoperative imaging studies lead to poorly planned diagnostic attempts. No structure in the anterior, middle, or posterior mediastinum should be biopsied (fine-needle aspiration or incisional biopsy) without confirmatory studies to eliminate the possibility that the lesion is of vascular origin.
- Standard mediastinoscopy should be performed with great care and only by those familiar with the anatomic position of the trachea, superior vena cava, azygos vein, and right and left pulmonary arteries as seen through the mediastinoscope. Needle aspiration should always be performed prior to biopsy. Compression of the innominate artery by overzealous upward lifting of the scope may tear the artery or dislodge atheromatous debris distally.
- Intracavitary cardiac masses should be biopsied preoperatively in patients with history of prior malignancy to prevent unnecessary and possibly harmful surgical procedures.
- Posterior neurogenic tumors must be assumed to have vertebral foraminal extension until conclusively ruled out to prevent incomplete excision or spinal cord injury.

KEY REFERENCES

Demmey TL. Tumors of the heart and pericardium. In Asiner JA, Arriagada R, Green M, et al., eds. Comprehensive Textbook of Thoracic Oncology. Baltimore: Williams & Wilkins, 1996, pp 681-710.
This is a current review of cardiac oncology.

Filly R, Blank N, Castellino RA. Radiologic distribution of intrathoracic disease in previously untreated patients with Hodgkins disease and non-Hodgkins lymphoma. Radiology 120:277-281, 1976.
This is a classic description of mediastinal diagnosis of Hodgkin's disease and non-Hodgkin's lymphoma.

Martini N, Yellin A, Binsbeng RJ, et al. Management of non–small cell lung cancer with direct mediastinal involvement. Ann Thorac Surg 58:1447-1451, 1994.
This article reviews the mediastinal extensions of lung cancer.

Shields TW. The mediastinum and its contents. In Shields TW, ed. Mediastinal Surgery. Philadelphia: Lea & Febiger, 1991, pp 33-35.

Walsh GC. General principles and surgical considerations in the management of mediastinal masses. In Roth JA, Ruckdeschel JC, Weisenburger TH, eds. Thoracic Oncology. Philadelphia: WB Saunders, 1995, pp 445-467.

The text by Shields and the chapter by Walsh (in the Roth textbook) provide classic descriptions of mediastinal surgery.

Wood DE, Thomas CR, eds. Mediastinal Tumors, Update 1995. New York: Springer-Verlag, 1995.

This is a current review of the management of mediastinal tumors.

SUGGESTED READINGS

Adams GA, Shochat SJ, Smith EI, et al. Thoracic neuroblastoma: A pediatric oncology group study. J Pediatr Surg 28:372-377, 1993.

Allen MS, Wright CD, Heitmiller RF. In Wood DE, Thomas CR, eds. Mediastinal Tumors, Update 1995. New York: Springer-Verlag, 1995.

Bloom NA. Tumors of the mediastinum. In Beattie EJ, Bloom ND, Harvey JC, eds. Thoracic Surgical Oncology. New York: Churchill Livingstone, 1992, pp 237-250.

Carlens E. Mediastinoscopy: A method of inspection and tissue biopsy in the superior mediastinum. Chest 36:343, 1959.

Elk B, Lynch M, Balk M, et al. Role of transesophageal echocardiography in the management of two patients with bronchogenic carcinoma invading the left atrium. Am J Cardiol 76:1101, 1995.

Ginsberg RJ, Rice TW, Goldberg M, et al. Extended cervical mediastinoscopy—The best procedure for staging left upper lobe tumors. J Thorac Cardiovasc Surg 94:673, 1987.

Hood RM. Mediastinum. In Hood RM, ed. Techniques in General Thoracic Surgery, 2nd ed. Philadelphia: Lea & Febiger, 1993, pp 185-193.

Kirklin JW, Barratt-Boyes BG. Cardiac tumors. In Kirklin JW, Barratt-Boyes BG. Cardiac Surgery, 2nd ed. New York: Churchill Livingstone, 1993, pp 1635-1653.

Lee RB, Miller JI. Mediastinal paragangliomas. In Wood DE, Thomas CR, eds. Mediastinal Tumors, Update 1995. New York: Springer-Verlag, 1995, pp 63-78.

Osada H, Aoki H, Yokote K, et al. Dumbbell neurogenic tumor of the mediastinum: A report of three cases undergoing single staged complete removal without thoracotomy. Jpn J Surg 21:224-228, 1991.

Wain JC. Neurogenic tumors of the mediastinum. In Wood DE, Thomas CR, eds. Mediastinal Tumors, Update 1995. New York: Springer-Verlag, 1995, pp 71-78.

Thymus

The thymic gland lies within the superior anterior mediastinum. The frequency of both benign and malignant tumors of the thymus and the association with myasthenia gravis mandates additional in-depth and separate discussion of the thymus. The most common tumor of the anterior superior mediastinum, thymoma, is unusual in that mitotic figures are infrequent and malignancy is determined not by histology but clinically by depth of invasion. Even when judged malignant, thymic tumors follow a relatively benign course.

The thymus contains several cell types. The term thymoma has been reserved for tumors arising from its epithelial components. Originally proposed by Bell in 1917, "a thymoma may now be defined as a tumor, benign or malignant, probably derived from thymic epithelium." This restriction was reiterated by Rosai and Levine, who stated that the definition of thymoma be limited to "neoplasms of thymic epithelial cells regardless of presence or absence of a lymphoid component."

Histologically, thymomas consist of varying degrees of thymic epithelial cells and lymphocytes. This has resulted in various classifications based on ratios of the cell types. The following schema has been proposed based on the most prevalent epithelial cell type and the pattern of lymphoid infiltration:

1. Cortical thymoma: Lymphocytes are the predominate cell types, and many are blastic.
2. Medullary thymoma: Predominant cell types are medullary epithelial cells, with lymphocytes.
3. Mixed thymoma: Have cortical and medullary epithelial cells, and lymphocytes vary in number; therefore subtypes are mixed common type, mixed cortical predominant, and mixed medullary predominant.

Medullary (epithelial cell predominant) and mixed types are more frequently benign (noninvasive), with good long-term survival and prognosis. The cortical (lymphocyte cell predominant) and predominant cortical types are generally malignant (invasive), with poor long-term prognosis.

Tumor staging has evolved based on clinical assessment at the time of operation by the thoracic surgical oncologist and less so based on histology. In 1991 Masaoka et al. proposed the classification most often used and accepted as the standard staging system for thymomas.

Masaoka Staging Classification

Stage I — Macroscopically, completely encapsulated; microscopically, no capsular invasion

Stage II — Macroscopic invasion into surrounding fatty tissue, or microscopic capsular invasion

Stage III — Macroscopic invasion of adjacent organs (pericardium, great vessels, lung)

Stage IV — A: Pleural or pericardial dissemination

B: Lymphatic or hematogenous metastasis

The Thymic Tumor Study Group modified Masaoka's classification to account for completeness of resection. This is an important modification because most authors of large series report that extent of tumor invasion and completeness of resection are the most important prognostic factors.

Thymic Tumor Study Group Staging System

Stage IA — Encapsulated, noninvasive tumor; total excision

IB — Apparently encapsulated tumor; total excision but adhesions to mediastinal structures, indicating microscopic invasiveness seen at surgery

Stage II — Invasive tumor; total excision

Stage IIIA — Invasive tumor; incomplete excision

IIIB — Simple biopsy (when performing mediastinoscopy, thoracoscopy, or thoracotomy)

Stage IVA — Subpleural metastasis

IVB — Extrathoracic metastasis

The widespread use of chest CT for evaluation of myasthenia gravis has revealed an increasing number of previously undetected early thymomas. Approximately 20% of patients with myasthenia gravis have a thymoma. Forty percent to 60% of patients with thymomas have myasthenia when examined. Thus most thymomas are seen as stage I or stage II tumors.

Table 4-4   *Data From Thymoma Review*

Stage	No. of Cases	Recurrence (%)	Actuarial Survival (%)	
			5 Years	10 Years
I	133	1.5	89.2	86.9
II	34	12.5	71.9	59.9
III	53	29.7	71.3	64.3
IVA	21	25.0	59.4	39.6

Modified from Maggi G, Casadio C, Cavallo A, et al. Thymoma: Results of 241 operated cases. Ann Thorac Surg 51:152-156, 1991. Reprinted with permission from the Society of Thoracic Surgeons.

One third of thymomas will be classified as "malignant" due to invasion of nearby structures (stage III or stage IV). Pleural and pericardial implants constitute stage IV disease. This is a somewhat unusual and infrequent finding. Even less common is extrathoracic metastasis to bone, supraclavicular lymph nodes, liver, and spleen.

Recurrence is more common than metastasis and is most likely related to unrecognized and incomplete resection or understaging. Benign thymomas (stage I) recur at a rate less than 2%, usually in the mediastinum. Recurrence may also be due to unrecognized dissemination at the time of surgery or from tumor implants during operative manipulation. The recurrence rate for stage II tumor is approximately 10%, and 15% for totally resected stage III tumors. Patients with recurrence may undergo successful repeat operations, with expected actuarial survival of 66% at 5 years and 49% at 10 years.

The mean patient age at diagnosis is within the fourth decade; thymomas in children are uncommon. There is no geographic or race distinction. Males are affected slightly more often than females, but the difference is not statistically significant. When myasthenia gravis is known to exist, the patient is more often female. Approximately one third of patients have no symptoms. The remainder may complain of pain in the chest or back (24%) or cough (20%). More than 50% of patients without myasthenia gravis have no symptoms. Autoimmune diseases are commonly associated with thymoma, with myasthenia gravis being the most common, occurring in 60% of patients.

Table 4-5   *Conditions Associated With Thymoma*

Condition	Percentage of Patients
Myasthenia gravis	30-60
Cytopenia	15
Other nonthymic malignancies	12
Systemic lupus erythematosus	1
Rheumatoid arthritis	1
Pemphigus	1
Hemolytic anemia	1

Data from Levasseur P, Mesestrier M, Gaud C, et al. Thymomes et maladies associées. Rev Mal Respir 5:173-178, 1988; Souadjian JV, Enriquez P, Silverstein MN, et al. The spectrum of disease with thymoma. Coincidence or syndrome? Arch Intern Med 134:374-379, 1974.

SURGICAL ANATOMY

The thymus is a glandular bilobate structure with an isthmus, composed of an epithelial cell stroma and varying amounts of lymphoid cells. It occupies a position in the anterosuperior mediastinum. Beginning in the third week of fetal development, the thymus evolves as a portion of the third pharyngeal pouch along with the parathyroid glands and descends into the anterior mediastinum to rest on the anterior surface of the aortic arch. Thus in adult life aberrant thymic tissue may be found anywhere along this path of descent, particularly near the parathyroid glands, and infrequently at other sites, including neck, eardrum, pulmonary hilum, or posterior mediastinum. I have excised a thymoma from the inferior pulmonary ligament as well as the posterior mediastinum. The cells arising from the third pharyngeal pouch are epithelial cells and form the reticular framework, or medulla, to which the lymphoid cells migrate. During the third month of fetal life lymphocytes arising from the totipotential stem cells migrate to this epithelial stroma and undergo differentiation into T lymphocytes under the influence of thymic hormones. Thymus-derived lymphocytes, or T cells, are responsible for the cell-mediated portion of the immunologic defense system. The thymus is a large organ at birth and continues to grow into adolescence, reaching a volume of 40 gm. Thereafter it undergoes fatty infiltration, termed involution.

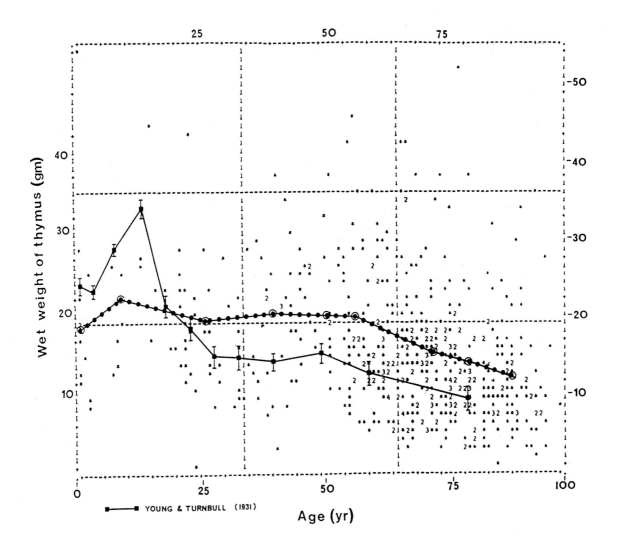

Congenital absence of the thymus may occur as part of DiGeorge syndrome, leading to profound immunoincompetence and early death.

The adult thymus is located posterior to the sternum, beginning superiorly at the lower aspect of the inferior thyroid poles and extending through the thoracic inlet to the level of the fourth costal cartilage.

Blood Supply

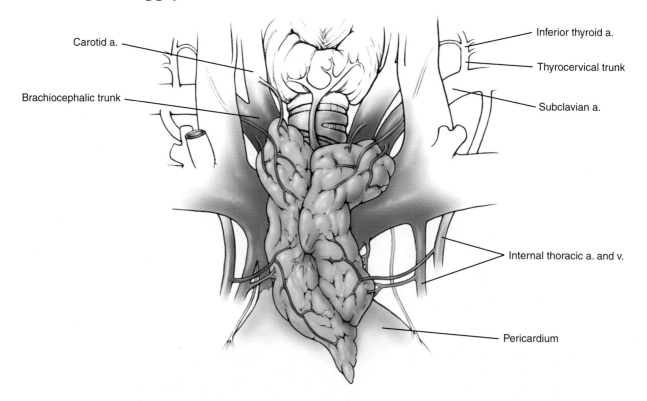

The arterial blood supply is derived from five sources. The major blood supply is from branches of the inferior thyroid artery and internal thoracic arteries. Smaller branches from the superior thyroid, subclavian, and carotid arteries constitute the remainder of the blood supply. These are easily controlled by ligation or clipping during resection.

The venous drainage of the thymus, like that of most other organs, is variable. The medial aspects of the right and left lobes are drained by separate 2 to 3 mm veins that join posteriorly and superiorly to form the great vein of Keynes. The vein of Keynes is a short, wide vein that travels superiorly and joins the anteroinferior surface of the left brachiocephalic vein. The lateral aspect of the right lobe drains directly into the superior vena cava, with the left lateral side draining into the left brachiocephalic vein. Smaller, short, friable veins drain the isthmus and posterior aspect of the gland. These veins drain directly into the innominate vein, and often cause problems during resection. Other unnamed and inconsistent branches drain the gland and flow into the internal thoracic veins, thyroid ima, and inferior thyroid veins.

Lymphatic Drainage

The lymphatic drainage of the thymus has been studied and discussed by multiple anatomists. The thymus lacks afferent lymphatic vessels. Efferent lymphatic vessels originate from the medulla and corticomedullary junction and travel superiorly through the supporting stroma to drain into the brachiocephalic, tracheobronchial, and internal mammary lymph nodes. The thymus derives innervation from the autonomic nervous system, the phrenic nerve, and the ansa hypoglossi. The sympathetic supply runs with the vasculature and originates from the stellate ganglion. The vagus nerve also sends out nerve trunks to the thymus.

SURGICAL APPLICATIONS
Resection of Thymic Gland Tumors

Access to the thymus is attained through three primary incisions: transcervic, partial median sternotomy, and complete median sternotomy. The transcervical approach is advocated as most applicable in patients undergoing thymectomy for myasthenia gravis with a small (<5 cm) thymoma or no tumor at all. A partial sternotomy, or T incision, combines a smaller transcervical incision with a vertical incision down to the fourth cartilage. This allows a partial vertical sternotomy, which exposes the entire thymus and superior mediastinum. This is the approach utilized by Miller et al. and me when performing thymectomy for myasthenia gravis without thymoma. This incision allows excellent exposure of the thymus and underlying vasculature for resection of moderate sized tumors. Tumors larger than 5 to 10 cm and those believed to be invasive should be resected through a complete median sternotomy to allow resection of the lateral-most aspects of the tumor. I have on occasion resected thymomas exceeding 10 cm through a right or left thoracotomy. This is not the preferred approach, because resection of the left lobe across the anterior mediastinum through a right thorocotomy is difficult, and it can be challenging to control the vascular supply of the left lobe. A transthoracic approach should be entertained only when the tumor is large, bulky, and predominantly on one side of the mediastinum. All thymic tissue must be resected.

Several basic principles of the surgical management of thymic tumors have been outlined by Wilkins:

1. Use of contrast-enhanced chest CT for characterization of tumor
2. Avoidance of needle or open biopsy to decrease risk for tumor implantation and spread
3. Complete median sternotomy for approach
4. Incision and opening of both pleural cavities for examination of the extent of tumor
5. Total thymectomy encompassing all thymic tissue
6. Extended radical resection for invasive tumors, including pericardium, pleura, lung parenchyma, phrenic nerve, and innominate vein when invaded
7. Partial pleurectomy (stripping) when pleural implants are noted

After complete median sternotomy, dissection is begun at the lower aspect of the uninvolved pole or the inferior margin if structural anatomy is distorted by tumor. Sharp and blunt dissection with scissors and cautery begins inferiorly and progresses superiorly and laterally.

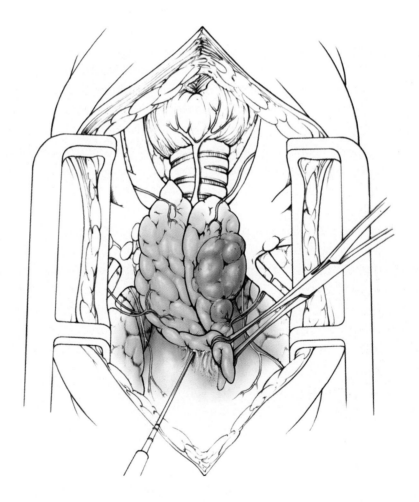

Tissue planes are usually easily separable. Dense adhesions imply probable extension of tumor through the capsule into pleura or pericardium (invasive thymoma). Either or both should be excised with the tumor en bloc. The opposite pole is dissected similarly, so that the entire mass is elevated superiorly as the innominate vein is approached. The great vein of Keynes may be encountered and should be ligated. Generally two to five veins directly enter the innominate vein. Each should be ligated or clipped.

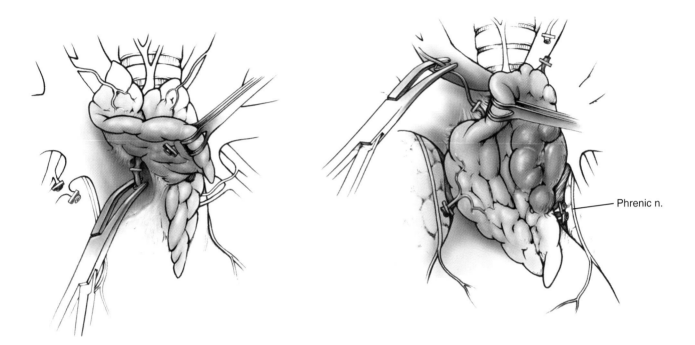

Phrenic n.

The dissection proceeds superiorly into the thoracic inlet and lower cervical region. The upper poles usually end inferior to the lower thyroid poles. The supporting ligamentous cord and the arterial supply should be ligated and divided. It is essential for all thymic tissue to be excised. All surrounding adipose and superior mediastinal lymph nodes should be excised, and an involved phrenic nerve should be resected when necessary. Care should be taken in patients with myasthenia gravis, which can contribute to respiratory insufficiency. It is justifiable and essential to resect all involved structures, based on low recurrence rate and extended survival with complete and total resection. The recurrence rate is less than 2% for stage I thymomas. In Wilkins' series, 20-year actuarial survival for stage I was 78%, for stage II 75%, and for stage III 21%. Other recurrence and survival data, as reported by Maggi et al., are equally favorable.

I have resected the phrenic nerve, lung parenchyma, innominate vein, and superior vena cava when indicated, without consequence. The innominate vein can usually be ligated without sequelae. The superior vena cava should be reconstructed.

Anatomic Basis of Complications

- Phrenic nerves: Due to their lateral location on the pericardium superior to the pulmonary hilum, the phrenic nerves are not infrequently involved by thymic tumors. It is unusual for both phrenic nerves to be involved. A single nerve can and should be resected if necessary for complete resection. Care should be taken in patients with myasthenia gravis.
- Recurrent laryngeal nerves: The recurrent laryngeal nerves are usually well lateral in the chest and posterior in the neck. Care should be taken if the thymic tumor involves the left lobe and extends down near the aortic arch.
- Innominate vein: The innominate vein is the vascular structure most often injured during thymectomy. Great care should be employed when ligating venous tributaries entering the innominate vein from the thymus, to prevent possible catastrophic bleeding. Caution should also be used when opening the sternal retractor so as not to create a stretching or traction tear of the innominate vein.

KEY REFERENCES

Bloom ND. Tumors of the mediastinum. In Beattie EJ, Bloom ND, Harvey JC, eds. Thoracic Surgical Oncology. New York: Churchill Livingstone, 1992, pp 239-243.
This chapter provides a good description of tumors in the thymus and mediastinum.

Cooper JD, Ali-Jilaihawa AN, Pearson FG, et al. An improved technique to facilitate transcervical thymectomy for myasthenia gravis. Ann Thorac Surg 45:242-247, 1988.
These authors describe a technique in which a specially designed retractor permits improved visualization of the anterior mediastinum.

Glatstein E, Levinson B. Malignancies of the thymus. In Roth JA, Ruckdeschel JC, Weisenburger TH, eds. Thoracic Oncology. Philadelphia: WB Saunders, 1995, pp 468-479.
This chapter explains in detail malignancies of the thymus.

Kaiser LR, Martini N. Clinical management of thymomas. The Memorial Sloan-Kettering experience in thoracic surgery: Frontiers and uncommon neoplasms. In Martini N, Vogt-Monkopf, eds. International Trends in General Thoracic Surgery. St Louis: Mosby, 1989, p 5.

The Memorial Sloan-Kettering experience with thymomas is presented.

Miller JI, Mansour K, Hatcher C. Median sternotomy T incision for thymectomy in myasthenia gravis. Ann Thorac Surg 34:473-474, 1982.

These authors describe their technique using a small T incision and partial sternotomy.

Wilkins EW. Thymoma surgical management. In Wood DE, Thomas CR, eds. Mediastinal Tumors, Update 1995. New York: Springer-Verlag, 1995, pp 11-18.

This is a recent review of thymoma management.

SUGGESTED READINGS

Batata MA, Martin N, Huvos AG, et al. Thymomas: Clinicopathologic features, therapy and prognosis. Cancer 34:389-396, 1974.

Bell ET. Tumors of the thymus in myasthenia gravis. J Nerv Dis 45:130-140, 1917.

Blalock A, Mason MF, Morgan HT, et al. Myasthenia gravis and tumors of the thymic region. Ann Surg 110:544-546, 1939.

Bretel JJ. Staging and preliminary results of the Thymic Tumor Study Group. Thymic tumors. In Sarrazin R, Vroussos C, Vincent J, eds. Fourth Cancer Research Workshop. Basel: Karger, 1989 pp 156-164.

Frist W, Thirumalai T, Doehring CB, et al. Thymectomy for the myasthenia gravis patient: Factors influencing outcome. Ann Thorac Surg 57:334-338, 1994.

Givel JC, ed. Surgery of the Thymus. Berlin: Springer-Verlag, 1990.

Maggi G, Casadio C, Cavallo A, et al. Thymoma: Results of 241 operated cases. Ann Thorac Surg 51:152-156, 1991.

Masaoka A, Monden Y, Nakalara K, et al. Follow-up study of thymomas with special reference to their clinical stages. Cancer 68:1984-1987, 1991.

Pollack A, EI-Naggar AK, Cox JD, et al. Thymoma: The prognostic significance of flow cytometric DNA analysis. Cancer 69:1702-1709, 1992.

Rosai J, Levine GD. Tumors of the Thymus. Atlas of Tumor Pathology, Fascile, Second Series. Washington, D.C.: Armed Forces Institute of Pathology, 1976, pp 34-161.

Verley JM, Hollmann KH. Thymoma: A comparative study of clinical stages, histologic features, and survival in 200 cases. Cancer 55:1074-1078, 1985.

Wilkins EW, Castleman B. Thymoma: A continuing survey at Massachusetts General Hospital. Ann Thorac Surg 28:252-256, 1979.

Cervical and Thoracic Trachea

The trachea and main stem bronchi, although not anatomically distinct from the remainder of the respiratory system, are less often affected by malignant processes, but lesions in this area present a considerably more formidable surgical challenge than malignancies of the lung parenchyma. Thoracic surgical pioneers such as Grillo, Pearson, and Mathisen have defined tracheal anatomy and formulated surgical approaches that are anatomically based. It is from their early work and from my own experience that this section is based.

Unlike the more commonly seen parenchymal bronchogenic carcinoma, tracheal tumors are relatively rare, occurring at an estimated rate of 2.7 new cases per million per year. Tracheal lesions may be categorized into three groups: primary malignant, primary benign, and secondary malignant. The presentation of tracheal tumors is often insidious and delayed. The most frequent complaint is dyspnea. Wheezing often develops and frequently leads to the mistaken diagnosis and treatment of adult-onset asthma. Stridor occurs as a relatively late sequelae, when at least 75% of the tracheal circumference is affected. Cough is a frequent complaint, and hemoptysis occurs in 33% of patients. When present at the carina or main stem bronchus level, the only symptoms or signs may be recurrent pneumonia. All of these subtle findings lead to delay in diagnosis if a high index of suspicion is not maintained.

Evaluation is radiographic and endoscopic. Posteroanterior and lateral chest radiographs often do not elucidate tracheal tumors. Overpenetrated cervical and upper thoracic views are frequently more revealing and may lead to more sophisticated radiologic endeavors. Conventional tracheal tomograms give additional information, but are of more historical interest, having been replaced by the ever increasingly sophisticated techniques of CT with three-dimensional reconstruction.

The radiographic technique I favor is helical CT. Scans can be obtained at sections as small as 3 mm, beginning at the vocal cords and extending to the takeoff of the upper lobe bronchi. This technique allows accurate determination of the proximal, distal, and lateral extent of a lesion. The degree of circumferential narrowing and extratracheal mediastinal spread can be determined. Invasion of nearby structures is also revealed. Relevant mediastinal lymph nodes may also be assessed. Our current method allows computer-generated three-dimensional reconstruction of the trachea. Utilization of these techniques allows an accurate operative strategy to be formed. MRI allows coronal and sagittal images to be produced, but these images are not superior to those obtained with helical CT and are certainly more costly. I have rarely

used MRI. Tracheobronchial barium contrast studies are of historical importance, but are not being performed in most centers doing tracheal surgery.

Endoscopic evaluation should follow radiographic imaging of the tumor.
The surgical oncologist must be facile with both flexible and rigid bronchoscopy. Many patients will have nearly obstructing lesions, and therefore flexible bronchoscopy outside the operative theater may be inadvisable. One must
be able to protect the patency of the airway at all times and be prepared to intubate the patient with the rigid bronchoscope or endotracheal tube if compromise occurs due to bleeding, swelling, or secretions. The flexible scope allows passage beyond a tumor in the trachea or major bronchi to obtain distal
mucosal biopsy specimens and thereby determines the extent of distal resection or defines unresectability. This is most important when the tumor is of an
adenoid cystic histologic type, because this tumor extends submucosally beyond visible gross tumor.

Video-assisted rigid bronchoscopy is my preferred endoscopic method. This
allows more precise measurement of distances from the vocal cords to the proximal aspect of the tumor, the distal aspect of the tumor, and the carina. Length
of the tumor and degree of circumferential narrowing can be determined. Photographic documentation is also performed. Carinal and main stem bronchial
lesions may require both methods, because navigating around lesions to determine distal extent and margins is essential. I often use the neodymium:ytterium-
aluminum-garnet (Nd:YAG) laser to temporarily palliate the airway until
definitive open surgical resection can be performed.

Primary malignant tumors of the trachea are more common than benign
tumors. The two largest series of surgically resected primary tracheal tumors
are from Massachusetts General Hospital (MGH) (198 patients) and the Center
for Surgery, Moscow (144 patients). Adenoid cystic carcinoma was the most
frequently encountered primary tumor (and primary malignant tumor) in both
series: MGH series, 80 of 198 patients (40.4%); Moscow series, 66 of 144 patients (45.8%). Squamous cell carcinoma was the second most common malignant tumor in each series: MGH, 70 of 198 (35.4%); Moscow, 21 of 144
(14.6%). Carcinoid tumors were the third most frequently seen tumors. Primary benign tumors were far less common: MGH, 10.6%; and Moscow,
16.6%. Many of these tumors are very rare and have been noted only one
time, making meaningful statements somewhat superficial. In each series, resection of these benign tumors was curative and was accomplished with low
mortality.

Secondary malignant tumors are those malignant processes involving
anatomically adjacent organs that invade the trachea by extension of the primary tumor. Those tumors arise from the lung, larynx, esophagus, and thyroid
gland.

Table 4-6   *Frequency of Tracheal Tumors*

	Boston Grillo, Mathisen (n = 198)	Moscow Perelman (n = 144)
Malignant tumors		
Adenoid cystic	80	66
Squamous cell	70	21
Spindle cell squamous	2	—
Adenocarcinoma	1	1
Adenosquamous carcinoma	1	—
Small cell carcinoid	1	3
Melanoma	1	—
Atypical carcinoid	1	—
Plasmacytoma	—	3
Intermediate tumors		
Carcinoid	10	20
Mucoepidermoid	4	1
Benign processes		
Squamous papilloma	5	2
Pleomorphic adenoma	2	—
Granular cell tumor	2	—
Chondroma	2	—
Neurilemoma	—	5
Hemangioma	1	4

Data adapted from Mathisen DJ. Tracheal tumors. Chest Surg Clin North Am 6:875-898, 1996; Perelman MI, Koroleva N, Birjukov J, et al. Primary tracheal tumors. Semin Thorac Cardiovasc Surg 8:400-402, 1996.

SURGICAL ANATOMY

The adult trachea is 10 to 12 cm long, depending on patient age, sex, and race. Beginning at the cricoid cartilage (C6 in the supine patient), it extends to the carina (T4 in the supine patient). The area from the undersurface of the vocal cords to the superior aspect of the cricoid is considered the subglottic area. The trachea is composed of C-shaped cartilages anteriorly and laterally. The posterior aspect of the trachea, the membranous trachea, is flat and pliable, opposed to and therefore directly anterior to the esophagus. The anterior cartilages and posterior membranous trachea are in a unique configuration that provides strength and patency while allowing dynamic physiologic changes during respiration. The trachea is composed of 20 to 22 of these C rings, with approximately 2.1 rings per centimeter. The tracheal length may vary as much as 1.5 to 2.5 cm during respiration and swallowing.

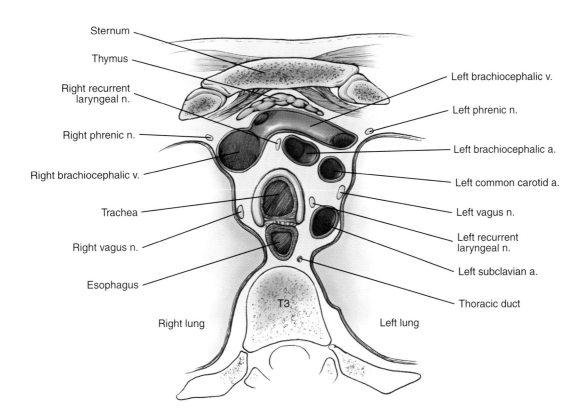

The cervical trachea is relatively unprotected and vulnerable from the cricoid cartilage to the sternal notch. It parallels the vertebral column more so than the sternum, traveling posteriorly to lie deep within the posterior mediastinum posterior to the cardiac structures. The angle between the sternum and trachea approaches 90 degrees at the thoracic inlet and increases with age as kyphosis progresses. This has significant operative ramifications as the cervical trachea (50% of the tracheal length) may be exposed through a properly placed transverse cervical collar incision. The proximal cervical trachea is posterior to the thyroid isthmus, inferior thyroid veins, and thyroid ima artery when present. The sternothyroid and sternohyoid muscles, cervical fascia, and inconsistent crossing branches of the anterior jugular veins are superficial to these structures. The right and left lobes of the thyroid gland cover the lateral aspects of the proximal cervical trachea. The cervical esophagus is directly posterior to the membranous trachea. One of the vital structures in this area is the recurrent laryngeal nerves. The recurrent nerves are small cord-like structures found in the tracheoesophageal groove. They are difficult to identify, and therefore the area of the tracheoesophageal groove should be avoided during dissection.

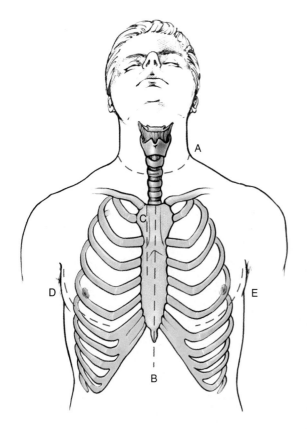

The second part of the trachea begins at or below the sternal notch. This is an arbitrary division used in planning a surgical approach for resection. At the level of the sternal notch the trachea begins to dive posteriorly and deep as it follows the vertebral column. Access for resection is better obtained through a partial median sternotomy, full median sternotomy, or right posterolateral thoracotomy.

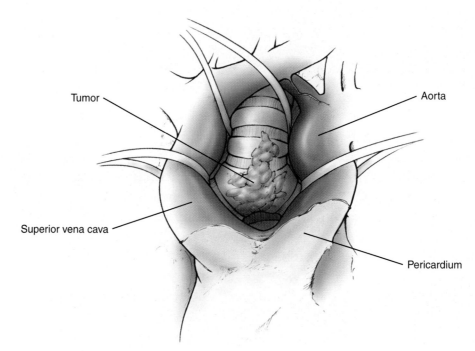

Anteriorly and to the right laterally are the innominate artery and left innominate vein. The left carotid and subclavian arteries and the left vagus and phrenic nerves are to the left and lateral of the proximal thoracic trachea. Two centimeters more distal the anterior surface of the thoracic trachea is crossed by the aortic arch. The superior vena cava comes to oppose the right lateral aspect of the trachea at this point, and the esophagus begins to deviate from the midline to the left posterolateral aspect of the thoracic trachea. As the trachea travels deeper into the chest and emerges from underneath the aortic arch, the azygous vein is encountered on the right as it travels anteriorly to empty into the superior vena cava. Great caution should be exercised in this area during resection or mediastinoscopy, because the azygous vein is easily injured by traction tears or inadvertent biopsy. Finally, the most distal aspect of the thoracic trachea passes posterior to the bifurcation of the main pulmonary artery. The trachea ends at the carina, which is deep to the posterior pericardium. The area may be approached anteriorly by mobilizing the superior vena cava and ascending aorta laterally and then incising the posterior pericardium.

Blood Supply

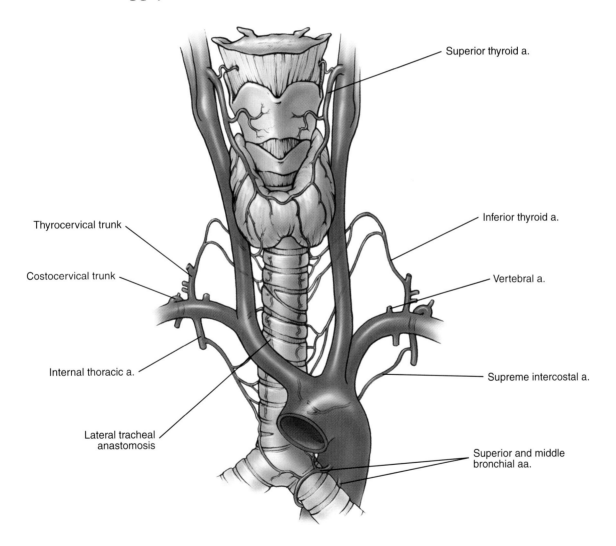

The major arterial supply to the cervical trachea is the inferior thyroid artery. Grillo and Miura are credited with defining the upper vascular supply in 1966 when they injected barium sulfate into the inferior thyroid artery. They revealed that the inferior thyroid artery gives rise to three branches, which travel medially to the lateral wall of the trachea where they coalesce to form a lateral longitudinal artery just anterior to the tracheoesophageal groove. This finding was substantiated when Salassa et al. performed a cervical dissection in 21 human cadavers. They documented several anatomic patterns of the inferior thyroid artery. Most commonly the artery arose from the thyrocervical trunk of the subclavian artery and traveled posteriorly to the common carotid artery, then divided into three branches. These branches coalesced to form a longitudinal artery that gave off small branches to the membranous portion of the trachea between cartilages. This pattern of three branches occurred more than half of the time. The next most common patterns consisted of two branches in 35% and one branch in 12%. The first branch typically supplies the lower cervical trachea; the second branch supplies the area of the trachea between the first and third arterial branches, and a portion of the cervical esophagus; and the third, most superior of the three branches, supplies the cervical trachea underlying the thyroid gland.

The thoracic tracheal arterial supply is much more inconsistent and involves more arterial sources. The innominate and subclavian arteries remain the parent source. The supreme intercostal artery was revealed by Salassa et al. to be the main source of arterial supply in 38% of their cadavers. Branches originating from the subclavian proximal to the vertebral artery ostia were the major sources in 31% of cadavers. As in the cervical region, these arteries arrive on the lateral aspect of the trachea from their superior origin and form the lateral longitudinal artery of the trachea. Finally, the right internal mammary artery was the main arterial supply in 13% and the innominate artery in 19% of cadavers. All cervical and thoracic tracheal supply sources approach the trachea laterally and form lateral longitudinal anastomoses about 0.5 cm anterior to the tracheoesophageal groove. These vessels of the longitudinal network are 1 to 2 mm in diameter. This network gives off two branches, the anterior and posterior transverse intercartilaginous arteries. These vessels enter between the cartilage rings and form a capillary plexus in the submucosa. The posterior membranous trachea is supplied by small tracheal branches from primary esophageal vessels. The cartilaginous rings receive their blood supply by diffusion of nutrients via the submucosal plexus. The posterior membranous portion of the trachea is composed of fibroelastic tissue and smooth muscle that is responsible for the changing diameter of the trachea and is sometimes called the trachealis muscle.

Venous drainage is from the submucosa through ever enlarging channels that eventually reach the inferior thyroid veins. Tracheal lymphatic vessels drain into cervical, peritracheal, and tracheobronchial lymph node chains. The trachea is supplied by sympathetic and parasympathetic fibers.

Histologically the tracheal mucosa is composed of pseudostratified ciliated columnar epithelium and mucus-producing goblet cells. Microvilli containing brush cells are also present.

SURGICAL APPLICATIONS

Bronchoscopy

The general surgical oncologist and thoracic surgical oncologist must be knowledgeable regarding both flexible and rigid bronchoscopy. Each has its advantages and may often complement the other.

An advantage of flexible fiberoptic bronchoscopy is that it can be performed in the awake patient after application of topical lidocaine administered by nebulizer. Intravenous sedation with short-acting benzodiazepines and synthetic narcotics is advantageous because the cooperative patient is more easily examined. Each of these agents may be reversed at the completion of the procedure by administration of flumazenil (Romazican) and naloxone (Narcan), respectively.

The bronchoscope may be attached to a video system for magnification and photographic documentation or used for standard direct vision. The bronchoscope may be introduced through the nares or orotracheally. I find it easier to pass the scope through the nares, thus avoiding the posterior tongue and thereby reducing the gag reflex.

The first structures visualized are the epiglottis and the laryngeal complex. Both form and movement of the vocal cord should be analyzed. The scope is passed down through the vocal cords into the subglottic area, noting the diameter. Advancement to the carina is then accomplished, noting any endotracheal tumor or deformity and documenting its length, reduction of tracheal diameter, and distances from the vocal cords and carina. The right and left bronchi are then examined. The flexible scope may be passed all the way down to the lobar and segmental bronchi. The flexible scope may be used to visualize anatomic details or obtain biopsy specimens or for laser destruction of airway tumors.

Rigid bronchoscopy requires a general anesthetic and paralysis. The surgeon should be prepared to intubate with the rigid scope should the airway collapse during relaxation. A video-assisted bronchoscope is far superior to the traditional, poorly lit direct vision scope. I use the Dumon-Harrell ventilating bronchoscope (Bryan Corp., Worchester, Mass.). The patient is placed in the supine position with the neck hyperextended, eyes shielded, and teeth protected. The scope is introduced posterior to the base of the tongue and advanced forward into the posterior pharynx to view the epiglottis. The epiglottis is lifted anteriorly with the tip of the scope to allow vocal cord examination. Passage through the vocal cords is facilitated by rotation of the scope 90 degrees. The subglottic area and proximal, middle, and distal trachea may then be examined. The experienced endoscopist can pass the scope to the level of the segmental bronchi. The rigid scope can be used for both mechanical and Nd:YAG laser destruction of tumor as a temporizing maneuver to open the airway prior to resection or as palliation in the high-risk surgical candidate. On occasion, the flexible scope may be introduced through the rigid scope to reach the more distal airway.

Incisions for Tracheal and Major Bronchial Resections

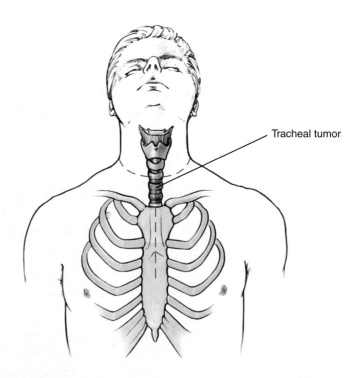

Tracheal tumor

The trachea can be approached through a multitude of incisions. It is best to divide the trachea into cervical and thoracic divisions to plan the surgical approach. Fully half of the trachea, the cervical trachea, can be adequately exposed through a cervical collar incision with the patient supine. When a transverse roll is placed underneath the shoulders and the head hyperextended, an additional 2 to 4 cm of upper thoracic trachea may be visualized. A partial or complete median sternotomy may be added for further exposure of the upper or middle thoracic portions of the trachea.

A complete median sternotomy allows access to the carina. It is unusual and generally unnecessary to approach the carina from an anterior direction for oncologic purposes. This approach is most often used for management of carinal trauma or closure of a postoperative bronchopleural fistula after pneumonectomy.

Through a complete median sternotomy the anterosuperior aspect of the pericardium is opened. The reflections of the pericardium are removed from the great vessels with the electrocautery. The superior vena cava is released from its pericardial attachments and freed from the underlying right main pulmonary artery and retracted with tapes laterally to the right. The ascending aorta is freed from pericardial reflections and the underlying right main pulmonary artery and retracted with tapes laterally to the left. The right main pulmonary artery may need to be mobilized and retracted inferiorly. The posterior pericardium is then incised to reveal the carina. Mobilization maneuvers can also be performed through this incision.

The traditional right posterior lateral thoracotomy is the incision of choice for exposure of the carina and thoracic trachea. This approach allows adequate exposure of the lower half of the trachea and carina. Vertebral kyphosis increases with age, bringing more of the cervical trachea below the thoracic inlet into the chest. Allen has shown that large differences in the amount of extrathoracic trachea occur between flexion and extension. Thus, with profound flexion in the younger patient, the cricoid cartilage may be brought very near the thoracic inlet, making more of the lower cervical and upper thoracic trachea accessible through a posterolateral thoracotomy. When this approach is utilized, a standard skin incision is made, the latissimus muscle is mobilized and divided, and the serratus anterior muscle is mobilized, reflected anteriorly, and spared. I have not chosen to perform tracheal resection and reconstruction through a vertical muscle-sparing incision. The fifth intercostal space may be utilized, or the fourth if the lesion is in the upper thoracic trachea.

The left posterolateral thoracotomy is infrequently utilized for tracheal and carinal resection because of the limited exposure related to the presence of the aortic arch and descending aorta. Occasionally this incision and approach are utilized for a sleeve resection involving the left main stem bronchus.

Resection and Reconstruction of Cervical Trachea

Primary and secondary tumors involving the upper half of the trachea are most easily approached through a collar incision. The patient is prepared and draped for a median sternotomy in case additional exposure of the upper thoracic trachea is required. Through the collar incision, superior and inferior subplatysmal flaps are formed. The midline of the sternohyoid and sternothyroid is identified and incised and the muscles retracted laterally with stay sutures or neuro hooks. The thyroid isthmus is divided as necessary. The anterior and lateral aspects of the trachea are now exposed from the cricoid to the sternal notch.

Mobilization of the trachea is essential for achieving a tension-free anastomosis after resection. All fascial and areolar tissue attachments are freed from the anterior surface down to and including the anterior surface of the carina and main stem bronchi. Great care must be exercised in the region of the innominate vessels to avert vascular injury. The posterior mobilization is more easily performed after proximal transection. The lateral attachments, or "tissue stalks," should be left undisturbed to prevent injury to the longitudinal tracheal artery and recurrent nerves. The site of proximal transection should have been previously determined through bronchoscopy and CT; thus the site of the proximal incision on the trachea and the length of the resection should be predetermined. Final determination is now performed by having the first assistant pass a fiberoptic bronchoscope proximal to the tumor. The surgeon then passes an 18-gauge needle through the anterior wall of the trachea at the incision site. The bronchoscopist will determine the correctness of the chosen site and adequacy of the margin.

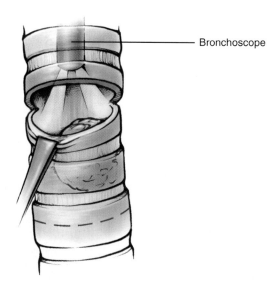

Bronchoscope

The trachea is divided anterior to posterior. The distal transection site is determined by direct inspection. A sterile malleable wire–reinforced endotracheal tube is passed into the remaining distal trachea for ventilation during the reconstruction.

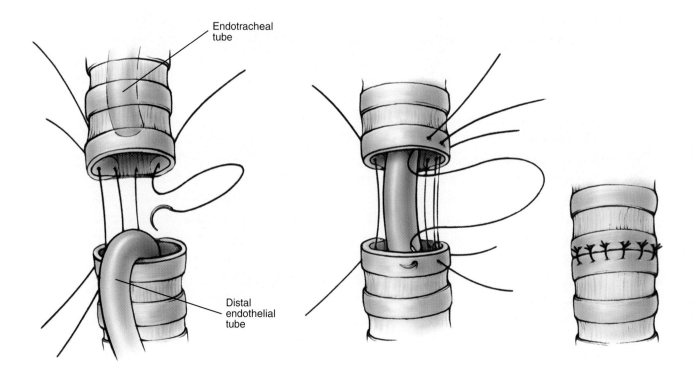

Endotracheal tube

Distal endothelial tube

When proper ventilation is ensured, the membranous portion of the remaining tracheal segment is sharply and bluntly separated from the underlying esophagus. The reconstruction may now be performed. It is essential that the end-to-end tracheal anastomosis be performed with no tension, which on occasion will require additional release maneuvers such as the hilar and laryngeal release described by Heitmiller. When the tumor is an adenoid cystic carcinoma, frozen-section analysis of multiple areas proximally and distally must be performed, because this tumor has the propensity to extend in the submucosa far beyond grossly recognizable tumor. After confirming free margins, the anastomosis is begun.

Two 0 silk sutures are placed through the lateral cartilage of the proximal and distal segment 2 cm from the cut end. Hemostats are placed on these "traction sutures," which are then crossed and used to pull the segments toward each other. The membranous trachea is brought together utilizing interrupted 2-0 Vicryl sutures with knots tied on the outside. All sutures are placed first, then tied in order to be under the least possible tension. The distal endotracheal tube is removed prior to tying the anterior suture line, and the original endotracheal tube, which was left in place in the proximal trachea, is advanced through the partially completed anastomosis into the distal trachea. The endotracheal tube placement is confirmed and ventilation resumed. The lateral and anterior portions of the anastomosis are completed in similar fashion, utilizing interrupted sutures with knots tied on the outside. The lateral stay sutures are now tied to further reduce the tension. The strap muscles are reapproximated, the platysma is reapproximated, and the skin is closed. The patient's neck is brought to maximal flexion and the chin sutured to the anterior chest wall for 7 to 10 days. All attempts are made at extubation to prevent suture line disruption by the endotracheal tube.

Resection and Reconstruction of Thoracic Trachea

Tumors in the thoracic portion of the trachea, not including the carina, are most easily approached through a right posterolateral thoracotomy. A left double-lumen endotracheal tube and single-lung ventilation should be utilized. Mediastinoscopy should be performed immediately prior to the anticipated resection. This accomplishes two objectives. First, paratracheal lymph nodes are sampled. When the tumor is parenchymal in origin, this nodal group remains an N2 group and should preclude further resection except under investigational multimodality protocol situations for stage IIIA bronchogenic carcinomas. When the tumor is primary to the intrathoracic trachea, paratracheal lymph nodes are N1 lymph nodes and may be considered a relative contraindication, depending on the overall clinical situation. Second, mediastinoscopy also serves the purpose of dividing tissue in the pretracheal plane down to the carina and left main stem bronchus. This maneuver enhances mobilization. The parietal pleura overlying the trachea is identified and incised. The right vagus nerve is mobilized posteriorly and the superior vena cava anteriorly. The azygous vein is occluded with a suture at its entrance into the superior vena cava and divided at the chest wall after ligation. The length of the intervening section is maintained in this fashion and allows the vein to be used as an onlay tissue graft covering of the tracheal anastomosis. The proximal trachea, carina, and right and left main stem bronchi are further mobilized and encircled with cotton tapes. Division of the right inferior pulmonary ligament and right hilar release allows additional mobilization. The lateral aspects of the trachea are once again avoided.

The sites of proximal and distal division are determined as described for cervical resection. The tracheal anastomosis in the thorax is sometimes facilitated by placement of sutures first in the left lateral wall, because this is now the deepest aspect. The membranous portion, anterior aspect, and finally the right lateral aspect are closed with interrupted Vicryl sutures with knots tied on the outside. The endotracheal tube is managed as previously discussed. The "azygous vein flap" may now be sutured over the anastomosis to separate it from the surrounding structures. A longitudinal pericardial flap may be formed and used for the same purpose.

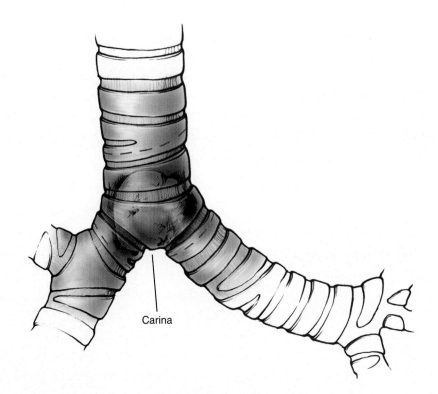

Carina

Tumors at the carina or proximal main stem bronchi without involvement of the lung parenchyma are uncommon. Those tumors that are relatively small and endobronchial may be resected utilizing a carinal resection or sleeve pneumonectomy. Such resections require great experience and clinical judgment, and must be approached on an individual basis.

Reconstruction After Carinal Resection

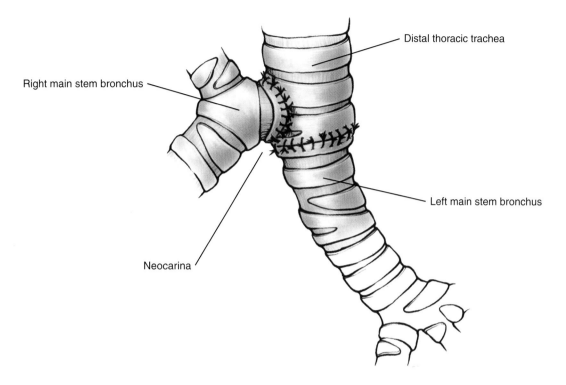

The right main stem bronchus is anastomosed end to side to the distal thoracic trachea. The end of the left main stem bronchus is then anastomosed to the distal end of the thoracic trachea. Resection and reconstructive techniques are beyond the scope of this text. Mathisen provides an excellent description of these techniques in his work "Carinal Reconstruction: Techniques and Problems."

Anatomic Basis of Complications

- The surgical oncologist must recognize that the longitudinal tracheal artery is present laterally and is the vital blood supply of the trachea. Disruption will lead to possible anastomotic failure.
- The recurrent laryngeal nerves run laterally in the tracheoesophageal groove. Failure to avoid this area may lead to unilateral or bilateral vocal cord paralysis.
- When a lower cervical tracheal resection is performed, the reconstruction may lie in close proximity to the transversely running innominate artery. A muscle or pericardial flap should be interposed between the tracheal anastomosis and the innominate artery to prevent tracheal–innominate artery fistula.

KEY REFERENCES

Allen MS. Surgical anatomy of the trachea. Chest Surg Clin North Am 6:627–635, 1996.
This article describes the anatomy of the trachea and highlights how these anatomic details affect the surgical procedures.

Grillo HC, Mathisen DJ. Primary tracheal tumors: Treatment and results. Ann Thorac Surg 49:69–77, 1990.
This 26-year study from Massachusetts General Hospital was conducted on 198 patients with primary tracheal tumors.

Mansour KA, Lee RB, Miller JI. Tracheal resections: Lessons learned. Ann Thorac Surg 57:1120–1125, 1994.
This is a 19-year experience from Emory University of the lessons learned from tracheal resections.

Mathisen DJ. Tracheal tumors. Chest Surg Clin North Am 6:875–898, 1996.
This article updates the Massachusetts General Hospital series.

Perelman MI, Koroleva N, Birjukov J, et al. Primary tracheal tumors. Semin Thorac Cardiovasc Surg 8:400–402, 1996.
This article reports the 33-year study of 144 patients who underwent surgery for primary tumors of the trachea at the Russian Academy of Medical Sciences in Moscow.

Pearson FG, Thompson DW, Weissberg D, et al. Adenoid cystic carcinoma of the trachea. Experience with 16 patients managed by tracheal resection. Ann Thorac Surg 18:16, 1974.
This article reports the experience in Toronto treating 16 patients with adenoid cystic tumors of the trachea.

Weber AL, Grillo HC. Tracheal tumors: A radiological, clinical, and pathologic evaluation of 84 cases. Radiol Clin North Am 16:227–301, 1978.
This article offers a superb description of the evaluation of a patient with a tracheal tumor.

SUGGESTED READINGS

Grillo HC, Suen HC, Mathisen DJ, et al. Resectional management of thyroid carcinoma invading the airway. Ann Thorac Surg 54:3–8, 1992.

Heitmiller RF. Tracheal release maneuvers. Chest Surg Clin North Am 6:675–682, 1996.

Lee RB. Traumatic injury of the cervicothoracic trachea and major bronchi. Chest Surg Clin North Am 7:285–303, 1997.

Mathisen DJ. Carinal reconstruction: Techniques and problems. Semin Thorac Cardiovasc Surg 8:403–413, 1996.

Miura T, Grillo HC. The contribution of the inferior thyroid artery to the blood supply of the human trachea. Surg Gynecol Obstet 123:91–102, 1966.

Salassa JR, Pearson BW, Payne WS. Gross and microscopical blood supply of the trachea. Ann Thorac Surg 24:100–107, 1977.

Zanni P, Melloni G. Surgical management of thyroid cancer invading the trachea. Chest Surg Clin North Am 6:777–790, 1996.

Lung

In 1998, 1,228,600 new cancer cases will be diagnosed. Prostate cancer will predominate in men (184,500 new cases), and breast cancer will be the most frequent new cancer in women (178,700 new cases). Lung cancer will be diagnosed in 171,500 patients (91,400 men, 80,100 women).

Table 4-7   *Estimated Incidence and Mortality for Cancers in Men, 1998**

Cancer	Incidence	Mortality
Prostate	184,500 (29%)	39,200
Lung and bronchus	93,100 (15%)	91,400
Colon and rectum	60,600 (10%)	27,900
All sites	627,900	294,200

Adapted from Landis SH, Murray T, Bolden S, et al. Cancer statistics in 1998. CA Cancer J Clin 48: 6-29, 1998.
*Excludes carcinoma in situ or basal and squamous cell skin cancers.

Table 4-8   *Estimated Incidence and Mortality for Cancers in Women, 1998**

Cancer	Incidence	Mortality
Breast	178,700 (30%)	43,500
Lung and bronchus	80,100 (13%)	67,100
Colon and rectum	67,000 (11%)	28,600

Adapted from Landis SH, Murray T, Bolden S, et al. Cancer statistics in 1998. CA Cancer J Clin 48: 6-29, 1998.
*Excludes carcinoma in situ or basal and squamous cell skin cancers.

The most sobering statistic, however, is that lung cancer is the most common cause of cancer death in both sexes (93,100 deaths in men, 67,500 deaths in women), far exceeding both prostate and breast cancer. Lung cancer deaths in women surpassed death due to breast cancer more than a decade ago, in 1987. In 1998 lung cancer was responsible for 25% of all cancer deaths in women. This frightening epidemic has gone largely unrecognized by the public, due in part to the public paranoia regarding the acquired immunodeficiency syndrome (AIDS) epidemic.

Lung cancer is a relatively new disease, a disease of the twentieth century, due to environmental pollution from industry and more commonly tobacco use. The first recognized correlation between the environment and pulmonary malignancies occurred in 1879 when Haerting and Hesse reported that 75% of deaths among the Schneeberg miners of the Black Forest in Germany were due to pulmonary tumors. The first clinical report of a primary pulmonary malignancy was authored by G.H. Bayle in 1810, who described a left hilar pulmonary mass with lymph node, liver, and subcutaneous tissue metastases.

The motivational causes prompting the development of thoracic surgery were trauma and infection (i.e., tuberculosis and empyema). Development of thoracic surgical oncology was delayed by the slow development of endotracheal intubation, positive pressure ventilation, and inhalation anesthetics. The first successful lobectomy for malignancy in which there was anatomic dissection and ligation of the hilar structures was by H.M. Davies, an English surgeon who resected the right lower lobe. Prior to this, mass ligation of the hilar structures was performed. The first successful pneumonectomy for lung cancer was performed by Ewarts A. Graham in a 48-year-old fellow physician. The hilar structures were mass ligated and the bronchus closed with catgut. The year was 1933, and the patient survived 30 years despite metastasis to regional lymph nodes. The reader is referred to Kittle's description of the history of thoracic surgical oncology for an excellent in-depth discussion.

Significant improvements have been made in cardiorespiratory assessment, perioperative staging, and perioperative care. Belief that removal of the entire lung, pneumonectomy, was superior to lobectomy led to mortality rates of 40% to 50% from the 1930s to the late 1950s. By 1983 Ginsberg et al. were reporting a 30-day operative mortality of 3.9% in a series of 2500 consecutive resections for lung cancer. Most recently in 1998, Wada et al. reported a 30-day operative mortality of 1.3% in 7099 consecutive resections for lung cancer (January to December 1994). Despite the marked improvements in perioperative care and marked reduction in operative mortality, there has been no significant improvement in 5-year survival for resectable non–small cell lung cancer in the past 40 years. Currently, 5-year survival approximates 40%, not significantly different from Pearson's report in 1985, in which he pointed out that 5-year survival at the beginning of his career was 23%. Our failure to progress is largely due to inaccuracy of preoperative clinical staging, lack of uniform performance of operative staging, lymph node dissection, and largely ineffective postoperative adjuvant therapy. The recent introduction of neoadjuvant chemotherapy and chemotherapy plus radiation therapy holds true promise for improving 5-year survival for lung cancer patients with locoregional lymph node metastasis from primary lung cancer. Only continued vigilance in perioperative care, improved accuracy of perioperative and intraoperative staging, and institution of multimodality protocols as treatment strategy will lead to meaningful improvement in 5-year survival.

STAGING OF LUNG CANCER

Early classification and categorization of the different histologic types of lung cancer evolved and culminated into the classification scheme proposed by the World Health Organization in 1981. Clinically the thoracic surgical oncologist is faced with a more practical division of these various lung cancers into two biologically diverse subgroups: small cell lung carcinomas and non–small cell lung carcinomas. Small cell lung carcinomas are believed to be biologically aggressive, frequently having locoregional nodal metastasis and distant organ metastasis at the time of discovery. The role of surgery in small cell lung carcinoma is often limited to diagnosis and staging, and chemotherapy plus radiation therapy is considered the best therapeutic option. The role of surgery is somewhat controversial but distinctly present. Urschel and Kohman have discussed the surgical management of peripheral and central small cell lung carcinomas, respectively.

The thoracic surgeon is most often called on to intervene and manage pulmonary malignancy due to non–small cell lung carcinomas. The most frequently encountered non–small cell lung carcinomas are (1) squamous cell carcinoma, (2) adenocarcinoma, (3) large cell carcinoma, (4) adenosquamous carcinoma, and (5) carcinoid tumors; the first three are the most common. All authors note a decrease in the predominance of squamous cell carcinoma and an increased number of adenocarcinomas. There is also an alarming change in the male:female ratio, from historical ratios of 3.4:1 in the 1970s to 1.1:1 in 1998. Fraire provides an excellent current review of lung cancer pathology.

Accurate radiologic noninvasive and surgical invasive staging is essential to determine operability in patients with apparently favorable and resectable lesions. Accurate staging allows prognostic determination of 5-year survival for patients with stage I and stage II disease, identifies patients with stage IIIA disease who might benefit from neoadjuvant chemotherapy and radiation therapy trials prior to resection, and eliminates patients with stage IV disease with distant metastasis who generally will not benefit from surgical resection. Accurate staging determines the extent of disease within the individual patient, allowing the patient to be grouped with patients with similarly staged disease for purposes of providing conventionally proved therapeutic options or providing access to experimental multimodality therapeutic protocols when effective therapeutic options have not been established for that patient's lung cancer stage.

World Health Organization
Classification of Lung Tumors

Epithelial tumors
  Benign
    Papillomas
      Squamous cell
      "Transitional"
    Adenomas
      Pleomorphic ("mixed tumor")
      Monomorphic
      Other
  Dysplasia
  Carcinoma in situ
  Malignant
    Squamous cell carcinoma
    Variant: Spindle cell (squamous) carcinoma
    Small cell carcinoma
      Oat cell
      Intermediate cell type
      Combined oat cell
    Adenocarcinoma
      Acinar
      Papillary
      Bronchoalveolar
      Solid carcinoma with mucus formation
    Large cell carcinoma
      Giant cell
      Clean cell
    Adenosquamous carcinoma
    Carcinoid tumor
    Bronchial gland carcinoma
      Adenoid cystic
      Mucoepidermoid
      Other
    Other

TNM Description

Primary Tumor (T)

TX   Primary tumor cannot be assessed, or tumor proved by the presence of malignant cells in sputum or bronchial washings but not visualized at imaging or bronchoscopy

T0   No evidence of primary tumor

Tis   Carcinoma in situ

T1   Tumor ≤3 cm in greatest dimension, surrounded by lung or visceral pleura, without bronchoscopic evidence of invasion more proximal than the lobar bronchus[*] (i.e., not in the main bronchus)

T2   Tumor with any of the following features of size or extent:
>3 cm in greatest dimension
Involves main bronchus, ≥2 cm distal to the carina
Invades the visceral pleura
Associated with atelectasis or obstructive pneumonitis that extends to the hilar region but does not involve the entire lung

T3   Tumor of any size that directly invades any of the following: chest wall (including superior sulcus tumors), diaphragm, mediastinal pleura, parietal pericardium; or tumor in the main bronchus <2 cm distal to the carina, but without involvement of the carina; or associated atelectasis or obstructive pneumonitis of the entire lung

T4   Tumor of any size that invades any of the following: mediastinum, heart, great vessels, trachea, esophagus, vertebral body, carina; or tumor with a malignant pleural or pericardial effusion,[†] or with satellite tumor nodule(s) within the ipsilateral primary tumor lobe of the lung

Regional Lymph Nodes (N)

NX   Regional lymph nodes cannot be assessed

N0   No regional lymph node metastasis

N1   Metastasis to ipsilateral hilar lymph nodes, and intrapulmonary nodes involved by direct extension of the primary tumor

N2   Metastasis to ipsilateral and/or subcarinal lymph node(s)

N3   Metastasis to contralateral mediastinal, contralateral hilar, ipsilateral or contralateral scalene, or supraclavicular lymph node(s)

Distant Metastasis (M)

MX   Presence of distant metastasis cannot be assessed

M0   No distant metastasis

M1   Distant metastasis present[‡]

From Mountain CF. Revisions in the international system for staging lung cancer. Chest 111:1710-1717, 1997.

[*]The uncommon superficial tumor of any size with its invasive component limited to the bronchial wall, which may extend proximal to the main bronchus, is also classified T1.

[†]Most pleural effusions associated with lung cancer are due to tumor. However, in a few patients multiple cytopathologic examinations of pleural fluid show no tumor. In these cases, the fluid is non-bloody and is not an exudate. When these elements and clinical judgment dictate that the effusion is not related to the tumor, the effusion should be excluded as a staging element and the patient's disease should be staged T1, T2, or T3. Pericardial effusion is classified according to the same rules.

[‡]Separate metastatic tumor nodule(s) in the ipsilateral nonprimary tumor lobe(s) of the lung are also classified M1.

Stage Grouping TNM Subsets⋆

Stage	TNM Subset
0	Carcinoma in situ
IA	T1 N0 M0
IB	T2 N0 M0
IIA	T1 N1 M0
IIB	T2 N1 M0
	T3 N0 M0
IIIA	T3 N1 M0
	T1 N2 M0
	T2 N2 M0
	T3 N2 M0
IIIB	T4 N0 M0
	T4 N1 M0
	T4 N2 M0
	T1 N3 M0
	T2 N3 M0
	T3 N3 M0
	T4 N3 M0
IV	Any T, Any N M1

From Mountain CF. Revisions in the international system for staging lung cancer. Chest 111:1710-1717, 1997.
⋆Staging is not relevant for occult carcinoma, designated TX N0 M0.

The TNM system for staging lung cancer is based on anatomic criteria, as are most other malignancies (T = tumor size, N = presence or absence of regional lymph node metastasis, and M = presence or absence of distant metastasis). Originally staging proposals for lung cancer were formed in the middle to late 1950s by the American Joint Committee for Cancer Staging and End Results Reporting (AJCC) and the International Union Against Cancer (UICC). Over the years differences in survival were noted among some of the subset groups, leading the AJCC and the UICC to form a single system in 1985, which was presented at the Fourth World Congress on Lung Cancer by the task force chairman, Clifton F. Mountain, M.D. This universally accepted system was recently revised and published in June 1997. This system is the presently accepted staging system for lung cancer. The revised international system for staging lung cancer was formulated to address the heterogeneity of end results (i.e., survival) within the stage groupings and to provide for greater specificity in stage classification while disrupting the current system as little as possible.

Clinical staging is accomplished by noninvasive means (plain chest radiography, genography, CT, nuclear MRI, radionuclide scanning, positron emission tomography) and invasive means (rigid and fiberoptic bronchoscopy, mediastinoscopy, mediastinotomy, fine-needle aspiration biopsy, video-assisted thoracoscopy, thoracotomy). Detailed descriptions and virtues of these various investigational maneuvers are not within the format of this text but are contained in texts by Roth et al. and by Aisner et al.

STAGE-BASED TREATMENT OF LUNG CANCER

Surgical therapy remains the mainstay of treatment for stage I and stage II bronchogenic carcinoma. Neoadjuvant chemotherapy and chemotherapy–radiation therapy followed by surgical resection have improved survival in patients with stage IIIA disease, but the chemotherapeutic agents and sequencing of chemotherapy, radiation therapy, and surgical resection remain debatable. At the time of this writing, randomized, multicenter, cooperative trials are nearing completion. It is hoped that analysis of data from these trials will provide some illumination and allow standardization of treatment of stage IIIA lung cancer. Stage IIIB lung cancer has been treated largely with chemotherapeutic agents and radiation therapy. Stage IV disease has a similar prognosis and treatment options.

Stage I non–small cell lung carcinomas are tumors less than 3 cm in diameter not invading the visceral pleura, with no nodal metastasis (stage IA). Stage IB tumors are >3 cm, invading the visceral pleura or involving the main stem bronchus >2 cm distal to the carina. If postobstructive atelectasis or pneumonitis develops, the tumor is considered stage IB. These tumors should be resected by lobectomy with a mediastinal lymphadenectomy. Lobectomy results in superior survival, compared with wedge resection or segmental resection. Five-year survival for pathologically staged IA non-small cell lung carcinomas is 67%, and for IB is 57%.

Stage II non–small cell lung carcinomas consist of stage IIA (T1 N1 M0) and IIB (T2 N1 M0 and T3 N0 M0) tumors. The N1 designation is defined as metastasis to ipsilateral peribronchial or ipsilateral hilar lymph nodes and intrapulmonary nodes involved by direct extension of the primary tumor. This stage is defined by the presence of N1 nodal metastasis, which has significant implications for survival. Stage IIA (T1 N1 M0) has a pathologic 5-year survival rate of 55%, and stage IIB (T2 N1 M0) has a 5-year survival rate of 39%. Also added to stage IIB in the revised staging system are T3 N0 tumors. T3 tumors are any size tumor that invade the chest wall, diaphragm, mediastinal pleura, or parietal pericardium, and tumors <2 cm distal to the carina without involving the carina. Tumors causing complete atelectasis or obstructive pneumonitis of the entire lung are T3. T3 N0 M0 tumors have a similar pathologic survival rate of 38%. Surgical treatment is generally lobectomy with en bloc resection of chest wall, diaphragm, or pericardium. Pneumonectomy or sleeve resection is performed for tumors of the hilum or tumors of the main stem bronchus.

Stage III non–small cell lung carcinoma designates those tumors with metastasis to N2 lymph nodes, ipsilateral mediastinal, or subcarinal lymph nodes, or N3 lymph nodes contralateral mediastinal, contralateral hilar, ipsilateral or contralateral scalene, or supraclavicular lymph nodes. This stage also includes T4 tumors: tumors of any size that invade the mediastinum, heart, great vessels, trachea, esophagus, vertebral body, or carina. Tumors producing pleural or pericardial effusions or those with satellite tumor nodules within the ipsilateral primary tumor lobe are T4 lesions. Five-year survival for this stage is <25%. Improved survival up to 35% to 40% has been seen with the addition of neoadjuvant chemotherapy for stage IIIA, N2 disease. Surgical management requires lobectomy, pneumonectomy, or complex radical resection with extensive lymphadenectomy. Note the poor survival of T3 lesions when there is local lymph node metastasis. Stage IIIB tumors are defined as T4 tumors with N0 to N3 nodal status. Five-year survival is poor at 7%, although some small series have reported better survival for carefully selected T4 N0 M0 lesions. Stage IIIB also includes tumors with N3 metastasis (T1 to T4). Survival is an abysmal 3%. Surgical resection is not an option for N3 disease, and only an option for very select T4 N0 lesions.

Stage IV non–small cell lung carcinoma is defined as lesions with distant metastasis. Five-year survival is poor, 1%. Occasionally a patient with solitary brain metastasis or adrenal metastasis may be a surgical candidate. Reported series are small and anecdotal, with 5-year survival approximating 15%.

SURGICAL ANATOMY
Bronchopulmonary Segments

Early surgical endeavors to resect pulmonary malignancies involved mass ligation of the hilum and pneumonectomy, as described by Graham. This technique quickly was abandoned as careful identification of the arterial and venous structures of the hilum were appreciated and understood, thereby allowing development of techniques of lobectomy to preserve lung parenchyma unaffected by tumor. The anatomic unit of the lung is termed the bronchopulmonary segment, defined as that portion of the lung that can function independently, a segmental branching of a major lobar bronchus with its own pulmonary arterial supply and venous drainage.

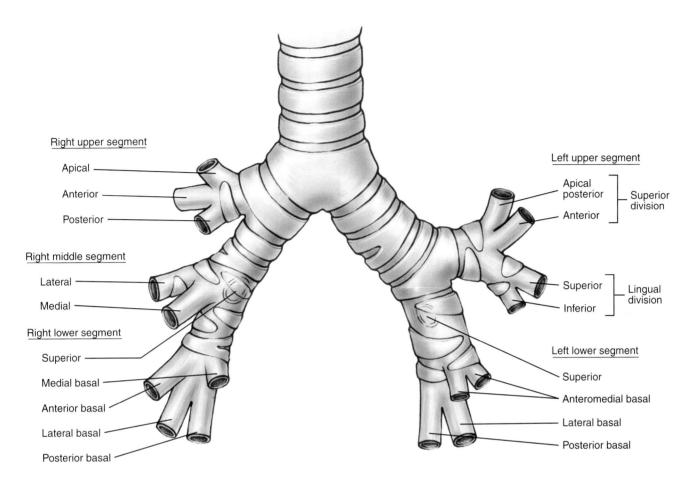

Right upper segment
Apical
Anterior
Posterior

Right middle segment
Lateral
Medial

Right lower segment
Superior
Medial basal
Anterior basal
Lateral basal
Posterior basal

Left upper segment
Apical posterior — Superior division
Anterior
Superior — Lingual division
Inferior

Left lower segment
Superior
Anteromedial basal
Lateral basal
Posterior basal

The lung is generally composed of 18 segments (10 on the right, eight on the left). The right lung has more parenchymal mass and is composed of three lobes: the upper, middle, and lower lobes, which are separated by two fissures. The major fissure runs obliquely from posterior to anterior, beginning at the level of the fifth rib posteriorly, following the course of the sixth rib, and ending at the diaphragm near the sixth costochondral junction. The horizontal fissure separates the upper lobe from the middle lobe, beginning in the oblique fissure in the midaxillary line at the level of the sixth rib and running anteriorly to the fourth costochondral junction. Within the right upper lobe are three bronchopulmonary segments: apical, posterior, and anterior. The right middle lobe is composed of a medial and lateral segment. The right lower lobe is composed of five segments: superior, medial basal, anterior basal, lateral basal, and posterior basal. Within the segments the course of the bronchus is most consistent. The segmental pulmonary artery follows the course of the bronchus but is more variable. The bronchus and pulmonary artery are centrally located within the segment, but the pulmonary veins course along the plane formed by adjacent segments, draining those adjacent segments. The pulmonary veins form the boundaries of the segments.

The left lung is composed of eight bronchopulmonary segments, four in the upper lobe and four in the lower lobe. The left upper lobe consists of an apical posterior, anterior, and two lingular segments (the superior lingular and inferior lingular segments). The upper lobe is separated from the lower lobe by a single obliquely running fissure that starts at about the level of the fourth rib and proceeds anteriorly and inferiorly to end near the sixth or seventh costochondral junction. The lingular segments of the upper lobe are anatomically equivalent to those of the right middle lobe. The left lower lobe is composed of the remaining four segments: superior, anteromedial basal, lateral basal, and posterior basal.

Accessory fissures do occur, producing unusual or anomalous lobulations. These fissures usually are found where the planes separating bronchopulmonary segments are located. Such lobes have been termed the posterior accessory, inferior accessory, and left middle lobe. Rarely an accessory segmental bronchus arises from the trachea. This bronchus usually goes to the apical segment of the right upper lobe.

Right Hilum

Knowledge and familiarity of the anatomic spatial relationships between the bronchus, pulmonary artery, and pulmonary veins is essential for pulmonary resection. Centrally located tumors may require intrapericardial control of the vascular structures. The most superior and posterior structure of the right hilum is the right main stem bronchus, which emanates from the carina (at the level of the T4 vertebra) and travels inferior to the azygous vein before dividing into the right upper lobe lobar bronchus approximately 1 to 2 cm from the origin of the right main stem bronchus and the bronchus intermedius. The bronchus intermedius is 1.5 to 2 cm long and terminates in the right middle lobe bronchus anteriorly and the right lower lobe bronchus posteriorly and slightly inferiorly. Each of the lobar bronchi give rise to segmental bronchi named for the bronchopulmonary segments.

The main pulmonary artery arises from the right ventricular outflow tract and divides within the cradle of the aortic arch into the right and left main pulmonary arteries. The right pulmonary artery passes to the right hilum posterior (deep) to the ascending aorta and posterior to the superior vena cava, toward the right lung parenchyma. It gives off its first branch, the truncus anterior, before entering the lung. The right pulmonary artery is anterior and inferior to the right main stem bronchus.

The third major hilar structure proceeding in an inferior direction is the right superior pulmonary vein. The tributary pulmonary veins originate between bronchopulmonary segments draining adjacent segments. Variations are not infrequent. Three branches from the right upper lobe (apical anterior, anterior inferior, and posterior) are joined by a fourth major branch that drains the middle lobe. This inferior-most venous tributary is composed of two smaller branches draining the right middle lobe. Occasionally the right middle lobe vein drains directly into the left atrium, and rarely the right inferior pulmonary vein. The right superior pulmonary vein enters the pericardium to empty into the left atrium. A predominance (approximately two thirds) of the vein is intrapericardial. A common pulmonary vein draining all three lobes occurs in 3% of patients. The right superior pulmonary vein is anterior and slightly inferior to the first branch of the pulmonary artery, obscuring the continuation of the pulmonary artery as it becomes interlobar.

The right inferior pulmonary vein is the inferior-most structure of the right hilum, lying inferior and posterior to the superior vein. This vein is composed of two tributaries draining the right lower lobe: the superior segmental vein and the common basal vein. The bronchus intermedius is superior and anterior to the right inferior pulmonary vein.

Anterior to the hilum on the lateral pericardium is the intrathoracic phrenic nerve. Posterior to the hilum is the vagus nerve and the esophagus.

Left Hilum

The most superior structure in the left hilum is the left pulmonary artery. The left pulmonary artery is shorter than the right pulmonary artery and passes inferior to the aortic arch to lie anterior and superior to the remaining hilar structures. The left pulmonary artery is tethered to the aortic arch by the ductus arteriosus remnant, the ligamentous arteriosum. The left recurrent nerve is located lateral to the ligament as it courses around the aorta to travel superiorly. The truncus anterior is the first branch of the left pulmonary artery, a much shorter vessel than its right counterpart. It supplies the anterior segment of the left upper lobe. Directly inferiorly and slightly anterior to the left pulmonary artery is the left main stem bronchus. At the carina the left main stem bronchus passes to the left under the aortic arch. It is longer and more acutely angled than the right main stem bronchus. It travels 4 to 6 cm before giving off its first branch, the left upper lobe bronchus. The left upper lobe bronchus bifurcates after 1.5 cm into a superior branch and an inferior or lingular branch. The superior bronchus subsequently divides into apical posterior and anterior segmental bronchi. The lingular branch divides into superior and inferior segmental bronchi after 1 to 2 cm. A short distance, less than 1 cm, beyond the left upper lobe orifice the left lower lobe bronchus gives off the superior segmental bronchus. The basal bronchus extends an additional 1 to 1.5 cm to bifurcate into an anteromedial basal segmental bronchus and a common segmental bronchus to the lateral and posterior basal segments.

Directly anterior to the left main stem bronchus is the superior pulmonary vein, the most anterior structure of the left hilum. The left superior pulmonary vein is anterior and inferior to the left pulmonary artery. The left superior pulmonary vein is formed by three intersegmental veins: the apical posterior, anterior, and lingular. The lingular branch is solitary 50% of the time, but has a superior and inferior branch 50% of the time. It occasionally drains into the inferior pulmonary vein. The left inferior pulmonary vein is the most inferior structure of the left hilum, inferior and posterior to the left superior pulmonary vein. It is composed of two tributaries: the superior and inferior basal veins. As the left pulmonary veins are invested by pericardium, they join to form a common trunk before entering the left atrium in up to 25% of patients.

The esophagus and left vagus are posterior to the left hilum. Anomalies of the pulmonary arteries, veins, and bronchi are described in textbooks of congenital heart surgery.

Blood Supply and Nerve Supply

The bronchial system has its own systemic arterial blood supply. This arterial supply is variable, more constant on the right than left, and generally arises from the anterolateral aspect of the descending aorta within 2 to 3 cm distal to the left subclavian artery takeoff. Origin of the bronchial arteries may be an intercostal artery and, infrequently, the subclavian or innominate artery. A common origin of the left and right bronchial arterial supply exists in 20% of patients.

The right bronchial artery arises in common with an intercostal artery from the descending thoracic aorta between T5 and T6 in the majority of cases, courses anteriorly along the anterolateral aspect of the vertebral column, and crosses the esophagus to end near the origin of the right main stem bronchus. The left bronchial artery arises from the descending aorta in the great majority of cases, but is more variable in its course to the left main stem bronchus. It usually travels posterior to the trachea toward the origin of the left main stem bronchus. As the right and left bronchial arteries enter the membranous bronchi, they form a communicating arc around the bronchus anteriorly and posteriorly with multiple intercommunicating branches that follow the arborization of the bronchus. Anastomosis occurs with the pulmonary artery distally.

A dual venous system exists to drain the bronchi. Tributary segmental veins coalesce and eventually empty into the pulmonary venous system. This accounts for the majority of venous drainage. The bronchial veins are present in the bronchial mucosa and also externally. Approximately one third of the venous tributaries form larger veins, which flow into a perihilar venous plexus that eventually empties into the azygous system on the right and the hemiazygous system on the left.

The sympathetic plexus and the parasympathetic plexus via the vagi supply nerve rami to both lungs that control the smooth muscle of the bronchi, the bronchial arteries, and the bronchial glands. The nerves reach the hilum, where an anterior plexus is formed about the pulmonary artery and a posterior plexus around the bronchi. From these sites the nerve branches pass into the lung parenchyma, where periarterial plexuses (nonmyelinated) and peribronchial plexuses (myelinated and nonmyelinated) are formed.

SURGICAL APPLICATIONS
Posterolateral Thoracotomy

Posterolateral thoracotomy remains the most popular access route into the thoracic cavity for pulmonary resection. It previously has been mentioned for distal tracheal and right main stem bronchus resections. The patient is positioned on a beanbag in the lateral position. It is essential to have proper protection and cushioning of pressure points to prevent injuries due to positioning. Pillows are placed above and below the flexed lower leg. The upper leg is rested on the underlying pillow and kept straight. The patient is then secured in position by deflating the beanbag and using adhesive tape over the hips. A soft pliable roll is placed under the axilla to prevent pressure on the brachial plexus. The lower arm may be extended straight on an arm board or flexed at the elbow and placed next to the head. The upper arm is cushioned on an arm sling or brought up and suspended in a right angle to the thorax, thus rotating the scapula forward. A warming blanket, arterial and central venous monitoring, Foley catheter, and single-lung ventilation utilizing a double-lumen endotracheal tube or bronchial blocker are standard.

The incision is begun at the anterior axillary line and extended posterolaterally 2 to 3 cm inferior to the scapular tip and then superiorly paralleling the vertebral spines and vertebral border of the scapula. This is approximately the course of the fifth rib. The electrocautery is used to deepen the incision through the subcutaneous tissues until the aponeurosis of the latissimus muscle is identified. The latissimus muscle is divided. The inferior border of the trapezius muscle is mobilized posteriorly, and occasionally it may need to be incised. The serratus anterior muscle is reflected off the anterior chest wall and retracted anteriorly; the posterior edge may be removed from its rib insertion for increased exposure. Ribs are palpated from the superior first rib downward to the fifth rib. Any interspace from third to tenth may be entered, but the fifth interspace provides the best exposure of the hilar structures. It is generally unnecessary to remove a rib. The thoracolumbar fascia and paravertebral muscles are elevated with the electrocautery and retracted; they need not be divided. After the intercostal space is chosen, the three layers of intercostal muscles and the deep parietal pleura are divided along the upper border of the lower rib, utilizing the electrocautery and avoiding the intercostal neurovascular bundle. A medium rib spreader is placed anteriorly and a large rib spreader is placed posteriorly within the interspace to separate the ribs and expose the thoracic contents.

Limited or Muscle-Sparing Thoracotomy

The limited or muscle-sparing thoracotomy is my preference for exposure of the thoracic contents. It provides excellent exposure of the intrathoracic contents for most resections, with as little disturbance of chest wall muscles and therefore chest wall mechanics as practical. It can be performed with less risk in patients with marginal pulmonary function and heals with an acceptably cosmetic result. A vertical incision is begun at the base of the axilla in the mid-axillary line and extended inferiorly to the level of the eighth or ninth rib. Subcutaneous tissues are divided until the anterior edge of the latissimus muscle is identified. A latissimus myocutaneous flap is elevated and retracted posteriorly, then carried inferiorly or deeply to the vertebral spinous processes. The posterior edge of the serratus muscle is reflected with the electrocautery; it may be necessary to sever the muscle from its posterior rib insertions. The fifth intercostal space is identified and entered. A suction drain is placed underneath the latissimus flap after closure of the incision, because a seroma frequently develops (20% of cases).

Median Sternotomy Incision

The median sternotomy incision is occasionally utilized for pulmonary resection and has the advantage of causing the least disturbance of pulmonary mechanics postoperatively. The incision begins in the midline at the suprasternal notch and extends inferiorly to just below the xiphi sternum. The electrocautery is used to divide the subcutaneous tissues down to and including the medial aspect of the superficial pectoral fascia. Distally (caudally) the linea alba is divided in the midline. The pectoral fascia and anterior periosteum of the sternum are divided with the electrocautery. Two venous structures are remarkably constant: one at the suprasternal notch, identified as the jugular arch connecting the left and right anterior jugular veins (sometimes called the transternal vein), and a venous branch crossing the midline just above the xiphoid. These veins should be anticipated and clipped or ligated to prevent unnecessary and sometimes torrential blood loss. The sternum is divided in the midline with a reciprocating electric or air-powered saw, such as the Sarnes sternal saw. The footpad of the saw should be hooked beneath the suprasternal notch and the saw brought inferiorly left to right or the blade reversed and the saw placed inferiorly and brought superiorly right to left, which I prefer. Care should be exercised to keep the footpad in close contact with the posterior table of the sternum to prevent injury to the underlying structures or inadvertent pleural injury. An oscillating saw allows more precise control of the depth of penetration of the sternal saw and should be used when prior sternotomy has been performed or when the surgeon suspects that tumor abuts the posterior sternal table. Hemostasis of the anterior and posterior periosteum is obtained with discreet use of the electrocautery. Bone wax may be used sparingly to seal the bleeding marrow. Sterile towels are placed along the sternal edges, and a sternal retractor is placed in the incision. This approach provides excellent hilar exposure for right-sided pneumonectomy or lobectomies of the right upper, middle, and lower lobes. Control and division of the right inferior pulmonary vein are sometimes difficult during right lower lobectomy due to the posterior position of the right inferior pulmonary vein. Left upper lobectomy may also be performed. Left pneumonectomy and left lower lobectomy are often difficult, somewhat dangerous, and frequently impossible because the left inferior pulmonary vein underlies the left ventricle, and retraction or manipulation of the heart causes hypotension and arrhythmias. Finally, this approach is preferred for bilateral metastectomy by wedge excision for pulmonary metastasis.

Pulmonary Resection

Lobectomy and pneumonectomy are the most frequently performed resections for pulmonary malignancy. Wedge resection and segmentectomy do not have the same long-term survival as lobectomy for similarly staged lesions. In-depth description of bronchoplastic parenchymal-sparing procedures and other thoracic surgical procedures is beyond the scope and purpose of this text; the interested reader is referred to Kaiser and Aretz's *Atlas of General Thoracic Sugery* or Urschel and Cooper's *Atlas of Thoracic Surgery* for supplemental reading.

Lobectomy did not become the standard anatomic dissection for lung cancer until Churchill et al. reported the Massachusetts General Hospital series in 1950. Lobectomy is the preferred treatment for peripheral stage I, stage II, and selected stage IIIA lung cancers. After the pleural space is entered, the entire lung and pleura are inspected for synchronous tumors or metastasis not evident on preoperative imaging studies, and the feasibility of lobectomy is determined. If complete resection encompassing all tumor is possible, the inferior pulmonary ligament, anterior and posterior mediastinal pleurae, and all adhesions are divided with the electrocautery. The inferior pulmonary ligament (station 9) and periesophageal (station 8) lymph nodes are excised for pathologic staging so as not to be forgotten during the later formal lymph node dissection. Division of the pleurae facilitates hilar and lymph node dissections. Generally the pulmonary vein or veins are ligated or stapled first to maintain the "no touch technique," preventing tumor cell embolization. The fissure is then entered and completed with a linear stapler. The pulmonary artery branches are divided with ligatures or staples (3.5 mm vascular staples). Finally, the bronchus is mobilized and stapled with a 3.5 or 4.8 mm stapling device. The surgeon should take care not to devascularize the bronchus and avoid compromising the main stem bronchus or remaining lobar bronchi with a stapled bronchial closure. The bronchial stump may also be hand sewn. Margins are checked for tumor with frozen-section analysis. Many surgeons prefer ligation of pulmonary artery branches first to avert congestion of the lung by blood retention, believing that manipulation of the tumor rarely releases viable tumor cells into the venous outflow.

Right Upper Lobectomy

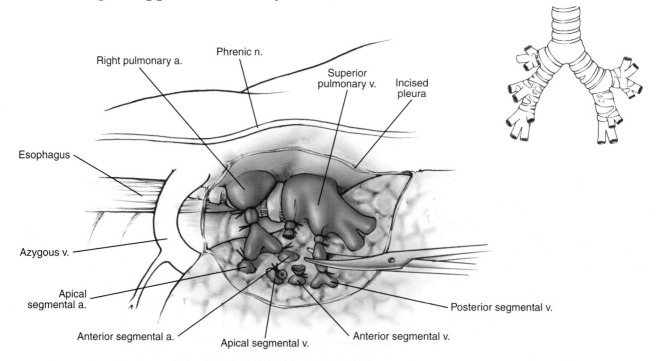

The right upper lobe is most frequently resected. After division of the anterior mediastinal pleura, the right superior pulmonary vein is identified and its tributaries, the apical anterior, inferior, and posterior veins, are encircled with silk ligatures. Great care must be used in identifying and sparing the venous tributary from the right middle lobe as it enters the superior vein. If it has been previously determined that all tumor will be encompassed by the lobectomy, these branches may be doubly ligated and divided. The truncus anterior is the first and usually the largest branch of the right pulmonary artery and may be the only pulmonary artery branch in 10% of patients. It bifurcates within 1 to 1.5 cm. It should be encircled at the origin and, after the bifurcation, doubly ligated and divided. The right pulmonary artery proceeds on into the lung parenchyma, giving off one (60%), two (29%), or three (1%) ascending branches that originate along the anterosuperior border of the pulmonary artery and enter the inferior surface of the right upper lobe. These branches are most easily dissected and ligated through the completed major and minor fissure. The posterior ascending artery is the most common, occurring in 88% of patients. After the vasculature is divided, the lung is retracted medially and the bronchus to the upper lobe exposed as it originates from the lateral wall of the right main stem bronchus, approximately 2 cm from the origin of the right main stem bronchus. Its anterior and posterior surfaces are dissected sharply and bluntly. The bronchial arterial supply to the remaining lung and bronchus should be disturbed as little as possible to avert bronchial stump breakdown. The bronchus is then stapled (4.8 mm staples) and margins of the specimen examined. The surgeon should remember that rarely (1%) an anomalous apical segmental bronchus will arise from the trachea or right main stem bronchus. When the

minor fissure is complete, the right middle lobe should be placed in its anatomically correct position and secured to the right lower lobe to avert possible torsion.

Right Middle Lobectomy

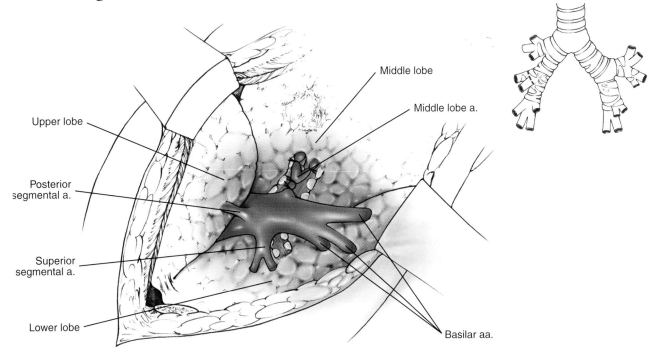

Right middle lobectomy is performed less often than other lobectomies. It is
sometimes performed as part of a bilobectomy when the minor fissure is crossed
by tumor, necessitating right upper-middle lobectomy, or when the tumor is
anterior and crosses the major fissure, necessitating right middle-lower lobectomy. It may be necessary to perform a bilobectomy when N1 lymph nodes
(stations 12, 13, and 14) are involved from a lower lobe tumor. Involvement of
the bronchus intermedius dictates bilobectomy of the right middle and lower
lobes.

 The right middle lobe receives one or two branches from the pars intralobares. These branches are most easily found by dissection at the minor fissure–
major fissure junction. The second artery is encountered first when proceeding
in this direction, emanating from the anteromedial surface opposite the branch
to the superior segment of the right lower lobe. This artery is doubly ligated
and divided. The first branch to the right middle lobe is larger and the next
branch of the pulmonary artery after the truncus anterior. It is found on the
anteromedial surface opposite the ascending branch to the right upper lobe.
This artery usually has a wide base of origin, and care in ligation and division
should be exercised to avert fracture of the delicate pars intralobares. Division
of this branch will expose the solitary right middle lobe bronchus, which travels
approximately 1.5 to 2 cm before branching into middle and lateral segmental
bronchi. The bronchus is stapled and divided. The remaining structure to be

dissected, ligated, and divided is the anteriorly placed right middle lobe vein formed by medial and lateral intrasegmental tributaries and draining into the right superior pulmonary vein. It is usually the most inferior branch of the superior vein and may be ligated first or last. One or both of the fissures may need to be completed with a linear stapler to finish the lobectomy.

Right Lower Lobectomy

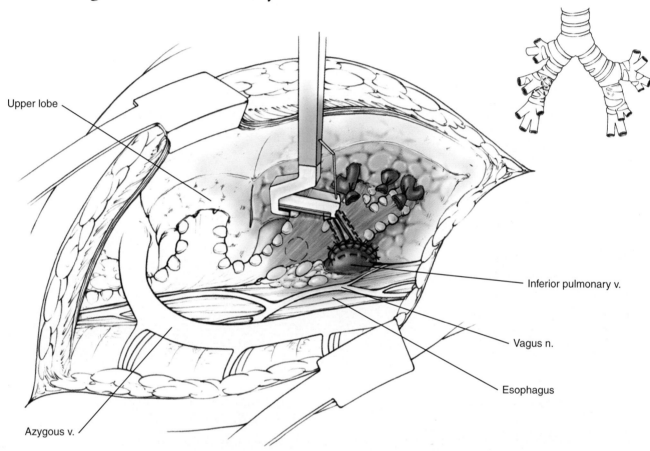

Right lower lobectomy is begun similarly to right middle lobectomy by dissecting in the central portion of the major fissure or at the junction of the two fissures. I find it easier to begin at the junction of the two fissures, identifying the right middle lobe artery followed by the basilar arteries. The most posterior branch of the pars intralobares is the branch to the superior segment of the right lower lobe. More than 75% of the time the posterosuperior segment is supplied by one artery, the remainder of the time by two. This branch or branches are doubly ligated and divided, providing better access to the basilar branches. The basal segmental arterial supply is variable, consisting of one to three branches arising from the inferior aspect of the pulmonary artery. One branch supplies the anterior and medial segments. The pars intralobares then terminates by dividing into lateral and posterior basal segmental arteries. The basilar branches can frequently be stapled after dividing the posterosuperior branch. Two intrasegmental vessels, the superior and common basal veins, form the inferior pulmonary vein. There tends to be a greater extrapericardial segment of this vein, allowing it to be doubly stapled and divided. The final structure to be divided is the right lower lobe bronchus, which originates at the termination of the bronchus intermedius. It divides into a superior segmental bronchus opposite and anterior to the middle lobe bronchus. The four basal segmental bronchi are the medial basal (most proximal), anterior basal, and then a common segmental bronchus to the lateral and posterior segments. Great care must be taken before dividing the bronchus to ensure that the right middle lobe bronchus is not compromised. Because the bronchus intermedius terminates abruptly, the distance between the right middle and lower lobe orifices is minimal. When the superior segment bronchus takes off high or early it may be necessary to close this bronchus and the basilar bronchus separately.

Left Upper Lobectomy

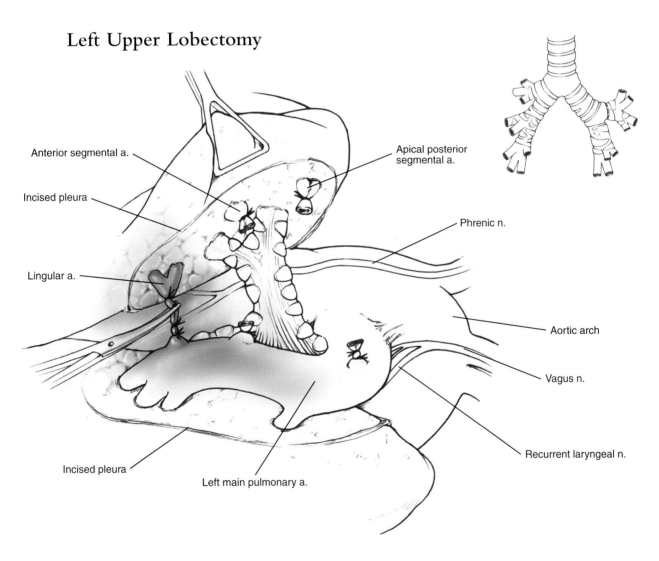

Left upper lobectomy is frequently the most challenging of all pulmonary resections for two reasons: (1) the presence of the left recurrent nerve in the aortopulmonary window is near the dissection and lymphadenectomy, and (2) the lingular, anterior posterior, and anterior segmental vessels are short and broad based, making inadvertent traction tears not infrequent. Injury to the fragile pulmonary artery may be difficult to repair, forcing the surgeon to perform a pneumonectomy to prevent blood loss.

As on the right side, the mediastinal pleura surrounding the hilum and the inferior pulmonary ligament are divided with the electrocautery. After it has been determined that the tumor can be resected totally by lobectomy, the upper lobe is retracted superiorly and the lower lobe inferiorly, exposing the major fissure. Dissection is begun posteriorly and directed anteriorly to expose and mobilize pulmonary artery branches to the lingula. The major fissure is completed by division with a linear stapler. Dissection is then gently advanced cephalad to mobilize and isolate first the posterior branch, then the anterior branch. The anterior branch is often the shortest artery and therefore most easily injured by traction. Some authors advocate ligation of the segmental arteries at this point; however, I have found that division of the left superior pulmonary vein prior to division of the segmental arteries is safer and facilitates exposure of the anterior segmental artery. The lung is retracted posteriorly and slightly inferiorly to expose the anterior hilum and the superior pulmonary vein. The superior pulmonary vein is generally formed from three intrasegmental veins: the anterior, apical posterior, and lingular veins. These structures are doubly ligated and divided or stapled if sufficient extrapericardial vein exists. Division of the vein exposes the underlying truncus anterior. Circumnavigation of the vein must be carefully and deliberately performed to prevent injury to the underlying segmental artery.

Attention is then turned to the major fissure. The lingular branch or branches may be doubly ligated and divided. The next branches to be ligated are the posterior segmental branches (none to five in number), which are small and emanate from the medial inside curve of the pulmonary artery. The apicoposterior branch is now ligated. The short anterior segmental artery is ligated and divided. The last structure to be divided is the left upper lobe bronchus. The left upper lobe bronchus arises much more distally down the left main stem bronchus than its right counterpart. It immediately splits into the lingular orifice and common trunk to the anterior and apicoposterior segments. The bronchus is sharply and bluntly skeletonized and divided with a 4.8 mm stapling device.

Left Lower Lobectomy

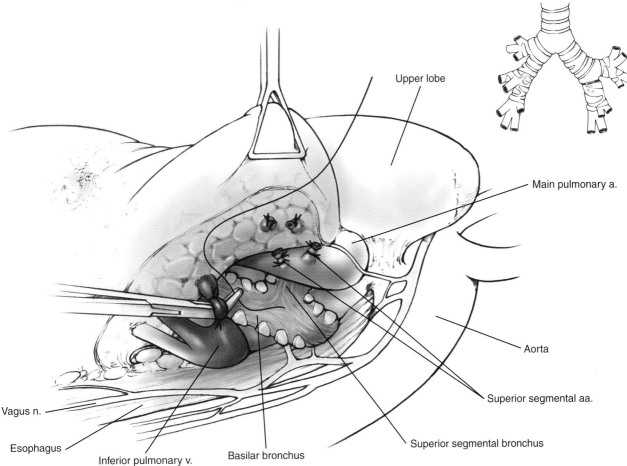

Left lower lobectomy is by far the easiest to perform. The inferior pulmonary vein is formed by two intrasegmental branches: the superior segmental and common basal. Sufficient extrapericardial length usually exists for stapling the main inferior vein. The major fissure is now entered to expose the superior segmental artery (generally a single artery, double in 25% of patients). After giving off the superior segmental artery the left pulmonary artery terminates in two to four basilar arteries, usually one to the anterior medial segment and a second supplying the posterior and lateral segments. These arteries are doubly ligated and divided. The lower lobe bronchus is now easily visible. The lower lobe bronchus originates at the termination of the left main stem bronchus. It quickly bifurcates into a posterior lateral segmental bronchus to the superior segment and, 1 to 2 cm distally, a common basal bronchus that then bifurcates (80%) or trifurcates. The bronchus is divided with a 4.8 mm stapler to complete the resection.

Right and Left Pneumonectomy

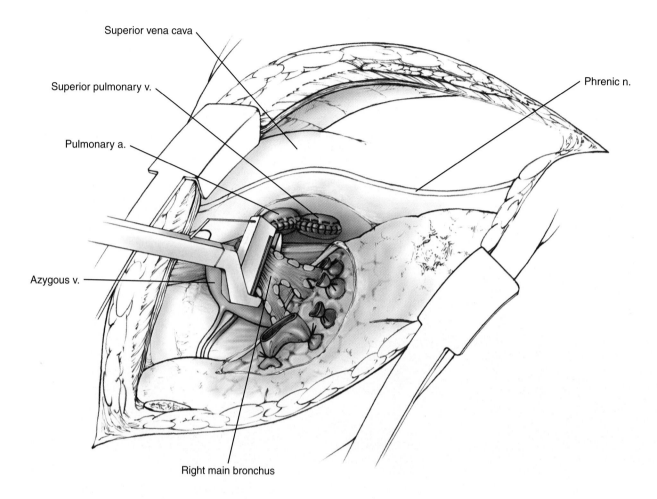

Superior vena cava

Superior pulmonary v.

Pulmonary a.

Azygous v.

Phrenic n.

Right main bronchus

Early attempts at pulmonary resection for malignancy began with an attempt to remove the whole lung containing the tumor. Multiple methods were tried, but not until 1933 did a patient survive the early postoperative period. By 1940 pneumonectomy had become the accepted technique for removing resectable pulmonary malignancies, despite mortality ranging from 15% to 20%. Presently the indications for pneumonectomy are (1) centrally located lung cancer, (2) lung cancer crossing major fissures, or (3) lung cancer not amenable to lobectomy. Mortality is approximately 6%.

The surgical approach is most often posterolateral thoracotomy. Once the extent of the disease is established and resectability ensured, the inferior pulmonary ligament and mediastinal pleura surrounding the hilum are divided with an electrocautery. The pulmonary artery and pulmonary veins are skeletonized. Which vessels are addressed first is dictated by the size and location of the tumor, and the surgeon should be flexible. If practical and safe, the veins are divided first. The inferior veins on both the left and right are generally the most accessible. The lung is retracted first superiorly to dissect the inferior surface, then anteriorly and superiorly to dissect the posterior surface, and finally posteriorly to dissect the anterior surface. The vein is then doubly stapled and divided. The superior veins are divided similarly. Great care must be exercised because the superior veins are closely approximated and often adherent to the underlying pulmonary artery. Inadvertent injury to the truncus anterior may be associated with audible blood loss. When a tumor is palpated within the veins, the dissection should be carried intrapericardially and the veins divided with a cuff (1 to 2 mm) of atrium. The pulmonary artery is divided next by first dividing the truncus anterior. This allows greater length to be obtained for stapling the main pulmonary artery. The pulmonary artery is doubly stapled and divided, taking care not to produce a traction injury. When the tumor is closely adherent to the pulmonary artery it may be necessary to divide the pericardium anteriorly to gain additional length. Further additional length on the left can be obtained by dividing the ligamentum arteriosum, carefully averting traction on or injury to the left recurrent nerve. On the right the superior vena cava can be mobilized and the artery divided medial to the superior vena cava. An initial maneuver that should be performed is to encircle the artery with a vascular tape prior to mobilization. This allows vascular control, which may be lifesaving if the artery is injured.

The main stem bronchus is most often divided last. The bronchus should be divided as proximal as possible, disrupting the bronchial arterial supply as little as possible. The carina should be identified and the bronchus divided with a 4.8 mm stapler or divided and closed with absorbable sutures placed anterior to posterior. The bronchus is then tested by insufflation of the airway to 35 cm static peak airway pressure. I prefer to cover the bronchus with autogenous tissue: pericardium, pericardial fat, pleura, intercostal muscle, or on the right the divided azygous vein. A 28 Fr chest tube is tunneled into the chest to allow positioning of the mediastinum and as a possible monitor of blood loss. When the patient is turned to the supine position, the remaining lung is hyperexpanded with positive pressure and the chest tube clamped. The chest tube is removed in 24 hours. Some authors prefer not to use a chest tube and aspirate approximately 1000 ml of air to bring the mediastinum back to the midline. Other surgeons prefer to use a balanced drainage system.

Mediastinal Lymph Node Dissection

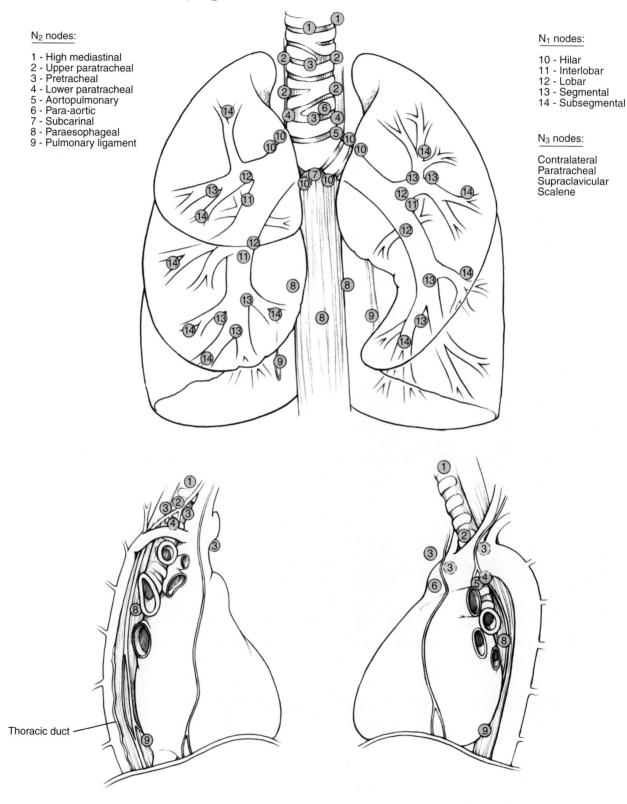

N₂ nodes:

1 - High mediastinal
2 - Upper paratracheal
3 - Pretracheal
4 - Lower paratracheal
5 - Aortopulmonary
6 - Para-aortic
7 - Subcarinal
8 - Paraesophageal
9 - Pulmonary ligament

N₁ nodes:

10 - Hilar
11 - Interlobar
12 - Lobar
13 - Segmental
14 - Subsegmental

N₃ nodes:

Contralateral
Paratracheal
Supraclavicular
Scalene

Thoracic duct

Perhaps the most important part of pulmonary resection and probably the least often correctly performed is proper lymph node dissection. Two chest tubes are placed: a right-angle tube into the apex and a straight tube posteriorly. The bronchial stump should be checked under water to 35 cm of static peak airway pressure.

It is essential that the surgeon know the drainage pattern to the various lymph node groups from each lobe. The regional nodal stations and their designated numbers are illustrated. Basic dissection technique requires that the lymph nodes be left intact and therefore are usually dissected as part of an en bloc fatty tissue specimen that includes the lymph nodes. Small blood vessels and lymphatic vessels should be ligated rather than cauterized to prevent postoperative bleeding and exudation of lymph.

Right upper lobectomy should be combined with dissection of lymph nodes in the superior mediastinum and right peritracheal and subcarinal areas. Metastasis from right upper lobe tumors involves the right upper lobe peribronchial, lobar, and intralobar hilar superior mediastinal nodes. Metastasis to nodes of the middle and lower lobes from a right upper lobe tumor is uncommon.

Resection of the middle lobe for middle lobe tumors should be accompanied by dissection of the hilar, subcarinal, and right peritracheal lymph nodes. Middle lobe tumors more frequently metastasize to the sump lymph nodes. Therefore it may be necessary to perform a bilobectomy to resect the entire nodal drainage system.

Right lower lobe tumors metastasize to the subcarinal area and the peritracheal area. They also tend to metastasize to sump nodes around the middle lobe. Therefore, as with right middle lobe tumors, bilobectomy may be necessary to encompass all lymph nodes affected.

Dissection of the right mediastinal lymph nodes generally involves resection of the right peritracheal lymph nodes in the 2R and 4R areas, the pretracheal lymph nodes (station 3), and the subcarinal lymph nodes (station 7).

An incision is made with an electrocautery parallel to the trachea and superior vena cava. The azygous vein may be divided if lymph nodes are enlarged or access is difficult. The underlying fat pad containing the right peritracheal lymph nodes is then excised using sharp and blunt dissection, clipping lymphatic vessels and blood vessels as necessary. The pretracheal (station 3) and tracheobronchial angle (station 4) are taken with this lymph node pad. The dissection is carried up to the level of the right subclavian artery. Care should be taken to avoid the right recurrent laryngeal nerve and the right phrenic nerve.

The subcarinal lymph nodes are dissected by entering the subcarinal space. Dissection is begun at the edge of the right main stem bronchus and carried to the carina, then 2 cm down the left main stem bronchus. All attempts should be made to not crush the lymph nodes. Special lymph node forceps can be used to hold the fat pad that contains the lowest subcarinal lymph nodes (station 7) and the contralateral left main bronchial lymph nodes (station 10). The bronchial artery to the right main stem bronchus may frequently need to be ligated and divided.

On the left side the left upper lobe tumors drain into the sump nodes between the lobes (stations 11 and 12). Pretracheal lymph nodes (station 3) may also be sites of metastasis. All peribronchial lymph nodes (station 4L) should also be taken. It is unnecessary to resect the paraesophageal (station 8) or pulmonary ligament (station 9) lymph nodes. However, I frequently do, because it adds little time or morbidity to the procedure. Subcarinal lymph nodes are resected similarly to those on the right. Resection of the left upper lobe should also include resection of periaortic (ascending aorta or phrenic) lymph nodes (station 6) and subaortic (aortopulmonary window) lymph nodes (station 5). Great care should be taken in dissecting the aortopulmonary window lymph nodes, as the left recurrent nerve is just lateral to the ligamentum arteriosum. In this area I prefer to identify the nerve first, then resect the fat and lymph nodes within the aortopulmonary window without using the electrocautery.

Tumors of the lower lobe generally metastasize to the pulmonary ligament nodes (station 9), paraesophageal nodes (station 8), and subcarinal lymph nodes (station 7). Therefore it is necessary to resect these nodal areas.

Anatomic Basis of Complications

- Most frequently occurring error is injury to the truncus anterior branch of the pulmonary artery on the left side. This short, friable artery is easily injured by traction. Every effort should be made to produce as little tension on the artery as possible during its dissection and mobilization to avert injury.
- The left recurrent nerve is easily injured during dissection of the aortopulmonary window lymph nodes. This can be prevented by knowing the course and location of the recurrent nerve. The electrocautery should not be used in this area, and extreme care should be maintained during the dissection to prevent inadvertent injury from traction.
- The surgeon should have adequate knowledge of the intrapericardial anatomy of the pulmonary arteries and pulmonary veins if control of these vascular structures is needed in the event of their injury during dissection of large tumors.
- Resection of the right upper or lower lobe may leave the right middle lobe bronchus in a precarious or compromised position. The right middle lobe bronchus must not be injured or narrowed during bronchial resection of the right upper or lower lobe. Compromise of the right middle lobe bronchus leads to atelectasis and eventual infection of the lobe that is difficult to manage.

KEY REFERENCES

Baye GH. Recherches sur la Phthrisie Pulmonaire. Paris Gabon, 1810, pp 24-34.
This is a classic antique paper.

Churchill ED, Sweet RH, Sutton L, et al. The surgical management of carcinoma of the lung. A study of cases treated at the Massachusetts General Hospital from 1930-1950. J Thorac Cardiovasc Surg 20:349-356, 1950.
This article is a major historical landmark presentation from the Massachusetts General Hospital.

Davies HM. Recent advances in the surgery of the lung and pleura. Br J Surg 1:228, 1913.
This paper from 1913 presents the state of the art at that time.

Ginsberg RJ, Hill LD, Eagan RT, et al. Modern 30-day operative mortality for surgical resections in lung cancer. J Thorac Cardiovasc Surg 86:654-658, 1983.
This paper from 1983 reported the "modern" operative mortality rates for surgical resection.

Ginsberg RJ, Rubenstein LC. Randomized trial of lobectomy versus limited resection for T1N0 nonsmall cell cancer (Lung Cancer Study Group). Ann Thorac Surg 60:615-623, 1995.
This paper established the value and importance of adequate resection.

Graham EA, Singer J. Successful removal of an entire lung for carcinoma of the bronchus. JAMA 101:1371, 1933.
This is a classic description of the first successful removal of the entire lung.

Haepting GH, Hesse W. Der Lungenkrebs, die Bergkrankheit in den Schneeberger Gruben. Vrtjschr Gerlichti Med 30:296, 31:102, 1879.
This German paper from 1879 is an historical note.

Landis SH, Murray T, Bolden S, et al. Cancer statistics in 1998. CA Cancer J Clin 48:6-29, 1998.
This is the 32nd annual compilation of cancer incidence, mortality, and survival data for the United States and around the world. It is published by the Department of Epidemiology and Surveillance of the American Cancer Society.

Mountain CF. A new international staging system for lung cancer. Chest 89:225S-233S, 1986.
This article provides an explanation of the staging system.

Mountain CF. Revisions in the international system for staging lung cancer. Chest 111:1710-1717, 1997.

The revisions to the staging system are explained in this article.

Pearson FG. Lung cancer: The past 25 years. Chest 89:200S-205S, 1986.

This keynote address at the Fourth World Conference on Lung Cancer summarizes the last 25 years of lung cancer treatment.

Wada H, Nakamura T, Nakamoto K, et al. Thirty-day operative mortality for thoracotomy in lung cancer. J Thorac Cardiovasc Surg 115:70-73, 1998.

This current research effort from Japan could be used as a standard when discussing operative outcomes.

SUGGESTED READINGS

Aisner J, Arriagada R, Green M, et al., eds. Comprehensive Textbook of Thoracic Oncology. Baltimore: Williams & Wilkins, 1996.

Fraire AE. Pathology of lung cancer. In Aisner J, Arriagada R, Green MR, et al., eds. Comprehensive Textbook of Thoracic Oncology. Baltimore: Williams & Wilkins, 1996, pp 245-275.

Ginsberg RJ. Alternative (muscle-sparing) incisions in thoracic surgery. The first International Symposium of Thoracoscopic Surgery. Ann Thorac Surg 56:752-754, 1993.

Kaiser LR, Aretz TA. Atlas of General Thoracic Surgery. St Louis: Mosby, 1997.

Kittle FC. History of thoracic surgical oncology. In Beattie EJ, Bloom N, Harvey J, eds. Thoracic Surgical Oncology. New York: Churchill Livingstone, 1992, pp 1-11, 1992.

Kohman LJ. Is there a place for surgery in central small cell lung cancer? Chest Clin North Am 7(1):105-112, 1997.

Rice TW. Anatomy in thoracic surgery. In Pearson FG, Deslauries J, Ginsberg RJ, et al., eds. New York: Churchill Livingstone, 1995, pp 355-369.

Roth JA, Ruckdeschel JC, Weisenberger TH, eds. Thoracic Oncology, 2nd ed. Philadelphia: WB Saunders, 1995.

Urschel HC, Cooper JD. Atlas of Thoracic Surgery. New York: Churchill Livingstone, 1995.

Urschel JD. Surgical treatment of peripheral small cell lung cancer. Chest Clin North Am 7(1):95-103, 1997.

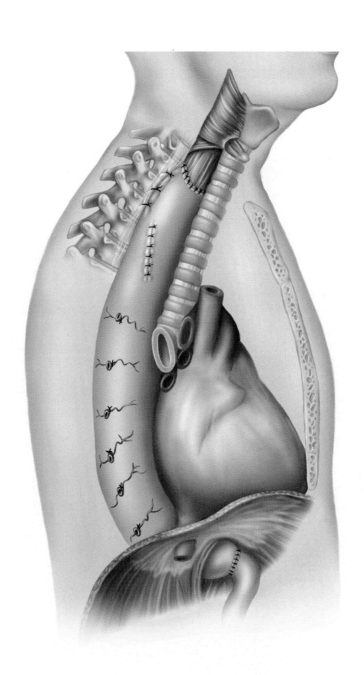

Esophagus and Diaphragm

Panagiotis N. Symbas, M.D., and Nikolas P. Symbas, M.D.

Surgical Applications

Esophagus

Diaphragm

Esophagus

A variety of benign or malignant tumors may arise in the esophagus. Benign tumors may be epithelial, such as polyps, adenomas, papillomas, and cysts, or non-epithelial, such as leiomyomas, fibromas, fibromyomas, and lipomas. The malignant esophageal tumors include the various sarcomas and melanomas and the most common tumors, that is, squamous cell carcinomas and adenocarcinomas.

Carcinoma of the esophagus constitutes approximately 2% of all reported cancers. In the United States, squamous cell carcinoma accounts for 70% of all esophageal tumors, with an incidence of approximately 6 per 100,000 persons. Affected persons most often are between 50 and 70 years of age, and the disease is three to five times more common in men than in women. Esophageal carcinoma should be suspected in any patient with persistent dysphagia, particularly in those older than 40. The diagnosis is established at esophagography and esophagoscopy. During esophagoscopy, esophageal washing for cytologic examination should be obtained, in addition to a biopsy specimen of the esophageal lesion. After the diagnosis of esophageal carcinoma is established, a complete workup, including thoracoabdominal computed tomography (CT), should be performed. In patients with upper and middle third esophageal carcinoma, bronchoscopy should be performed to exclude tumor invasion of the trachea or left main bronchus.

The most common benign tumor of the esophagus is the leiomyoma, comprising 60% to 80% of all benign neoplasms, followed in order of frequency by cysts, lipomas, fibromas, and vascular or neurogenic tumors. Esophageal adenomas, papillomas, granular cell tumors, myxofibromas, and lymphangiomas are rare.

Treatment of both benign and malignant lesions of the esophagus is surgical excision whenever feasible. The type and extent of resection are tailored to the type of lesion.

SURGICAL ANATOMY

The esophagus is a muscular tube connecting the pharynx and stomach. It originates at the lower border of the cricoid cartilage at the level of the sixth cervical vertebra, descends behind the trachea, through the neck, the posterior mediastinum, and the esophageal hiatus, and terminates in the cardia of the stomach opposite the twelfth thoracic vertebra. In general, the axis of the esophagus is straight except for three minor deviations from the midline. The first is toward the left at the base of the neck, the second toward the right at the level of the seventh thoracic vertebra, and the third, the most prominent angulation to the left, is located just above the esophagogastric junction. The length of the esophagus varies with age, sex, and body habitus. In adults, when it is measured using the nostrils or the incisor teeth as a landmark, the length is 13 to 16 cm to the cricoid cartilage, 23 to 26 cm to the tracheal bifurcation, and 36 to 48 cm to the gastric opening.

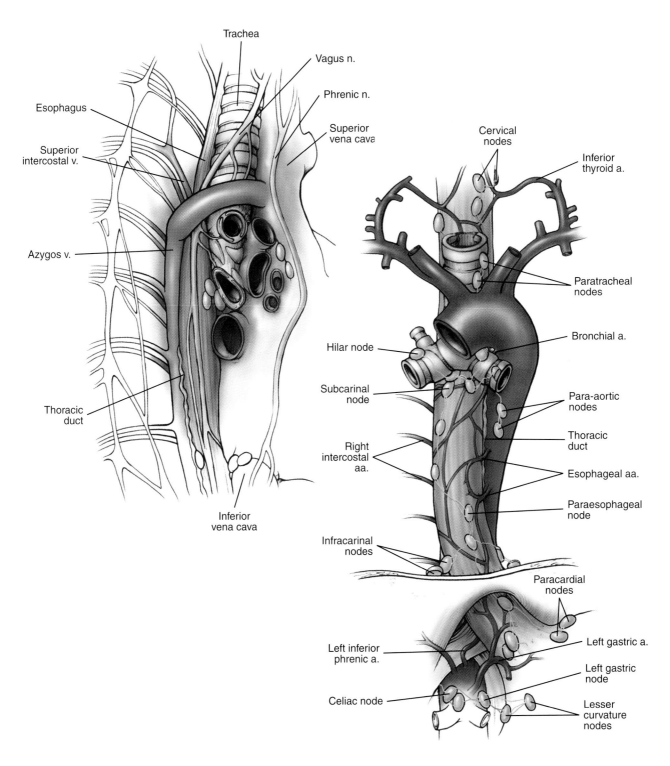

The esophagus is surrounded by many vital structures, making radical en bloc resection of carcinoma virtually impossible. Anterior to the esophagus are the trachea, aortic arch, right pulmonary artery, left main bronchus, pericardium, anterior vagal trunk, and esophageal hiatus. The posteriorly located important structures are the posterior vagal trunk, the anterior wall of the descending aorta, the thoracic duct obliquely from T7 and T4, and the right posterior intercostal arteries. Right laterally situated vital organs are the azygos vein and right main bronchus, and left laterally are the aortic arch, the left recurrent laryngeal nerve, the thoracic duct from T4 to C7, and the descending thoracic aorta. Planned or accidental injury to any of these structures accounts for the major complications during and after esophagectomy.

In the mediastinum the esophagus is enveloped by loose connective tissue that connects it to the neighboring structures and allows great mobility. Within this connective tissue are vessels, nerve fibers, and lymphatic channels and nodes. This anatomic characteristic permits, in selected cases, the so-called blunt esophageal resection. Such resection is not feasible and is hazardous when extraesophageal tumor extension or postinflammatory dense adhesions are present.

The structure of the esophagus parallels that of the rest of the digestive tube, except for lack of a serosal layer. The outer layer of the esophagus, the muscularis externa, consists of a longitudinal and a circular layer. The longitudinal layer represents one sheet of multiple flat and delicate muscle bundles that completely wrap the esophageal wall. The muscle fibers of the circular layer at no place form closed rings, but are circles with superimposed ends. Between these two layers of the muscularis externa are the myenteric ganglia of Auerbach, which, together with those of Meissner's plexus in the submucosa, coordinate esophageal movement.

The mucosal layer consists of nonkeratinizing squamous epithelium. Underneath it is the lamina propria, which contains loose connective tissue, a network of capillaries and lymphatic vessels, and mucus-producing tubular glands. The next layer of the mucosa is the muscularis mucosa, which is composed mainly of bundles of longitudinal smooth muscle. The submucosal layer contains collagenous elastic fibers and blood vessels, nerves, and mucus-producing glands. The collagenous fibers of this layer, together with the muscularis mucosa, are the main structures that provide strength to the esophageal suture line.

The squamous epithelium of the distal esophagus may be destroyed when gastroesophageal regurgitation is present. Cephalad migration of the columnar gastric lining then reepithelizes the injured area. The resulting columnar epithelial lining of the distal esophagus, extending at least 3 cm above the gastroesophageal junction, is Barrett's esophagus. Barrett's esophagus has been diagnosed in 27 patients per 100,000 population, but was found in 375 per 100,000 population at autopsy. In 5% to 10% of patients, the columnar epithelium of Barrett's esophagus becomes dysplastic, which may progress to carcinoma. The true incidence of carcinoma arising from benign Barrett's esophagus is not known, but the estimated risk ranges from 30 to 169 times the risk in the normal population. The overwhelming majority of patients in whom carcinoma develops are middle-aged white men. Because of the greater risk for malignancy, close surveillance of patients with Barrett's esophagus is recommended. The best type of surveillance is not known, but yearly follow-up, increased to every 3 months when dysplasia is discovered, has been found effective to detect early malignancy.

Blood Supply

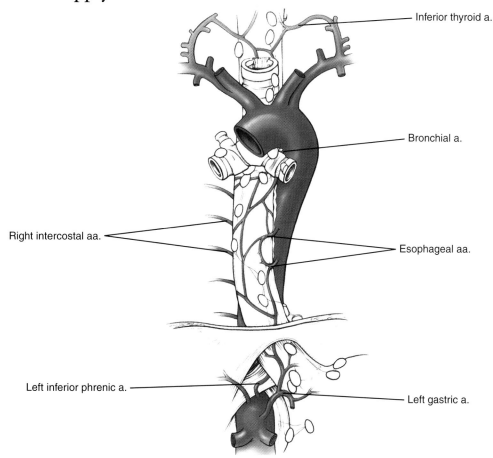

Six pathways provide most of the blood supply to the esophagus. The three most important are the inferior thyroid arteries, the bronchial arteries, and the left gastric artery, followed by the esophageal arteries, which arise from the descending aorta, the right intercostal arteries, and the left inferior phrenic artery. All of these vessels supply the muscularis externa before reaching the submucosa, where they join plexuses of vessels that extend throughout the length of the esophagus. This submucosal vascular network provides blood to the extramural branches. As a result, ligation of an extramural vessel and mobilization of a short esophageal segment do not compromise the viability of the related esophageal wall. Also, failure of an anastomosis between the esophagus and another conduit usually is not due to the blood supply of the esophagus but to that of the visceral substitute.

Lymphatic Drainage

The esophageal lymph drains from the lymphatic capillaries and the collecting channels to the subadventitial and the mediastinal trunks and then to the regional nodes. The lymphatic capillaries are in the submucosal layer and form longitudinally arranged collecting channels. This lymphatic arrangement perhaps permits the intramural spread of carcinoma along the longitudinal axis of the esophagus. Intramural microscopic spread of carcinoma has been shown to occur cephalad 3 to 6 cm from the tumor in about 65% of cases and 10 cm in the rest, and caudally about 4 cm from the tumor.

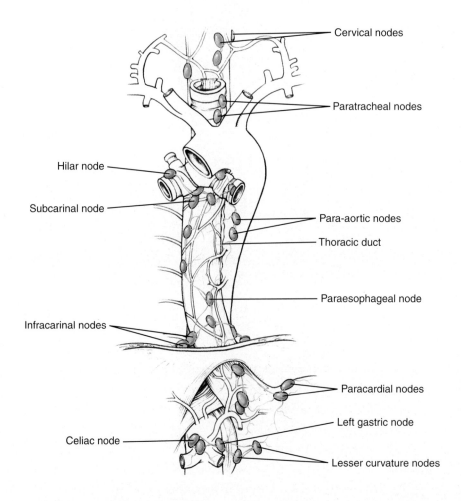

The lymphatic trunks drain into the periesophageal, subcarinal, peritracheal, cervical, paracardial, left gastric, and celiac axis nodes. Lymph flow from the upper third of the esophagus is primarily to the upper mediastinal and cervical nodes. Lymph drainage from the middle third of the esophagus is to the upper mediastinal and cervical nodes and to the abdominal nodes, and lymph flow from the lower third is to the abdominal nodes. As a result, carcinoma of the upper third of the esophagus usually metastasizes to the cervical nodes, carcinoma of the middle third to the cervical and the celiac axis nodes, and carcinoma of the lower third to the celiac axis nodes.

Nerve Supply

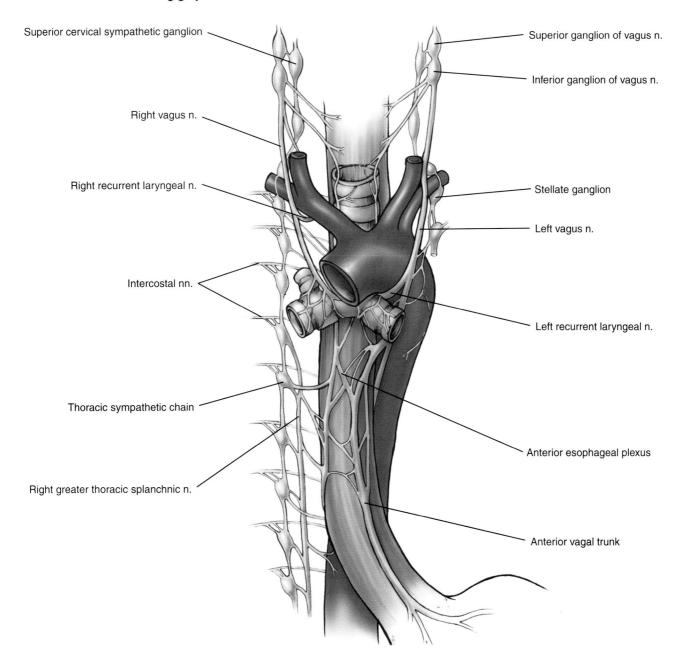

Superior cervical sympathetic ganglion

Right vagus n.

Right recurrent laryngeal n.

Intercostal nn.

Thoracic sympathetic chain

Right greater thoracic splanchnic n.

Superior ganglion of vagus n.

Inferior ganglion of vagus n.

Stellate ganglion

Left vagus n.

Left recurrent laryngeal n.

Anterior esophageal plexus

Anterior vagal trunk

The esophagus is innervated by sympathetic nerves from the cervical and thoracic chains and by parasympathetic nerves from the vagus nerves. During esophagectomy, because of their anatomic location, both vagus nerves are severed. This compelled vagectomy is considered to cause gastric atony and lack of pyloric relaxation, resulting in poor emptying of the gastric pouch. For this reason, pyloromyotomy or pyloroplasty is performed after esophagectomy by some surgeons and by us to assist gastric emptying; others claim that the incidence of poor gastric emptying is not greater without these procedures.

CARCINOMA OF THE ESOPHAGUS

The type of treatment of carcinoma of the esophagus depends on the stage of the disease and the overall medical status of the patient. If patients are unable to tolerate a major surgical procedure because of coexisting medical conditions and there is no evidence of metastasis to the liver, radiation therapy with or without chemotherapy is administered. In patients with preoperative evidence of liver metastasis and major dysphagia, treatment includes insertion of an endoesophageal prosthesis or mechanical dilation. A passage may be cored through the tumor under endoscopic vision, but with significant risk for perforation. Insertion of an endoesophageal prosthesis may also be used to protect from aspiration of saliva or food in the patient with a tracheoesophageal or bronchoesophageal fistula.

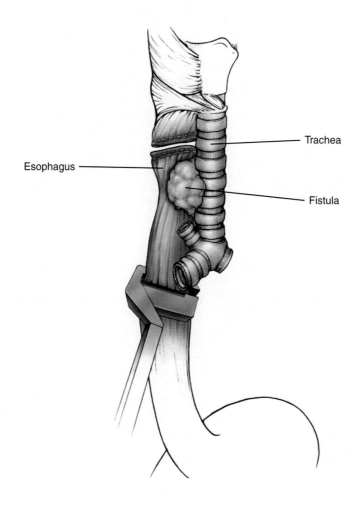

Trachea

Esophagus

Fistula

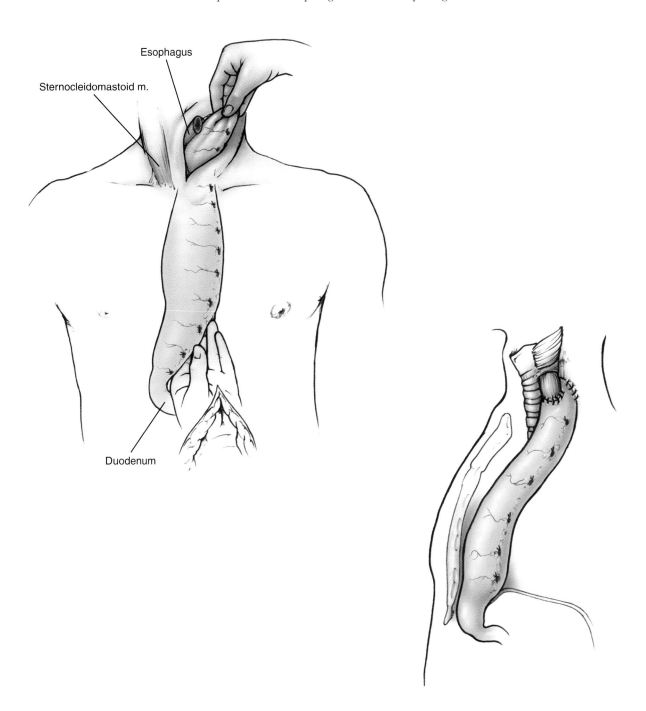

Esophagus

Sternocleidomastoid m.

Duodenum

Occasionally exclusion of the fistula, esophagectomy, or esophagogastrostomy, followed by radiation therapy may be used in highly selected patients with tracheoesophageal fistula. In patients without evidence of liver metastasis or other distal metastasis, resection of the carcinoma is the treatment of choice, with or without preoperative radiation therapy and chemotherapy.

There is no unanimity as to the best operation for removal of a cancer of the esophagus. Each surgeon has a preferred procedure for resecting carcinomas in various locations in the thoracic esophagus. The most commonly used surgical approach for the resection of carcinoma of the thoracic esophagus incorporates two incisions, a right thoracotomy and upper midline laparotomy with or without a cervical incision. Less commonly used approaches are the left thoracotomy and the transhiatal dissection through an upper midline abdominal and a cervical incision.

Preoperative or postoperative radiation therapy had been added to surgical treatment of esophageal carcinoma, but no improvement has been noted in either median or 5-year survival.

During the last several years, preoperative treatment with combined radiation therapy and chemotherapy has been used widely, most frequently radiation plus 5-fluorouracil (5-FU) and mitomycin or cisplatin. At present the precise benefit of preoperative treatment of esophageal carcinoma with the combination of radiation and any of the chemotherapeutic agents has not been clearly established; more prospective studies are needed.

SURGICAL APPLICATIONS
Esophagectomy Through Right Thoracotomy

Right thoracotomy with upper midline laparotomy allows easy resection of the esophagus and esophagogastrostomy at any site on the upper trunk. The patient is placed in the left decubitus position with the arms extended in front. A towel roll is used to prop the right upper trunk from the table at about 50 degrees, and the lower part of the trunk is positioned on the table as flat as possible and secured with beanbag weights (Vac-bag) and tape. The table is then rotated to the right or until the abdomen is brought into the horizontal plane, insofar as possible.

An upper midline vertical incision is made from the xiphoid process to the umbilicus and the liver is inspected for evidence of metastasis. If liver metastasis is present and the patient has significant esophageal obstruction, an endoesophageal prosthesis is inserted. When no hepatic metastasis is found, mobilization of the stomach is begun. The omentum and the transverse colon are lifted and the lesser omental space is entered. Once this space is identified, the greater omentum along the greater curvature of the stomach is divided and ligated about 2 cm from the artery to prevent inadvertent injury to it. The triangular ligament of the liver and the peritoneum overlying the esophageal hiatus are incised.

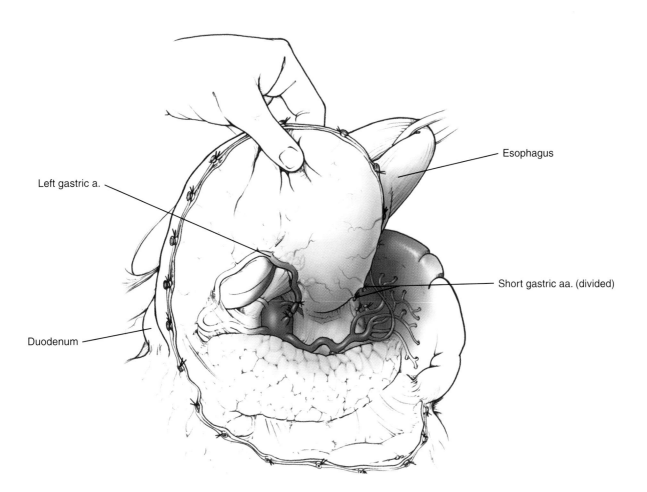

Left gastric a.

Esophagus

Short gastric aa. (divided)

Duodenum

The distal esophagus is encircled with tape. Traction on it and on the stomach toward the right facilitates exposure of the short gastric vessels. These are then double ligated and divided, while special care is taken to protect the spleen and the gastric wall from injury. After the entire greater curvature of the stomach is mobilized, the stomach is retracted to the right and the left gastric vessels are exposed, double ligated, and divided. The remaining gastrohepatic ligament is then incised toward the hiatus and the pylorus, carefully protecting the right gastroepiploic artery and the hepatic artery, portal vein, and common bile duct. The esophageal hiatus is widened to about four fingerbreadths by incising its right side radially, if needed. With downward traction on the encircling rubber drain, the distal esophagus is mobilized as far as possible into the mediastinum. A Kocher maneuver is done, incising the parietal peritoneum, and the duodenum is mobilized medially as far as possible. A pyloromyotomy is performed, ensuring that the entire pylorus muscle is divided, or a pyloroplasty is performed. The pylorus is opened longitudinally and the incision is extended into the distal pylorus and the proximal duodenum. The incision is closed transversely in two layers, the mucosal layer reapproximated with continuous absorbable suture and the seromuscular layer with interrupted silk sutures.

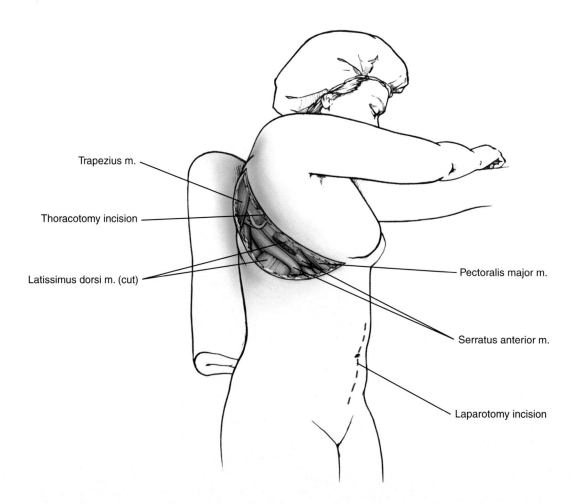

The operating table is then rotated to the left until the patient is returned to the lateral decubitus position. A right thoracotomy is made, and the pleural space is entered through the fourth or fifth intercostal space. The right lung is deflated, and ventilation is maintained only through the left lung during the entire endothoracic portion of the procedure. The inferior pulmonary ligament is divided, the right lower lobe is retracted upward and medially, and the distal esophagus, which usually has been mobilized previously during the transhiatal dissection, is encircled with a rubber drain. The azygous vein is ligated and divided and the mediastinal pleural is incised. When the carcinoma appears to have penetrated the full thickness of the esophageal wall, the parietal pleura overlying the esophagus is resected with it.

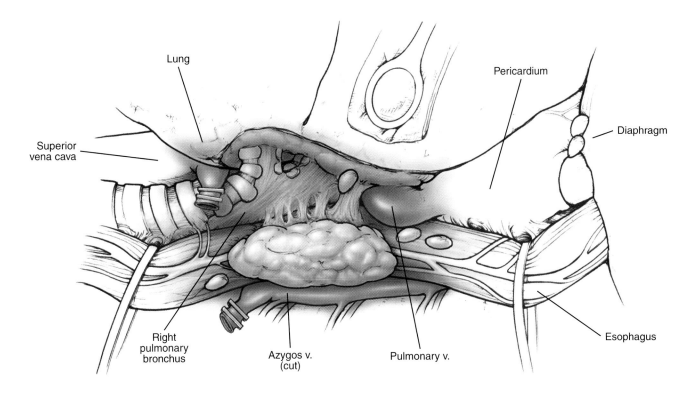

A segment of the esophagus cephalad to the tumor is dissected and encircled with tape. Gentle traction on both tapes laterally and on the heart and lung medially provides good exposure, and the esophagus is freed with sharp and blunt dissection after the esophageal vessels are ligated with surgical clips and divided. During the dissection, any noticeable lymph nodes are removed with the esophagus. If the tumor is adherent to the trachea, special care is exercised so that the tracheal lumen is not inadvertently entered. After 10 to 12 cm of the esophageal segment cephalad to the tumor is dissected free along with the remaining esophagus, the stomach is delivered through the hiatus into the right pleural space, keeping its lesser curvature exactly to the right side and paying special attention not to twist it. When the anastomosis is planned to be done with staples, as we usually do, the esophagus is transected about 8 to 10 cm cephalad from the tumor.

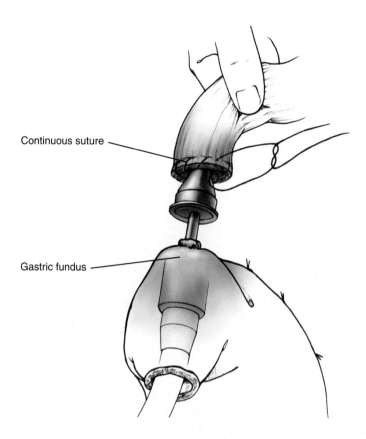

Continuous suture

Gastric fundus

A purse-string suture, about 1 cm in diameter, is placed at the tip of the gastric fundus. In addition, a 3-0 polypropylene over-and-over purse-string suture is placed through all layers of the circumference of the esophageal end, about 2 mm from the cut edge.

The specimen is transected distal to the gastroesophageal junction, along the lesser curvature so that the resected specimen encompasses the esophagus, the periesophageal tissue and nodes, the cardia, and part of the lesser curvature and its regional nodes. The cartridge end of the EEA stapling device with the anvil removed is inserted through the gastric opening and gently advanced until the central rod is at the center of the purse-string suture. A small opening is made and the rod is passed through. The purse-string suture is tied snugly around the rod and the ends are cut close to the knot so that they will not be in the way of the circular blade. The anvil is then screwed securely onto the rod, and the wing nut at the handle end of the instrument is turned counterclockwise until maximum separation of the anvil and cartridge is achieved. The anvil is gently inserted into the esophageal lumen, and the purse-string suture is tied snugly and cut close to the knot. The anvil and cartridge are brought together by turning the wing nut clockwise. The view window on the shelf of the instrument indicates when the segments have been apposed. The entire circumference of the planned anastomosis is inspected for good apposition of the esophageal and gastric walls with no intervening foreign material or other tissue. The safety catch is released, and the handle is squeezed firmly until it is fully closed. As the tissue is cut and the staples are fired, resistance will be felt.

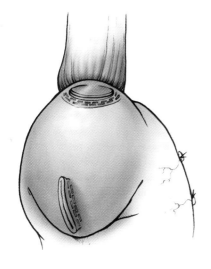

The cartridge and anvil are separated by three and one-half counterclockwise turns of the wing nut. The instrument then is rotated 180 degrees, both clockwise and counterclockwise, several times until it is disengaged from the anastomosis. The anvil is detached to inspect the two tissue cylinders.

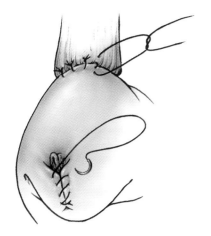

The gastric opening at the gastroesophageal junction is then stapled and oversewn with running over-and-over polypropylene sutures, and the suture line of the anastomosis is enforced with vertical interrupted mattress silk sutures.

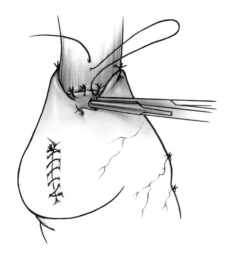

If sufficient length of the stomach is left, four to six sutures are placed to further reinforce the suture line by invaginating the suture line into the stomach. These sutures are placed about 2 cm from the suture line on the gastric wall and on either the esophageal wall or the mediastinal pleura.

When manual esophagogastrostomy is planned, the stomach just distal to the gastroesophageal junction, and the esophagus cephalad to the carcinoma, is divided with a stapler (GIA).

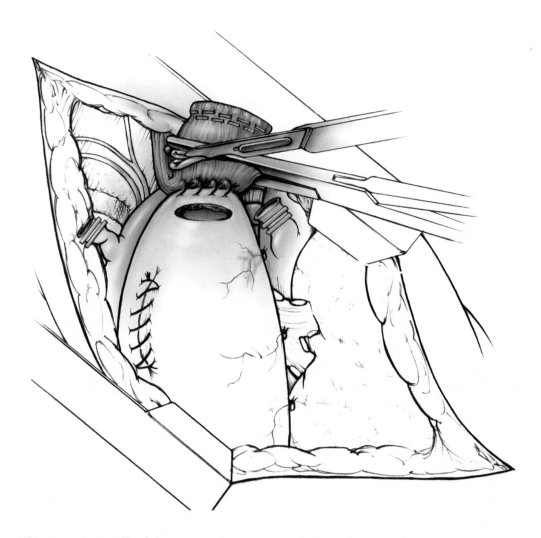

The anterior wall of the stomach, 3 to 4 cm below the tip of the fundus, is then sutured to the posterior wall of the esophagus with interrupted sutures. The sutures are placed slightly obliquely to encompass the muscle bundles and the submucosa of the esophagus and through the seromuscular layer of the stomach. After completion of the posterior suture line the stapled esophageal end is cut off 2 to 3 mm distal to the anastomosis and an appropriate opening is made in the gastric wall 2 to 3 mm from the suture line to match the spread esophageal opening.

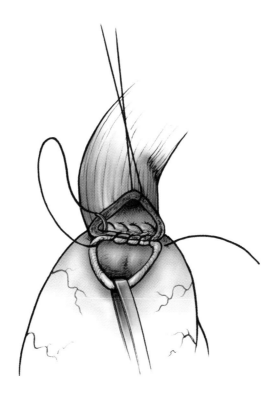

The posterior gastric and esophageal mucosae first, and then the anterior mucosae, are reapproximated with running over-and-over or interrupted absorbable sutures, with the knots tied inside the esophagus. The placement of the sutures should be such that there is good mucosa-to-mucosa coaptation. Just after completion of the posterior mucosal suture line a nasogastric tube is advanced about 10 cm into the stomach and secured to the nose with a strip of adhesive tape. The anterior suture line is then completed with interrupted silk sutures placed through the muscularis and submucosal layers of the esophagus and the seromuscular layer of the stomach.

When excision of the tumor with adequate margin and intrathoracic esophagogastrostomy cannot be done because of the close proximity of the tumor to the inlet of the chest, dissection of the esophagus is done in the cervical region. It is then ligated and divided with a GIA stapling device, and the specimen is removed after transecting the stomach at least 3 to 5 cm distal to the gastroesophageal junction. The stomach is positioned along the posterior mediastinum and secured high in the neck to the vertebra fascia, leaving sufficient length of fundus free to be pulled later in the neck. The edge of the hiatus is tacked to the gastric wall with a few interrupted silk sutures to prevent subsequent herniation of the intestine, and jejunostomy is performed. The laparotomy and thoracotomy are closed, and the pleural space is drained with two chest tubes, one placed anterior into the apex and one inferiorly along the diaphragm. The patient is positioned supine on the table, with the head turned to the left.

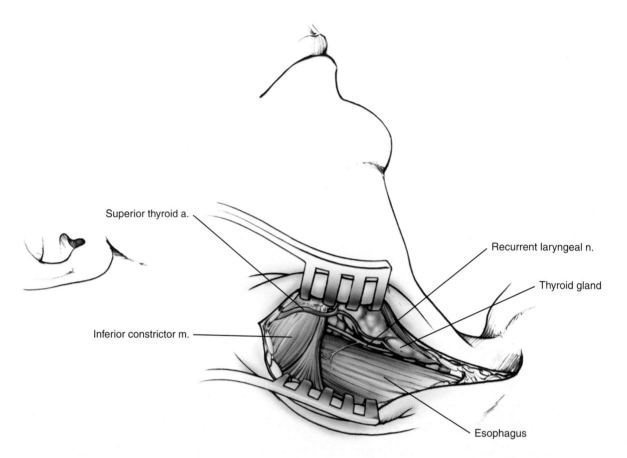

A cervical incision is made parallel to the anterior border of the sternocleido-mastoid muscle, beginning just below the cricoid cartilage and ending at the suprasternal notch. The platysma and omohyoid muscles are divided, the carotid sheath is gently retracted laterally, and the esophagus is exposed. A tube previously inserted transnasally into the esophagus greatly facilitates palpation and location of the esophagus. The esophagus is first dissected posteriorly from the vertebral fascia. Then with the finger hugging the esophagus, and with blunt dissection, it is carefully separated from the membranous portion of the trachea, paying attention to not injure it or the recurrent pharyngeal nerve.

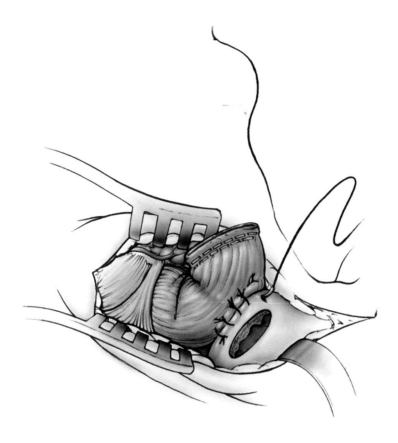

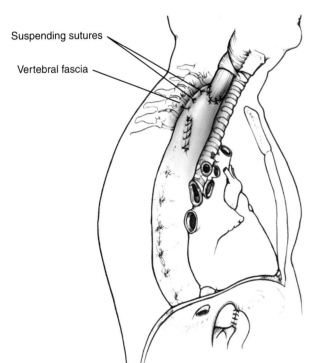

Suspending sutures

Vertebral fascia

The transected end of the esophagus is delivered into the cervical incision, as well as the tip of the gastric fundus. Esophagogastrostomy is then done manually as described.

Esophagectomy Through Left Thoracotomy

This approach is mainly applicable with carcinoma of the distal esophagus, particularly of the gastroesophageal junction, and when esophagogastrostomy can be done safely below the aortic arch. With the patient in the right lateral decubitus position, a left posterolateral thoracotomy through the seventh intercostal space is performed.

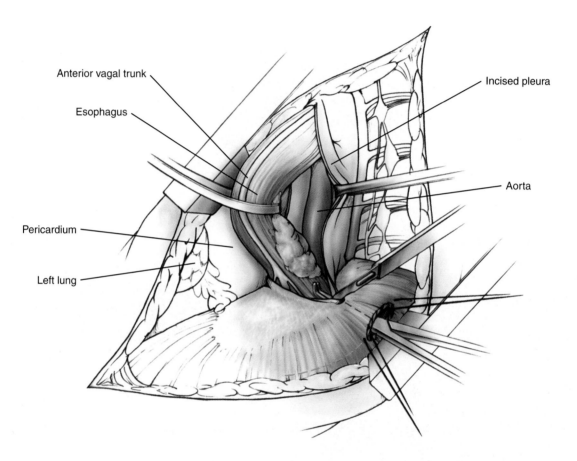

The left lung is collapsed and retracted medially and the mediastinal pleura between it and the aorta is incised. This incision is extended into the posterolateral segment of the diaphragm while protecting the intra-abdominal organs from injury. When additional exposure is needed for mobilization of the stomach, the diaphragmatic incision can be extended curvilinearly anteriorly, leaving a diaphragmatic rim attached to the chest wall. A segment of the lower esophagus is mobilized and encircled with tape. With gentle traction on the tape, the esophagus is freed up 10 to 12 cm from the tumor margin. Then through the diaphragmatic incision the stomach is dissected free, and pyloromyotomy or pyloroplasty is performed (see pp. 279 and 281). The tumor with adequate cephalad and caudal margins is resected along with all the visible nodes, and esophagogastrostomy is performed with the use of a stapling device or manually as described.

Esophagectomy Without Thoracotomy

Resection of the esophagus without thoracotomy is performed through an upper midline laparotomy, from the xiphoid process to the umbilicus, and a left cervical incision parallel to the anterior border of the sternocleidomastoid muscle. This approach is mainly applicable for the resection of carcinomas of the distal esophagus and the cardia. The major advantages of this approach are elimination of thoracotomy and its consequences, mainly pulmonary complications and impairment of pulmonary functions, and perhaps shortening of the operating time.

With the patient supine, an upper midline laparotomy extending from the umbilicus to the xiphoid process is made. The stomach and gastroesophageal junction are dissected free, and a Kocher maneuver and pyloromyotomy or pyloroplasty are performed as described. A tape is passed around the distal esophagus, and the esophageal hiatus is enlarged by dividing the right crus.

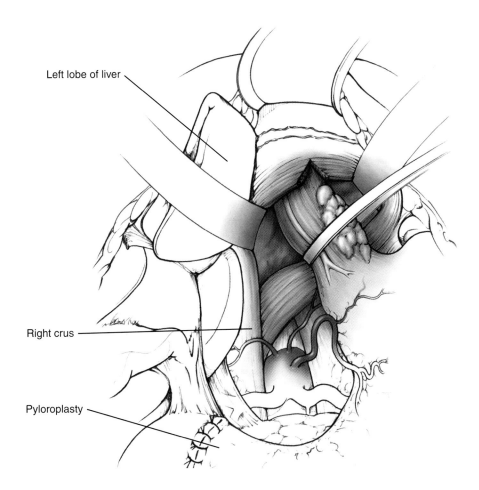

Left lobe of liver

Right crus

Pyloroplasty

With two malleable retractors placed in the hiatus, the diaphragm is retracted upward, medially, and laterally and the posterior mediastinum is exposed. With traction on the tape, the esophagus is freed from the surrounding structure with blunt and sharp dissection, and the esophageal arterial branches are ligated with liga clips and divided.

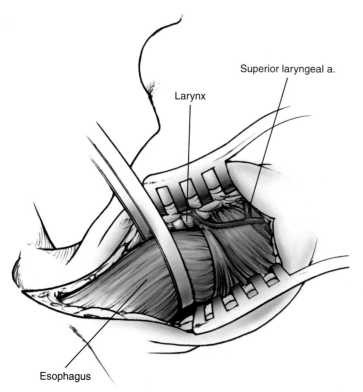

Larynx

Superior laryngeal a.

Esophagus

A left cervical incision parallel to the anterior border of the sternocleidomastoid muscle is made, and the cervical esophagus is dissected free and encircled with tape as described. With traction of the cervical esophagus, manual blunt downward dissection of the esophagus is first done posteriorly, then anteriorly, with extreme care to prevent tearing of the membranous portion of the trachea.

With traction of both the proximal and distal esophagus, its midportion, the area at the tracheal bifurcation, is dissected bimanually by inserting one hand through the hiatus and the other through the cervical incision. The dissection is first done posteriorly and then anteriorly, with intermittent brief periods of dissection to avoid prolonged displacement and compression of the heart. Arrhythmias and hypotension may occur while the surgeon's hand displaces the heart. These complications can be minimized or prevented by sufficiently replenishing the patient's blood volume before this phase of the esophageal dissection and by making each dissection period short. The bimanual dissection is continued until the fingers of the two hands meet.

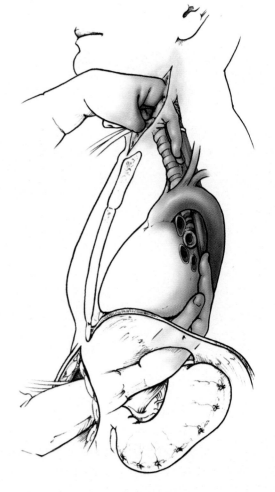

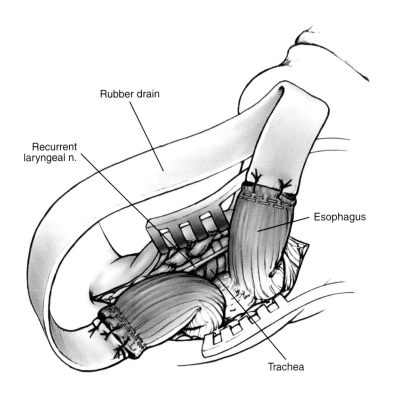

Rubber drain

Recurrent
laryngeal n.

Esophagus

Trachea

The esophagus is then transected with a GIA stapling device at the inlet of the chest. The ends of a long rubber drain are sutured to each end of the transected esophagus. The specimen is pulled into the abdominal incision and the esophagus is removed after it is stapled and divided distal to the gastroesophageal junction.

The abdominal end of the rubber drain is sutured to the tip of the gastric fundus. The esophageal bed is sufficiently widened to allow easy delivery of the stomach into the mediastinum and neck. This is done manually or with a half sponge stick passed through the cervical and abdominal incisions. The mediastinum is thoroughly inspected for bleeding, and by gently pulling on the cervical end of the rubber drain and mainly by manual pushing of the stomach into the mediastinum, the tip of the gastric fundus is brought into the neck incision. While this is done, special attention should be paid to prevent rotation of the stomach.

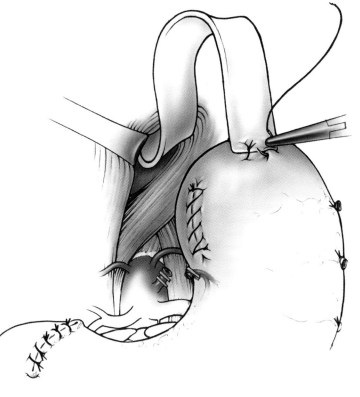

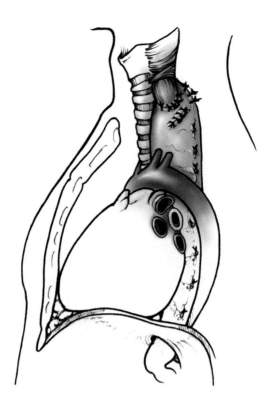

The stomach is secured with two or three sutures to the vertebral fascia and esophagogastrostomy is performed manually as described previously.

Postoperative Management

After surgery the nasogastric tube is connected to low-grade suction to prevent distention of the stomach. Due to the extensive operative area, encompassing both the abdominal and thoracic cavities, patients usually sequestrate fluids. As a result, in the first 24 to 48 postoperative hours they require a significant volume of fluids. This extravascular fluid is usually mobilized the second, third, or fourth postoperative day, sometimes causing pulmonary congestion and decreased partial pressure of arterial oxygen (PaO_2). Enhancement of diuresis, good pulmonary toilet, and assisted ventilation, if needed, will correct these changes. Chest radiographs should be obtained daily for the first 4 or 5 postoperative days to monitor any pulmonary changes and assess drainage of the stomach and the status of the mediastinum. When no abnormality is observed and the postoperative course is uncomplicated, an esophagogram is obtained on the seventh postoperative day to determine the integrity of the esophagogastrostomy suture line and emptying of the stomach.

Results

The overall results of treatment of esophageal carcinoma are discouraging, mainly because of late discovery and treatment of the disease. Five-year survival appears to depend mainly on the stage of the disease rather than the superiority of any operative technique. In large studies the reported 5-year survival for stage I disease was 60% to 70%, compared with 5% to 6% for stage IV disease. Although the earlier reported surgical mortality for esophagectomy and esophagogastrostomy has been as high as 30% to 40%, the current mortality in our and other institutions is 4% to 5%.

BENIGN TUMORS OF THE ESOPHAGUS
Benign Tumor Resection

The method of excision of benign esophageal lesions depends on their site and type. Pedunculated intraluminal lesions with a narrow base are removed endoscopically with a diathermy loop, whereas sessile intraluminal tumors are resected through vertical esophagotomy. Intramural tumors usually can be removed without entering the esophageal lumen, through posterolateral thoracotomy or with the use of video-assisted thoracoscopy.

For resection of sessile intraluminal and intramural tumors the esophagus is exposed through the appropriate incision according to the site of the lesion. Tumors of the cervical esophagus are removed through a longitudinal skin incision along the anterior border of the sternocleidomastoid muscle or through a collar incision starting two fingerbreadths above the sternal notch, to the right of the midline, and extending into the left supraclavicular fossa, parallel to the clavicle. The platysma and the omohyoid muscles are divided, the carotid sheath is retracted laterally, and the esophagus is exposed and carefully dissected from the membranous portion of the trachea and encircled with tape. Tumors of the upper or middle third of the thoracic esophagus are excised through a right posterolateral thoracotomy at the fourth or fifth intercostal space. Tumors of the lower third of the esophagus are resected through a left posterior lateral incision through the sixth or seventh intercostal space.

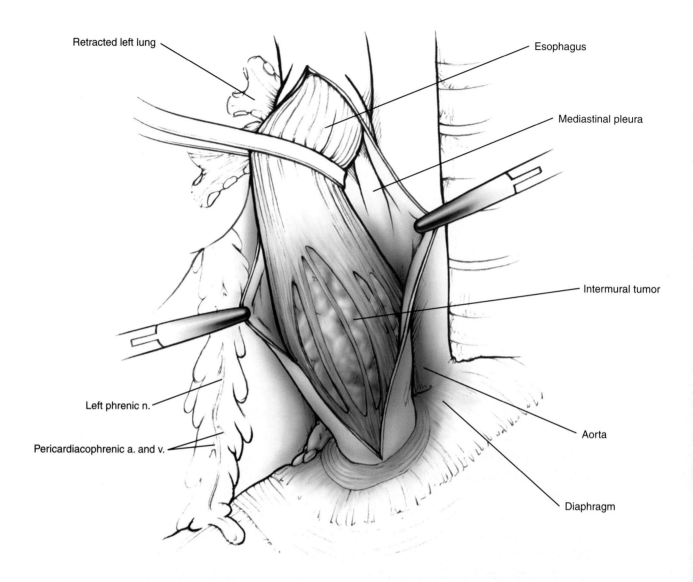

Retracted left lung

Esophagus

Mediastinal pleura

Intermural tumor

Left phrenic n.

Pericardiacophrenic a. and v.

Aorta

Diaphragm

After the site of the tumor is exposed, the overlaying mediastinal pleura is incised vertically and the esophagus above the site of the mass is encircled with
tape. Intermural tumors are usually covered with a thin muscular layer and can
be seen or palpated easily. The muscle fibers are split apart, and the tumor is
exposed. With blunt dissection, the tumor is carefully separated from the surrounding tissue, paying particular attention not to injure the mucosa. This is
usually easily accomplished, because most tumors are encapsulated and are not
firmly adherent to the mucosa, unless endoscopic biopsy of the tumor has been
previously done, in which case mucosal injury is unavoidable.

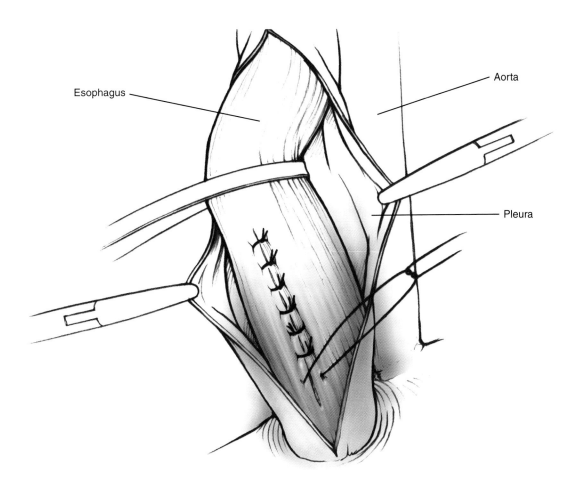

After the tumor is removed, the muscularis is reapproximated with interrupted silk sutures. When mucosal injury occurs, the defect is first repaired with interrupted sutures and the muscularis is approximated. Sessile tumors of the mucosa are removed through a longitudinal esophagotomy opposite the site of the tumor. The mass is then removed with a healthy tissue margin of several millimeters. The created mucosal defect is closed with interrupted sutures.

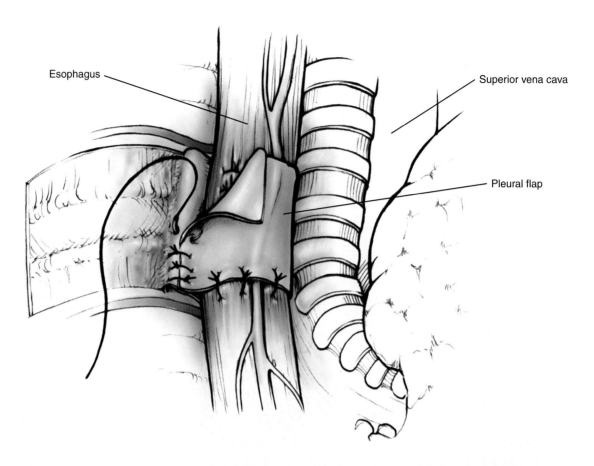

Esophagus

Superior vena cava

Pleural flap

The muscle fibers are approximated with interrupted sutures, and the esoph-ageal suture line is covered with a parietal pleura pedicle flap by wrapping it around the esophagus.

Excision of intramural tumors of the thoracic esophagus also can be done under video-assisted thoracoscopy. The patient is placed in the left lateral de-cubitus position with a roll under the right upper torso to widen the left in-tercostal spaces. Four same size ports are placed in a rhomboidal configuration. The position of the ports depends on the site of the tumor. For lesions of the upper and middle thirds of the esophagus, the trocars are placed distal to the lesion. The first port is inserted in the seventh or eighth intercostal space at the midaxillary line; a second trocar is inserted in the sixth or seventh intercostal space anteriorly to the anterior axillary line; and the other two ports are placed in the fifth and fourth intercostal spaces at the posterior and anterior axillary lines, respectively. For tumors of the distal third of the esophagus, the first trocar is positioned in the fourth intercostal space at the anterior axillary line, the second in the fifth intercostal space behind the posterior axillary line, and the other two as seems desirable along the sixth intercostal space. With sharp and blunt dissection the tumor is removed through a conventional thoracotomy as described.

Anatomic Basis of Complications

MAJOR

- Injury of the recurrent laryngeal nerve causes paralysis of a vocal cord.
- Injury of the thoracic duct results in chylothorax.
- Severance of the vagus nerve causes gastric atony and lack of pyloric relaxation.

MINOR

- Injury of the intercostal nerve may result in chronic chest pain.

KEY REFERENCES

Earlam R, Cunha-Melo JR. Oesophageal squamous cell carcinoma: I. A critical review of surgery. Br J Surg 67:381, 1980.

Squamous cell carcinoma of the esophagus was analyzed by review of data for 83,783 patients reported in 122 papers. The mean operative mortality was 29%, and the 1-year survival was 18%.

Ellis FH Jr. Treatment of carcinoma of the esophagus or cardia. Mayo Clin Proc 64:945, 1989.

From 1970 to 1988, 310 patients with cancer of the esophagus were treated surgically. Two hundred seventy-five underwent resection, with resectability rate of 88.7%. Surgical mortality was 2.2%; overall 5-year survival rate was 20.8%, and median survival time was 17.9 months.

Muller JM, Erasmi H, Stelzner M, Zieren U, Pechlmaier H. Surgical therapy of oesophageal carcinoma. Br J Surg 77:845, 1990.

Treatment outcomes from 1201 papers on surgical treatment of esophageal cancer were reviewed. Tumor stage was found to be the primary determinant of outcome. The data did not indicate that any particular operative technique was superior with respect to long-term survival.

Wu YK, Huang KC. Chinese experience in the surgical treatment of carcinoma of the esophagus. Ann Surg 190:361, 1979.

In a collective series of 5412 patients who underwent tumor resection in China, in the early years the operative mortality was more than 25%. By 1960 it declined to around 10%, and in the following years to 3% to 5%.

SUGGESTED READINGS

Blot WS, Devesa SJ, Kneller RW, et al. Rising incidence of adenocarcinoma of the esophagus and gastric cardia. JAMA 265(10):1287, 1989.

Blot WJ, Frammens JF Jr. Geographic epidemiology of cancer in the United States. In Schotterfeld D, Fraumens J, eds. Cancer Epidemiology and Prevention. Philadelphia: WB Saunders, 1982, p 179.

Boyd DP, Hill LD. Benign tumors and cysts of the esophagus. Am J Surg 93:252, 1957.

Burgess HM, et al. Carcinoma of the esophagus. Clinicopathologic Study. Surg Clin North Am 31:965, 1951.

Dillow BM, Neis DD, Sellers RD. Leiomyoma of the esophagus. Am J Surg 120:165, 1970.

Drucker MH, Mansour KA, Hatcher CR Jr, et al. Esophageal carcinoma: An aggressive approach. Ann Thorac Surg 28:133-138, 1979.

Iizuka T, Isono K, Kakegawa T, et al. Parameters linked to 10-year survival in Japan of selected esophageal carcinoma. Chest 96:1005, 1989.

Lewis I. The surgical treatment of carcinoma of the esophagus with special reference to a new operation for growths of the middle third. Br J Surg 34:18, 1946.

Liebermann-Meffert D. Anatomy, embryology, and histology. In Pearson FG, Deslauriers J, Ginsberg RJ, et al., eds. Esophageal Surgery. New York: Churchill Livingstone, 1996, pp 1-25.

Liebermann-Meffert D, Allgower M, Schmid P, et al. Muscular equivalent of the lower esophageal sphincter. Gastroenterology 76:31-38, 1979.

Miller C. Carcinoma of thoracic esophagus and cardia. Br J Surg 49:507, 1962.

Moersch HJ, Herrington SW. Benign tumors of the esophagus. Ann Otol Rhinol Laryngol 53:800, 1967.

Oringer MB, Sloan H. Esophagectomy without thoracotomy. J Thorac Cardiovasc Surg 76:643, 1978.

Plachta A. Benign tumors of the esophagus. Am J Gastroenterol 38:639, 1962.

Seremetis MG, de Guzman VL, Lyons WS, et al. Leiomyoma of the esophagus. Ann Thorac Surg 16:308, 1973.

Shapiro AL, Robillard GL. The esophageal arteries. Ann Surg 131:171-185, 1950.

Steiger Z, Franklin R, Wilson RF, et al. Eradication and palliation of squamous cell carcinoma of the esophagus with chemotherapy, radiotherapy, and surgical therapy. J Thorac Cardiovasc Surg 82:713-719, 1981.

Sweet RH. Carcinoma of the thoracic midthoracic esophagus; Treatment by radical resection and high intrathoracic esophagogastric anastomosis. Ann Surg 124:653, 1946.

Symbas PN, McKeown PP, Hatcher CR Jr, et al. Tracheoesophageal fistula from carcinoma of the esophagus. Ann Thorac Surg 38:382, 1984.

Tanabe G, Baba M, Kuroshima K, et al. Clinical evaluation of the esophageal lymph flow system based on RI uptake of dissected regional lymph nodes following lymphoscintigraphy. Nippon Geka Gakkai Zasshi 87:315, 1986.

Diaphragm
SURGICAL ANATOMY

The diaphragm is a dome-shaped musculofibrous septum that separates the thoracic and peritoneal cavities. It originates from the dorsum of the xiphoid process, from the inner surface of the cartilage and adjacent portions of the last six ribs and from the first and second lumbar vertebrae. The motor nerve to the diaphragm is supplied by the right and left phrenic nerves. The right phrenic nerve enters the diaphragm through the central tendon just lateral to the inferior vena cava, and the left pierces the superior surface of the muscular portion of the diaphragm just lateral to the left border of the heart. Both nerves trifurcate, and the branches are distributed into the muscular portion of the diaphragm.

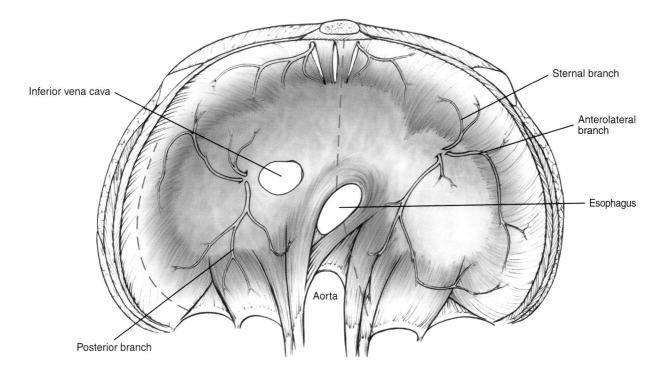

Inferior vena cava

Sternal branch

Anterolateral branch

Esophagus

Aorta

Posterior branch

Because of this topography of the nerves, when incision of the diaphragm is required to expose organs in the pleura or peritoneal cavity, a radial incision from the hiatus to the posterior chest wall or to the paraxiphoid region, or a curvilinear incision about 2 cm from the diaphragmatic attachment to the ribs, will result in the least impairment of diaphragmatic function.

CARCINOMA OF THE DIAPHRAGM

Diaphragmatic tumors may be primary or secondary, originating from an adjacent organ and invading the diaphragm. Primary tumors may be benign or malignant, but all secondary tumors are malignant. Neurofibromas, lipomas, angiofibromas, and mesothelial cysts are the most common benign tumors, and sarcomas are the main malignant tumors.

SURGICAL APPLICATIONS
Resection and Reconstruction

Treatment of these lesions is enucleation of benign tumors and wide resection of malignant tumors. With the patient in the lateral decubitus position, the diaphragm is exposed through a posterolateral thoracotomy at the seventh intercostal space. Benign lesions are enucleated, and the diaphragmatic defect is closed with interrupted 0 sutures. The malignant tumors are removed along with 3 cm margins of normal diaphragm around the tumor. The resultant diaphragmatic defect is repaired with interrupted sutures, if feasible, or for large diaphragmatic defects with nylon or Marlex mesh prostheses. Marlex is our material of choice. Pedicled autologous tissue such as muscle or preferably pericardium may also be used in selected cases for the repair of large diaphragmatic defects.

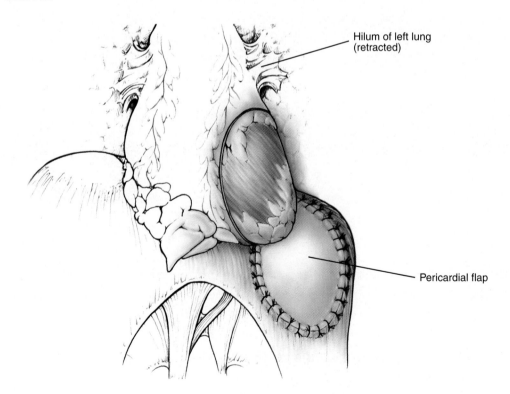

Hilum of left lung (retracted)

Pericardial flap

The pericardium is incised posterolaterally along the phrenic nerve and anterior to it, as well as anteriorly, up to the root of the great vessels. The created pedicle is left attached to the membranous portion of the diaphragm and sutured to the diaphragmatic defect with interrupted sutures.

KEY REFERENCES

Olafsson G, Raussing AS, Holen O. Primary tumors of the diaphragm. Chest 59:568, 1971.

An undifferentiated sarcoma of the diaphragm and 85 primary diaphragmatic tumors, including those reported by Weiner and Chou, are reviewed. Of those, 52 were benign and 33 were malignant. The most frequent benign tumors were cystic formations such as bronchial, mesothelial, and the teratoid cysts, and the most common malignant tumors were fibrosarcomas. Lower chest and epigastrial pain was the most frequent complaint.

Weiner MF, Chou WH. Primary tumors of the diaphragm. Arch Surg 90:143, 1965.

SUGGESTED READING

McClenathan JH, Okada F. Primary neurilemmoma of the diaphragm. Ann Thorac Surg 48:126, 1989.

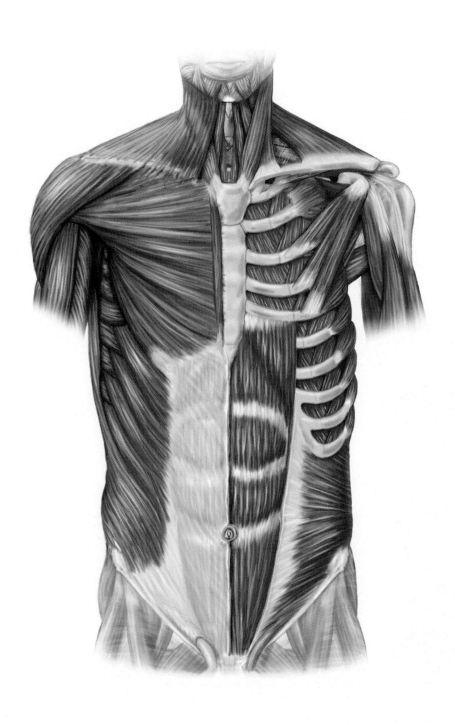

Chapter 6

Abdominal Wall

William S. Richardson, M.D., and Charles A. Staley, M.D.

Surgical Applications

*T*he anatomy of the abdominal wall is significant for the planning and performance of abdominal incisions and for placement of endoscopes and trocars.

SURGICAL ANATOMY

Topography

Landmarks

The abdomen is defined as that region of the trunk between the diaphragm above and the inlet of the pelvis below. The xiphoid process is the cartilaginous lower part of the sternum that is easily palpated in the depression where the costal margins meet in the upper part of the anterior abdominal wall. The costal margin is the curved lower margin of the thoracic wall that is formed in front by the cartilages of the seventh, eighth, ninth, and tenth ribs and behind by the cartilages of the eleventh and twelfth ribs. The iliac crest can be palpated along its entire length and ends in front at the anterior iliac spine and behind at the posterior superior iliac spine. The inguinal ligament, the rolled edge of the aponeurosis of the external oblique muscle, extends laterally to the anterior superior iliac spine and curves downward and medially to the pubic tubercle. The pubic tubercle is the small protuberance along the superior surface of the pubis. The symphysis pubis is the cartilaginous joint that lies in the midline between the bodies of the pubic bones. The midline of the abdominal fascia is called the linea alba and is formed by the fusion of the aponeuroses of the muscles of the anterior abdominal wall. The umbilicus lies in the linea alba and is the site of attachment of the umbilical cord in the fetus. The linea semilunaris is the lateral edge of the rectus abdominis muscle and crosses the costal margin at the tip of the ninth costal cartilage.

Abdominal Regions

For clinical purposes, it is customary to divide the abdomen into nine regions by two vertical and two horizontal lines. Each vertical line (midinguinal) passes through the midpoint between the anterior superior iliac spine and the symphysis pubis. The upper horizontal line, referred to as the subcostal plane, joins the lowest point of the costal margin on each side. The lowest horizontal line, referred to as the intertubercular plane, joins the tubercles on each iliac crest.

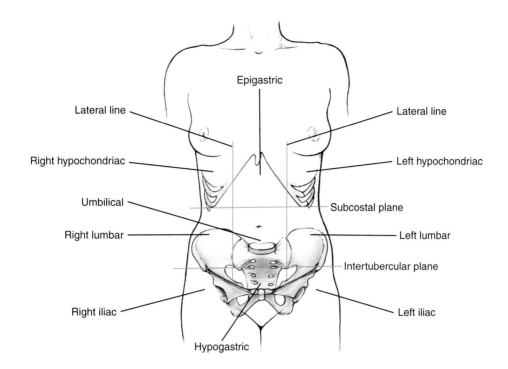

The upper abdomen includes the right hypochondric, epigastric, and left hypochondric regions. The middle abdomen includes the right lumbar, umbilical, and left lumbar regions. The lower abdomen includes right iliac, hypogastric, and left iliac areas.

Structure of Abdominal Wall

Superiorly, the abdominal wall is formed by the diaphragm, which separates the abdominal cavity from the thoracic cavity. Inferiorly, the abdominal cavity is continuous with the pelvic cavity through the pelvic inlet. Anteriorly, the abdominal wall is formed above by the lower part of the thoracic cage and below by the rectus abdominis, external oblique, and transversus abdominis muscles. Posteriorly, the abdominal wall is formed in the midline by the lumbar vertebrae and their intervertebral disks. Posterolaterally, the abdominal wall is formed by the twelfth ribs, the upper part of the body pelvis, the psoas muscles, the quadratus lumborum muscles, and the aponeuroses of the transversus abdominis muscles. Laterally, the abdominal wall is formed above by the lower part of the thoracic wall, including the lungs and pleura, and below by the external oblique, internal oblique, and transversus abdominis muscles.

Anterior and Lateral Abdominal Wall

The general layers of the anterolateral abdominal wall from the outside in are the skin, superficial fascia, deep fascia, abdominal muscles with their fascia, transversalis fascia, extraperitoneal fat, and parietal peritoneum.

Skin

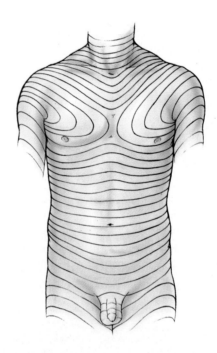

The skin is the outermost layer. The course of the connective bundles of the corium form lines of cleavage (Langer's lines of minimal tension) in the skin. These natural lines of cleavage in the skin are constant and run almost horizontally around the trunk. This is important clinically because an incision along a cleavage line will heal as a narrow scar, whereas one that crosses these lines will heal as a wide scar.

Superficial Fascia

The superficial fascia may be divided into a superficial fatty layer and a deep membranous layer. The fatty layer of superficial fascia is called Camper's fascia. The deeper portion of the subcutaneous tissue contains more fibrous elements and forms a membranous fascial layer called Scarpa's fascia.

Muscles of Anterior and Lateral Abdominal Walls

The muscles of the anterior and lateral abdominal walls include the external oblique, the internal oblique, the transversus, the rectus abdominis, and the pyramidalis muscles.

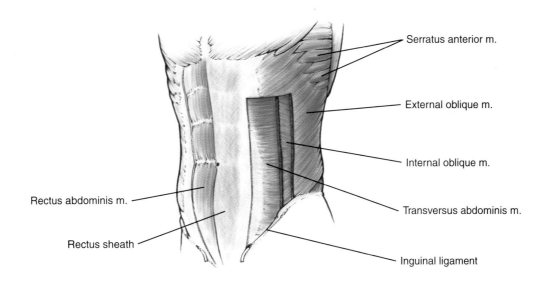

EXTERNAL OBLIQUE

The external oblique muscle is a broad, thin, muscular sheet that arises from the outer surfaces of the lower eight ribs and fans out to insert into the xiphoid process, the linea alba, the pubic crest, the pubic tubercle, and the anterior half of the iliac crest. A triangular defect in the external oblique aponeurosis, known as the superficial inguinal ring, lies immediately above and medial to the pubic tubercle. The spermatic cord (or round ligament of the uterus) passes through this opening and carries the external spermatic fascia (or the external covering of the round ligament of the uterus) from the margins of the ring. Between the anterior superior iliac spine and the pubic tubercle, the lower border of the aponeurosis is folded backward on itself, forming the inguinal ligament. The external oblique aponeurosis is different from the fascia of Gallaudet.

INTERNAL OBLIQUE

The internal oblique muscle is a broad, thin, muscular sheet that lies deep to the external oblique muscle. The majority of its fibers run at right angles to those of the external oblique muscle. It arises from the lumbar fascia, the anterior two thirds of the iliac crest, and the lateral two thirds of the inguinal ligament. The muscle fibers radiate as they pass upward and forward. The muscle is inserted into the lower borders of the lower three ribs and their costal cartilages, the xiphoid process, the linea alba, and the symphysis pubis. The internal oblique muscle has a lower free border that arches over the spermatic cord (or round ligament of the uterus) and then descends behind it to be attached to the pubic crest and the pectineal line.

Near their insertion, the lowest tendinous fibers are joined by similar fibers from the transversus abdominis muscle to form the conjoint tendon.

As the spermatic cord passes under the lower border of the internal oblique muscle, it carries with it some of the muscle fibers that are called the cremaster muscle.

TRANSVERSUS

The transversus abdominis muscle is a thin sheet of muscle that lies deep to the internal oblique muscle, and its fibers run horizontally forward. It arises from the deep surface of the lower six costal cartilages, lumbodorsal fascia, anterior two thirds of the iliac crest, and lateral third of the inguinal ligament. The muscle inserts into the xiphoid process, the linea alba, and the symphysis pubis.

RECTUS ABDOMINIS

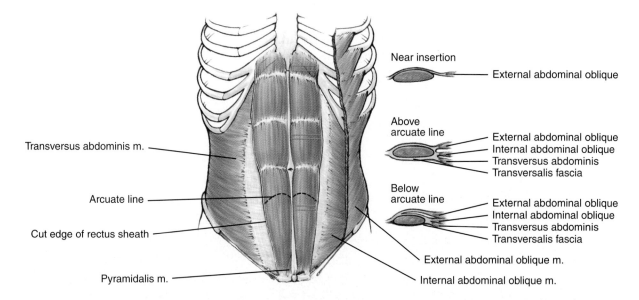

Near insertion — External abdominal oblique

Above arcuate line — External abdominal oblique / Internal abdominal oblique / Transversus abdominis / Transversalis fascia

Below arcuate line — External abdominal oblique / Internal abdominal oblique / Transversus abdominis / Transversalis fascia

Transversus abdominis m.

Arcuate line

Cut edge of rectus sheath

Pyramidalis m.

External abdominal oblique m.

Internal abdominal oblique m.

The rectus abdominis muscles are paired long strap muscles that extend vertically along the whole length of the anterior abdominal wall. They are broader above and lie close to the midline, separated from each other by the linea alba. The rectus abdominis muscle arises from two heads, from the front of the symphysis pubis and from the pubis crest. It inserts into the fifth, sixth, and seventh costal cartilages and the xiphoid process. When the rectus abdominis muscle contracts, its lateral margin forms a palpable and visible curved ridge known as the linea semilunaris. The anterior surface of the muscle is crossed by three tendinous intersections, at the tip of the xiphoid, at the umbilicus, and halfway between the two. These intersections are strongly attached to the anterior wall of the rectus sheath. The rectus abdominis muscle is enclosed between the aponeuroses of the external oblique, the internal oblique, and the transversus abdominis muscles, which form the rectus sheath.

The pyramidalis muscle is a triangular muscle, and many times is absent. When present, the muscle arises from the anterior surface of the pubis and inserts into the linea alba. It lies in front of the lower part of the rectus abdominis muscle.

RECTUS SHEATH

The rectus sheath is a long sheath that encloses the rectus abdominis muscle and pyramidalis muscle (if present) and contains the anterior rami of the lower six thoracic nerves and the superior and inferior epigastric vessels and lymphatic vessels. It is formed largely by the aponeuroses of the three lateral abdominal muscles.

Between the costal margin and the level of the anterior superior iliac spine, the aponeurosis of the internal oblique splits to enclose the rectus muscle; the external oblique aponeurosis is directed in front of the muscle, and the transversus aponeurosis is directed behind the muscle. Between the level of the anterior superior iliac spine and the pubis, the aponeuroses of all three muscles form the anterior sheath. The posterior sheath is absent, and the rectus muscle lies in contact with the fascia transversalis. Finally, in front of the pubis, the origin of the rectus muscle and the pyramidalis (if present) is covered anteriorly by the aponeuroses of all three muscles. The posterior wall is formed by the body of the pubis.

At the point the aponeuroses forming the posterior wall pass in front of the rectus at the level of the anterior superior iliac spine, the posterior wall has a free, curved lower border called the arcuate line. At this site the inferior epigastric vessels enter the rectus sheath and pass upward to anastomose with the superior epigastric vessels. The rectus sheath is separated from the rectus muscle on the opposite side by the linea alba.

Transversalis Fascia

The next layer of the abdominal wall is the transversalis fascia, which lines the abdominal cavity somewhat like the peritoneum. The transversalis fascia is thicker in the lower half of the abdomen, especially below the arcuate line, where the posterior rectus sheath is absent. The portion of the fascia beneath the rectus muscle is so closely attached to the overlying posterior rectus sheath that the rectus sheath, peritoneum, and the transversalis fascia form one layer. Lateral to the posterior rectus sheath the transversalis fascia is loosely attached to the transversus abdominis, quadratus lumborum, and psoas muscles. Thus this extraperitoneal plane can be dissected to expose the kidney, ureters, vena cava, and aorta.

Extraperitoneal Fat

This layer consists of loose areolar fibrous fatty tissue that lies between the overlying transversalis fascia and the underlying parietal peritoneum. The falciform ligament is a fold of the parietal peritoneum, which contains extraperitoneal fat and paraumbilical blood vessels.

Peritoneum

The parietal peritoneum is the innermost layer of the abdominal wall and is reflected onto the various viscera to form the visceral peritoneum. The peritoneum has little strength and can tear easily.

Blood Supply

Cutaneous arteries, which are branches of the superior and inferior epigastric arteries, supply the area near the skin in the midline. Branches from the intercostal, lumbar, and deep circumflex iliac arteries supply the skin over the flank.

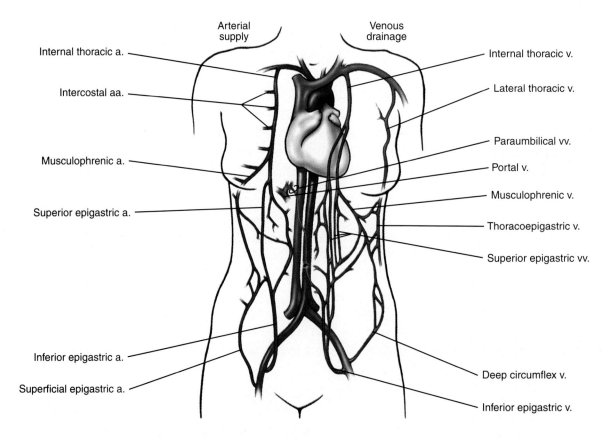

The venous blood is collected into a network of veins that radiates out from the umbilicus. The network is drained above into the axillary vein via the lateral thoracic vein and below into the femoral vein via the superficial epigastric vein. The lumbar veins drain the midabdominal and flank areas. A few small veins, the paraumbilical veins, connect the network through the umbilicus and along the ligamentum teres to the portal vein. They form an important portosystemic venous anastomosis.

The anterolateral abdominal wall receives its arterial blood supply from the last six intercostal and four lumbar arteries, the superior and inferior epigastric arteries, and the deep circumflex iliac arteries. The lower six intercostal arteries and the four lumbar arteries pass forward between the muscle layers and supply the lateral part of the abdominal wall.

The superior epigastric artery, one of the terminal branches of the internal thoracic (mammary) artery, enters the upper part of the rectus sheath between the sternal and costal origins of the diaphragm. It descends behind the rectus muscle, supplying the upper central part of the anterior abdominal wall, and anastomoses with the inferior epigastric artery.

The inferior epigastric artery is a branch of the external iliac artery just above the inguinal ligament. It runs upward and medially along the medial side of the deep inguinal ring and passes through the transversalis fascia to enter the rectus sheath anterior to the arcuate line. After ascending behind the rectus muscle to supply the lower central part of the anterior abdominal wall, the inferior epigastric artery anastomoses with the superior epigastric artery.

The deep circumflex iliac artery is a branch of the external iliac artery just above the inguinal ligament. It runs upward and laterally toward the anterior superior iliac spine and then continues along the iliac crest to supply the lower lateral part of the abdominal wall.

Lymphatic Drainage

The cutaneous lymph vessels above the level of the umbilicus drain upward into the anterior axillary lymph nodes. The vessels below this level drain downward into the superficial inguinal nodes. The deep lymph vessels follow the arteries and drain into the internal thoracic, external iliac, posterior mediastinal, and para-aortic (lumbar) nodes.

Nerve Supply

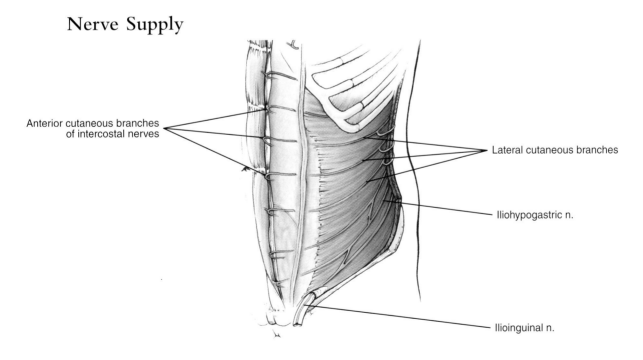

The cutaneous nerve supply to the anterior abdominal wall is derived from the anterior rami of the lower six thoracic and first lumbar nerves. The dermatome of T7 is situated in the epigastrium just over the xiphoid process, T10 includes the umbilicus, and L1 lies just above the inguinal ligament and the symphysis pubis.

Each nerve passes forward in the interval between the internal oblique and transversus abdominis muscles to supply the skin of the anterior abdominal wall, the muscles, and the parietal peritoneum. The lower six thoracic nerves then pierce the posterior wall of the rectus sheath to supply the rectus muscle and the pyramidalis. Each nerve then terminates by piercing the anterior wall of the rectus sheath and supplies the skin. The first lumbar nerve does not enter the rectus sheath but gives off contributions to both the iliohypogastric nerve, which pierces the external oblique aponeurosis above the superficial inguinal ring, and the ilioinguinal nerve, which emerges through the inguinal ring. Both the ilioinguinal and iliohypogastric nerves end by supplying the skin just above the inguinal ligament and the symphysis pubis.

SURGICAL APPLICATIONS
Incisions

The importance of selecting the proper incision for a cancer operation cannot be underestimated. A badly placed incision without the option for extension may compromise the ability for a complete and margin-free tumor resection. The incision must give ready and direct access to the anatomy to be investigated and provide adequate space to perform the indicated operation. Once the proper incision is made, exposure of the operative field is maximized by carefully placed retractors and correct positioning of the operative table. The incision should be extendible in the direction that will allow for the possible enlargement of the scope of the operation.

Abdominal incisions can be roughly divided into vertical and transverse incisions. All abdominal incisions have some degree of pulmonary physiology impairment. In the 1940s it was noted that pulmonary complications occurred four times more frequently in patients with a vertical, compared with transverse, abdominal incisions. Also, upper abdominal incisions were shown to have marked effects on pulmonary physiology. However, with the use of epidural catheters and patient-controlled anesthesia for postoperative pain, the effect of the various incisions on pulmonary function has been minimized.

Upper Midline Incision

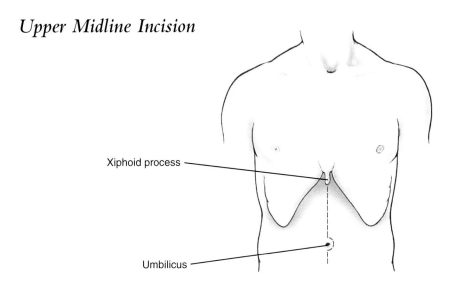

An upper midline incision is a preferred approach of some surgeons for operations involving the stomach. The incision can be extended upward to remove the xiphoid process and provides an excellent operative field for total or partial gastrectomy. It can be extended downward around the umbilicus if necessary. The incision can be made quickly, destroys no nerves, transects no muscles, and is easy to close. The incision is made through the skin from the xiphoid to a few centimeters above the umbilicus. The linea alba is identified, and the decussation of fibers indicates the midline. Dividing the linea alba exposes the extraperitoneal fat, which can be thinned out to reveal the peritoneum. Two clamps are placed on the peritoneum, and upward traction is applied while it is divided to avoid injury to underlying bowel. The falciform ligament is divided and tied.

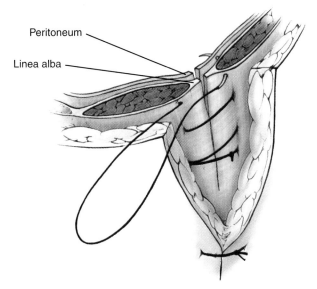

After the intended operation is completed, the incision is closed. There are many acceptable ways to close this abdominal incision. We generally close this incision with a No. 1 nonabsorbable running suture approximating the linea alba and peritoneum in one layer. Stitches are traditionally placed at least 1 cm in from the edge of the linea alba and move along at a distance of 1 cm. If there is any question about the integrity of the fascia, large interrupted nylon retention sutures can be placed to prevent evisceration.

Lower Midline Incision

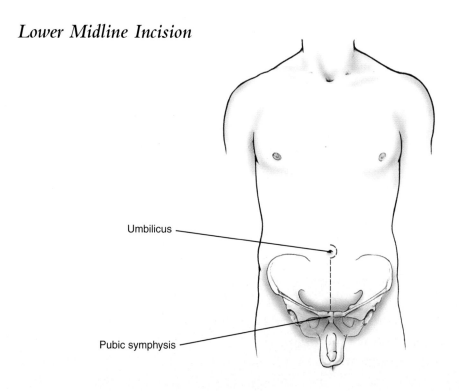

A lower midline incision is commonly used for operations to resect pelvic tumors and for surgery on the rectosigmoid colon and other viscera in the pelvis. A urinary bladder catheter is placed before making an incision to prevent injury to the bladder. An incision is made through the skin and subcutaneous tissue to expose the linea alba, which is narrow below the umbilicus. Often it is easier to divide the fascia in the midline high near the umbilicus and then continue inferiorly to the symphysis pubis. The peritoneum is carefully opened, making sure not to injure underlying bowel. The perivesicle fat is divided out laterally to prevent damage to the bladder. After the operative procedure is completed, the anterior fascia is closed with a No. 1 nonabsorbable suture in a continuous method, which distributes the tension along the suture line evenly.

Transverse Abdominal Incision

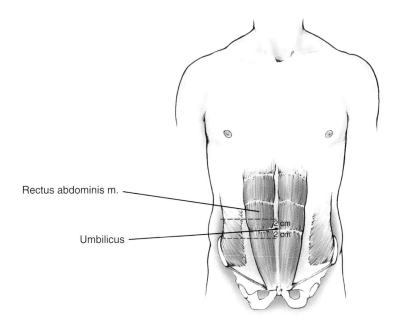

Rectus abdominis m.

2 cm
2 cm

Umbilicus

A transverse abdominal incision may be used at any level on the abdominal wall and may be made on the right or left. It takes longer to make and is more tedious to close. A transverse midabdominal incision can be used as an alternative to a vertical midline incision for colon surgery. The skin incision is made either 2 cm above or below the umbilicus, depending on where the lesion is located. Dissection is carried down through the subcutaneous tissue to expose the anterior rectus sheath and the external oblique muscle aponeurosis. The anterior rectus sheath is incised and the muscle transected. The external oblique muscle is split in the direction of its fibers. The epigastric vessels are clamped within the rectus muscle to prevent postoperative bleeding. The posterior rectus sheath and peritoneum are incised transversely to open the abdominal cavity. Moving out laterally, the internal oblique and transversus abdominis muscles are split in the direction of their fibers. The incision can be extended either way for more exposure. After the operation the peritoneum, transversalis fascia, internal oblique, and posterior rectus fasciae are closed with a continuous 0 absorbable suture. Finally, the external oblique fascia and the anterior rectus fasciae are closed in the same layer with No. 1 nonabsorbable suture.

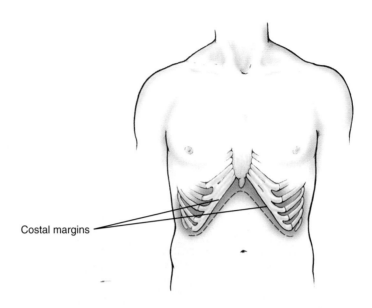

Costal margins

The bilateral subcostal incision gives excellent exposure to the pancreas, liver, and stomach. An incision is made two fingerbreadths below the right and left costal margins. The right external oblique and right anterior rectus fasciae are incised. The right rectus muscle is transected. The posterior rectus fascia and peritoneum are incised to enter the abdomen. The falciform ligament is divided and ligated. The remaining abdominal wall muscles on the right are divided from medial to lateral. The left rectus muscle and left abdominal wall muscles are divided from medial to lateral. After the operation is completed, the abdomen is closed in two layers. The transversus, internal oblique, and posterior rectus sheaths are closed with No. 1 nonabsorbable suture in a continuous fashion. The external oblique and anterior rectus fasciae and the linea alba are closed in another layer in the same continuous fashion.

Diagnostic Laparoscopy

Laparoscopy is being increasingly used as an important staging modality in a variety of abdominal malignancies. Recent reports have demonstrated that laparoscopy enhances clinical staging for gastric, hepatobiliary, and pancreatic cancer. Laparoscopy can help assess the stage of the primary tumor and detect low-volume peritoneal disease unappreciated on computed tomography (CT) scans. The ability of laparoscopic staging to avoid unnecessary exploration clearly identifies its role in gastric and pancreatic cancer. At laparoscopy, 20% to 25% of patients will be found to have advanced unresectable disease. Patients with gastric cancer without symptoms of obstruction or bleeding who are found to have unsuspected peritoneal disease at laparoscopy are spared open laparotomy. With the success of endoscopic biliary stent placement, a patient with pancreatic cancer found to have unsuspected peritoneal disease at laparoscopy is spared open laparotomy if there are no symptoms of gastric outlet obstruction.

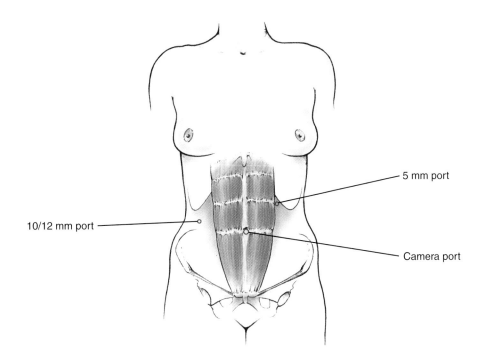

A diagnostic laparoscopy is performed with general anesthesia. It is our personal preference to use an open technique to gain access to the abdomen with a 10 mm Hasson cannula. Both 0- and 30-degree laparoscopes are used to explore the abdomen. About 250 ml of normal saline solution is instilled into the peritoneal cavity and then aspirated for cytologic examination. If present, intraperitoneal adhesions are divided. One or two 5 mm operating ports may be necessary for biopsy and for taking down adhesions. Any peritoneal nodules are biopsied. The liver is inspected while placing the patient in the reverse Trendelenburg position. A 10/12 mm port can be placed in the right upper quadrant for laparoscopic ultrasonography if it is available. For gastric tumors, the degree of wall penetration, local extension, volume, and fixation can be assessed. Currently trials are under way to examine the role of laparoscopic ultrasonography for detection of small liver lesions and assessment of resectability of pancreatic cancers. Diagnostic laparoscopy is a safe, sensitive, and cost-effective method for detecting occult metastatic disease in patients with gastric, hepatobiliary, or pancreatic cancer.

Laparoscopic Jejunostomy and Gastrostomy

For patients without extensive previous abdominal surgery and who need only a gastrostomy or feeding jejunostomy, a laparoscopic approach may spare them an open procedure. Many companies make laparoscopic gastrostomy and jejunostomy kits.

There are many methods of placing a feeding jejunostomy. One method is to place a Hasson cannula through a small incision below the umbilicus. The patient is placed in the Trendelenburg position. A 5 mm working port is placed in the right middle quadrant. The omentum is reflected superiorly to expose the ligament of Treitz.

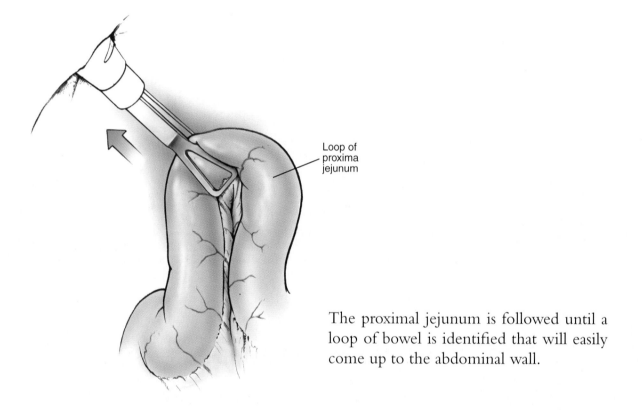

Loop of proxima jejunum

The proximal jejunum is followed until a loop of bowel is identified that will easily come up to the abdominal wall.

A small transverse incision is made in the abdominal wall and the jejunum is exteriorized. The jejunostomy tube is brought through the skin just below the skin incision and inserted into the jejunum in the standard fashion. The jejunum is tacked to the abdominal wall, and the incision is closed.

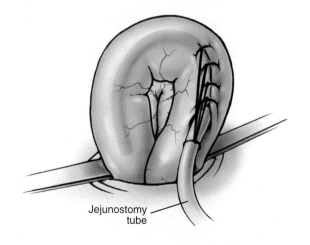

Jejunostomy tube

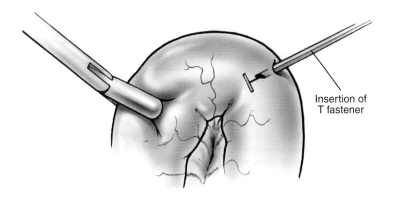

Insertion of T fastener

Another method, described by Way et al., is to use a percutaneous technique with T fasteners to pull the jejunum up to the abdominal wall.

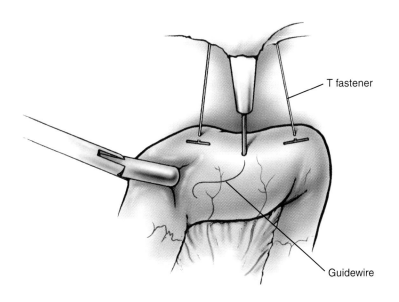

T fastener

Guidewire

A percutaneous introduction needle is then used to cannulate the jejunum, and a wire is passed into the bowel. Air can be insufflated into the bowel to confirm intraluminal placement of the needle before passing the wire. A series of dilators are passed under direct vision. The peel-away dilator is placed and the wire and dilator removed.

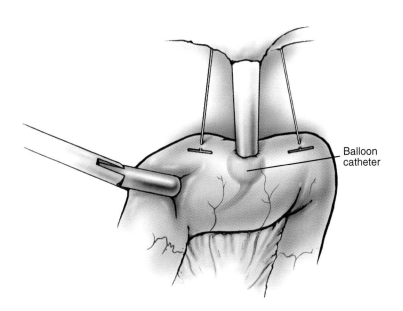

Balloon catheter

The jejunostomy is placed, and the balloon is inflated with 3 to 5 ml of saline solution. The jejunostomy is pulled snug to the abdominal wall. The T fasteners are tied securely to each other. The tube is irrigated to check its patency.

To perform a gastrostomy a Hasson cannula is placed through a small incision at the umbilicus. The laparoscope is placed through this cannula and the stomach is identified. A 5 mm working port is placed under direct vision in the right middle quadrant. The body of the stomach is brought up to the abdominal wall with a grasper to identify placement of the tube. A needle is placed percutaneously through the identified point for the tube and then into the anterior wall of the body of the stomach. Using the Seldinger technique, a wire is placed through the needle and into the body of the stomach. A series of dilators are inserted over the wire, followed by the gastrostomy tube. The balloon is inflated in the gastrostomy tube. The stomach is then tacked up to the abdominal wall with 3-0 silk intracorporeal sutures or with T fasteners, as described for the jejunostomy. Another option to secure the stomach to the abdominal wall is to take a 3-0 nylon suture on a Keith needle, place it through the skin, grasp it with a needle holder inside the abdomen, and place it through the stomach wall near the tube and then back out through the skin. The suture is tied extracorporeally over a cotton roll.

Laparoscopic Ileostomy and Colostomy

One hundred thousand patients undergo stoma surgery in the United States annually. Complications can be minimized by carefully selecting the stoma site, through adequate mobilization, avoiding tension on the bowel and maintaining the blood supply to the exteriorized segment. Many of these patients have end-stage cancer, and sparing them an open procedure could decrease their chances for complications. An ileostomy and transverse or sigmoid colostomy can all be done using a laparoscopic technique.

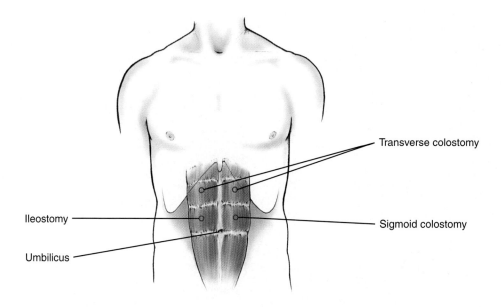

For optimal placement of stomas, enterstomal nurses mark the sites before surgery.

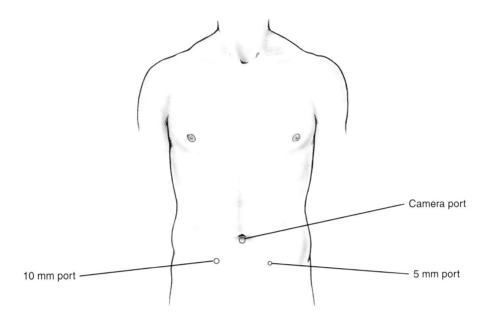

The operative technique for ileostomy involves placing a Hasson cannula in the usual periumbilical position after the induction of general anesthesia and placement of a Foley catheter and nasogastric tube. A laparoscopic Babcock clamp is used to grasp the small intestine through a 10 mm port placed through a preoperatively marked stoma site. A 5 mm port can be placed in the left lower quadrant if further dissection is required. The ileocecal valve is identified, and the distal ileum is followed proximally until a loop of bowel is identified that can be exteriorized without tension.

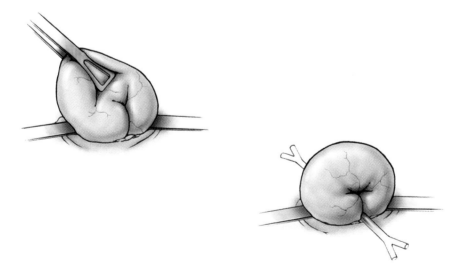

The bowel is brought out through a small incision, and the stoma is matured using the standard open Brooke method.

A transverse or sigmoid colostomy can be accomplished using a laparo-scopic approach. Most of these are loop colostomies done for palliation of downstream obstruction.

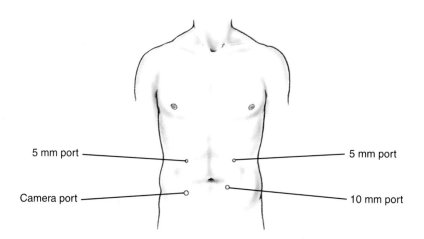

5 mm port —   — 5 mm port

Camera port —   — 10 mm port

For a transverse colostomy, the laparoscope is placed through a 10 mm Hasson cannula in the middle right quadrant. One or two 5 mm ports are placed to enable grasping the greater omentum in a cephalad direction.

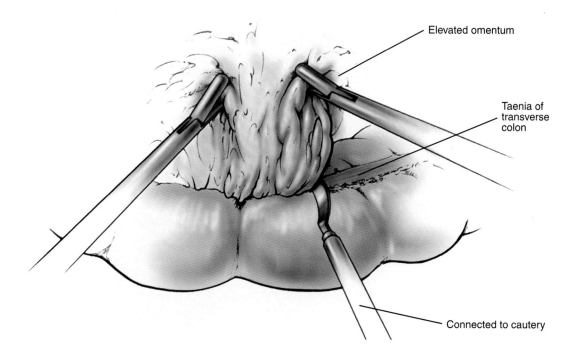

Elevated omentum

Taenia of transverse colon

Connected to cautery

With the weight of the transverse colon acting as countertraction, the omentum is dissected off the colon and brought up as the colostomy. This dissection is done through a 10 mm port placed through the stoma site.

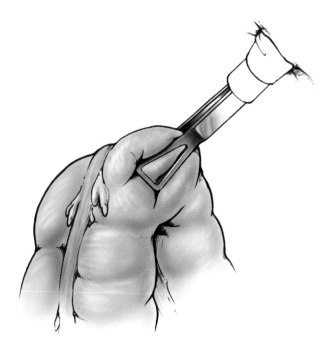

When the bowel has been sufficiently mobilized, it is brought up through the port site for the stoma. A similar technique is used for sigmoid colostomy. The Hasson cannula is placed in the umbilicus or middle right quadrant. The sigmoid colon is identified and mobilized along the white line of Toldt. A 10 mm port is placed through the stoma site for retraction of the colon.

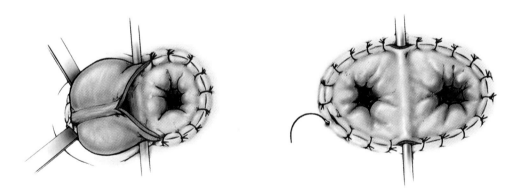

Once the mobilization is complete, a small incision is made around the port, the bowel is externalized, and the colostomy is matured.

Laparoscopic Colectomy

Since the first successful laparoscopic cholecystectomy in 1987, there has been progressive advancement of other laparoscopic procedures. Laparoscopic colon resection is especially attractive because it may offer benefits such as those described for laparoscopic cholecystectomy, including reductions in postoperative pain, narcotic requirements, duration of ileus, and duration of hospital stay. Early reports have demonstrated that patients undergoing laparoscopic colectomy regain bowel function sooner and are ready for discharge sooner than patients having an open procedure. The shorter period of postoperative ileus in laparoscopic colectomies is thought to be due to less bowel handling and less narcotic use. Laparoscopic colectomy is more challenging than cholecystectomy because several operative fields are involved, a larger specimen is taken, and intestinal anastomosis must be performed. A learning curve of 30 to 40 procedures has been described. One disadvantage of laparoscopic colectomy is the lack of tactile sense. However, technology such as laparoscopic ultrasonography to evaluate the liver, ureteral stents to help identify the ureters, and the dexterity glove, which through a 7 cm incision allows the surgeon to insert a hand through the abdominal wall for palpation and assistance with the laparoscopic procedure, all help to overcome this problem. The current indications for laparoscopy-assisted colectomy are segmental resection for colorectal polyps and diverticular disease. The role of laparoscopic colectomy in cancer is currently under intense investigation, and the procedure should be done only in a clinical protocol setting. Although there are no absolute selection criteria, thin patients with no previous surgery are considered ideal candidates for laparoscopic colectomy. The procedure in contraindicated in obese patients, patients who have had multiple intra-abdominal operations, and patients with severe cardiac or respiratory disease, or complex and advanced disease such as complicated diverticulitis, or bulky colon cancer. Lesions of the right, left, or sigmoid colon are amenable for laparoscopic resection. Transverse colon lesions are more difficult to resect because of the many omental attachments. Lesions larger than 15 cm are more easily resected because of the difficulty of transecting the distal rectum laparoscopically. Preoperative bowel preparation is the same for both open and laparoscopic colectomy.

Right Colectomy

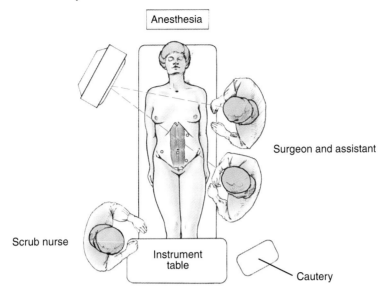

For resection of the right colon, the patient is placed supine on a beanbag. A nasogastric and Foley catheter are placed. After the induction of general anesthesia, the beanbag is secured around the patient, especially at the shoulders, and the abdomen is prepared and draped in the usual fashion. The surgeon and assistant operate from the patient's left side. A small periumbilical incision is made and the Hasson cannula inserted. Alternate sites can be used to enter the abdomen for those patients who have had previous surgery. The abdomen is insufflated with carbon dioxide to a pressure of 10 to 12 mm Hg. Higher pressures are associated with subcutaneous emphysema after the retroperitoneal dissection.

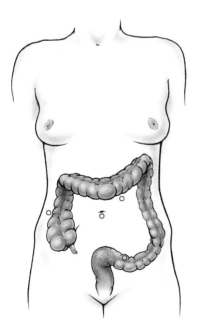

Additional 10 to 12 mm cannulas are placed. It is important to use cannulas with threads to prevent the cannulas from coming out during operative manipulation. Thorough exploration is performed, inspecting the liver, omentum, and peritoneum for metastatic disease. The 30-degree angled laparoscope is placed in the upper left paramedian cannula. The patient is placed in the Trendelenburg position with the left side down.

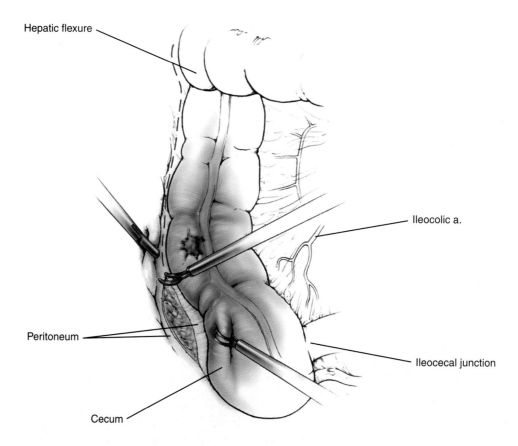

Hepatic flexure

Ileocolic a.

Peritoneum

Ileocecal junction

Cecum

The cecum is mobilized by grasping it with a Babcock clamp while the assistant provides countertraction on the adjacent peritoneal reflection. The white line of Toldt is incised with scissors, beginning at the cecum and progressing up to the hepatic flexure. After this dissection is completed, the right ureter can be identified. After the colon along the right gutter is mobilized, the laparoscope is moved to the left lower paramedian cannula. The patient is placed in reverse Trendelenburg position with the left side down.

The same technique, with a Babcock clamp on the colon and a grasper on the adjacent peritoneum, is used to mobilize the hepatic flexure. During this dissection the duodenum is visualized and injury is prevented. Continuing more medially, the omentum is dissected from the colon using electrocautery or vascular clips. After full mobilization of the right colon is complete, the colon is held up on tension to assess dissection of the mesentery. With the colon on tension, the ileocolic vessels should be easily identified.

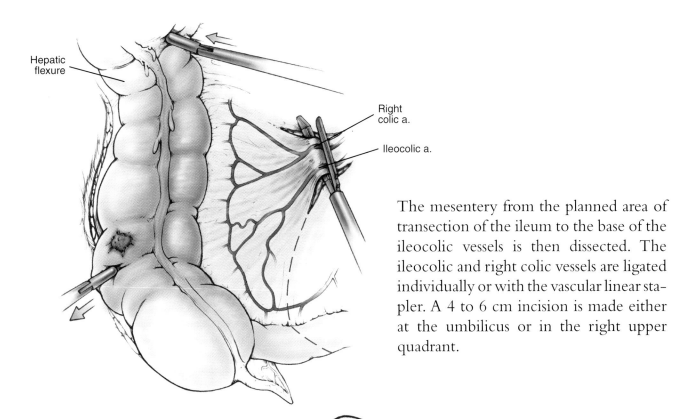

Hepatic
flexure

Right
colic a.

Ileocolic a.

The mesentery from the planned area of transection of the ileum to the base of the ileocolic vessels is then dissected. The ileocolic and right colic vessels are ligated individually or with the vascular linear stapler. A 4 to 6 cm incision is made either at the umbilicus or in the right upper quadrant.

The bowel is exteriorized and transected. The anastomosis is done in a standard fashion, and the mesentery is either closed entirely or left wide open. The bowel is returned to the abdominal cavity and the incision closed. The pneumoperitoneum is reestablished to check for hemostasis. The cannulas are removed under direct vision. The fasciae at the cannula site are closed with 0 absorbable suture.

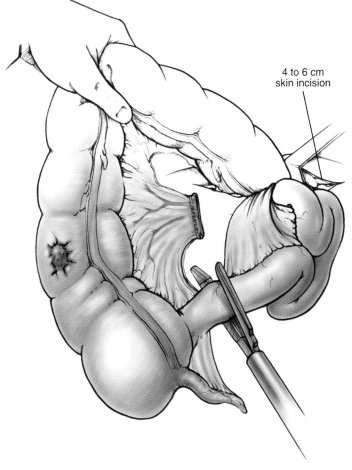

4 to 6 cm
skin incision

Left Colectomy

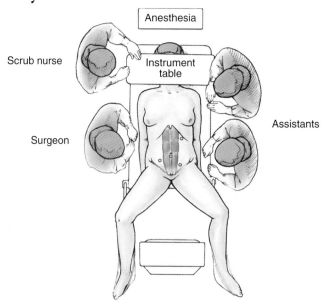

The surgeon and assistant operate from the patient's right side. After induction of general anesthesia, an infraumbilical Hasson cannula is placed, and the pneumoperitoneum is established.

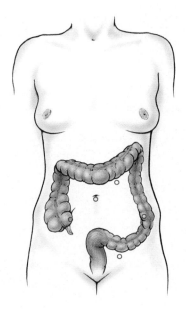

Other 10 to 12 mm cannulas are placed under direct vision. To mobilize the left colon the patient is placed in the Trendelenburg position with the right side down. The laparoscope is inserted in the right paramedian cannula. A Babcock clamp is used to retract the colon cephalad and to the patient's right.

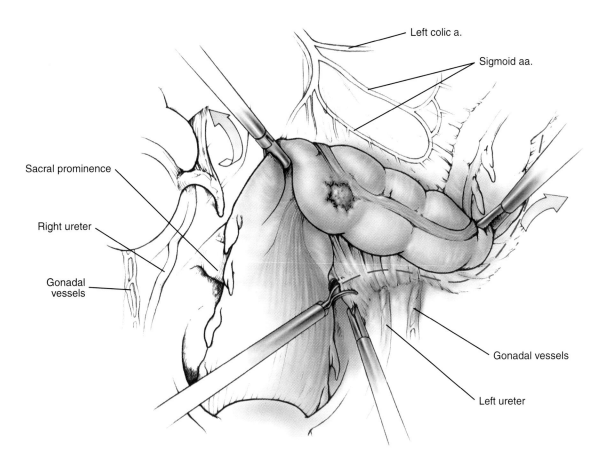

While the assistant retracts opposite the peritoneal attachments, the surgeon incises the left lateral peritoneal reflection from the sigmoid colon to the upper descending colon. If the ureter cannot be identified, the procedure should be converted to an open laparotomy. Lighted or infrared stents can facilitate identification of the left ureter. With the left colon mobilized to the splenic flexure, the laparoscope is placed in the right lower paramedian site. The patient is placed in the reverse Trendelenburg position with the right side down. While retracting the splenic flexure, the omentum is dissected from the colon.

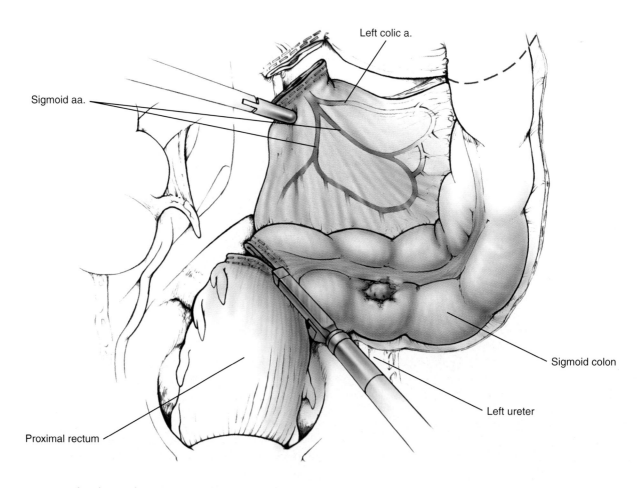

The bowel is retracted toward the abdominal wall and the sigmoidal and left colic vessels are divided using clips, EndoLoops, or a vascular linear stapler. A 4 to 6 cm incision is made at the left cannula to exteriorize the mobilized left colon. An extracorporeal anastomosis is done in the standard fashion, and the abdominal incision is closed.

Sigmoid Colectomy and Low Anterior Resection

For resection of the sigmoid colon and upper rectum, the patient is placed in the lithotomy position. The surgeon operates from the patient's right side. After the induction of general anesthesia, an infraumbilical Hasson cannula is placed, and the pneumoperitoneum is established.

Other 10 to 12 mm trocars are placed. The patient is placed in the Trendelenburg position with the right side down. The laparoscope is inserted in the left upper quadrant cannula. The left and sigmoid colons are mobilized as described.

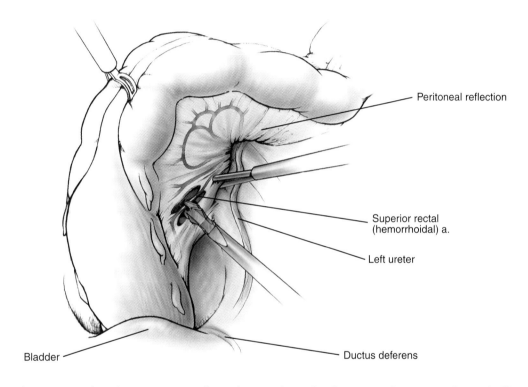

The sigmoid colon is grasped with a Babcock clamp and retracted medially. Countertraction is placed on the adjacent peritoneum, and the peritoneal reflection is incised with scissors. The ureter is identified in the left gutter. If the ureter cannot be identified, conversion to an open laparotomy is necessary. If the lesion is not transmural or is a polyp, intraoperative sigmoidoscopy may be necessary to find the lesion. To avoid intestinal distention, a laparoscopic bowel clamp is placed on the proximal left colon.

If a lower distal bowel transection is needed, the peritoneal reflection is incised circumferentially around the rectum and dissection is continued distally. A point at least 2 cm distal to the tumor is identified. A 60 mm linear stapler is inserted into an 18 mm cannula, which is exchanged for one of the smaller lower abdominal cannulas. The distal colon is transected with the stapler. The proximal colon is retracted toward the abdominal wall. The mesentery and the superior hemorrhoidal vessels are ligated with clips, electrocautery, or a vascular linear stapler. The proximal bowel is exteriorized through a 4 to 6 cm transverse incision around the left midabdominal cannula.

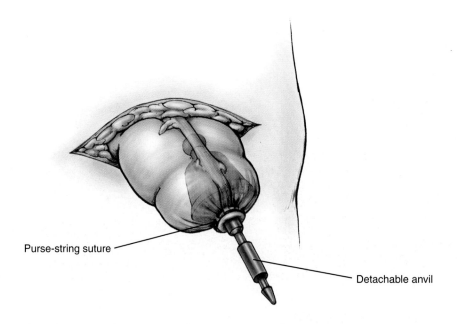

Purse-string suture

Detachable anvil

The proximal bowel is resected and the bowel diameter sized for a circular stapling device. A 2-0 monofilament purse-string suture is used to secure the anvil in the proximal bowel. The anvil and bowel are returned to the abdomen and the incision sutured closed.

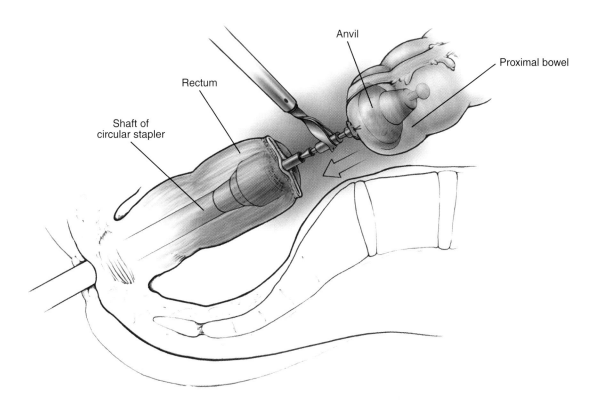

After reestablishment of the pneumoperitoneum, the anvil is attached to the stapler, which is introduced through the anus. After firing the stapler the proximal and distal tissue doughnuts are inspected. Proctoscopy is done to inspect the anastomosis for bleeding and intactness.

Anatomic Basis of Complications

MAJOR

• Inadequate closure of the anterior fascia may result in a dehiscence or evisceration.

MINOR

• Inadequate ligation and identification of the epigastric blood vessels during a transverse abdominal incision may result in a postoperative rectus sheath hematoma.

KEY REFERENCES

Conlon KC, Karpeh MS Jr. Laparoscopy and laparoscopic ultrasound in the staging of gastric cancer. Semin Oncol 23:347-351, 1996.

This study looked at the role of staging laparoscopy in patients with gastric cancer. Occult metastatic disease not seen on CT scan was found by laparoscopy in 25% to 30% of these patients.

Elftmann TD, Nelson H, Ota DM, et al. Laproscopic-assisted segmental colectomy: Surgical techniques. Mayo Clin Proc 69:825-833, 1994.

These authors reviewed surgical techniques for successful laparoscopic colon surgery. Morbidity and mortality were comparable to those for open procedures.

Gagner M. Laparoscopic adrenalectomy. Surg Clin North Am 76:523-537, 1996.

This article is a review of operative techniques and indications for laparoscopic adrenalectomy. Laparoscopic adrenalectomy can be done safely for a wide range of endocrine disorders.

Rege RV, Merriam LT, Joehl RJ. Laparoscopic splenectomy. Surg Clin North Am 76:459-463, 1996.

This article is a review of operative techniques and indications for laparoscopic splenectomy. Early results show the procedure can be done safely, and the reduced length in hospital stay is significant.

Wexner SD, Cohen SM. Port site metastases after laparoscopic colorectal surgery for cure of malignancy. Br J Surg 82:295-298, 1995.

This review of the literature examined the incidence of port site recurrences after laparoscopic colon surgery. The risk of port site recurrences supports the importance of randomized trials of laparoscopic colectomy.

SUGGESTED READINGS

Bîhm B, Milsom JW, Kitago K, et al. Use of laparoscopic techniques in oncologic right colectomy in a canine model. Ann Surg Oncol 2:6-13,1995.

Brown JP, Albala DM, Jahoda A. Laparoscopic surgery for adrenal lesions. Semin Surg Oncol 12:96-99, 1996.

Clemente CD. The abdomen. In Clemente CD, ed. Anatomy: A Regional Atlas of the Human Body. Baltimore: Urban and Schwarzenberg, 1987, pp 231-342.

Cuesta MA, Meijer S, Borgstein PJ, et al. Laparoscopic ultrasonography for hepatobiliary and pancreatic malignancy. Br J Surg 80:1571-1574, 1993.

Ellis H. Abdominal wall: Incisions and closures. In Schwartz SI, Ellis H, eds. Maingot's Abdominal Operations, 8th ed. Norwalk, Conn.: Appleton-Century-Crofts, 1985, pp 247-263.

Fernandez-Del Castillo C, Rattner DW, Warshaw AL. Further experience with laparoscopy and peritoneal cytology in the staging of pancreatic cancer. Br J Surg 82:1127-1129, 1995.

Fuhrman GM, Ota DM. Laparoscopic intestinal stomas. Dis Colon Rectum 37:444-449, 1994.

Greene FL. Laparoscopic staging of malignancies. In Arregui ME, Fitzgibbons RJ, Katkhouda N, et al, eds. Principles of Laparoscopic Surgery. New York: Springer-Verlag, 1995, pp 318-323.

Hall-Craggs ECB. The abdomen. In Hall-Craggs ECB, ed. Anatomy as a Basis for Clinical Medicine. London: Williams & Wilkins Waverly Europe, 1995, pp 220-281.

MacFadyen BV, Ricardo AE, Vecchio R. Ileostomy and colostomy. In MacFadyen BV, Ponsky SL, eds. Operative Laparoscopy and Thoracoscopy. Philadelphia: Lippincott-Raven, 1996, pp 711-727.

Reilly WT, Nelson H, Schroeder G, et al. Wound recurrence following conventional treatment of colorectal cancer. Dis Colon Rectum 39:200-207, 1996.

Schirmer BD. Laparoscopic colon resection. Surg Clin North Am 76:571-583, 1996.

Shackelford RT, Zuidema GD. Abdominal incisions. In Shackelford RT, Zuidema GD, eds. Surgery of the Alimentary Tract. Philadelphia: WB Saunders, 1981, pp 467-524.

Snell R. The abdomen: Part I. In Snell R, ed. Clinical Anatomy for Medical Students. Boston: Little, Brown, 1973, pp 145-165.

Unger SW, Edelman DS. Gastric and small bowel access for enteral feeding. In MacFadyen BV, Ponsky SL, eds. Operative Laparoscopy and Thoracoscopy. Philadelphia: Lippincott-Raven, 1996, pp 619-628.

Woodburne RT, Burkel WE. The abdomen. In Woodburne RT, ed. Essentials of Human Anatomy. New York: Oxford University Press, 1994, pp 417-512.

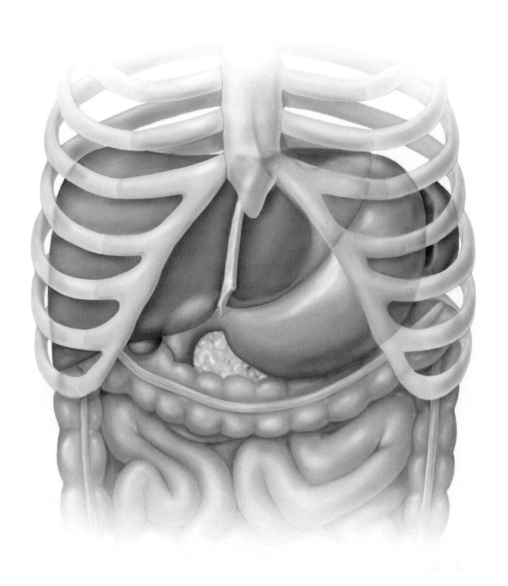

Chapter 7

Stomach

Charles A. Staley, M.D.

Surgical Applications

*I*t is estimated that gastric cancer, the eighth most common cause of cancer mortality, will account for 24,000 new cases each year. From 1930 to 1980 the incidence of gastric cancer decreased, but more recently the number of new cases has plateaued. Many environmental and dietary factors have been associated with an increased risk for gastric cancer, but more specifically, *Helicobacter pylori,* a gram-negative bacteria, has been implicated as a possible promotor agent. Ninty-five percent of gastric cancers are adenocarcinomas. The remaining 5% are lymphomas, carcinoids, and leiomyosarcomas. Clinically, gastric cancer lacks specific symptoms, which is why most patients have locally advanced or metastatic disease at presentation. Endoscopy with biopsy, computed tomography (CT), and endoscopic ultrasonography all aid in the diagnosis and staging of gastric cancer. Because of the limitation of CT in evaluation of peritoneal disease, diagnostic laparoscopy should be done before an open procedure in asymptomatic patients to avoid an unnecessary operation.

Proximal tumors of the cardia and midbody, which are increasing in occurrence, usually require total gastrectomy. Distal tumors, which account for 35% to 40% of all gastric tumors, necessitate subtotal gastrectomy with a 5 cm gross tumor margin. Splenectomy is not performed unless there is direct tumor adherence or invasion of the spleen. If splenectomy is contemplated, a pneumococcal vaccine should be given before surgery. Although the role of adjuvant and neoadjuvant therapy is still under investigation, surgical resection of gastric cancer remains the only potentially curative treatment. However, except for very rare early gastric cancers (T1 N0 M0), overall survival remains poor, with 5-year survival of only 15%.

In contrast to the decreasing incidence of gastric adenocarcinoma, the incidence of gastric lymphoma is steadily increasing. Gastric lymphomas account

Table 7-1 *Five-Year Survival Rate After Gastrectomy in the United States*

Tumor Stage	Five-Year Survival (%)
N0T1	90
N0T2	58
N0T3	50
N1	20
N2	10

Adapted from Noguchi Y, Imada T, Matsumoto A, et al. Radical surgery for gastric cancer: A review of the Japanese experience. Cancer 64:2055-2062, 1989. Copyright © 1989 American Cancer Society. Reprinted by permission of Wiley-Liss, Inc., a subsidiary of John Wiley & Sons, Inc.

for two thirds of all gastrointestinal lymphomas. The average patient age is 60 years, and they usually present with abdominal pain, weight loss, bleeding, and fatigue. Obstruction and massive bleeding are rare. Endoscopy establishes the diagnosis in 80% of cases. Treatment of gastric lymphomas varies among institutions, with some centers using surgery and others promoting chemotherapy and radiation. Overall, there seems to be a general trend toward treatment with aggressive chemotherapy alone, especially since the reported response rates are greater than 90%. Surgical resection is now reserved for patients with residual disease or recurrent disease or for patients in whom perforation, bleeding, or obstruction develop during treatment.

Many benign and malignant gastric cancers, along with a host of unresectable and metastatic intra-abdominal cancers, may require either a curative or palliative surgical procedure involving the stomach. Whether it is a palliative procedure such as a gastrostomy tube or gastrojejunostomy or a potentially curative gastric resection and lymphadenectomy, knowledge of the clinical anatomy and technical operative expertise in gastric surgery are imperative. Understanding the natural history and defining the patients for surgical intervention by appropriate clinical staging will minimize unnecessary surgery in patients with an overall poor survival.

TNM Staging System for Gastric Carcinoma

T1	Tumor invades lamina propria or submucosa
T2	Tumor invades muscularis propria or subserosa
T3	Tumor penetrates serosa
T4	Tumor invades adjacent organ structures
N0	No metastases in lymph nodes
N1	Metastasis in perigastric lymph nodes within 3 cm of primary tumor
N2	Metastasis in perigastric lymph nodes >3 cm from primary tumor or in lymph nodes along left gastric, common hepatic, splenic, or celiac arteries
M0	No evidence of distant metastasis
M1	Evidence of distant metastasis

From Beahrs O, Henson D, Hutter R, et al. Handbook of Staging of Cancer. Philadelphia: JB Lippincott, 1993, pp 80-87. Used with the permission of the American Joint Committee on Cancer (AJCC), Chicago, Ill.

SURGICAL ANATOMY
Topography

The stomach is the first abdominal organ of the digestive tract and acts as a reservoir for ingested food to begin both mechanical and chemical digestion. It lies principally in the left upper quadrant of the abdomen but terminates across the midline and frequently descends below the plane of umbilicus. The position of the stomach is variable, depending on body position, contents, and respiratory movements.

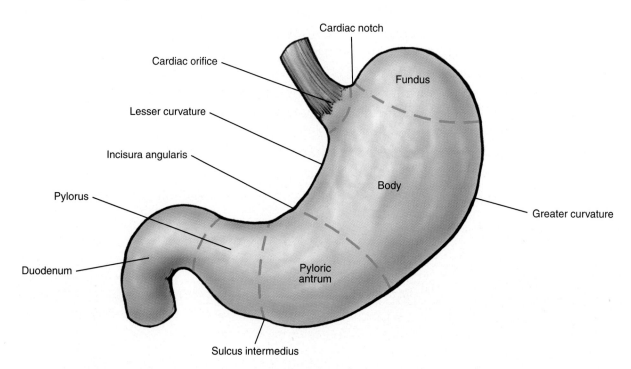

The anatomic regions of the stomach are divided into the cardia, fundus, body, and pylorus. The cardiac orifice marks the transition from the esophagus to the stomach. The cardia of the stomach is the portion immediately surrounding the esophageal opening and has a relatively stable location due to the esophageal attachments of the diaphragm and the peritoneal reflections (gastrophrenic ligament). At the esophagogastric junction a deep notch, defined as the cardiac notch, separates the esophagus and the fundus. The cardiac notch, together with decussating fibers of the diaphragm and circular fibers of the lower esophagus, forms a lower esophageal sphincter that prevents esophageal reflux under normal conditions. The fundus of the stomach expands upward, filling the dome of the diaphragm on the left side, and is limited below by the horizontal plane of the cardiac orifice. The incisura angularis, a sharp indentation about two thirds of the distance along the lesser curvature, marks a vertical separation between the body of the stomach to its left and the pyloric portion of the stomach to its right and is used surgically as the proximal line of transection for antrectomy. The pyloric portion of the stomach consists of the pyloric antrum, pyloric canal, and a markedly constricted terminal pylorus, composed of a greatly thickened muscular wall constituting the pyloric sphincter. The thickened sphincter marks the termination of the stomach and its transition to the retroperitoneal duodenum, which is fixed to the posterior body wall.

Curvatures and Surfaces

The axis of the stomach is oblique and extends from the fundus downward to the right and ventral. The lesser curvature marks the right border of the stomach and extends from the esophagogastric junction along a concave curve to the right and terminates at the pylorus. The greater curvature is the left and inferior border of the stomach. It begins at the cardiac notch, follows the superior curvature of the fundus, and then the convex curvature of the body down to the pylorus. The greater curvature is four or five times longer than the lesser curvature.

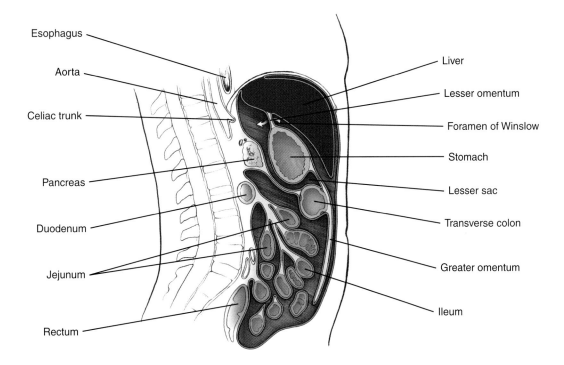

The rotation of the stomach during embryologic development creates a space, known as the lesser sac or omental bursa, between the stomach and the posterior abdominal wall. This space is bounded anteriorly by the stomach and lesser omentum, superiorly by the liver, inferiorly by the greater omentum (and its fusion to the transverse colon), and to the left by the spleen and its ligaments. On the right, the lesser sac opens into the greater sac through the epiploic foramen (of Winslow). The greater sac of the abdomen fills the remaining space within the peritoneal cavity.

Peritoneal Relations

The stomach is entirely covered by peritoneum except where the blood vessels course along the curvatures and except for a small triangular space behind the cardiac orifice. Here the stomach is left bare by the gastrophrenic peritoneal reflection. At the lesser curvature the two layers of peritoneum extend to the liver as the gastrohepatic portion of the lesser omentum. From the greater curvature the greater omentum spreads widely to the diaphragm as the gastrophrenic ligament, to the spleen as the gastrosplenic ligament, and to the transverse colon as the gastrocolic ligament.

Structure

The stomach wall is composed of four distinct histologic layers: the mucosa, submucosa, muscularis, and serosa. The mucosa is thrown into a series of coarse gastric folds known as rugae. These are oriented chiefly longitudinally along the lesser curvature. The submucosal layer is a loose, areolar, vascular layer. The muscular layer of the stomach is composed of an outer longitudinal and inner circular muscular layer, typical of the gastrointestinal tract, but also contains an internal oblique layer. The circular muscle is the dominant muscle layer of the stomach. The outer longitudinal layer is not so uniform as the circular layer, being concentrated particularly along the curvatures. The serosal layer is the peritoneum.

The gastric epithelium consists of a single layer of columnar cells. The stomach has specialized glands in the different regions of the stomach that vary in structure and function.

The cardiac glands are found in the region of the esophageal opening. Each gland is composed of a few branching tubules containing cells that secrete a form of mucus.

Fundic or gastric glands in the fundus and body of the stomach have long secreting tubules with short ducts opening into shallow gastric pits. Three types of cells line these tubules. The mucous neck cells in the upper part of the gland secrete mucus. The chief or zymogenic cells secrete pepsin, a proteolytic enzyme of the gastric juice. At intervals throughout the length of the tubule are large eosinophilic cells between the chief cells known as parietal cells, which are responsible for secretion of the hydrochloric acid in the gastric juice.

The pyloric glands are short, branched tubules opening into long duct-like gastric pits. The exact contribution of the pyloric glands to the gastric secretion is not known, although they resemble mucous neck cells. Gastrin, a hormone that increases acid production from the parietal cells and gastric motility, is secreted by the G cells in the pylorus of the stomach.

Blood Supply

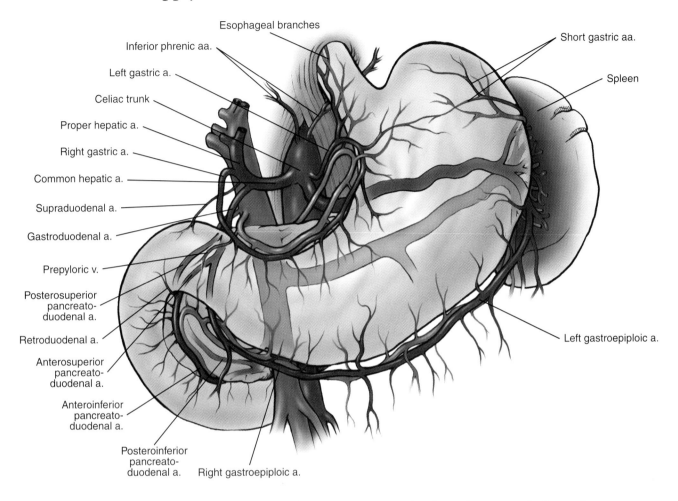

The blood supply to the stomach is extensive and is based on vessels from the celiac trunk. The four major vessels that supply the stomach are the right and left gastric and the right and left gastroepiploic arteries.

Celiac Trunk

The aorta passes through the aortic hiatus of the diaphragm into the abdominal cavity in front of the lower border of the twelfth thoracic vertebra. The celiac trunk and the superior mesenteric and inferior mesenteric arteries are the three principal ventral unpaired branches of the aorta and supply the majority of the gastrointestinal system.

The celiac trunk arises from the front of the abdominal aorta, just below the aortic hiatus and at the level of the upper portion of the first lumbar vertebra. Only 1 to 2 cm long, the celiac trunk passes forward above the upper margin of the pancreas and then divides behind the posterior body wall peritoneum into the left gastric, common hepatic, and splenic arteries. In the region of the celiac trunk lies the celiac lymph nodes and the celiac plexus of nerves and their ganglia.

Left Gastric Artery

The left gastric artery, the smallest branch of the celiac trunk, courses upward and to the left toward the cardiac end of the stomach. The vessel lies behind the body wall peritoneum in the floor of the lesser sac, where it frequently raises a fold of peritoneum, the left gastropancreatic fold. It reaches the stomach in the bare area behind the cardia, giving off esophageal branches that ascend along the esophagus to provide a portion of its arterial supply. The left gastric artery then turns onto the lesser curvature of the stomach between the layers of the hepatogastric ligament and follows this curvature as far as the pylorus, providing branches to both surfaces of the stomach, and anastomoses terminally with the right gastric artery.

Right Gastric and Right Gastroepiploic Arteries

The common hepatic artery arises from the celiac trunk, runs forward and to the right along the upper border of the pancreas, passes into the lesser omentum giving off the gastroduodenal artery, and continues to the liver as the proper hepatic artery. The gastroduodenal artery is a short, thick branch that takes its origin from the common hepatic artery at the upper border of the first part of the duodenum. It descends behind this portion of the duodenum and divides at its inferior border into the right gastroepiploic and anterosuperior pancreaticoduodenal arteries.

The right gastroepiploic artery passes from right to left along the greater curvature of the stomach between the layers of the gastrocolic ligament. It anastomoses with the left gastroepiploic artery to form a vascular arch along the greater curvature, from which pass gastric branches to both surfaces of the stomach and omental branches to the greater omentum.

The proper hepatic artery, which is the continuation of the common hepatic artery distal to the gastroduodenal artery, usually gives off the right gastric artery, and terminates by dividing into the right and left hepatic arteries. The small right gastric artery descends through the lesser omentum to the pyloric end of the lesser curvature of the stomach. It supplies branches to both surfaces of the pyloric portion of the stomach and anastomoses with the left gastric artery. The right gastric artery is most commonly a branch of the proper hepatic artery, but may arise from the left hepatic, gastroduodenal, or common hepatic arteries.

Left Gastroepiploic Artery

The splenic artery runs a highly tortuous course along the superior border of the pancreas, behind the peritoneum of the floor of the lesser sac. The left gastroepiploic artery arises from the splenic artery or an inferior terminal branch, passes toward the greater curvature of the stomach through the gastrosplenic ligament, and forms a vascular arcade with the right gastroepiploic artery. Its gastric and epiploic branches are distributed to both surfaces of the stomach and to the greater omentum.

The short gastric arteries are four or five small vessels that arise directly from the splenic artery and pass through the gastrosplenic ligament to reach the fundus of the stomach.

Veins

The veins of the stomach run parallel with the arteries and drain into the portal venous system.

The left gastric vein arises from tributaries on both surfaces of the stomach. It passes from right to left along the lesser curvature to the cardia, where it receives esophageal veins. The left gastric vein then turns to the right and descends in company with the left gastric artery, behind the posterior body wall peritoneum. Passing beyond the celiac arterial trunk, the left gastric vein ends in the portal vein. This circular course, first along the lesser curvature and then inferiorly on the body wall, is expressed in the old name "coronary vein."

The small right gastric vein is formed from the tributaries of both surfaces of the pyloric region of the stomach. It accompanies the right gastric artery between the layers of the lesser omentum and, passing from left to right, ends directly in the portal vein. A prepyloric vein ascends over the pylorus to the right gastric vein and is an anatomic landmark that enables the surgeon to identify the pylorus.

The right gastroepiploic vein accompanies the right gastroepiploic artery within the layers of the gastrocolic ligament. It receives tributaries from the inferior portions of both the anterior and posterior surfaces of the stomach and from the greater omentum. The vein crosses the uncinate process of the pancreas and ends in the superior mesenteric vein.

The left gastroepiploic vein completes the arch of veins along the greater curvature of the stomach and has the same pattern of drainage as the right gastroepiploic vein. It is directed to the left in the folds of the gastrocolic ligament. Entering the gastrosplenic ligament, the left gastroepiploic vein ends in the beginning of the splenic vein.

The short gastric veins, four or five in number, drain the fundus and the superior part of the greater curvature of the stomach. They pass between the layers of the gastrosplenic ligament toward the hilum of the spleen, where they terminate in the splenic vein.

Lymphatic Drainage

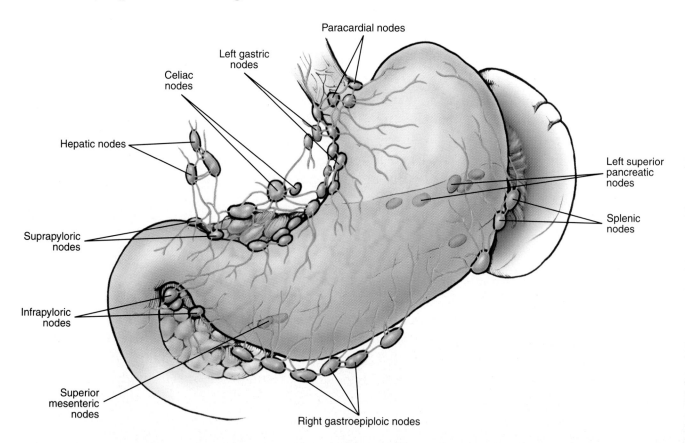

The lymphatic vessels of the stomach have a pattern similar to that of its arteries and veins. There are four major routes of lymphatic drainage from the stomach.

A large group of lymphatic vessels drain the surfaces toward the lesser curvature of the stomach to the left gastric nodes. These form a chain of 10 to 20 nodes extending from the angular notch of the stomach upward to the cardia. At the cardia a small group of five or six paracardiac nodes surround the esophagogastric junction. The left gastric nodes follow the left gastric blood vessels to the celiac nodes.

Another group of nodes drain the pyloric portion of the lesser curvature to the two or three right gastric nodes. These in turn run along the right gastric artery and drain into the hepatic nodes.

The left half of the stomach drains by lymphatic channels directed toward the greater curvature. Lymphatic vessels from the fundus and the upper portion of the body of the stomach follow the short gastric and left gastroepiploic blood vessels to the pancreatosplenic nodes. Three or four lymph nodes are situated along the posterosuperior border of the pancreas on the splenic blood vessels. The pancreatosplenic nodes drain the stomach, spleen, and pancreas and then drain into the celiac nodes.

Finally, from the lower portion of the left half of the stomach, lymphatic vessels drain to the six to 12 right gastroepiploic nodes, the efferents of which pass to the right to the pyloric nodes. The pyloric lymph nodes are six to eight nodes located in the angle between the first and second parts of the duodenum in close relation to the terminal division of the gastroduodenal artery. Their efferents pass along this artery to the hepatic nodes and then to the celiac nodes.

Lymph draining from the stomach by means of these various routes passes through the lymph node groups described and ultimately reaches the celiac nodes. The efferent channels of the celiac nodes help form, with efferents from the superior mesenteric nodes, the intestinal trunk.

Nerve Supply

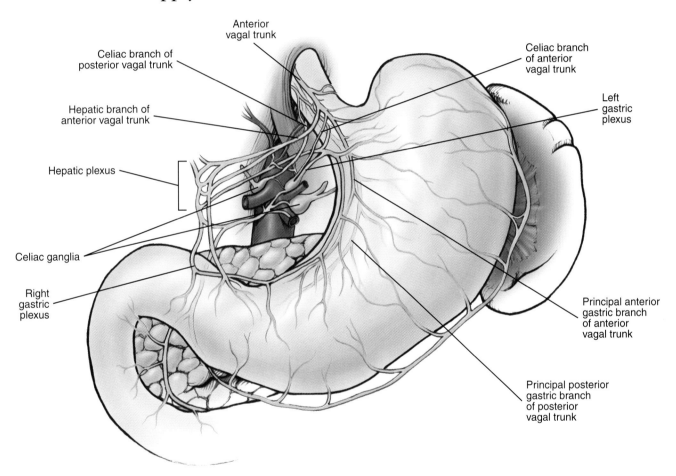

The nerves of the stomach are both parasympathetic by way of the vagus nerve and sympathetic by means of perivascular plexuses from the celiac plexus.

The right and left vagus nerves above the diaphragm coalesce to form the esophageal plexus. Just above the diaphragm the esophageal plexus divides into two nerve trunks that lie anterior and posterior to the esophagus, then pass through the esophageal hiatus of the diaphragm and down the lesser curve of the stomach.

Both vagus nerves supply gastric branches to the stomach that arise at the cardiac end of the stomach. Each anterior and posterior vagal trunk gives off one long branch, the principal nerves of the lesser curvature, also known as the nerves of Laterjet, which descend on the anterior and posterior surfaces of the stomach and terminate as a "crow's foot" on the pyloric antrum. In addition to the gastric branches, the anterior vagal trunk has a hepatic branch that passes from the stomach to the liver in the upper part of the hepatogastric ligament together with the hepatic branch of the left gastric artery. It also has a small branch that descends through the hepatogastric ligament to the pyloric portion of the stomach, duodenum, and pancreas. The posterior vagal trunk makes a major contribution to the celiac plexus by means of a celiac branch that follows the left gastric artery and vein.

The sympathetic nerve supply of the stomach is by perivascular plexuses (left gastric, hepatic, and splenic) that emanate from the celiac plexus. These are composed primarily of postganglionic sympathetic fibers, the cell bodies of which form the celiac ganglia. The preganglionic fibers reach the celiac ganglia by way of the greater thoracic splanchnic nerve from the fifth to the tenth thoracic cord segments.

The nerves to the stomach appear to have somewhat mixed functions. However, the parasympathetic innervation initiates or enhances muscular movements, and the sympathetic innervation is important in vasomotor control. The parasympathetic fibers exert the greater influence on the secretion of water and hydrochloric acid in the fundus and body; the sympathetic innervation has the major influence in the secretion of enzymes in the stomach.

SURGICAL APPLICATIONS
Gastrostomy

There are a number of indications for operative placement of gastrostomy tubes, but they are generally used for gastric decompression or short-term external tube feedings. Long-term enteral feeding through a gastrostomy tube should be avoided because of increased risk for pulmonary aspiration. Patients with carcinomatosis or bowel obstructions requiring extensive lysis of adhesions or patients undergoing long elective abdominal operations may benefit from placement of a gastrostomy tube rather than prolonged use of a nasogastric tube. The advantages of a gastrostomy tube include the following: (1) it is vastly more comfortable than a nasogastric tube, (2) it allows the patient more mobility, and (3) it does not interfere with respirations or pulmonary toilet. In older patients with underlying pulmonary diseases, a gastrostomy tube may prevent some potentially lethal postoperative complications.

The most widely used temporary gastrostomy is the Stamm gastrostomy. It is performed quickly, easily, and safely and provides excellent venting of the stomach. The stomach is identified and grasped along the greater curvature with two Babcock clamps. A point is chosen on the middle anterior surface of the stomach where it will easily be sewn to the abdominal wall without any tension. A large (20 to 28 Fr) Malecot or Silastic Foley catheter is brought through a small puncture site in the left upper quadrant, away from the costal margin.

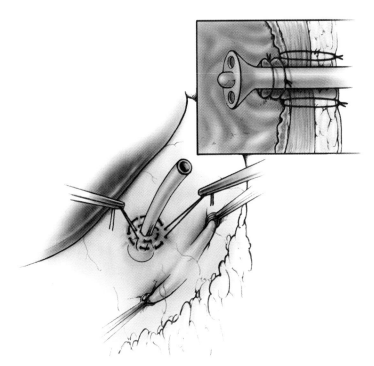

Two concentric 2-0 silk purse-string sutures are placed in the anterior body wall of the stomach. An opening is made in the stomach through the center of the inner purse-string suture using the electrocautery. The gastrostomy tube is inserted into the stomach, and the inner purse-string suture is securely tied. While pushing down on the catheter or directly applying downward pressure on the ends of the inner purse-string suture, the outer purse string is tied. The two purse-string sutures form a snug seal and serosal lining for the tube tract. The gastric wall surrounding the tube is sutured to the abdominal wall in all four quadrants to prevent retraction and leakage. The catheter is secured to the skin with a 3-0 nylon suture.

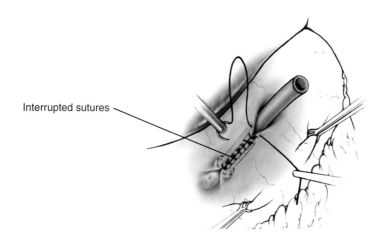

Interrupted sutures

In cases in which the stomach cannot come up to the abdominal wall because of severe adhesions or after a partial gastric resection, a Witzel gastrostomy can be done.

In this method, a single purse-string suture is placed, the tube is positioned through the gastric wall, and a tunnel is fashioned along the anterior gastric wall with 3-0 silk sutures. The gastrostomy tube penetrates the stomach at a distance from the point where it exits the abdominal wall to minimize leakage around the tube.

Postoperatively, the gastrostomy tube is placed to drain by gravity and is irrigated on every shift to avoid occlusion by mucus or other debris. The tube should be left in place for a minimum of 2 to 3 weeks to allow a tract to form between the stomach and the skin, thus preventing intra-abdominal leakage when removed.

Complications from gastrostomy placement are rare but can include leakage and retraction of the stomach from the abdominal wall. Small leaks can be treated conservatively with adequate drainage and nasogastric decompression of the stomach. Major leaks or retraction require repeat operation and repair.

Resection of Smooth Muscle Tumors

The most common benign tumor of the stomach in autopsy studies is a leiomyoma. These tumors are usually found incidentally, but can be a source of upper gastrointestinal tract bleeding or epigastric abdominal pain or can cause obstruction if located in the pylorus. Leiomyomas arise most commonly from the muscularis propria and may not be visualized by endoscopy, as would a mucosal lesion. Abdominal CT scans can be useful in determining an operative strategy for resection. Generally, if they are less than 5 cm in size and the histologic picture (low mitotic index) suggests a benign tumor, it is characterized as a leiomyoma (Applebaum's criteria). Lesions larger than 5 cm should be considered malignant sarcomas. The operative technique for a benign leiomyoma is exploration through an upper midline incision and a partial gastrectomy with a 2 cm margin. If the tumor is along the greater curvature, the omentum is removed from the stomach near the tumor.

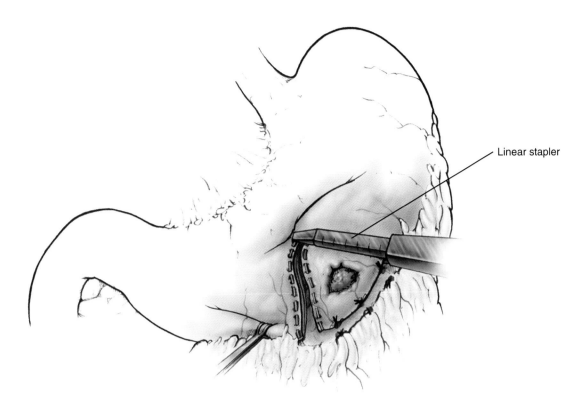

Linear stapler

The resection can be done using a linear stapler or by hand, with a standard two-layer closure. If stapled, the staple line is oversewn with a row of 3-0 silk Lembert sutures. Lesions along the lesser curvature are resected in a similar manner. However, if the resection is in the antral area, a pyloromyotomy should be performed to guard against gastric outlet obstruction from vagal nerve injury.

A Heineke-Mikulicz pyloroplasty is perhaps the most commonly performed pyloroplasty and is begun by placing two silk stay sutures at the cephalad and caudal portions of the pylorus.

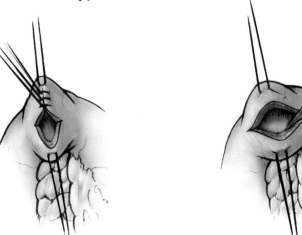

With gentle traction upward on the stay sutures, the pylorus is opened longitudinally and closed transversely with interrupted 3-0 silk sutures. In cases of prepyloric lesions, subtotal gastrectomy should be performed. For malignant sarcomas, the majority of which are leiomyosarcomas, gastric resection is performed, leaving a tumor-free margin. In resectable disease, tumor grade appears to be the single most important prognostic factor. There is no improvement in local control or overall survival with an extended gastric resection compared with lesser resections encompassing all gross disease. Adjuvant radiation therapy is often added to higher grade sarcomas analogously to soft tissue sarcomas.

Gastrojejunostomy

Gastrojejunostomy is indicated for patients with unresectable gastrointestinal cancers such as pancreatic, duodenal, or distal gastric cancers with evidence of impending or symptomatic mechanical gastric outlet obstruction. For patients with unresectable pancreatic or ampullary malignancies, a gastrojejunostomy is often combined with a biliary bypass. The procedure can be performed through either an upper midline or bilateral subcostal incision. Once exploration confirms unresectablility of the primary tumor and near obstruction of the distal stomach or duodenum, the most dependent area of the greater curvature of the stomach is identified.

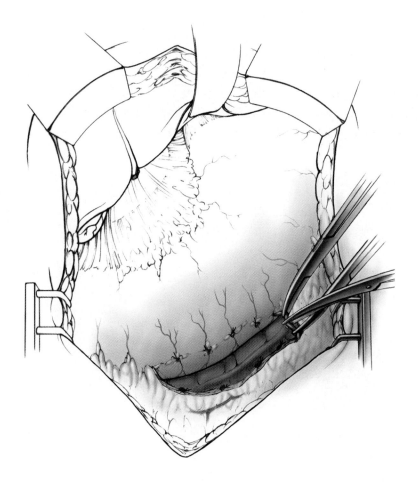

The omentum along this area is dissected from the greater curvature, and the lesser sac is entered. The next decision is whether to perform the anastomosis in an antecolic or retrocolic fashion. The retrocolic gastrojejunostomy generally empties better than the antecolic gastrojejunostomy but theoretically could be obstructed by tumors invading the transverse mesocolon. For these potentially obstructing tumors, an anticolic anastomosis is recommended.

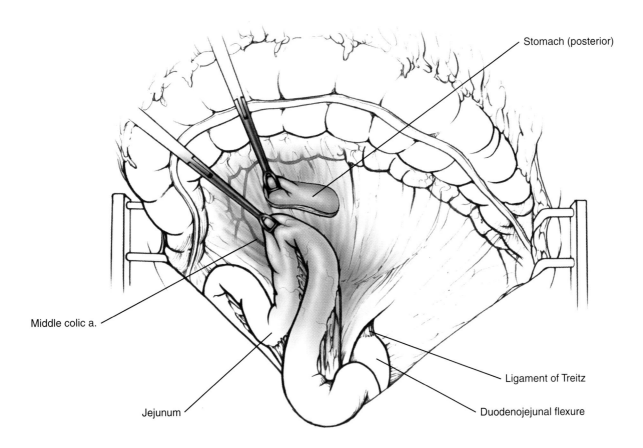

To perform the retrocolic anastomosis, the ligament of Treitz is identified, and a proximal loop of jejunum is brought up through an incision in an avascular area of the transverse mesocolon. A side-to-side anastomosis is made with an inner layer of 3-0 absorbable sutures and an outer layer of Lembert 3-0 silk interrupted sutures. To minimize the risk for afferent loop syndrome or afferent loop herniation, the afferent loop is brought up to the more proximal stomach, minimizing the length of this segment of jejunum.

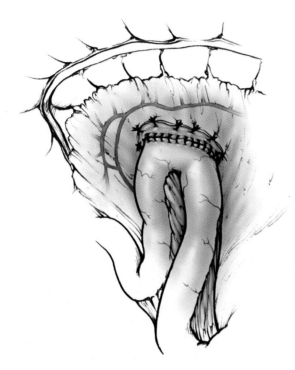

The gastrojejunostomy is then sutured to the rent in the transverse mesocolon on the gastric side to prevent obstruction of the anastomosis or bowel herniation.

An antecolic anastomosis is done in a similar fashion. However, the loop of jejunum is brought anterior to the colon, and the same side-to-side two-layer anastomosis is accomplished. A gastrostomy tube and feeding jejunostomy tube are placed distal to the anastomosis to aid in postoperative feeding and gastric decompression.

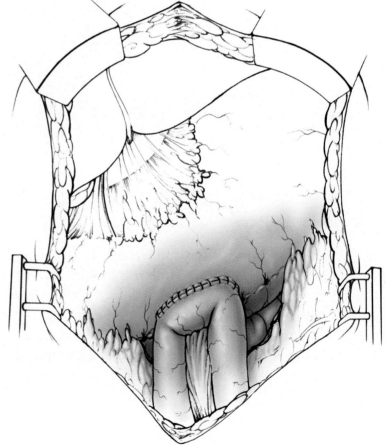

Subtotal Gastrectomy

Subtotal gastrectomy with R2 lymph node dissection can be performed through either an upper midline or a bilateral subcostal incision. A Goligher retractor is placed for exposure. The abdomen is completely explored to look for occult metastatic disease, and the primary tumor is assessed for resectability. The left lateral segment of the liver is mobilized by incising the left triangular ligament and folding the lobe underneath itself with gentle pressure from a self-retaining retractor.

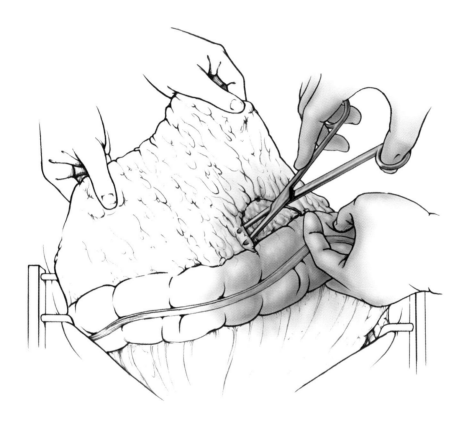

The stomach is exposed, and the lesser sac is entered by dissecting the greater omentum from the transverse colon. This dissection is facilitated by gentle opposing traction of the omentum and colon and is easier to begin over the left transverse colon.

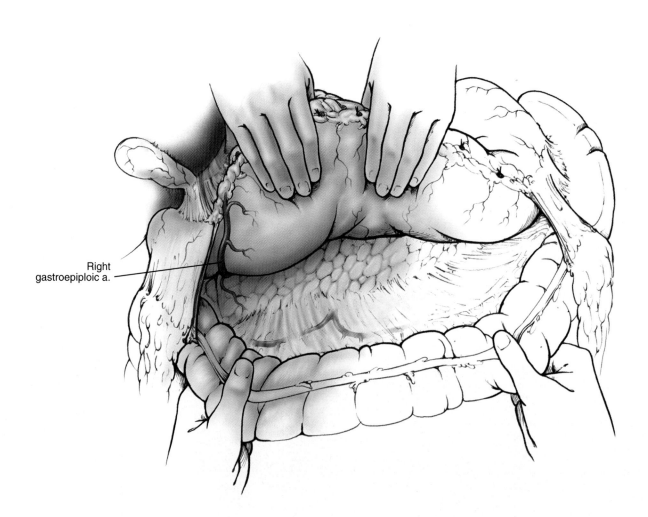

Right
gastroepiploic a.

The peritoneum overlying the cephalad portion of the transverse mesocolon
is dissected up, with care not to injure the middle colic vessels. In some patients
this plane of dissection is not possible because of fusion of the peritoneum.
When possible, this plane of dissection is continued past the base of the mesocolon to the inferior edge of the pancreas. The peritoneum and fatty tissue
over the pancreas are dissected in a cephalad fashion.

Once the lesser sac is entered, the dissection continues along an avascular
plane, moving to the patient's right until the right gastroepiploic vessels are
identified and ligated. To mobilize the duodenum and pylorus, a Kocher maneuver is performed by dividing the retroperitoneal attachments to the duodenum. The attachments between the gallbladder and duodenum are released
and the hepatoduodenal ligament is transected, exposing the porta hepatis.

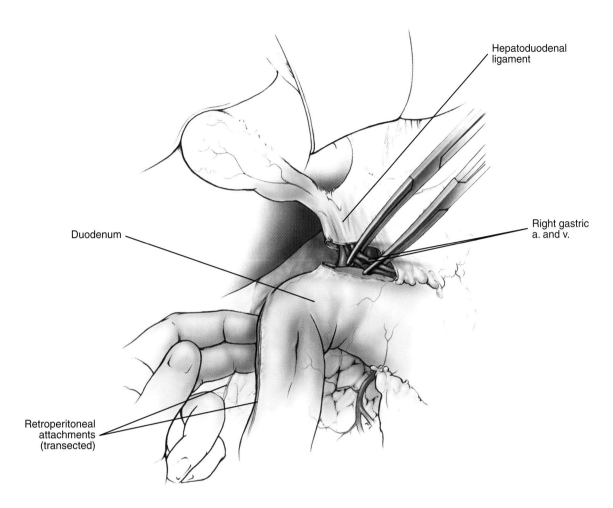

The right gastric vessels are identified and ligated. The pylorus and the first portion of the duodenum are mobilized just enough to achieve a tumor-free margin and safe closure of the duodenum.

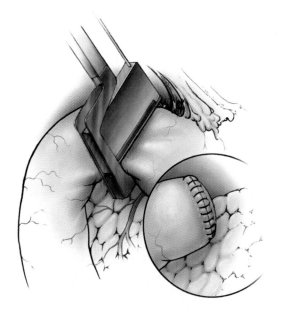

The duodenum is transected with a stapling device just 2 cm distal to the pylorus. The staple line is over-sewn with a row of interrupted 3-0 silk Lembert sutures.

The lesser omentum is taken down from its attachments to the liver along with the lymph node tissue inferior to the hepatic artery and along its course down to the celiac trunk. It is important to remember that an aberrant or accessory left hepatic artery may originate from the left gastric artery and reside in the lesser omentum. The aberrant artery should be preserved along with the main left gastric artery.

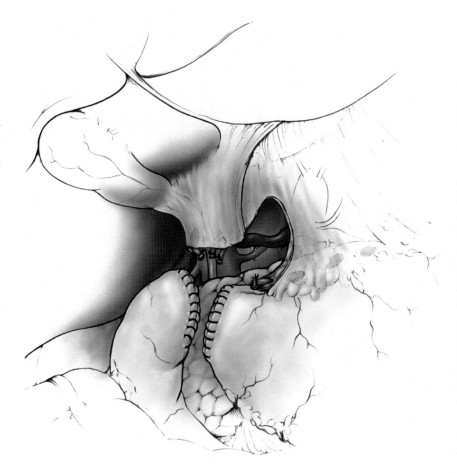

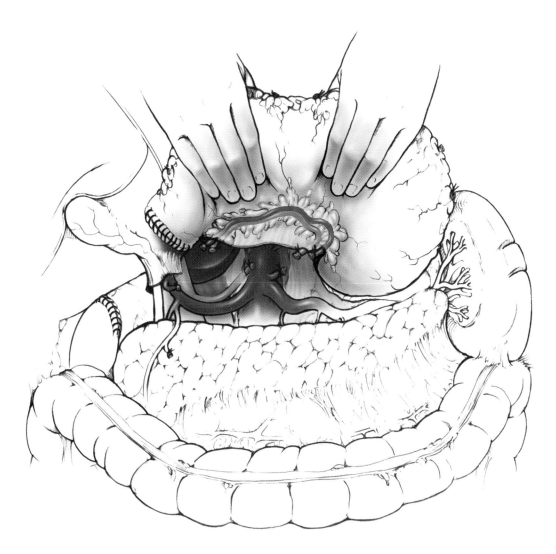

The stomach and omentum are then retracted cephalad, exposing the left gastric artery, which is doubly ligated at its origin and divided. The R2 nodes
around the celiac axis are dissected with the specimen along the aorta from the
celiac trunk to the superior border of the pancreas to the left along the splenic
vessels. The proximal line of gastric transection is chosen about 5 cm from the
tumor. The lesser and greater omentum are dissected from the stomach at the
proximal transection site.

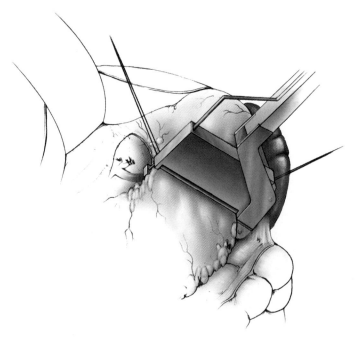

The proximal stomach is transected with a 90 mm stapling device. Studies have shown no benefit of total gastrectomy compared with subtotal gastrectomy as long as a tumor-free margin is achieved. After histologic confirmation of disease-negative resection margins, reconstruction is begun.

To prevent tension on the anastomosis, I prefer to use a retrocolic or anticolic Roux-en-Y gastrojejunostomy. A loop of proximal jejunum is identified and transected with a stapling device at about 20 cm from the ligament of Treitz. The jejunal limb is mobilized so that the distal limb reaches the proximal stomach. A 50 cm distal limb is measured and marked with a stitch. A side-to-side jejunojejunostomy is performed with either a two-layer hand-sewn or stapled method. The distal limb is either brought up through the mesocolon or in front of the colon, and an end-to-side gastrojejunostomy anastomosis is made using a two-layer technique of 3-0 running absorbable sutures for the inner layer and interrupted 3-0 silk Lembert sutures on the outside. An alternate technique is to use either an anticolic or retrocolic Billroth II loop gastrojejunostomy. However, with a large subtotal resection, many times there is not enough length on the loop for a tension-free anastomosis.

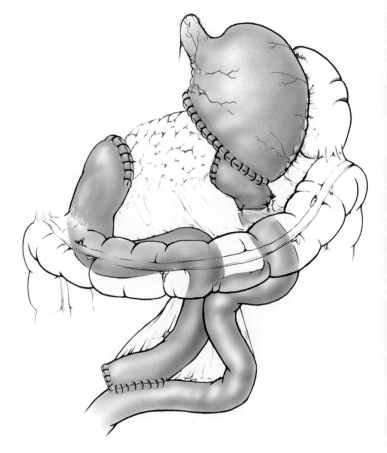

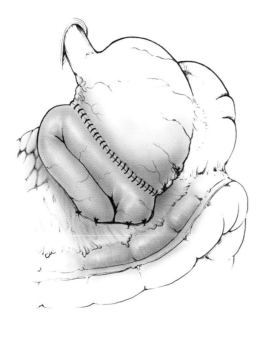

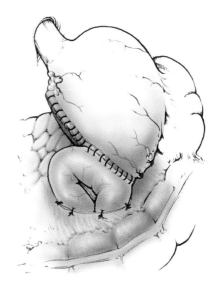

For a loop gastrojejunostomy, either a Polya or Hofmeister technique can be performed, based on personal preference. Whether the jejunal loop is placed isoperistaltic or antiperistaltic is not important functionally, but, more important, the jejunal loop should be oriented for the anastomosis in a way that minimizes tension, angulation, or undesirable twisting of the small bowel. Difficult duodenal closures should be drained with a closed suction drain. A feeding jejunostomy is placed for early postoperative feeding.

Potential complications after subtotal gastrectomy include intra-abdominal bleeding, delayed gastric emptying, pancreatitis, duodenal stump leakage, and anastomotic leakage. After the perioperative period, some of the so-called postgastrectomy syndromes can be devastating to the patient. These syndromes include afferent loop syndrome, bile gastritis, and dumping syndrome.

Radical Lymphadenectomy

Lower third lesions   Middle third lesions   Upper third lesions

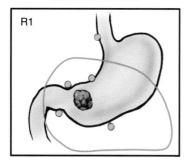 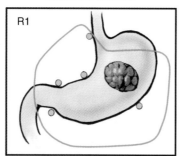 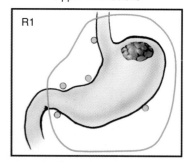

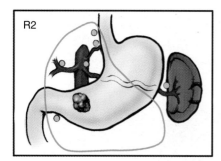 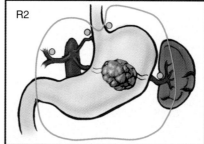 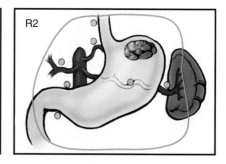

The role of a radical lymphadenectomy in the treatment of stomach cancer was introduced in 1981 by Kodama et al., who promised a survival benefit for those patients undergoing R2 lymphadenectomy as opposed to standard resection. An R2 extended nodal dissection includes the next echelon of draining nodes, most of which are in the area of the celiac trunk. Western studies have not been able to duplicate the survival benefit of the R2 dissection, although there does appear to be differences between the biology of gastric cancer in Japan and in Western countries. The role of R2 dissections remains controversial, but the morbidity and mortality among patients after R1 or R2 lymphadenectomy are similar. Prospective trials are currently under way in an attempt to definitively resolve the controversy over the role of radical lymphadenectomy in gastric carcinoma.

Total Gastrectomy

Total gastrectomy can be performed by extending the proximal dissection of the subtotal gastrectomy described previously.

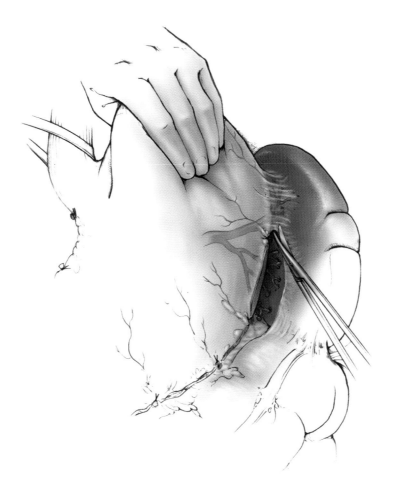

After the omentum is mobilized off the transverse colon, and dissection of the duodenal region and R2 lymphadenectomy are complete, the dissection is continued along the greater curvature, dividing the gastrosplenic ligament and each of the short gastric vessels. During this dissection, the surgeon needs to avoid excessive traction, which could result in a capsular tear of the spleen. Studies have shown no benefit to removing the spleen during gastrectomy unless there is direct tumor invasion. The dissection along the lesser omentum is extended up to the esophagus.

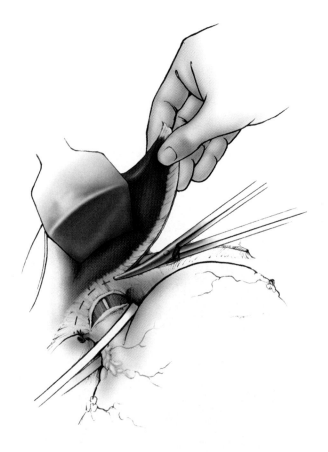

With the left lateral lobe of the liver retracted medially, the esophagus is identified by palpation of the nasogastric tube, and the peritoneum along its intra–abdominal portion is divided. A Penrose drain is placed around the esophagus to aid in the dissection. The vagus nerves are identified and divided above the esophagogastric junction.

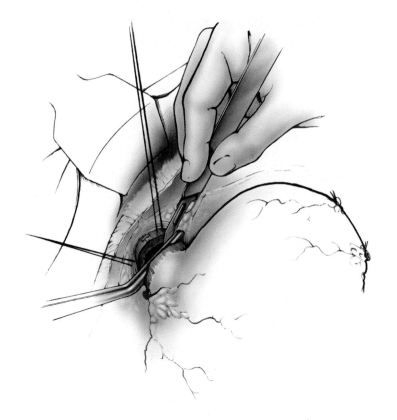

The esophagus is divided, and frozen-section pathologic evaluation is done because of the frequency of unsuspected proximal lymphatic infiltration of tumor.

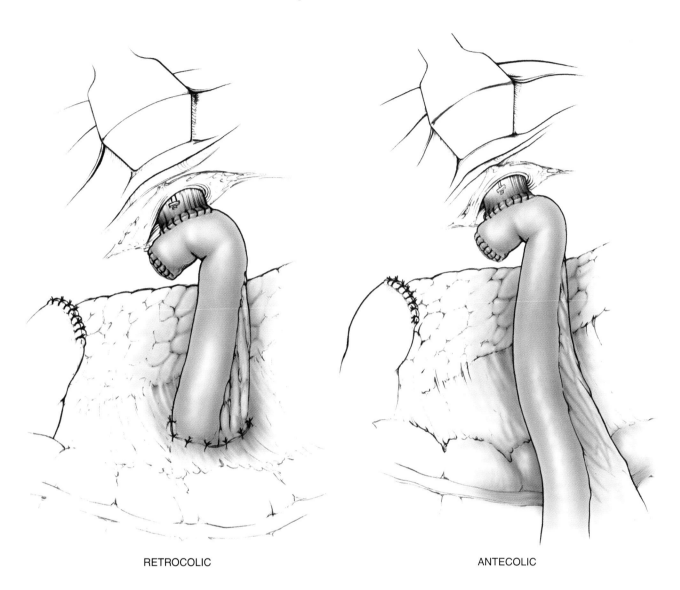

RETROCOLIC   ANTECOLIC

After removal of the specimen and disease-free margins are confirmed histologically, a Roux-en-Y end-to-side esophagojejunostomy is performed. Stay
sutures are placed on the lateral aspects of the esophagus. The Roux limb is
then brought up either retrocolic or antecolic. A point 8 to 10 cm from the
end of the Roux limb is then used for the end-to-side anastomosis, which can
be done either with the circular stapling device or a two-layer hand-sewn anastomosis.

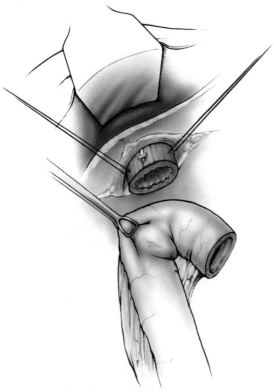

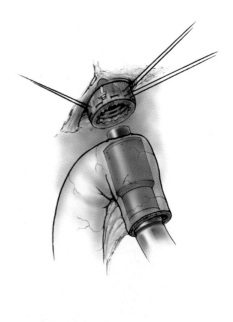

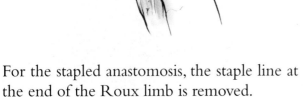

For the stapled anastomosis, the staple line at the end of the Roux limb is removed.

The appropriate sized circular stapler is introduced through the Roux limb.

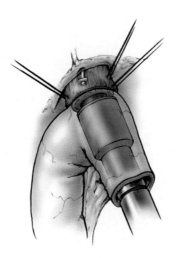

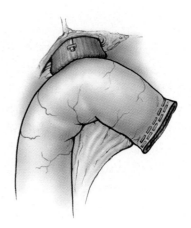

A 2-0 Prolene purse-string suture is placed in the end of the esophagus, and the anvil of the circular stapler is inserted into the esophagus. The purse-string suture is tightened and the stapler engaged.

After removing the stapler, the end of the jejunal limb is closed with a linear stapler. The nasogastric tube is placed down the efferent limb.

There are many modifications of the reconstruction of a total gastrectomy.

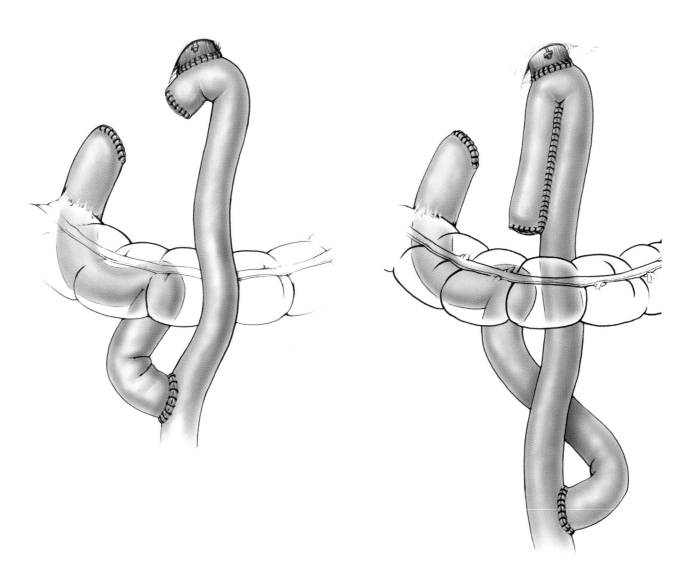

Some surgeons have advocated the use of a jejunal pouch (Hunt-Lawrence pouch), which can be created by performing a side-to-side jejunojejunostomy just below the esophagojejunostomy to act as a food reservoir. This pouch can be created using either a hand-sewn or stapled technique. However, there is no objective evidence that these pouches provide nutritional benefits over a standard Roux-en-Y esophagojejunostomy. A feeding jejunostomy is placed for early postoperative feeding. A closed suction drain is placed near the esophago-jejunostomy.

Extended Gastrectomy

Large gastric tumors may locally invade adjacent organs, and the operating surgeon must be prepared to resect these organs en bloc if necessary. Bulky tumors along the posterior wall of the antrum or body may extend into the pancreas or retroperitoneal structures. When this occurs, the distal pancreas and spleen should be removed en bloc with the stomach. The splenic flexure of the colon is mobilized to gain better exposure of the spleen. The retroperitoneal and colonic attachments to the spleen are divided. The spleen and distal pancreas are elevated and brought to the midline.

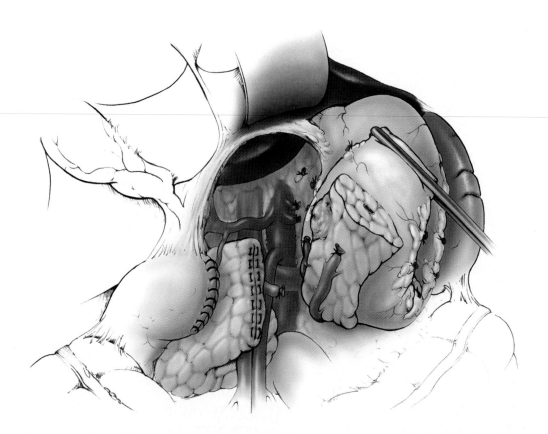

The splenic vein and artery are ligated. The pancreas is divided at the level of the mesenteric vessels. The residual pancreas requires ligation of the pancreatic duct with a 5-0 Prolene suture and closure of the pancreatic stump with 3-0 Prolene mattress sutures. A closed suction drain is placed near the pancreatic closure.

On occasion gastric carcinoma can locally also invade the left lateral lobe of the liver. This represents direct tumor invasion, not metastatic disease. An umbilical tape is placed around the porta hepatis if inflow occlusion is needed.

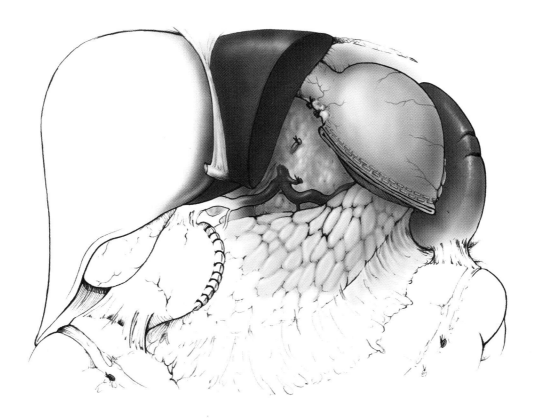

Overlapping large 0 chromic liver sutures are used for hemostatic control along the liver transection line. The liver tissue is then divided with at least a 1 cm gross margin using the ultrasonic dissector or the electrocautery unit. The remainder of the gastrectomy is done in the standard fashion.

Large tumors along the greater curve of the stomach may invade either the transverse colon mesentery or the transverse colon itself, and may require en bloc resection of the stomach and transverse colon. Given an adequate mechanical and antibiotic bowel preparation, a primary colon resection is performed with reanastomosis of the colon.

Anatomic Basis of Complications

MAJOR

- Too much traction on the gastrosplenic ligament may result in splenic injury, requiring splenectomy.
- Division of an aberrant left hepatic artery in the lesser omentum from the left gastric artery may cause ischemia or necrosis of the left lobe of the liver.
- Breakdown of the duodenal stump closure will result in intra-abdominal abscess formation and sepsis.

MINOR

- Pancreatitis can develop from dissection along the gland.
- Delayed gastric emptying will result in intermittent nausea and vomiting.
- Afferent loop syndrome can develop due to mechanical obstruction of an afferent loop of jejunum.

KEY REFERENCES

Behrns K, Dalton R, van Heerden J, et al. Extended lymph node dissection for gastric cancer. Surg Clin North Am 72:433-443, 1992.

> *These authors review Japanese and Western staging systems for gastric cancer. Through screening programs the Japanese identify more early gastric cancer, and their overall survival rate is better than that for the United States. The value of extended lymph node dissection has not been clearly defined.*

Cady B, Rossi R, Silverman M, et al. Gastric adenocarcinoma. Arch Surg 124:303-308, 1989.

> *This article reviews the natural history and outcome of 211 patients with gastric cancer from 1967-1982. Despite operative intervention, overall survival was 21%.*

Gouzi J, Huguier M, Fagniez P, et al. Ann Surg 209:162-166, 1989.

> *This multicenter trial compares postoperative mortality and 5-year survival of patients undergoing total gastrectomy vs. subtotal gastrectomy. Postoperative mortality was low in both groups; overall survival was the same in both groups. Total gastrectomy offers no benefit over subtotal gastrectomy.*

Kodama Y, Sugimachi K, Soejima K, et al. Evaluation of extensive lymph node dissection for carcinoma of the stomach. World J Surg 5:241-248, 1981.

> *This article reviews extensive regional lymph node dissection with gastric resection for the treatment of gastric adenocarcinoma. The authors suggest a benefit with radical lymphadenectomy with curative gastric resections.*

Smith J, Brennan M. Surgical treatment of gastric cancer. Surg Clin North Am 72:381-399, 1992.

This article presents a overall review of the diagnosis, preoperative staging, and surgery of gastric cancer. Only 30% of patients with gastric cancer will have disease that is resectable with a curative intent. Patients with proximal tumors had a poorer survival rate compared with that in other locations.

SUGGESTED READINGS

Ajani JA, Ota DM, Jessup JM, et al. Resectable gastric carcinoma. Cancer 68:1501-1506, 1991.

Beahrs O, Henson D, Hutter R, et al. eds. Handbook for Staging of Cancer. Philadelphia: JB Lippincott, 1993, pp 80-87.

Boddie AW, McBride CM, Balch CM. Gastric cancer. Am J Surg 157:595-606, 1989.

Bozzetti F, Bonfanti G, Bufalino R, et al. Adequacy of margins of resection in gastrectomy for cancer. Ann Surg 196: 685-690, 1982.

Brady MS, Rogatko A, Dent L, et al. Effect of splenectomy on morbidity and survival following curative gastrectomy for carcinoma. Arch Surg 126:359-364, 1991.

Cady B. Subtotal gastric resection. In Cady B, Daly J, eds. Atlas of Surgical Oncology. St Louis: Mosby–Year Book, 1993, pp 221-239.

Dougherty MJ, Compton C, Talbert M, et al. Sarcomas of the gastrointestinal tract. Ann Surg 214:569-574, 1991.

Grobler NG. The stomach. In Grobler NG, ed. Textbook of Clinical Anatomy. New York: Elsevier/North Holland Press, 1977, pp 267-283.

Jesseph J. Gastrostomy. In Nyhus L, Baker R, eds. Masters of Surgery. Boston: Little, Brown, 1992, pp 633-638.

Jewkes A, Taylor E, Fielding J, et al. Radical total gastrectomy for carcinoma. In Nyhus L, Baker R, eds. Masters of Surgery. Boston: Little, Brown, 1992, pp 721-730.

Kriplani AK, Kapur ML. Laparoscopy for pre-operative staging and assessment of operability in gastric carcinoma. Gastrointest Endosc 37:441-443, 1991.

Lawrence M, Shiu MH. Early gastric cancer. Ann Surg 213:327-334, 1991.

Lightdale CJ. Endoscopic ultrasound in the diagnosis, staging and follow-up of esophageal and gastric cancer. Endoscopy 24:297-303, 1992.

Morgan BK, Compton C, Talbert M, et al. Benign smooth muscle tumors of the gastrointestinal tract. Ann Surg 211:63-66, 1990.

Noguchi Y, Imada T, Matsumoto A, et al. Radical surgery for gastric cancer: A review of the Japanese experience. Cancer 64: 2053-2062,1989.

Pacelli F, Doglietto GB, Bellantone R, et al. Extensive versus limited lymph node dissection for gastric cancer: A comparative study of 320 patients. Br J Surg 80:1153-1156, 1993.

Romanes GJ. The stomach. In Romanes GJ, ed. Cunningham's Textbook of Anatomy. Oxford, England: Oxford University Press, 1981, pp 445-454.

Smith JW, Shiu MH, Kelsey L, et al. Morbidity of radical lymphadenectomy in the curative resection of gastric carcinoma. Arch Surg 126:1469-1473, 1991.

Snell R. The abdomen: Part II. In Snell R, ed. Clinical Anatomy for Medical Students. Boston: Little, Brown, 1973, pp 175-191.

Thirlby RC. Gastrointestinal lymphoma: A surgical perspective. Oncology 7:29-34, 1993.

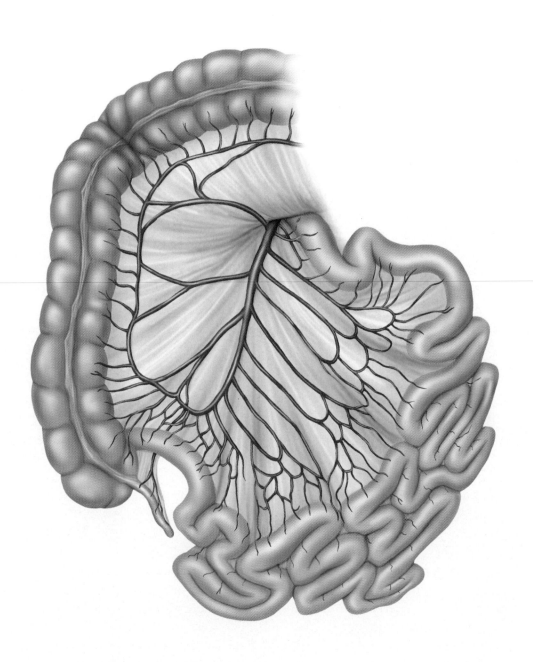

Chapter 8

Small Bowel and Mesentery

John E. Skandalakis, M.D., Ph.D., Gene Colborn, M.D., Ph.D., and Lee J. Skandalakis, M.D.

Surgical Applications

Resection of Small Bowel
Resection of Jejunum and Ileum
Anastomosis
Resection of Mesentery

*B*enign and malignant tumors of the jejunoileum are rare (Sarr). Approximately 1200 new small intestine adenocarcinomas are diagnosed in the United States each year, compared with 8000 esophageal carcinomas, 24,000 gastric carcinomas, and 150,000 colorectal carcinomas (Fuller et al.). Therefore, despite its length and the large absorptive mucosal stroma, only around 1% of all gastrointestinal malignancies develop in this anatomic area. Both benign leiomyomas and leiomyosaromas occur, and primary lymphomas and metastatic melanomas to the small bowel are other neoplastic sources of bleeding, intussusception, or obstruction.

SURGICAL ANATOMY
Topography

The intestinal wall is composed of a serosa of visceral peritoneum (muscularis obliquus externa) with longitudinal and circular muscle, a submucosa of connective tissue, and a mucosa of connective tissue, smooth muscle (lamina muscularis mucosae), and epithelium. The plicae circulares of the small intestine are most obvious in the jejunum. The jejunal villi are more distinct, long, tongue-shaped, or finger-like projections, compared with the ileal villi, which are shorter and blunter and disappear gradually toward the ileocecal valve.

Almost a century ago, Halsted pointed out the importance of the submucosal connective tissue in holding sutures. Fear of perforating the mucosa with a stitch makes seromuscular sutures seem safer, but the integrity of an anastomosis is greater if the submucosa is included.

The serosa surrounds the jejunum and ileum completely. Together with the muscular coat, the serosa is the well-known stroma for the application of seromuscular sutures during surgical procedures. The muscular coat is formed by the inner circular and outer longitudinal layers. It should be considered, at least surgically, one layer. It is responsible for intestinal motility and contains the myenteric plexus of Auerbach as well as ganglia for nonmyelinated nerve fibers.

The submucosa is the home of the very rich network of neuronal elements of Meissner's plexus, as well as arteries, veins, and lymphatic vessels. It also hosts Peyer's patches of isolated and confluent masses of lymphatic nodules in the antimesenteric side of the ileum.

Sixty percent of the length of the gastrointestinal tract is composed of small bowel. This small intestine performs 90% of absorption.

Blood Supply

The superior mesenteric artery arises from the aorta below the origin of the celiac trunk. About 1% of persons have a combined celiacomesenteric trunk. The celiac, superior, and inferior mesenteric arteries are the remnants of the paired vitelline arteries of the embryo. The superior mesenteric artery continues beyond the ileal border to supply Meckel's diverticulum, if one is present.

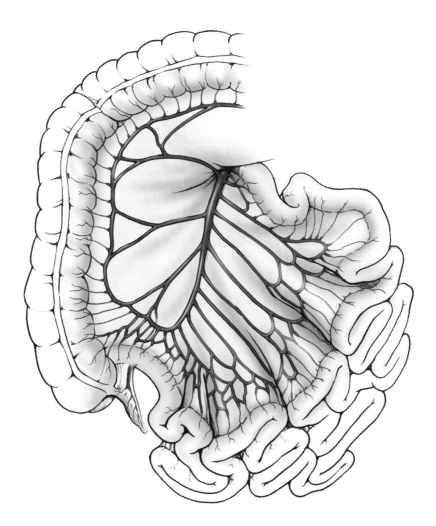

On average, the left side of the superior mesenteric artery gives origin to five intestinal arteries above the origin of the ileocolic artery and 11 arteries below that level. The intestinal vessels branch a few centimeters from the border of the intestine to form a series of arterial arcades. These arcades connect the intestinal arteries with one another. Their number increases from one to three in the proximal jejunum to three to five in the ileum. From the arches of these arcades the vasa recta arise and pass without branching into the intestinal wall. There they branch but do not anastomose before piercing the muscularis externa. This provides the most oxygenated blood to the mesenteric side of the bowel wall and the least to the antimesenteric border. There is a plexus of vessels in the submucosa from which short vessels reach the mucosa and villi. This is the only area of anastomosis distal to the arcades in the mesentery.

The vascular arches form the primary anastomoses of the arterial supply. A complete channel may exist from the posteroinferior pancreatoduodenal artery, which is parallel with the intestine and joins the marginal artery (of Drummond) of the colon. In some persons the pathway is incomplete, usually at the end of the ileum. From the arches of the arcades, numerous arteries (the vasa recta) arise and pass (without cross-communication) to enter the intestinal wall.

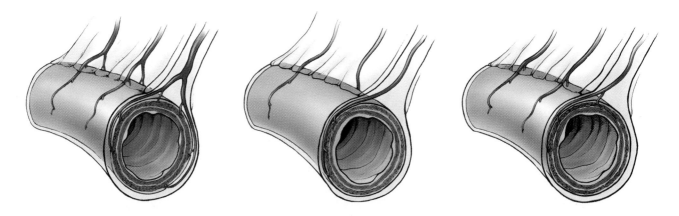

The vasa recta may divide into two short vessels to the mesenteric side of the intestine and two long vessels that supply the rest of the intestinal wall. More frequently a single long vessel supplies one side of the intestine, alternating with a vessel supplying the other side. A single long and short vessel may serve one side only. Other combinations of paired or single, and long and short vessels are possible.

The vasa recti branch, but do not anastomose, beneath the serosa before piercing the muscularis externa. There is no collateral circulation between the vasa recti or their branches at the surface of the intestines. This configuration provides the best supply of oxygenated blood to the mesenteric side of the intestine and the poorest supply to the antimesenteric border.

If we accept that there is no collateral circulation beyond the terminal arcades (in other words, no communication between the vasa recti or within the intramural network), the blood supply of the antimesenteric border of the small bowel is relatively poor.

Within the intestinal wall, the arteries form a large plexus in the submucosa. From this plexus short vessels reach the lamina propria to supply a network of capillaries around the intestinal crypts, and longer arteries supply the cores of the intestinal villi. Thus there are two regions of anastomoses of intestinal arteries: the extramural arches between intestinal arteries and the intramural submucosal plexus.

One or more small veins originate near the tip of each intestinal villus and travel outward, receiving contributions from a plexus of veins around the intestinal glands. They enter the submucosal plexus. This is drained through the muscular layer by larger veins traveling with the arteries in the mesentery to reach the superior mesenteric vein. These intestinal veins are interconnected by venous arcades that are similar to but less complex than the accompanying arterial arcades.

Nerve Supply

The innervation of the jejunum and ileum is by the autonomic system. However, pain secondary to small bowel disease is referred to the ninth, tenth, and eleventh thoracic nerves, and usually is periumbilical.

Lymphatic Drainage

Lymphatic vessels (lacteal vessels) arise in the cores of the intestinal villi and form plexuses at the base of the villi, the base of the crypts, the muscularis mucosa, the submucosa, and between the circular and longitudinal layers of the muscularis externa. This series of plexuses is drained by large lymphatic vessels that travel in the mesentery with the arteries and veins. The lymph flows to nodes residing between the leaves of the mesentery. More than 200 small mesenteric nodes lie near the vasa recta and along the intestinal arteries. Drainage from these is finally to the large, superior mesenteric lymph nodes at the root of the mesentery. Efferent vessels from these and the celiac nodes form the intestinal lymphatic trunk. This trunk passes beneath the left renal artery and ends in the left lumbar lymphatic trunk (70%) or the cisterna chyli (25%).

Small Bowel Lymphatic Pathways

Intramural
- Lacteal vessels
- Mucosal vessels
- Submucosal plexus
- Subserosal plexus

Extramural
- Vasa recti
- Lymph nodes along mesenteric vessels
- Lymph nodes along superior mesenteric artery and celiac artery
- Cisterna chyli

Neoplasms

From the gastroduodenal junction to the ileocecal junction, the small bowel is the home of rare benign and malignant tumors (Coit). Because of the differences in anatomic topography of the duodenum and the jejunoileum, the surgical techniques for treatment of duodenal and jejunoileal tumors are discussed separately.

Comparison of Jejunum and Ileum

Jejunum	Ileum
Wall thicker	Wall thinner
Lumen larger	Lumen smaller
Fat on mesentery	Fat on ileum and mesentery
Prominent plicae circulares	Less prominent plicae
Single line of arterial arcades	Several lines of arterial arcades
Aggregate lymph nodules (Peyer's patches) sparse	Aggregate lymph nodules frequent

Table 8-1   *Distribution of Malignant Tumors of the Small Bowel by Site in 27 Series*

Tumor Type	Duodenum	Jejunum	Ileum	Total (%)
Adenocarcinoma	634	454	301	1389 (44)
Carcinoid	60	92	781	933 (29)
Lymphoma	34	183	276	493 (15)
Sarcoma	61	159	148	368 (12)
Total (%)	789 (25)	888 (28)	1506 (47)	3183 (100)

From Coit DG. Cancers of the gastrointestinal tract. In DeVita VT Jr, Hellman S, Rosenberg SA, eds. Cancer: Principles and Practice of Oncology, 5th ed. Philadelphia: Lippincott-Raven, 1997, p 1133.

Table 8-2   *Distribution of Benign Tumors of the Small Bowel by Site in 13 Series*

Tumor Type	Duodenum	Jejunum	Ileum	Total (%)
Leiomyoma	24	64	47	135 (37)
Polyp/Adenoma	34	17	17	68 (19)
Lipoma	11	13	30	54 (15)
Hemangioma	1	10	26	37 (10)
Fibroma	4	7	12	23 (6)
Other	27	8	13	48 (13)
Total (%)	101 (27)	119 (33)	145 (40)	365 (100)

From Coit DG. Cancers of the gastrointestinal tract. In DeVita VT Jr, Hellman S, Rosenberg SA, eds. Cancer: Principles and Practice of Oncology, 5th ed. Philadelphia: Lippincott-Raven, 1997, p 1132.

In our own reviews of benign and malignant tumors (Skandalakis et al. and Blanchard et al.) we found that malignant tumors of the small bowel were adenocarcinoma (30% to 50%), leiomyosarcoma (10% to 20%), and lymphoma (10% to 15%). Carcinoid tumors were found in association with other tumors in 15% to 30%.

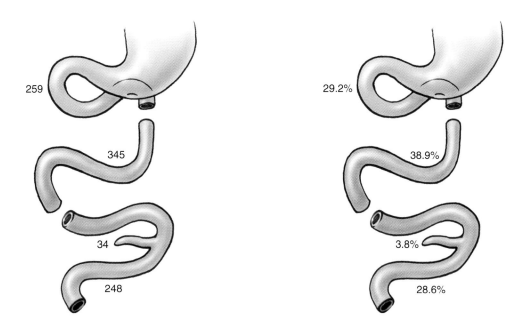

Of the 1052 cases of intestinal leiomyomas, the sites were specified in 886 cases (as noted above) and could not be determined in 166 cases.

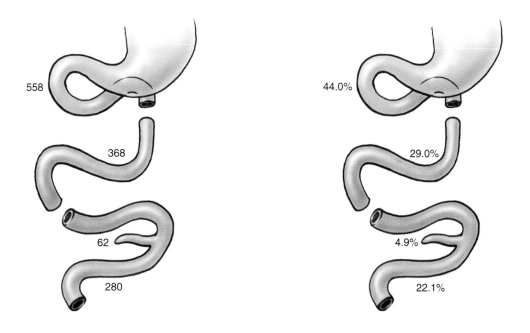

Of the 1655 cases of intestinal leiomyosarcoma, the sites were specified in 1268 cases (as noted above) and could not be determined in 387 cases.

We join other authors in strongly advising that leiomyoma of the gastrointestinal tract be treated as a malignant tumor because of the difficulty of diagnosis by frozen- or permanent-section analysis. This enigmatic presentation dictates radical surgery, even though the disease may be benign. Similarly, because of the possibility of malignancy, sessile villous adenoma should be treated with segmental resection, not enterotomy and excision.

The number of carcinoid tumors from several locations have been compared in Table 8-3. It will be seen that per inch many more tumors occur in both the appendix and Meckel's diverticulum than in the duodenum and small intestine.

Table 8-3   *Relative Frequency of Carcinoid Tumors Reported in the Intestinal Tract*

Organs	Length (inches)	No. of Tumors[*]	Tumors per Inch of Length
Duodenum	10	43	4.3
Jejunum	96	49	0.5
Ileum	144	813	5.6
Meckel's Diverticulum	2	33 (1650)[†]	16.5 (825.0)[†]
Appendix	3	1340	446.6

From Singhabhandhu B, Gray SW, Krieger H, Gerstmann KE, Skandalakis JE. Carcinoid tumor of Meckel's diverticulum: Report of a case and review of literature. J Med Assoc Ga 62:84-89, 1973.
[*]Number reported up to 1966.
[†]The diverticulum is present in 2% of patients; hence, 33 × 50 = 1650 for those patients with a diverticulum.

Table 8-4   *Incidence of Carcinoid Tumors of Meckel's Diverticulum by Age and Sex[*]*

Age (yr)	Male	Female
20-29	1	—
30-39	2	—
40-49	3	1
50-59	13	5
60-69	10	2
70-79	7	1
80-89	1	—
Not stated	2	1
	39	10

From Singhabhandhu B, Gray SW, Krieger H, Gerstmann KE, Skandalakis JE. Carcinoid tumor of Meckel's diverticulum: Report of a case and review of literature. J Med Assoc Ga 62:84-89, 1973.
[*]In one case, sex was not stated.

National Cancer Institute (NCI) studies spanning the period from 1950 to 1991 reported 1570 cases of carcinoid tumor of the appendix (Modlin and Sandor). In our world literature review from 1875 to 1996 of smooth muscle (stromal) tumors, we found only five cases of leiomyosarcoma of the appendix (Blanchard et al.).

Intussusception and Its Relationship to Neoplasia

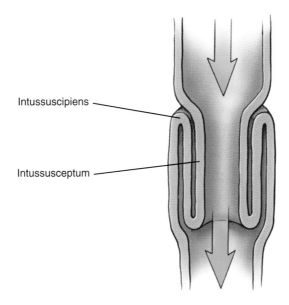

An intussusception is created when a proximal segment of intestine (the intussusceptum) invaginates into the portion of intestine immediately distal to it (the intussuscipiens). In adults, our "two thirds" rule can be applied:
* Two thirds are from known causes.
* Of these, two thirds are due to neoplasms.
* Of those caused by neoplasms, two thirds of the neoplasms will be malignant.

SURGICAL APPLICATIONS

With benign or malignant lesions, segmental resection is preferable to wedge resection as performed for simple diverticulum.

Resection of Small Bowel

In resecting a segment of the proximal part of the jejunoileum, remove 20 cm of healthy small bowel on each side of the lesion, as well as a V-like mesenteric excision. In performing a resection of the terminal ileum, a right-sided colectomy is the appropriate procedure, because of the anatomic lymphatic pathway. Remember to measure and record the remaining small bowel after resection.

Resection of Jejunum and Ileum

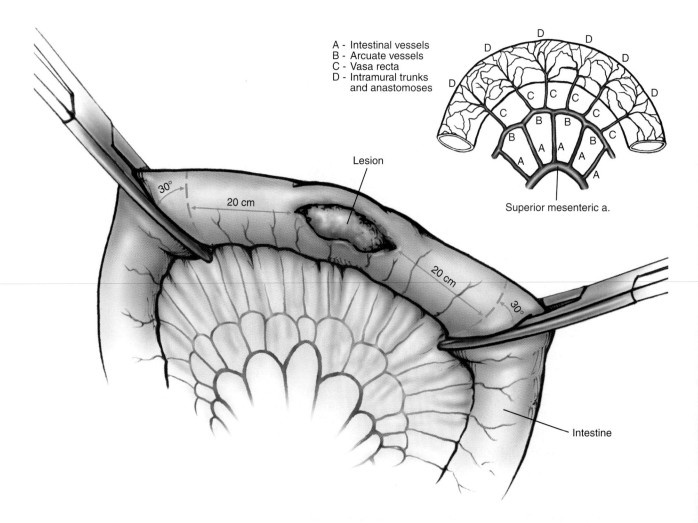

A - Intestinal vessels
B - Arcuate vessels
C - Vasa recta
D - Intramural trunks
    and anastomoses

Lesion

Superior mesenteric a.

30°

20 cm

20 cm

30°

Intestine

Jejunal or ileal resection may be done in response to pathologic entities of the small bowel, such as benign or malignant tumors with or without intestinal obstruction or intussusception. A midline vertical incision is made, and the area is explored. The intestinal segment is isolated, and the loop of intestine with the tumor is brought out of the abdomen together with sufficient length proximal and distal to the area to be resected. The exposed segment and the general peritoneal cavity are protected with warm laparotomy pads. Noncrushing clamps are applied obliquely 20 cm from the tumor on each side. In addition, straight Kocher clamps are applied on each side on the specimen side. A V-type incision is made with a knife in the mesentery, incising only the visceral peritoneum.

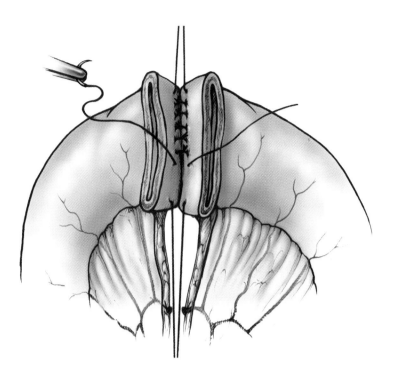

The mesenteric vessels are isolated with care, and the intestinal segment with the tumor is transected proximally and distally. The specimen is removed, and both cut edges are covered with warm laparotomy pads to prevent possible contamination. The anastomosis may be end-to-end, side-to-side, or any appropriate variation.

Anastomosis

To prepare a long loop of jejunum for anastomosis, the following steps can be used, after securing the duodenojejunal junction and drawing the proximal jejunum out of the abdomen:

1. The peritoneum is incised halfway between the root and the mesenteric border. It is elevated from the selected loop. Fat and lymph nodes are removed to within 1 to 2 cm from the wall of the intestine.
2. The jejunal vessels are skeletonized of connective tissue, nerve fibers, and lymphatic vessels, separately freeing the arteries and veins, with careful exposure of the vascular arcades.

The exposed blood vessels are again covered with peritoneum. At the same time, the anatomy of the jejunal arteries and their arcades is examined to determine the feasibility of dividing the necessary number of arteries (usually three or four) required for mobilization of a loop of adequate length. If needed, the root of the mesentery is divided as necessary to gain length.

Open-Lumen Stapling Technique

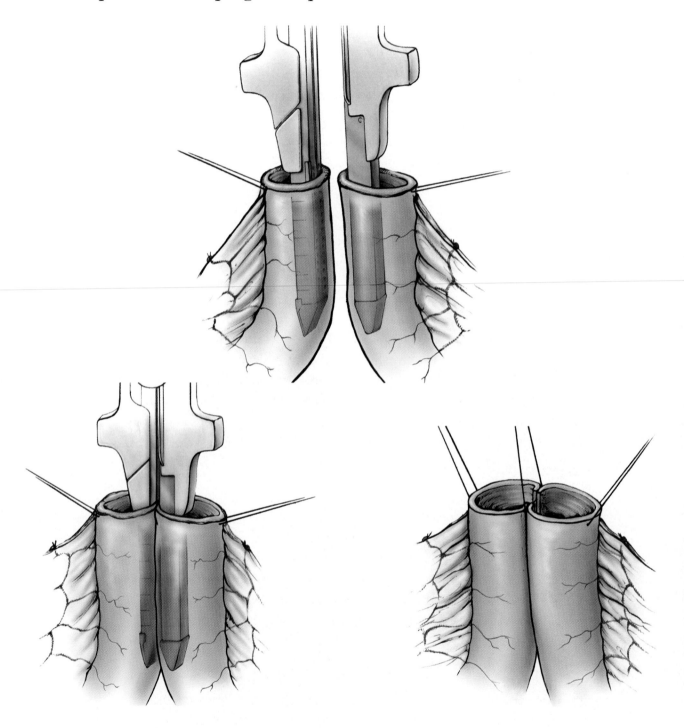

The anastomosis is done on the antimesenteric border with a GIA 55 or 75 stapler. Traction sutures are placed at the mesenteric and antimesenteric borders of both bowel lumina. The antimesenteric borders of the proximal and distal bowel loops are approximated. GIA forks are inserted into proximal and distal lumens. The bowel ends should be aligned evenly on the GIA forks. The instrument is then closed and the staples fired. The knife in the GIA divides between two double staple lines, creating a stoma.

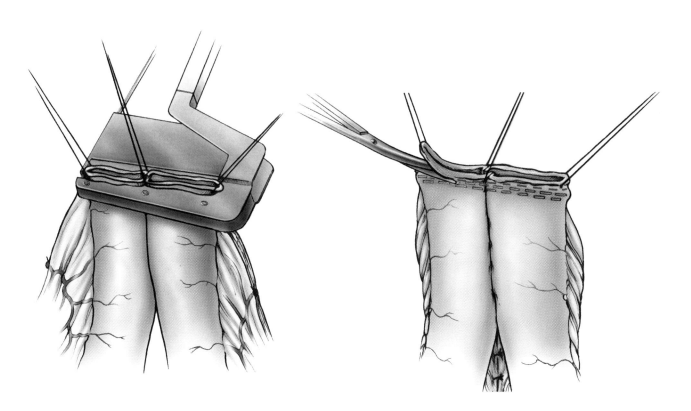

Allis clamps or through-and-through sutures including all the layers of the stomas of the proximal and distal loop are now placed. The apposition of the walls of the proximal and distal limb should be complete. A TA-55 device is used to close the opening between the two limbs by carefully incorporating all the layers of the loops. The redundant bowel is excised with a knife or scissors before removing the device.

Resection of Mesentery

Primary tumors of the mesentery are uncommon. The most common tumors of the mesentery and omentum are metastatic, arising from primary malignant tumors of anatomic entities within the peritoneal cavity (e.g., ovaries).

The primary treatment for mesenteric tumors is surgical excision. The radicality of the operation depends on whether the tumor is benign or malignant, its size, its location, and the degree of invasion to neighboring anatomy. A V-like excision of the mesentery, including the corresponding loop or loops of the small bowel, is the treatment of choice. When resection is not possible, radiation therapy is an alternative.

Anatomic Basis of Complications

VASCULAR INJURY

- Vascular injury to the superior mesenteric artery must be repaired at once. Injury to the mesentery and one or more of the intestinal arteries requires ligation. It will also add to the length of devitalized segment of intestine and hence the length of resection needed. Any line of resection must be so placed as to minimize injury to the blood supply. As many vascular arches and vasa recta as possible must be preserved.

- Hematomas at the anastomotic site will cause ischemia, necrosis, and perforation. Hematomas are most common at the junction of the mesentery with the anastomotic site. Here mesenteric vessels can be occluded, producing local ischemia.

ORGAN INJURY

- The abdominal cavity should be well packed before any enterotomy or enterostomy to prevent contamination and future infection, with resulting intraperitoneal or abdominal wall abscess.

- Leakage at the suture line is the result of poor technique and will be followed by a fistula or general peritonitis. Care in closing the mesentery at the suture line without damage to blood vessels, and prevention of tension on the anastomosis reduces the possibility of leakage.

- An inadequate stoma will result in stasis of intestinal contents and possible obstruction. A slightly oblique line of resection will help enlarge the anastomotic opening and preserve the blood supply to the antimesenteric border.

- Tension and torsion at the anastomosis must be prevented. The surgeon must be sure that any tension or torsion has not been merely transferred to a more distal or proximal site. The resection of an intestinal obstruction does not preclude the presence of another obstruction distal to the anastomosis. This is of great importance in surgery to treat intestinal atresias in infancy.

KEY REFERENCES

Blanchard DK, Budde JM, Hatch GF III, Wertheimer-Hatch L, Hatch KF, Davis GB, Foster RS Jr, Skandalakis JE. Smooth muscle (stromal) tumors of the small intestine. World J Surg (in press).
This is a collective review of the Emory University experience of smooth muscle tumors of the small bowel.

Coit DG. Cancers of the gastrointestinal tract. In DeVita VT Jr, Hellman S, Rosenberg SA, eds. Cancer: Principles and Practice of Oncology, 5th ed. Philadelphia: Lippincott-Raven, 1997, pp 1128-1143.
This chapter is a beautiful presentation of malignant tumors of the gastrointestinal tract.

Fuller RD, Chaudhuri B, Chaudhuri PK. Adenocarcinomas and sarcomas of the small intestine. In Wastell C, Nyhus LM, Donahue PE, eds. Surgery of the Esophagus, Stomach, and Small Intestine, 5th ed. Boston: Little, Brown, 1995, pp 878-886.
This is a review of epithelial and nonepithelial tumors of the small bowel.

Sarr MG. Small intestinal neoplasms. In Greenfield LJ, Mulholland MW, Oldham KT, et al., eds. Surgery: Scientific Principles and Practice. Philadelphia: JB Lippincott, 1993, pp 753-763.
This is an excellent review of the Mayo Clinic experience with intestinal neoplasms.

Skandalakis JE, Gray SW, Shephard D, et al. Smooth Muscle Tumors of the Alimentary Tract: Leiomyomas and Leiomyosarcomas. A Review of 2525 Cases. Springfield, Ill.: Charles C Thomas, 1962.
This is a major review of the world literature on leiomyomas and leiomyosarcomas. It includes 2525 cases up to 1961. An updated collective review will appear in World Journal of Surgery in 1998.

SUGGESTED READINGS

Backman L, Hallberg D. Small-intestinal length. Acta Chir Scand 140:57, 1974.

Herbsman H, Wetstein L, Rosen Y. Tumors of the small intestine. Curr Probl Surg 17:121, 1980.

Koltun WA, Pappas TN. Anatomy and physiology of the small intestine. In Greenfield LJ, ed. Surgery: Scientific Principles and Practice. Philadelphia: JB Lippincott, 1993.

Levine LA. Stepladder incision technique for lengthening of bowel mesentery. J Urol 148(2 Part 1):351-352, 1992.

Michels NA, Siddharth P, Kornblith PL, et al. The variant blood supply to the small and large intestines: Its import in regional resections. J Int Coll Surg 39:127, 1963.

Modlin IM, Sandor A. An analysis of 8305 cases of carcinoid tumors. Cancer 79:813-829, 1997.

Noer RJ, Derr JW, Johnston CG. The circulation of the small intestine: An evaluation of its revascularizing potential. Ann Surg 130:608, 1949.

Rosenberg JC, DiDio LJA. Anatomic and clinical aspects of the junction of the ileum with the large intestine. Dis Colon Rectum 13:220, 1970.

Thirlby RC. Optimizing results and techniques of mesenteric lengthening in ileal pouch–anal anastomosis. Am J Surg 169:499, 1995.

Vaez-Zadeh K, Dutz W. Ileosigmoid knotting. Ann Surg 172:1027, 1970.

Wilson JM, Melvin DB, Gray CF. Primary malignancies of the small bowel: A report of 96 cases and review of the literature. Ann Surg 180:175, 1974.

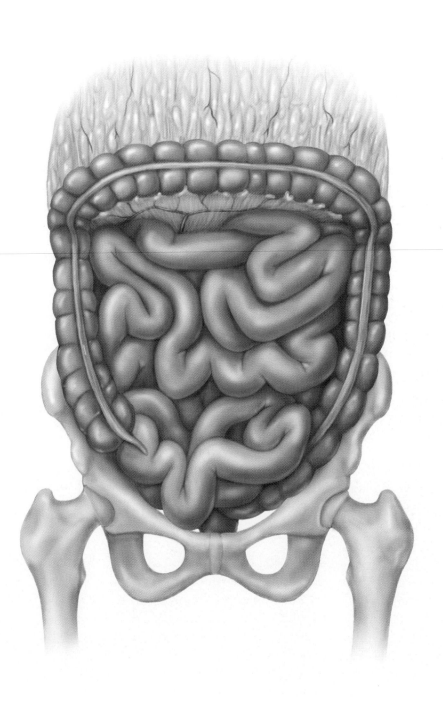

Chapter 9

Colon and Appendix

George Barnes, Jr., M.D.

Surgical Applications

Colon cancer is the most common intra-abdominal malignancy requiring surgical therapy, with an estimated 90,000 cases diagnosed per year. Ninety percent to 95% of colon tumors are adenocarcinomas; less frequent types include carcinoids, stromal tumors (formerly leiomyosarcomas), lymphomas, and undetermined lesions. Approximately 75% are diagnosed in a localized or regional metastasizing stage and are thereby amenable to surgical cure. Surgical resection, in combination with standard techniques that have changed little over the past three decades, remains the cornerstone of curative therapy. Significant improvements have been made in preoperative preparation and the increased use of gastrointestinal staplers.

Tumor location continues to be the major determinant of the type and extent of colon resection, influencing the degree of resection based on the arterial, venous, and lymphatic drainage of the affected colon segment. The primary tumor location relative to adjacent organs also decides resectability in locally advanced cases. An appropriate response to these factors demands detailed knowledge of surgical anatomy in the planning and execution of colon resections.

Colon
SURGICAL ANATOMY
Topography

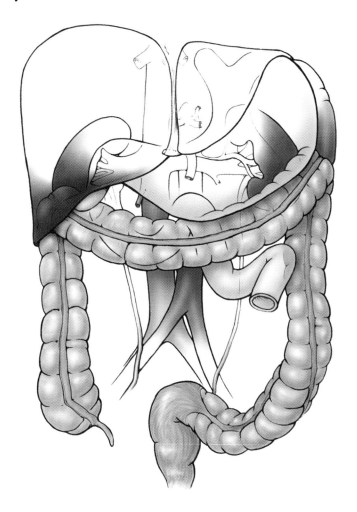

The colon is 120 to 200 cm long, surrounds the small intestine in the peritoneal cavity, and has a variant course within the abdominal cavity depending on its intraperitoneal or extraperitoneal location. Oncologic implications for potential patterns of treatment failure can be found in the peritoneal location of the colon. Recurrent intraperitoneal tumors often present as peritoneal seeding.

The diameter of the colon diminishes gradually from 7.5 cm at the cecum to 2.5 cm at the sigmoid colon. External anatomic characteristics of the colon that distinguish it from the small bowel include taenia coli, haustral sacculations of the bowel wall, appendix epiploicae, and the attachment of the greater omentum to the transverse colon.

Derived portions of midgut and foregut constitute the colon's developmental division. The embryologic origin of the colon segments is significant in that their blood supplies follow the superior mesenteric–midgut and inferior mesenteric–hindgut supply relationships. Therefore traditional colectomies are based on the vascular supply of the subsegments of the colon. Anatomic segments of the colon on which colectomies are based include the cecum, ascending colon, transverse colon, descending colon, and sigmoid colon.

Cecum

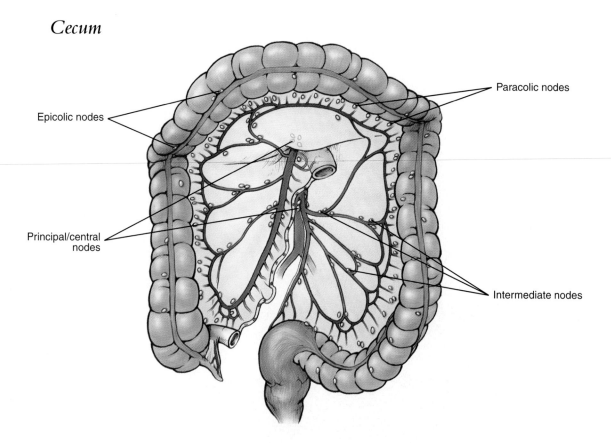

The cecum is the colon segment that originates after the ileocecal valve. It is located in the right iliac fossa and has the widest transverse diameter of all the colon segments, 7.5 cm. It is mobile, completely covered with visceral peritoneum, and lies below the latter half of the inguinal ligament. The ileocecal valve is located medially at the cecum's junction with the terminal ileum, and it acts as a sphincter to regulate the emptying of ileal contents into the cecum. Normally this valve relaxes in response to food entering the stomach (gastroileal reflux) and is incompetent in 30% of individuals.

The ileocecal valve's anatomic location has important management implications for patients with distal colon cancers. A closed-loop obstruction can arise due to the presence of a functional ileocecal valve proximal to an obstructing colon cancer, thereby increasing the potential for cecal rupture. The cecum has clinically important anatomic relationships with the right ureter, which rests posteriorly on the psoas muscle and the lateral abdominal wall.

Ascending Colon

The ascending colon is found distal to the cecum and proximal to the hepatic flexure and thereby has important anatomic relationships to the liver, duodenum, right kidney, and ureter as it posteriorly transverses the psoas muscle. This colon segment varies in length from 12 to 20 cm and is completely covered, except posteriorly, by visceral peritoneum. At the undersurface of the liver, where the ascending colon turns medially and posteriorly, it is defined as the hepatic flexure.

The ascending colon is laterally attached to the parietal peritoneum along the white line of Toldt, an area that represents an embryonic fusion plane between the visceral and parietal peritoneum. Since it is a fusion plane that is relatively avascular, the white line of Toldt is an important surgical landmark for identifying the point of peritoneal division for colon mobilization.

Transverse Colon

The transverse colon extends from the hepatic flexure to the splenic flexure, with important anatomic relationships including the stomach, tail of pancreas, spleen, and left kidney. It is completely invested with peritoneum and has a long mesentery known as the transverse mesocolon, defining it as the colon's most mobile portion. Spanning 40 to 50 cm, this segment is fixed at the hepatic and splenic flexures and attached at the greater curvature of the stomach by the gastrocolic omentum. The discovery of locally advanced lesions in this segment can present technically challenging resections because of its increased mobility and the potential to involve numerous adjacent organs.

Descending Colon

The descending colon extends from the splenic flexure to the sigmoid colon on the left side of the peritoneal cavity, forming important posterior anatomic relationships to the kidney, ureter, and iliac vessels at the pelvic brim. This segment is narrower and longer by 35 cm than the ascending colon. Save for its posterior area, where it is fixed to the fascia covering the quadratum lumborum muscle, the descending colon is covered with visceral peritoneum.

Sigmoid Colon

Originating at the pelvic brim, the sigmoid colon is located at the lower end of the descending colon and usually ends at the third sacral vertebrae of the rectosigmoid junction. It has long V-shaped mesentery, is very mobile, and is completely invested in visceral peritoneum. Because of its long mesentery and increased mobility the sigmoid colon has important anatomic relationships to the pelvic organs and the posterior ureter.

Blood Supply
Arteries

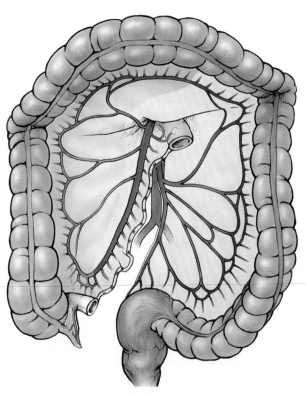

A colon segment's vascular supply is defined by its embryonic origins. The right colon and proximal transverse colon are derived from the midgut, a region supplied by the superior mesenteric artery, and the distal transverse colon and left colon are derived from the hindgut, supplied by the inferior mesenteric artery. These two arterial systems arborize along the mesenteric border of the colon, forming the marginal artery of Drummond. This marginal system is formed by tributaries from the ileocolic, right colic, middle colic, left colic, and sigmoid arteries and stretches from the ileocecal valve to the rectosigmoid colon. The terminal vessels that vascularize a limited area of bowel wall are supplied by these arteries. Collateralization is excellent along this system, serving as an important source of a segment's blood supply when a major vessel is occluded. The presence of these marginal arteries also allows the sacrifice of major vessels, facilitating the colon's mobilization for distal anastomosis.

Receiving its principal arterial supply from the superior mesenteric artery originating below the celiac axis, the right colon then exits from the retroperitoneum between the pancreas and third portion of the duodenum. The superior mesenteric artery also arises at the level of the first lumbar vertebra, from the anterior surface of the aorta, with major distribution through the ileocolic, right colic, and middle colic arteries.

The artery with the most consistent anatomic location in the superior mesenteric artery distribution is the ileocolic artery, which supplies the terminal ileum, appendix, and cecum while also contributing a superior branch to the marginal artery. Right colon resections often include this artery. It is important, however, to ensure that the remaining terminal ileum has an adequate blood supply for an anastomosis.

In terms of location, presence, and vessel of origin, the right colic artery is the most variable blood supply. It usually originates between the proximal middle colic and distal ileocolic branches of the superior mesenteric artery, then divides into ascending and descending branches that anastomose with the ileocolic and middle colic branches.

The middle colic artery is a major blood supplier to the colon and is an important surgical landmark when planning a colon resection because it is a demarcation point for the clinical definition of a right or left hemicolectomy. This artery arises at the entrance of the superior mesenteric artery into the small bowel mesentery at the inferior border of the pancreas. It then ascends into the transverse mesocolon, anastomosing with the right and left colon blood supplies through the marginal artery. A considerable portion of the transverse colon often becomes gangrenous when the middle colic artery is occluded.

The left colon arises embryologically from the hindgut, which receives its blood supply from the inferior mesenteric artery. This artery originates at the level of the third lumbar vertebra and supplies the distal transverse colon to the anus. It has a more consistent arterial distribution than does the superior mesenteric artery and is defined by three principal branches: the left colic, sigmoid, and superior hemorrhoid arteries.

The first branch of the inferior mesenteric artery is the left colic artery, which divides into ascending and descending branches as it passes upward. The ascending branch anastomoses with the branches of the middle colic artery, a system that supplies the distal transverse colon and splenic flexures. After supplying the descending colon, the descending branch joins branches of the sigmoid artery.

Originating from the inferior mesenteric artery, the sigmoid artery divides into ascending and descending collateral branches as it travels through the sigmoid mesocolon. The descending branch supplies the sigmoid colon; the ascending vessels merge with the marginal artery system. The terminal vessel of the inferior mesenteric artery is the superior hemorrhoid artery, supplying the rectum.

Veins

The colon's venous anatomy parallels the arterial supply of the corresponding midgut- or hindgut-derived segments. Drainage of the midgut-derived right colon is achieved by the superior mesenteric venous system, which includes the ileocolic, right colic, and middle colic veins. This configuration forms the superior mesenteric vein and empties into the portal venous system. Drainage of the left colon derived from the hindgut is accomplished by the inferior mesenteric venous system, which differs from the superior mesenteric venous system by joining the splenic vein before entering the portal vein. The descending and sigmoid colon segments are drained through the left colic and sigmoidal veins, respectively. A primary explanation for the high incidence of the liver as a site of failure in colon cancer is provided by the central portal venous drainage pattern of the colon.

Lymphatic Drainage

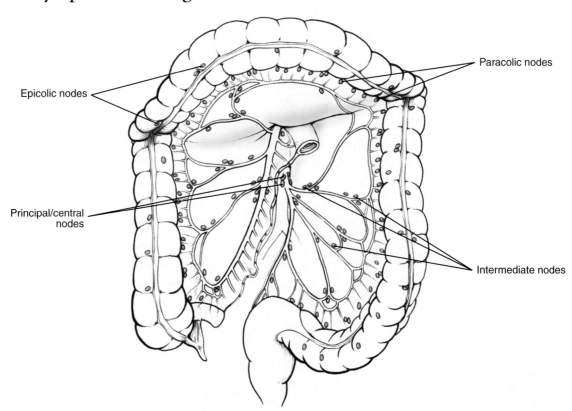

Organization of the lymphatic system is constant throughout the colon and is grouped into four primary nodal groups: the epicolic, paracolic, intermediate, and principal/central nodes. This complex originates as an extensive plexus between the lamina propria and muscularis mucosa, with its vessels coalescing and draining through the submucosa to the lymphatic follicles. Communicating through lymphatic channels that traverse the bowel wall, these follicles then drain to the bowel wall's epicolic nodes, the first distinct group of nodes. The paracolic nodes that follow are the most numerous of the colonic mesenteric nodes and are found between the bowel wall and the marginal artery of Drummond. From this level the lymphatic vessels follow the terminal arteries, from the marginal artery toward the major vessel supplying that particular segment. An intermediate group of nodes are encountered along the arterial trunks and are clustered at bifurcations. The principal/central group of nodes is found at the origin of the superior and inferior mesenteric arteries. These principal nodes empty into the para-aortic lymphatic channels and, eventually, into the cistern chyli.

Controversy surrounds the appropriate extent of lymphadenectomy in a routine colon resection, with the crux of the debate focusing on the need for high ligation of the segmental artery arising from the aorta vs. ligation of the named colon artery. The argument centers on whether the principal/central nodes should be resected or the resection should be limited to the intermediate nodal groups along the arteries supplying the particular segment. Retrospective conclusions are available to support either side, although no perspective data are currently available. In conclusion, the current routine for adequate lymph node dissection in colon cancer continues to include the intermediate nodal group.

Nerve Supply

Just as in the small intestine, the colon contains ganglia in both the submucosa and myenteric plexi. These plexi receive extrinsic innervation from the parasympathetic and sympathetic divisions of the autonomic nervous system, and the neural supplies are thought to parallel the vascular supply.

The sympathetic nerves consist of afferent and efferent fibers originating from the eleventh and twelfth thoracic and first and second lumbar nerves. The postganglionic efferent fibers follow the superior mesenteric artery as it branches to supply the right colon. In their journey to supply the left colon the afferent fibers pass through the sympathetic chain, into the ganglia, and on to the inferior mesenteric plexus.

The origins of the parasympathetic innervation to the colon are not so clear, although this innervation is generally perceived to arise from the vagus nerve to supply the right colon. Nerve fibers originating from the sacral segments of the spinal cord, S2, S3, and S4, contribute to the left colon's innervation.

SURGICAL APPLICATIONS

Surgical resection continues to be the primary therapeutic method for malignant tumors of the colon. The particular tumor's location determines the extent of resection, and the vascular supply and lymphatic drainage to the mesenteric segment define the limits of resection. These anatomic determinants have remained constant over the past three decades, with the only recent change to the procedure being the emphasis on preoperative preparation.

An important component of preoperative preparation is mechanical bowel preparation, which consists of administration of a polyethylene glycol electrolyte solution, oral nonabsorbable antibiotics, intravenous antibiotics, and correction fluid for electrolyte abnormalities. On completion of the essential preoperative steps, malignancy may be surgically approached with a right hemicolectomy, left or descending colectomy, transverse colectomy, sigmoid colectomy, or subtotal colectomy.

Colonoscopic Polypectomy

Nonneoplastic polyps are the colon's most common benign tumors, with estimates of their prevalence in the general population ranging from 1.6% to 12%, whereas neoplastic polyps, also known as adenomas, have a highly malignant potential. When adenomas are discovered during such procedures as colonoscopic or barium contrast studies, therapeutic action is required, with the malignant potential of each particular adenomatous colon polyp determining its appropriate treatment. Adenomatous polyps are characterized as tubular, villous, or tubulovillous. Although a higher percentage of villous polyps are cancerous, most malignant polyps are tubular or tubulovillous. Certainly all polyps should be viewed as possessing malignant possibility, although a polyp's risk for containing invasive cancer does increase as its size increases; most malignant polyps are 1 to 3 cm in diameter.

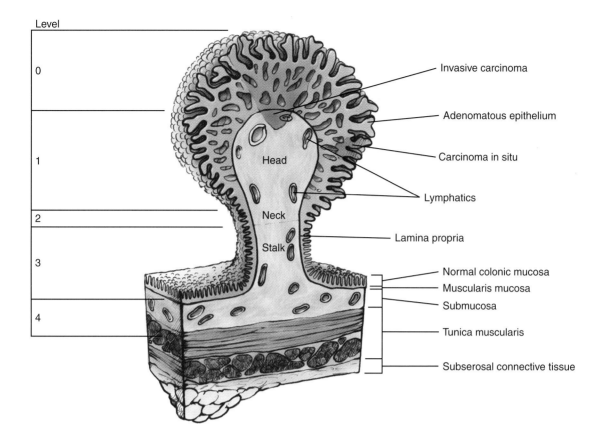

Colonoscopic polypectomy's increased usage has caused uncertainty regarding treatment recommendations for malignant polyps, an ambivalence that focuses on the ability to accurately predict the risk for an adverse outcome for a particular set of polyp characteristics. The prognosis for sessile polyps is worse than that for pedunculated polyps, proving that the morphologic features of a polyp are highly significant. The issue of depth of invasion within a polyp has also been examined and becomes critical in the muscularis mucosa because the lymphatic vessels are associated with its fibers. The internal level of polyp invasion also is important. The greatest risk for lymph node metastases occurs when invasion extends into the submucosa of the bowel wall, below the neck of the polyp, and above the muscularis propria. Other criteria associated with poor prognosis include lymphovascular invasion, grade III or poorly differentiated histologic findings, and a positive or uncertain margin.

The indications for colon resection following colonoscopic excision of a polyp are determined by the presence of residual disease risk. With malignant polyps that exhibit no level IV invasion, poorly differentiated elements, lymphovascular invasion, or positive margins, the risk is less than 1.5% for residual disease. Consequently, conservative follow-up is sufficient, with repeat colonoscopy at 3 months to rule out disease. For endoscopically resected polyps with these criteria that are pedunculated, colon resection is required. Malignant sessile polyps should be resected when discovered. Differentiation of the margin becomes difficult when polyps are resected piecemeal, making colon resection necessary.

Right Hemicolectomy

Tumors located in the appendix, cecum, or ascending colon often require a right hemicolectomy, the anatomic boundaries of which span the cecum to the proximal transverse colon. An extended right hemicolectomy includes the transverse colon, a segment located to the left of the middle colic artery.

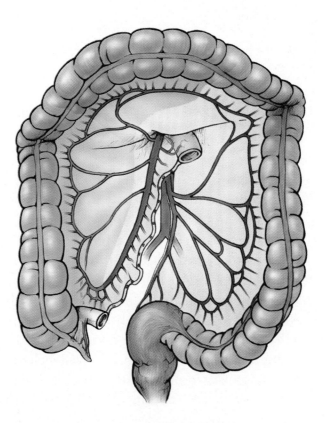

Although the abdominal incisions used to execute a right hemicolectomy may vary, with choices including a midline, paramedian, or transverse supraumbilical incision, the procedure always involves standard exploration on entering the abdominal cavity. Such examination is necessary to assess disease extent and subsequent resectability. Anatomic areas of interest with a right-sided lesion include other areas of the colon, liver, porta hepatis, mesenteric lymph nodes, ovaries, right ureter, duodenum, and peritoneal surfaces.

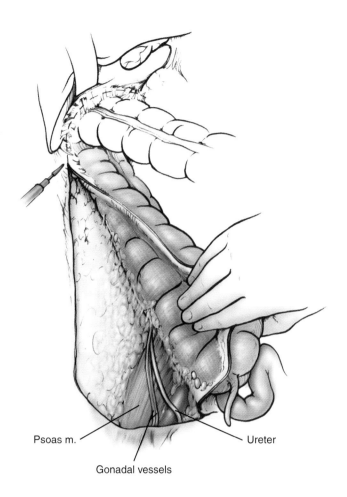

Psoas m.

Gonadal vessels

Ureter

A right hemicolectomy is initiated by mobilizing the colon from its lateral peritoneal wall attachments. The colon is then retracted medially, exposing the lateral peritoneal wall, or white line of Toldt. Electrocautery or scissors is used to sharply incise this peritoneal fold from the cecum to the hepatic flexure, and medial mobilization of the colon is accomplished through blunt finger and sharp dissection of the retroperitoneal attachments. Caution must be observed so as to identify and protect the right ureter, a tube posteriorly coursing along the psoas muscle, during the entire retroperitoneal mobilization.

The sharp and blunt dissection of the retroperitoneal plane is continued superiorly into the hepatic flexure, with the dissecting hand placed behind the hepatic flexure to isolate the hepatocolic ligament, which is divided sharply with the electrocautery. Mobilization of the right colon is completed when the hepatic flexure is freed superiorly from the liver and posteriorly from the duodenum.

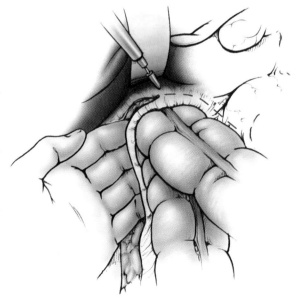

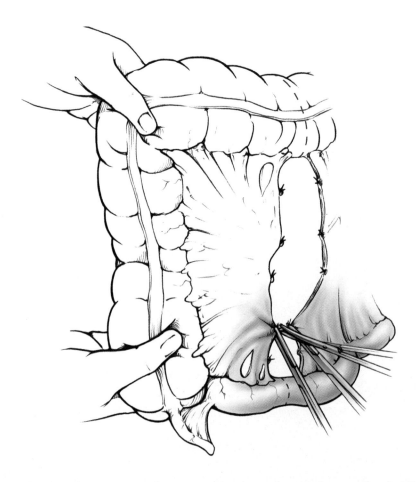

On mobilization, the extent of mesenteric resection is determined. The transection points of the distal colon and ileum are marked on the mesenteric borders by creating rents in the mesentery, and the corresponding mesentery is divided to the origins of the ileocolic and right colic arteries. The initiation and completion of a standard double clamping and mesentery ligation with 3-0 silk suture technique follows. This level of sacrificed mesentery ensures inclusion of the intermediate group of nodes.

The ileum is transected 10 to 15 cm from the ileocecal valve for cecal lesions, although a 4 cm ileal margin is sufficient if the tumor is distal to the cecum. The distal point of transection is proximal to the middle colic artery for a standard right hemicolectomy. Either a GIA stapler or intestinal clamps are used to divide and seal the bowel lumens. The omentum can then be mobilized from the right transverse colon through an avascular plane, provided it is not in proximity to the tumor.

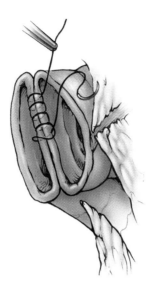

Restoration of gastrointestinal continuity is accomplished with either a hand-sewn or stapled anastomosis. The standard hand-sewn technique creates an end-to-end anastomosis between the ileum and transverse colon, which includes one or two layers depending on the use of an internal continuous layer. Connecting the bowel ends with a seromuscular row of posterior 3-0 nonabsorbable suture constitutes the basic two-layer technique. At this juncture the staple lines created by the GIA are open and noncrushing clamps are placed across the bowel lumens.

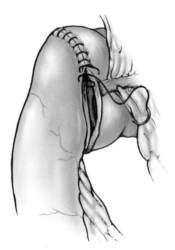

The interior continuous layer is a full-thickness absorbable locking suture, beginning posteriorly and running anteriorly as a Connell inverting suture. The anterior layers are then reinforced with a Lembert seromuscular suture, and the mesenteric defect is closed.

Due to both an associated decrease in operative time and less manipulation of the tissue used in the anastomosis, the use of staplers has gained popularity over the hand-sewn method. Despite this general preference, the two techniques have equivalent functional results and similar mobility-related complications.

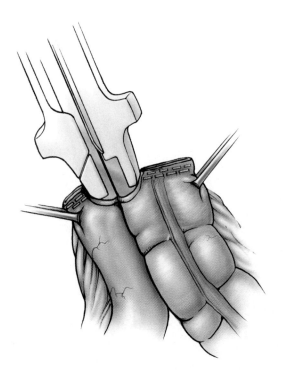

The stapled anastomosis begins by aligning the two ends of the bowel along the end of the antimesenteric borders, with noncrushing clamps applied proximally on the bowel lumens. The antimesenteric corner of the staple line is excised on both bowel ends, and the forks of the GIA instrument are inserted into the ileum and colon. On firing the instrument the internal staple line is checked for bleeding, and the resultant ileocolostomy edges are aligned using Allis clamps.

A TA-55 stapling instrument is used to close the opening. To complete the procedure, the staple lines are inspected, a 3-0 silk suture is placed at the base of the anastomosis, and the mesenteric defect is closed. Although routine drainage is not necessary for a right hemicolectomy, the anastomosis and the colon bed are then inspected for hemostasis. A No. 1 Prolene suture is used to close the abdomen in layers, and the skin is closed with clips or sutures.

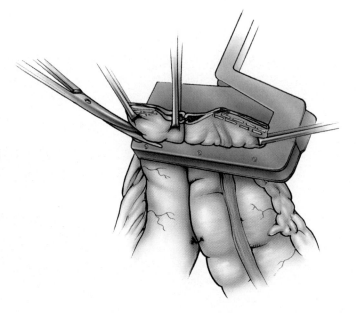

Left Hemicolectomy

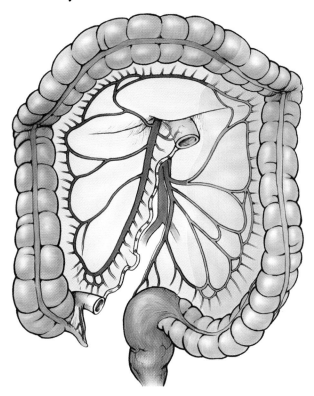

A tumor located in the descending colon requires a left hemicolectomy, a resection encompassing the splenic flexure to the proximal sigmoid. Because left-sided colon lesions are more likely to cause obstruction than right-sided lesions, preoperative assessment and bowel preparation are essential. These particular lesions are usually approached through a long vertical midline incision extending from the epigastrium to below the umbilicus, facilitating mobilization of the splenic flexure. Occasionally left paramedian incisions are used for colectomies.

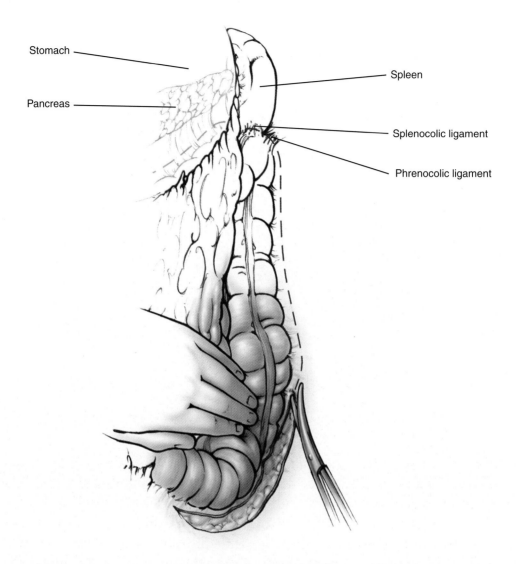

Standard exploration of the abdominal cavity, including examination of the colon and drainage of lymph nodes, liver, hypochondrium, and peritoneal surfaces, initiates the left hemicolectomy. At exploration the left colon is reflected medially, exposing the white line of Toldt. This lateral peritoneal fold is sharply incised using an electrocautery or scissors, and the opening is extended from the sigmoid colon to the splenic flexure. The splenic flexure is distracted inferiorly and the ileocolic ligaments sharply divided, and the left colon is mobilized medially from its retroperitoneal attachments with blunt and sharp dissection. Proximity of the lesion to the splenic flexure determines whether the gastrocolic omentum is mobilized off the transverse colon or is divided and included with the specimens. During the retroperitoneal dissection the left ureter is identified and protected.

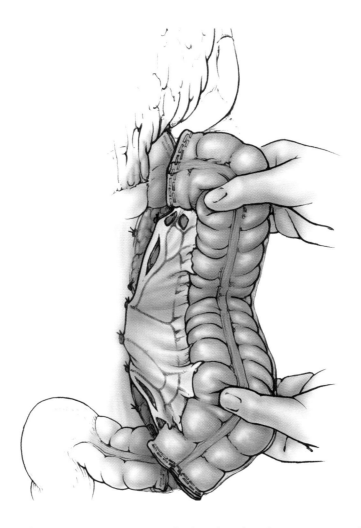

The left hemicolectomy specimen includes the distal transverse colon and the descending colon. Creating a window on the mesenteric border of the bowel wall in the mesocolon demarcates bowel resection. Terminal branches of the marginal artery supplying that segment are ligated if necessary, and the bowel lumens are divided and stapled with a GIA instrument. The distal point of transection is chosen and divided with a GIA instrument, and the extent of mesenteric resection is marked by incising the visceral peritoneal layer. The mesentery resection includes ligation of the left colic artery and proximal sigmoid artery at their origins. Prior to the resection, the ureter is again identified and packed out of the field. A standard clamp and ligation technique with 2-0 or 3-0 silk sutures completes the division.

An anastomosis between the transverse and sigmoid colons can be stapled or hand sewn. At the outset of stapling the two ends of the bowel lumens are aligned along the antimesenteric border using stay sutures, with two non-crushing clamps placed on the bowel wall proximal to the staple lines. The antimesenteric corners of the GIA staple lines are removed with scissors, and the forks of the GIA are inserted into the bowel lumen and the instrument fired. After inspection of the anastomosis the ostomy is closed with a TA-55 stapler.

A posterior 3-0 silk seromuscular layer initiates a hand-sewn anastomosis. Noncrushing clamps are placed on the bowel wall proximal to the staple lines, and the lumens are opened by excising the previously placed GIA staple line. The inner layer is completed by running an absorbable suture in both directions with a locking technique, closing the anterior wall. The placing of a 3-0 nonabsorbable Lembert suture layer completes the anterior anastomosis. On conclusion of either technique, the mesenteric defect is closed with a running or interrupted suture. The anastomosis, the left quadrant, and the retroperitoneum are inspected (drainage is unnecessary in this procedure), at which point a running No. 1 monofilament nonabsorbable suture is used to close the abdomen. The skin is then stapled or sutured.

Transverse Colectomy

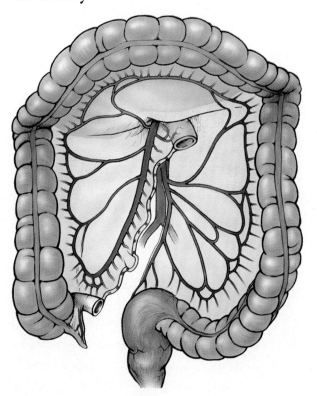

A transverse colectomy is most applicable to tumors located in the midtransverse colon, an area in proximity to the stomach, gastrocolic omentum, spleen, liver, and pancreas. Tumors located in the proximal hepatic flexure often can be managed by sacrificing the middle colic artery with an extended right hemicolectomy, although the distal transverse colon must then be carefully assessed for viability before creating an anastomosis. Occasionally the lesions of the distal transverse colon are managed with a resection encompassing the transverse and left colon proximal to the left colic artery. Such extensive resections are justified by concerns about both the viability of the splenic flexure and the distal transverse colon area's tenuous blood supplies. This particular area of the left colon is at risk because the marginal artery is its only blood supply, and the marginal artery's major contributor, the middle colic artery, is sacrificed in transverse colon resections.

Facilitating transverse colon resection requires complete mobilization of the right and left colons. The sharp and blunt dissection described for a standard hemicolectomy also mobilizes the right and left colons from their peritoneal attachments, followed by the mobilization of the hepatic and splenic flexures from their ligamentous attachments. The limits of mesocolon resection are then determined and marked, and the middle colic artery is identified and ligated at the base of the mesocolon. The colon-to-colon anastomosis is completed as described for left colon resection, using either a stapled or hand-sewn technique. A running or interrupted suture is used to close the mesentery defect, and the abdomen is closed with a No. 1 nonabsorbable monofilament suture. Clips or sutures are used to close the skin.

Sigmoid Colectomy

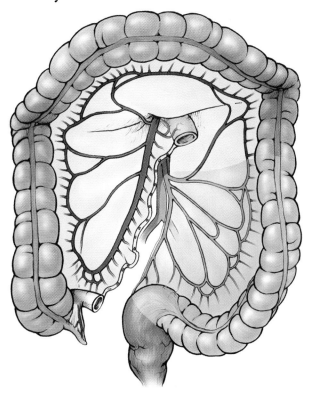

Lesions amenable to sigmoid resection, the margins of which extend from the lower portion of the descending colon to the level of the sacral promontory, incorporate the proximal or middle sigmoid colon. Tumors of this segment can obstruct due to small lumen size, and their long mesentery creates a greater propensity for involving adjacent organs. When a sigmoid tumor crosses the pelvic brim, additional problems can arise involving the bladder, ovaries, uterus, or distal ureter.

Sigmoid colon tumors can be approached through a standard midline incision, which allows enough length to mobilize the splenic flexure, thereby producing the new rectosigmoid anastomosis. The abdomen is explored as usual, as are the liver, colon, and small bowel. Drainage of the lymph nodes, bladder, ovaries, and uterus continues the procedure.

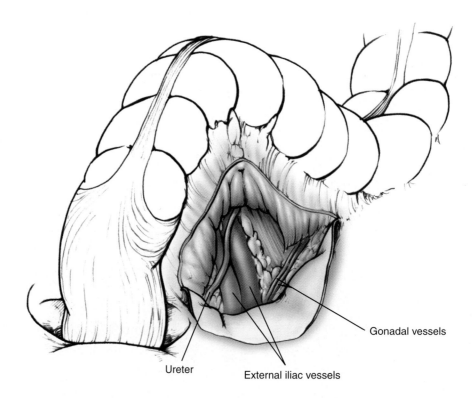

Gonadal vessels

Ureter

External iliac vessels

Mobilization of the left colon and splenic flexure from the lateral peritoneal wall is accomplished by medial retraction of the colon and a combination of blunt finger dissection and sharp dissection with an electrocautery or scissors. The sigmoid colon and the descending colon are retracted medially, and the left ureter is identified. It is most easily found as it crosses the left iliac artery. Remember that ureters may be multiple.

Determining the bowel wall's transection points is accomplished on mobilization, at which juncture mesenteric windows are created and the bowel is divided using the GIA instrument. The resection of proximal to middle sigmoid colon tumors includes the immediate nodes along the inferior mesenteric artery and sacrifice of the left colic and terminal sigmoid branches. The area of bowel resection extends from the mid-descending colon to the sacral promontory. The left colic artery can be spared with a distal tumor, in which case the superior hemorrhoidal arcade is resected. Such a bowel resection encompasses the distal descending colon to the rectosigmoid junction.

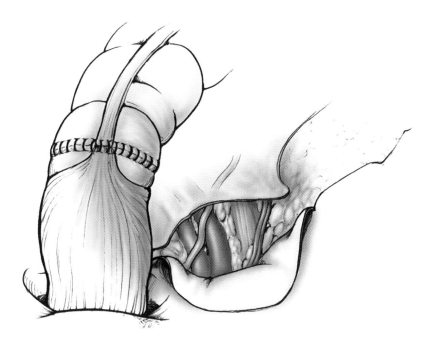

Restoration of bowel continuity is undertaken with an end-to-end anastomosis using either a hand-sewn or stapled technique. The hand-sewn technique involves either one or two layers. A two-layer approach aligns the colon ends with two stay sutures while a posterior seromuscular layer of 3-0 silk sutures is placed. Interior locking in combination with a 3-0 absorbable suture running in both directions composes the two-layer anastomosis, resulting in the anterior wall's complete inversion, after which the anterior wall is reinforced with a 3-0 Lembert suture technique. Optionally, a side-to-end anastomosis may be made, depending on whether the left colon mesentery is short. The diameter of the left colon provides additional length to prevent tension on the anastomosis.

A GIA instrument is used for the stapled anastomosis. The bowel is aligned with stay sutures, the staple lines are open at the antimesenteric corners, and the GIA forks are placed in the lumen and fired. After inspection of the area the opening is closed with a TA-55 stapler. Either a running or interrupted suture closes the mesenteric defect, a heavy nonabsorbable monofilament suture closes the fascia, and the skin is closed with a stapler or sutures.

Subtotal Colectomy

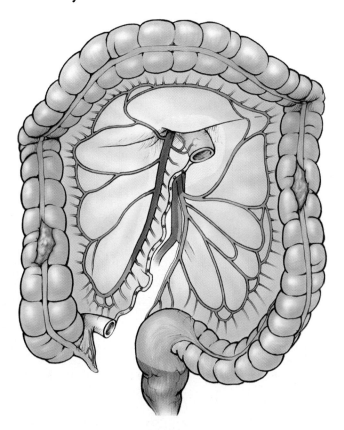

A subtotal colectomy consists of removal of the entire intraperitoneal colon, and is often required for inflammatory bowel disease, multiple polyps, and diverticulosis. Polyps associated with colon cancer occur in one third of these cases and, in some instances, are not amenable to colonoscopic removal, necessitating subtotal colectomy to encompass the disease. This procedure may also become necessary in the 5% of patients with a primary cancer and synchronous colon lesions or in the surgical treatment of transverse colon lesions when uncertainty arises concerning the adequacy of the remaining blood supply.

A standard midline incision initiates the subtotal colectomy. Prior to the resection, a complete abdominal exploration is undertaken to examine the liver, spleen, omentum, small bowel, pelvic organs, and entire colon. With sharp or blunt dissection the lateral peritoneal attachments of the right colon are mobilized. The colon itself is mobilized from the duodenum at the level of the hepatic flexure, and the hepatocolic ligament is sharply divided. If a transverse colon lesion is involved, the gastrocolic omentum is included with the specimen. The mobilization continues around the splenic flexure and along the lateral peritoneal reflections of the descending colon and is completed at the rectosigmoid junction.

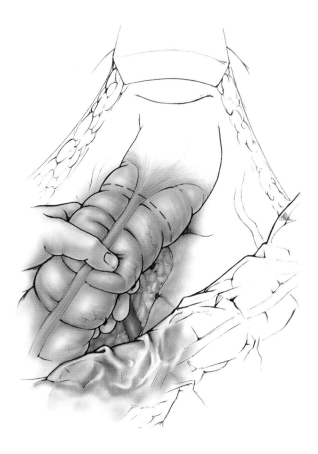

The margins for bowel transection are determined on complete mobilization. A GIA instrument is used to divide the terminal ileum 4 cm proximal to the ileocecal valve; the distal point of transection is usually at the rectosigmoid junction. Both the intermediate nodal group along the named segmental arteries and the resected arteries, including the ileocolic, right colic, middle colic, left colic, and sigmoid vessels, are included in the mesentery resection. This procedure may be extended for an associated benign condition such as diverticulosis, at which point the extent of such a resection can be modified according to operative findings.

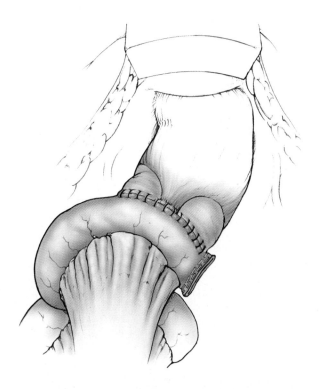

Restoration of gastrointestinal continuity requires an anastomosis between the ileum and the rectum, completed with a hand-sewn technique. The standard two-layer method is similar to that of the anastomosis of the ileum to the transverse colon. A posterior seromuscular layer is placed using a 3-0 silk suture, noncrushing clamps occlude the bowel lumens, and the staple lines are opened. The inner absorbable suture layer is introduced posteriorly, run in both directions until the anterior wall is closed, and reinforced with a 3-0 Lembert suture. For both hand-sewn and stapled techniques a running or interrupted suture is used to close the mesenteric defect; drainage is not necessary. The fascia is closed with a heavy nonabsorbable monofilament suture, and the skin is closed with clips or sutures.

Laparoscopic Colectomy

At present no prospective randomized trials have been published comparing the equivalency of laparoscopy with open colectomy to manage malignancy. Until such studies have been completed and conclusive data are compiled concerning patient outcome (e.g., 5-year survival, local or regional disease recurrence), laparoscopic colectomies should be limited to clinical trials.

Lymph Node Dissection

Surgical resection can offer a potential cure for colon cancer lymph node metastases that are diagnosed as local regional disease. An effective therapeutic component of such resection is regional lymph node dissection, although the extent or level of such dissection in relation to therapeutic effect remains controversial. Opinions are divided on whether dissection of the principal nodes or the central nodes improves the outcome, with current retrospective data to support both arguments. No conclusive randomized trial data supporting more radical node resection are available. Therefore present recommendations support routine resection of the intermediate nodes of the involved colon segment.

Appendix
SURGICAL ANATOMY
Topography

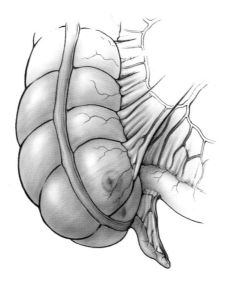

The vermiform appendix originates approximately 2.5 cm below the ileocecal junction at the posteromedial wall of the cecum, and its base is located at the convergence of the taenia coli onto the cecum. This blind tube varies from 2 to 20 cm in length, is freely mobile, and can be found in numerous positions, the most common being a retrocecal posture in the right iliac fossa. In cases of malrotation the appendix can also be found in the right upper quadrant or left iliac fossa. Its base projects to McBurney's point, an area on the abdominal wall one third of the distance between the right anterior superior iliac spine and the umbilicus.

Blood Supply

The mesoappendix is a triangular peritoneal fold running from the terminal ileum to the cecum's base. It carries the branch of the ileocolic artery known as the appendicular artery, single or paired.

Nerve Supply

The appendix is innervated by both the parasympathetic and sympathetic divisions of the autonomic nervous system, duplicating the innervation of the cecum. Parasympathetic innervation is thought to arise from the vagus nerve, and sympathetic innervation arises from the eleventh and twelfth thoracic and first and second lumbar nerves. Pain from the cecum and appendix is clinically referred to as McBurney's point.

Lymphatic Drainage

Lymphatic drainage from the appendix is encompassed in the right colon distribution.

SURGICAL APPLICATIONS

Malignant tumors arising from the appendix are rare, although when they do appear, carcinoids and adenocarcinomas are often the type diagnosed. Carcinoids are more common. In fact, the appendix is the most frequent site of carcinoid occurrence, and the incidence in surgically removed appendices is approximately 0.1%. Such tumors often are found incidentally during appendectomy.

The natural history of carcinoids reveals that malignant potential increases with size greater than 2 cm. Therefore the discovery of an incidental carcinoid in an appendectomy specimen requires a therapeutic decision. If the carcinoid is less than 2 cm in greatest dimension and is localized to the appendix, a simple appendectomy will usually suffice. A right hemicolectomy is recommended if the tumor is greater than 2 cm or if lymph node metastases are suspected.

Adenocarcinomas are more inclined to produce symptoms than carcinoids are. The common histologic variants are well-differentiated or mucus-producing tumors (malignant mucocele) or poorly differentiated adenocarcinomas. Both of these lesions can metastasize to regional nodes and distant sites. Adequate treatment requires a mesenteric resection encompassing the primary node's drainage system.

If the diagnosis of an adenocarcinoma is made incidentally, as in an appendectomy specimen, the need for future therapeutic intervention must be determined. In those few instances when a carcinoma is discovered early and is confined in situ, appendectomy and right hemicolectomy result in equivalent survival, although right hemicolectomy is recommended for pathologically confirmed invasion.

Transverse/Rockey-Davis Incision

Because preoperative diagnosis of a localized appendiceal tumor is unusual, the appendix is often approached through a more limited incision than that used for a suspected malignancy. The most common entrance technique used for routine appendectomy is a transverse/Rockey-Davis incision centered on McBurney's point, an area located one third the distance from the anterosuperior iliac spine on a line drawn to the umbilicus. The abdominal wall fascia and muscles are incised or split in the direction of the incision.

McBurney's Incision

A classic alternative to the transverse approach is McBurney's incision, the path of which runs obliquely through McBurney's point, is usually 8 to 10 cm in length, and extends to the lateral border of the rectus sheath. The abdominal wall fascia and muscles are then incised or split in the direction of the fibers. Although this method is often adequate, the transverse incision can be easily extended and gives superior exposure. An appendectomy can also be performed through a vertical midline incision if the diagnosis is uncertain or if a malignancy is suspected preoperatively.

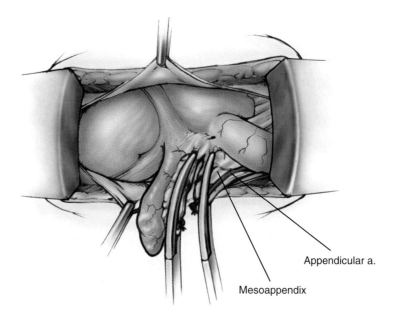

After the peritoneum is opened the appendix is identified by following the cecal taenia distally, and the cecum and appendix are delivered into the wound by gentle traction. Occasionally the lateral peritoneal reflection of the cecum is divided to improve exposure. These maneuvers should bring the cecum and appendix to the anterior abdominal wall, facilitating removal without vigorous retraction. Freed from any attachments, the mesoappendix can be identified, divided between clamps, and ligated to control the appendicular artery.

Appendectomy

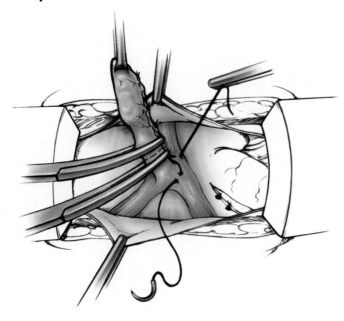

The appendiceal stump created by resection of the appendix can be treated by either inversion or simple ligation. Inversion follows ligation and amputation of the appendix above a hemostat placed on its base. The upper portion of a Z stitch is then placed as a Lembert suture in the cecum, distal to the base of the appendix. The suture is brought around the appendiceal base medially, and a lower Z stitch is placed below it at the base of the appendix and the cecum.

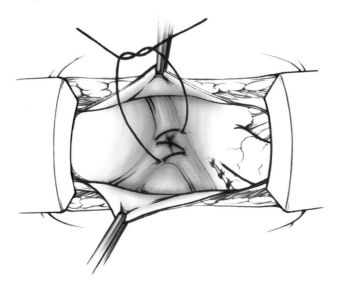

After amputation and inversion of the appendix and tying of the Z stitch, the procedure is completed. Simple ligation of the appendiceal stump is initiated by placing a crushing hemostat at the base. This clamp is moved 1 cm distally, and a ligature of 2-0 absorbable suture is placed in the groove and tied, at which point the appendix is transected above the clamp.

Anatomic Basis of Complications

- The risk of injury to the ureters increases if adequate exposure is not obtained before the mesentery is divided.
- Duodenal injury during mobilization of the right colon can occur due to its proximity to the hepatic flexure.
- Excessive traction on the descending colon before dividing the lineocolic ligaments can cause splenic capsule laceration.
- Sacrifice of mesentery involving the major collateral blood supply to a segment of bowel causes ischemia.
- Inadequate mobilization of colon length creates tension at an anastomosis and increases the risk of leakage.

KEY REFERENCES

Condon RE. Resection of the colon. In Zuidema GD, ed. Shackelford's Surgery of the Alimentary Tract. Philadelphia: WB Saunders, 1996, pp 207-224.
This is an excellent review of operations performed on the intraperitoneal colon. Fundamental principles and general techniques required for standard colon resections are described.

Docherty JG, McGregor JR, Akyol AM, et al. Comparison of manually constructed and stapled anastomoses in colorectal surgery. Ann Surg 221:176-184, 1995.
This prospective randomized trial compares stapled and sutured colorectal anastomoses. The authors conclude that suturing or stapling are equally effective in large bowel surgery.

Fazio VW, Tjandra JJ. Primary therapy of carcinoma of the large bowel. World J Surg 15:568-575, 1991.
This article puts forth the general principles of colon resection with curative intent. The authors present criteria for choosing the appropriate procedure according to tumor location and a description of the procedure.

Malssagne B, Valleur P, Serra J, et al. Relationship of apical lymph node involvement to survival in resected colon carcinoma. Dis Colon Rectum 36:645-653, 1993.
This prospective study explores the relationship between pathologic parameters such as apical nodes and survival. The authors suggest that apical lymph node involvement is a poor prognostic sign and that its intraoperative recognition might affect surgical decision making.

Romolo JL. Embryology and anatomy of the colon. In Zuidema GD, ed. Shackelford's Surgery of the Alimentary Tract. Philadelphia: WB Saunders, 1996, pp 3-16.
This chapter reviews colon development from the hindgut phase, including normal rotation and fixation phases. Anomalies associated with these phases of development are discussed. A concise overview of colon anatomy essential for performing colon resections concludes the chapter.

SUGGESTED READINGS

Abcarian H. Operative treatment of colorectal cancer. Cancer 70(Suppl 5):1350-1354, 1992.

Amaral JF, Bland KI, Copeland EM, et al. Surgery of tumors of the colon and rectum. In Bland KI, Karakousis CP, Copeland EM, eds. Atlas of Surgical Oncology. Philadelphia: WB Saunders, 1995, pp 501-529.

Bertagnolli MM, DeCosse JJ. Laparoscopic colon resection for cancer—An unfavorable view. Adv Surg 29:155-164, 1996.

Brief DK, Brener BJ, Goldenkranz R, et al. Defining the role of subtotal colectomy in the treatment of carcinoma of the colon. Ann Surg 213:248-252, 1991.

Cohen AM, Minsky BD, Schilsky RL. Cancer of the colon. In DeVita VT, Hellman S, Rosenberg SA, eds. Cancer Principles and Practice of Oncology, 5th ed. New York: Lippincott-Raven, 1997, pp 1144-1197.

Collier JG, Pollard SG. Right hemicolectomy and extended right hemicolectomy. In Calne R, Pollard SG, eds. Operative Surgery. Grower Medical Publishing, 1992, pp 5.61-5.64.

Daneker GW, Ellis LM. Colon cancer nodal metastasis: Biologic significance and therapeutic considerations. Surg Oncol Clin North Am 5:173-189, 1996.

Fazio VW. Surgery of colonic carcinoma: Technique and practice. Semin Colon Rectal Surg 2:36-43, 1991.

Kafka NJ, Coller JA. Endoscopic management of malignant colorectal polyps. Surg Oncol Clin North Am 5:633-661, 1996.

Nogueras JJ, Jagelman DG. Principles of surgical resection: Influence of surgical technique on treatment outcome. Surg Clin North Am 73:103-106, 1993.

Rombeau JL, Yu JC. Right and transverse colectomy. In Daly JM, Cady B, eds. Atlas of Surgical Oncology. St. Louis: Mosby–Year Book, 1993, pp 457-473.

Right and left colon resections. In Scott-Conner C, Dawson DL, eds. Operative Anatomy. Philadelphia: JB Lippincott, 1993, pp 462-476.

Watson CJ. Appendectomy. In Calne R, Pollard SG, eds. Operative Surgery. Grower Medical Publishing, 1992, pp 5.56-5.60.

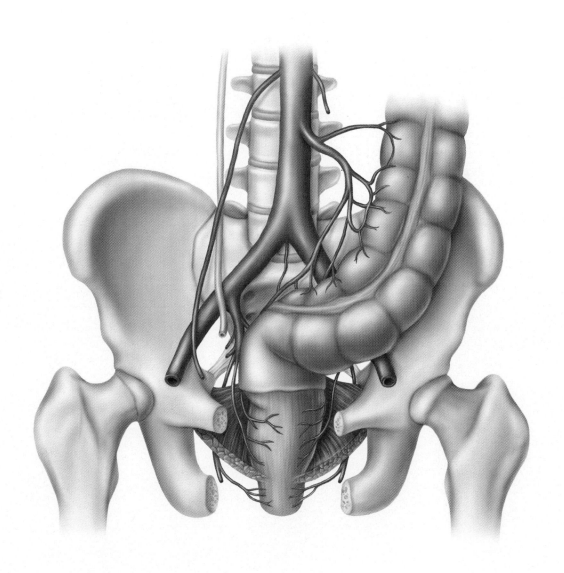

Chapter 10

Rectum

William C. Wood, M.D.

Surgical Applications

Low Anterior Resection

Coloanal Resection

Abdominoperineal Resection

Total Pelvic Exenteration

Per Anal Excision (or Transanal Excision)

Rectal tumors account for a significant part of a surgeon's practice. Thirty-four thousand new rectal tumors are diagnosed in the United States annually. These are more common in males than females, with a ratio of 1 to 0.73. The risk of adenocarcinoma of the rectum increases with each year of age. Other tumors also can develop in and about the rectum. These tumors raise both patient and surgeon concerns about tumor control and cure, and anxiety regarding the morbidity of rectal surgery. Fear of colostomy is mingled with fear of fecal or urinary incontinence and, for male patients, impotence. The rectum is an anatomic area for which a clear understanding of tumor biology and of precise anatomy significantly influences the results of surgical procedures.

In addition to adenocarcinoma of the mucosa-lined rectum, squamous cell carcinoma of the anus, basisquamous tumors, melanomas, sarcomas of the supporting structures, and retrorectal tumors all require detailed knowledge of the anatomy of the region and its surrounding and supporting structures. A benign tumor, villous adenoma of the rectum, often has areas of premalignant or frankly malignant change within it. Consequently, complete excision of these lesions may also be a technically demanding exercise requiring complete understanding of the anatomy of the region.

SURGICAL ANATOMY

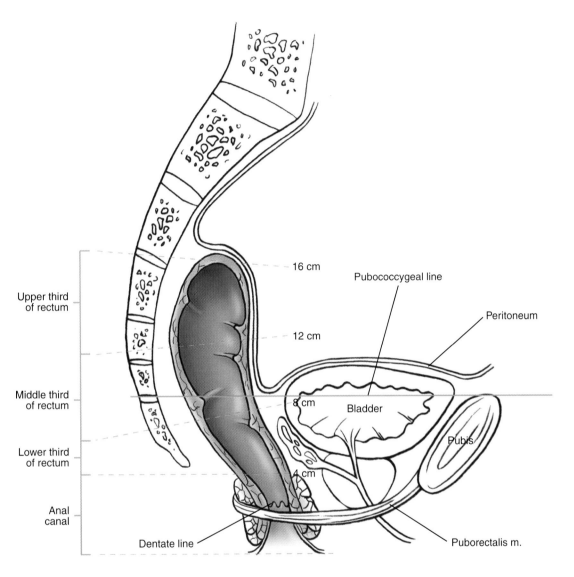

The anorectum is commonly visualized in terms of the "rule of four." The first 4 cm from the anal verge comprise the anal canal; the next three 4 cm sections make up the lower, middle, and upper thirds of the rectum. These dimensions are approximately correct when the rectum is either stretched from above or lifted with a rigid proctoscope. If the rectum is collapsed into the sacral hollow, however, these lengths are exaggerated, and 3 cm each would be a better estimate of the lower, middle, and upper thirds. These distances also correspond to the transverse folds of the rectum (valves of Houston): the left superior, right middle, and left inferior.

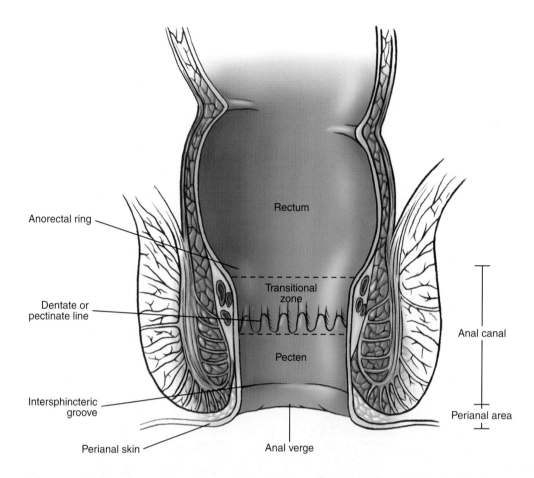

Three histologic patterns define the anal canal. The cutaneous zone of the perianal skin up to the anal verge (anocutaneous line) is covered by pigmented skin with hair follicles and sebaceous glands. Above the anal verge is the transitional zone, with modified skin containing no hair follicles, but with sebaceous glands. This lining extends to the pectinate line defined by the anal valves. Above that line begins the true mucosa of the anal canal. The pectinate line is a topographic feature formed by small mucosal pockets between the vertical folds of mucosa known as the anal columns of Morgagni. These extend upward from the pectinate line to the upper end of the surgical anal canal at the puborectalis sling. Their appearance derives from vertical bundles of the muscularis mucosae. The actual junction of stratified squamous and columnar epithelia is just above the pectinate line, and this is the true mucocutaneous junction. The pectinate line marks the transition from the visceral tissues above and the somatic tissues beneath.

Blood Supply

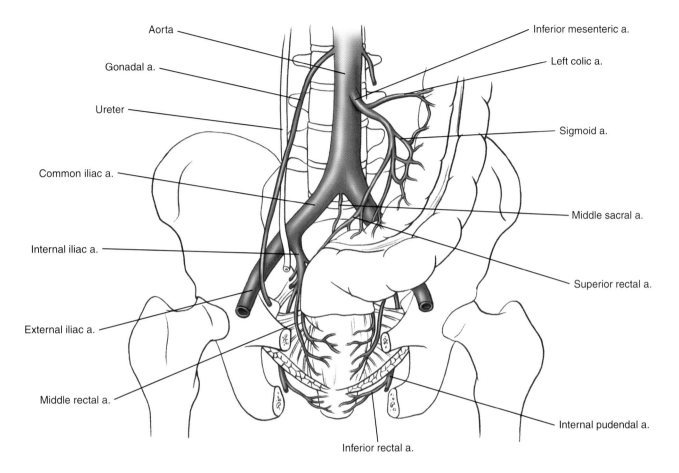

Arterial supply, but more significantly the venous and lymphatic drainage vessels and nerve supply, all change at the level of the pectinate line. The blood supply to the anorectum is derived from the superior rectal artery, the lowest extension of the inferior mesenteric artery. The middle and lower portions of the anorectum are supplied by branches of the hypogastric artery, specifically the middle rectal and inferior rectal arteries, which branch off the internal pudendal artery. The middle rectal artery is occasionally absent, and it has also been found to arise from the inferior vesicle or internal pudendal artery. This usually poses no problem to the surgeon.

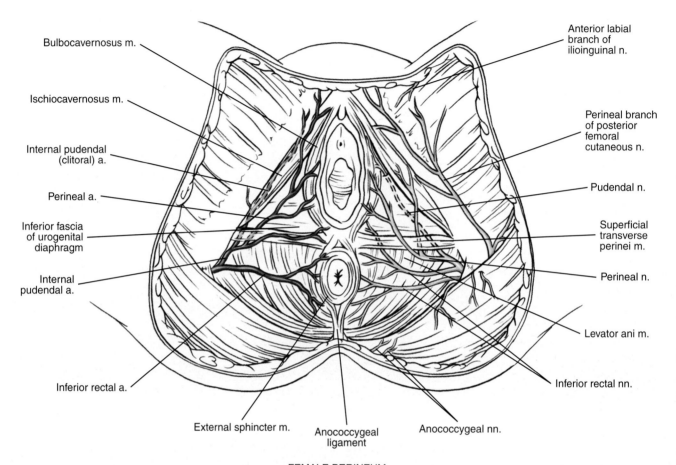

Bulbocavernosus m.

Ischiocavernosus m.

Internal pudendal (clitoral) a.

Perineal a.

Inferior fascia of urogenital diaphragm

Internal pudendal a.

Inferior rectal a.

Anterior labial branch of ilioinguinal n.

Perineal branch of posterior femoral cutaneous n.

Pudendal n.

Superficial transverse perinei m.

Perineal n.

Levator ani m.

Inferior rectal nn.

External sphincter m.

Anococcygeal ligament

Anococcygeal nn.

FEMALE PERINEUM

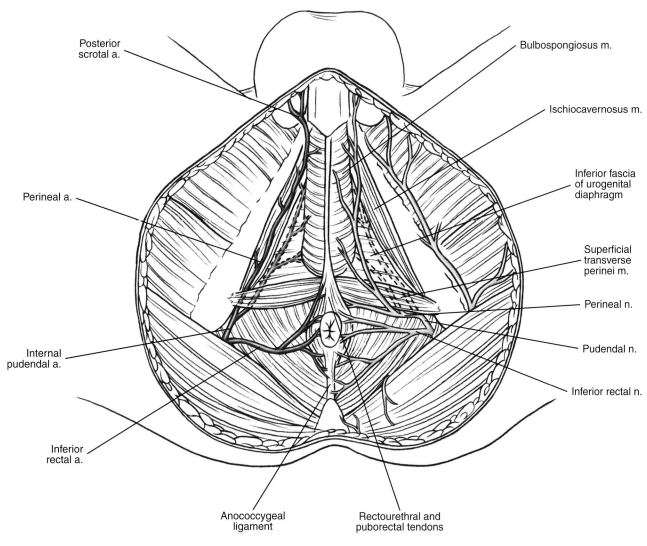

Posterior
scrotal a.

Perineal a.

Internal
pudendal a.

Inferior
rectal a.

Bulbospongiosus m.

Ischiocavernosus m.

Inferior fascia
of urogenital
diaphragm

Superficial
transverse
perinei m.

Perineal n.

Pudendal n.

Inferior rectal n.

Anococcygeal
ligament

Rectourethral and
puborectal tendons

MALE PERINEUM

The inferior rectal artery, which arises from the internal pudendal artery, may be confused because of varying origins of that vessel. It may arise in common with the obturator or the umbilical artery. The inferior rectal artery is not a dominant single trunk but a series of small unnamed branches that supply the lower part of the levator ani, the sphincter muscles, and the lower anorectum. These vessels and their relationship to the pudendal nerves and inferior rectal nerves are demonstrated in the female perineum and the male perineum.

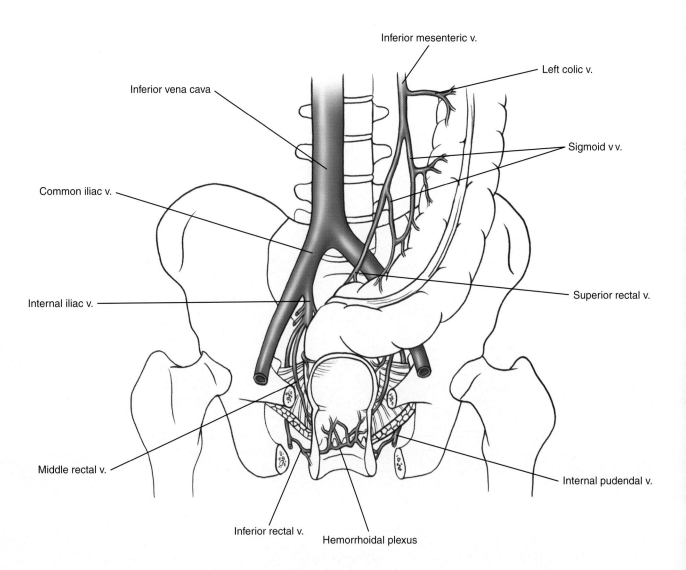

The inferior rectal (hemorrhoidal) veins beneath the pectinate line and levator sling drain into the internal pudendal veins and from there to the internal iliac vein. Just above the levators, the middle rectal veins follow the same drainage pattern.

Lymphatic Drainage

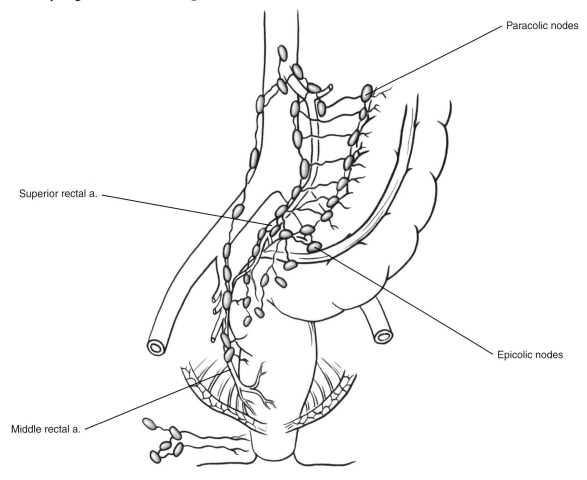

Lymphatic drainage parallels the venous drainage of the anorectum. This leads the lymphatic vessels from this region out along the levator sling to the pelvic sidewall. At the level of the superior rectal arteries, the venous and lymphatic drainage is portal and flows up to the inferior mesenteric vein. Below the pectinate line, the lymphatic plexus drains to the inguinal nodes. Consequently, the "watershed" of the extramural anorectal lymphatic vessels is at the pectinate line. The watershed for the intramural lymphatic vessels is higher, at the level of the middle valve. There are venous and lymphatic anastomoses between the lower branches draining with the systemic veins and the higher branches draining into the portal system.

Nerve Supply

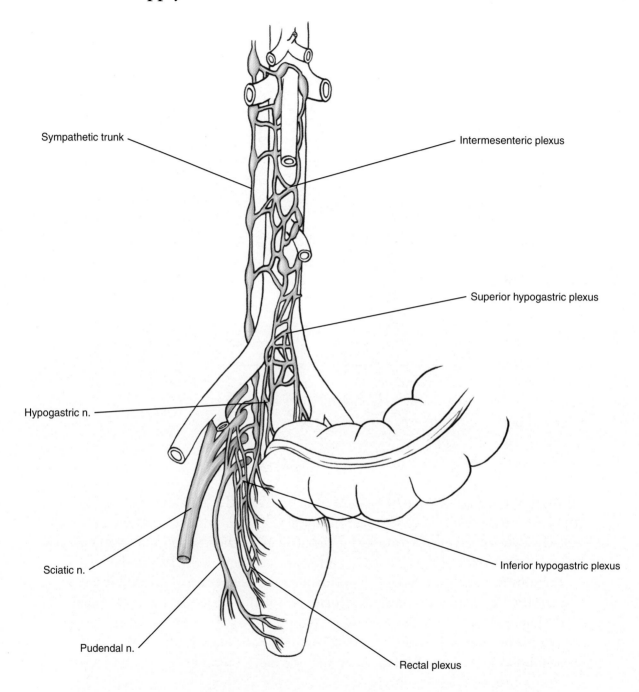

Sympathetic trunk

Intermesenteric plexus

Superior hypogastric plexus

Hypogastric n.

Sciatic n.

Inferior hypogastric plexus

Pudendal n.

Rectal plexus

Motor innervation of the internal rectal sphincter is sympathetic, causing contraction with parasympathetic fibers also supplied that inhibit contraction of this sphincter.

Parasympathetic afferent nerves carry sensations of rectal distention through the sacral plexus. The external rectal sphincter is supplied by an inferior rectal branch of the internal pudendal nerve and by a branch of the fourth sacral nerve. The parasympathetic pelvic splanchnic nerves and the sympathetic hypogastric nerves supply the wall of the lower rectum and together form the rectal plexus. The levator ani muscles are controlled by the third and fourth sacral nerves. Rectal continence is maintained by the pudendal and pelvic splanchnic nerves. The nerves that pass through the splanchnic nerves also supply the seminal vesicles and prostate gland in the male and the bladder. These are all at risk for injury that affects bladder and sexual function (see low anterior resection, p. 439, and abdominoperineal resection, p. 448).

The relation of the sphincteric muscles of the anus and the muscular pelvic floor and their separate innervations has remained a contentious area of surgical anatomy. A variety of schematic illustrations are used to define the functional aspects of muscular support and sphincter function. The inability to identify each of these structures in individual persons suggests that the external sphincter is one muscle mass and is not necessarily divided into layers and laminae, as may be found in some individuals. This external sphincter muscle mass retains skeletal attachment by the anococcygeal ligament to the coccyx. The perineal body is the anatomic location in the central perineum where there is a meeting of the anterior pelvic muscles (bulbospongiosus and superficial and deep transverse perinei muscles) and the external sphincter posteriorly. The superficial perineal muscle separates the anus from the vagina in the female and gives support to the perineum. The external sphincter muscle is supplied by the inferior rectal nerve and the perineal branch of the fourth sacral nerve. The internal sphincter muscle is merely a downward continuation of the circular smooth muscles of the inner muscular layer of the rectum that becomes thickened and rounded. The conjoined longitudinal muscle is the longitudinal muscle layer of the rectum, a continuation of the teniae coli above the peritoneal reflection that forms a coat descending between the internal and external sphincters and inserts on the perianal skin. It has been suggested that the role of the conjoined longitudinal muscle is to evert the anus during defecation. The levator ani muscle is a broad, thin muscle that forms the greater part of the pelvic floor and is supplied by the fourth sacral nerve. It is made up of the iliococcygeus, pubococcygeus, and puborectalis muscles. The significance of each of these elements in contributing to the support of the pelvic floor is contentious. The pudendal nerve supplies the latter two muscles, but there may also be a perineal nerve supply.

Fascial Support

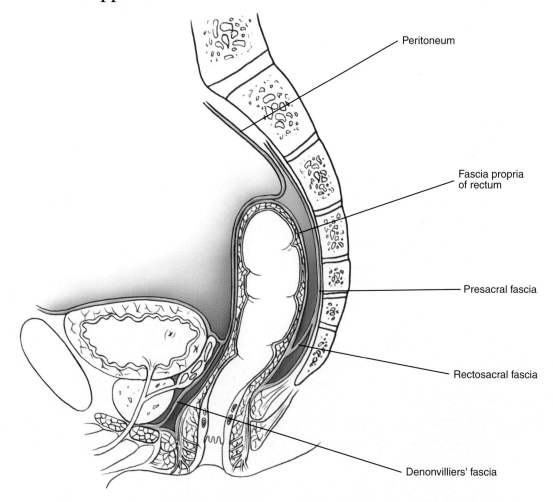

Peritoneum

Fascia propria
of rectum

Presacral fascia

Rectosacral fascia

Denonvilliers' fascia

In addition to the muscular floor of the pelvis, the anorectum is supported by fascial reflections. These are the anterior and posterior peritoneal reflections and, from about the S4 level of the sacrum, a rectosacral fascia that is a distinct supportive band of surgical importance. On the side of the rectum below the peritoneum is a condensation of fascia, known as the lateral ligaments or lateral stalks, that connect the rectum to the parietal pelvic fascia. The sacrum and coccyx are covered by the strong parietal pelvic fascia. In the presacral area, the parietal fascia covers the middle sacral vessels. The rectosacral fascia is also known as Waldeyer's fascia. Anteriorly, the rectum below the peritoneal reflection is covered with a visceral fascia that is relatively delicate, known as Denonvilliers' fascia. It separates the rectum from the vagina in the female and from the seminal vesicles and prostate gland in the male. These fascia are significant in resections of the rectum.

SURGICAL APPLICATIONS

For tumors of the anorectum, the tension lies between widely ablative procedures with generous margins and removal of broad areas of lymphatic drainage and the disability that such wide ablations produce. For lesions of the lower rectum, abdominoperineal resection, particularly at its most radical, achieves widespread resection, but at considerable cost. The loss of anal continence and the production of an abdominal colostomy are well managed by patients, particularly those who are taught by skilled enterostomal therapists. Nonetheless, the ability to treat tumors of the anorectum with equivalent benefit and preservation of anorectal continence, sexual function, and urinary continence is clearly the ideal. The procedures described have as their goals (1) control of the tumor and (2) preservation of function. These are not seen as competing goals; control of the tumor must never be compromised by any attempt to preserve function.

The procedures discussed include:

1. Low anterior resection
2. Coloanal resection
3. Abdominoperineal resection
4. Total pelvic exenteration
5. Per anal excision (or transanal excision)
6. Posterior approaches

The choice among these procedures for tumors of the anorectum is predicated on knowledge of tumor biology and the expected progress of both the tumor and the patient. An initial consideration is diagnosis and staging of the tumor, which requires an adequate biopsy specimen. It must be understood that a finding of severe dysplasia in a villous adenoma of the low rectum is common when other areas of the villous adenoma exhibit frank adenocarcinoma. The size of the tumor, both in its intraluminal and extraluminal extent, is a second consideration. Transrectal ultrasonography provides the ability to stage the extraluminal portion more effectively than had been previously available. Careful palpation, not only of the tumor for low rectal lesions but also for perirectal lymphadenopathy, is most important. Finally, the use of a rigid sigmoidoscope allows lifting the inferior margin of the tumor up into the pelvis for accurate determination of the level of the tumor, as well as assessing fixation or tethering of the tumor to the pelvic sidewall or anterior structures. Only when all of these have been accomplished can the optimal procedure be selected. For adenocarcinomas of the anorectum that are fixed, chemotherapy and radiation therapy should precede surgery. Tumors that are tethered probably also benefit from preoperative chemotherapy plus radiation therapy. Tumors of the middle or upper rectum are well managed with low anterior resection. The lymphatics draining the tumor as well as the tissues at risk can be excised and superior function preserved. For exophytic, smaller ($\leq$3 cm), low-grade lesions of the low rectum, per anal excision and radiation therapy afford control equivalent to that with abdominoperineal resection. For higher grade or ulcerative lesions of the low rectum, preoperative chemotherapy plus radiation therapy produces dramatic disease regression and complete regression in some patients. In tertiary care centers, coloanal anastomosis with a very low anterior resection to the level of the levator muscles and the pectinate line is being performed. It is not yet clear that this will afford the same level of control as abdominoperineal resection. Further studies will be needed to evaluate the degree of functional impairment associated with coloanal anastomosis and such low resection following chemotherapy plus radiation therapy and the extent of tumor control compared with that of abdominoperineal resection. Transsphincteric and posterior approaches have strong advocates but have never received the same degree of acceptance by the broad community of surgeons dealing with rectal tumors as have the other procedures, relative to the complications associated with these procedures. The fact that a few individuals have been their champions suggests that when frequently performed the complications and morbidity of these procedures may be lessened. Total pelvic exenteration is an appropriate procedure for well-staged, anteriorly fixed tumors with no evidence of disease outside the pelvis. The status of the ureters should be assessed with either excretory urography or computed tomography (CT) with contrast medium as part of the preoperative staging of rectal tumors with any degree of extraluminal extension. In female patients, if the anterior fixation is only to the uterus and vagina, posterior exenteration, sparing the bladder, may be performed. If the anterior fixation is also accompanied by lateral fixation to the pelvic sidewalls or posterior fixation to the sacrum, no advantage can be shown to pelvic exenteration, radically extirpating the bladder and urethra to gain anterior margin when it is not possible to obtain lateral or posterior margins around the tumor.

Low Anterior Resection

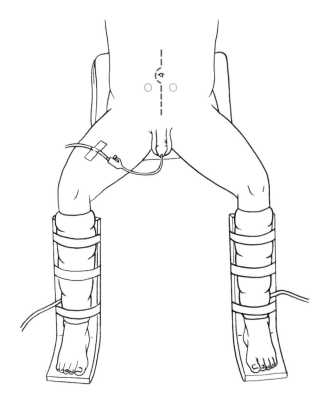

If the lower margin of the tumor cannot be elevated with a rigid proctoscope at least 3 cm above the most cephalad portion of the palpable anal sphincteric mechanism, low anterior resection is not an appropriate procedure. An indwelling urinary catheter should be placed in patients undergoing any anorectal surgery. For low anterior resection, the ideal position is the patient supine with legs in Allen or Lloyd-Davies stirrups. Elastic wraps or pneumatic sequential compression leggings are used to minimize the risk for deep venous thrombosis. A foam pad is used to elevate the sacrum and buttocks to provide easy access to the anus. When anything other than a very straightforward dissection is expected (e.g., in patients with prior pelvic surgery, pelvic radiation therapy, or recurrent tumors), ureteral stents minimize the risk for ureteral injury and facilitate pelvic dissection. After preparing and draping the abdomen and perineum, a midline incision is made from just above the umbilicus to the pubis.

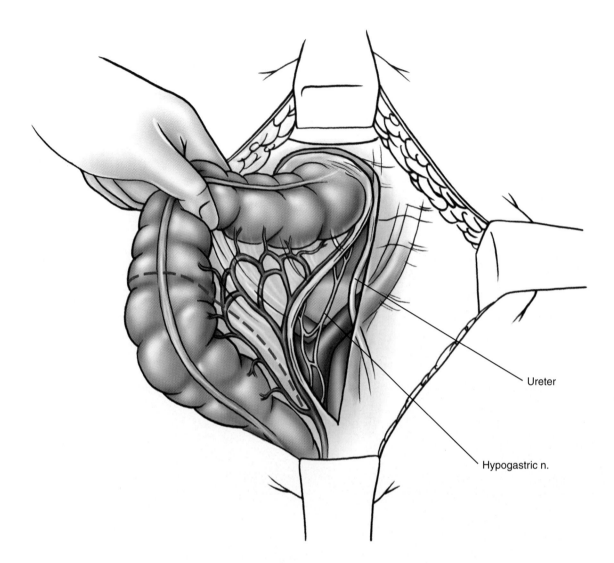

Ureter

Hypogastric n.

After careful exploration of the abdomen, the peritoneum is incised at the base
of the rectosigmoid mesentery downward to the lateral edge of the peritoneal
reflection onto the rectum. Developmental adhesions from the sigmoid colon
to the left pelvic sidewall are taken down; then the same peritoneal dissection
is performed on the left. The ureters are identified. Some surgeons prefer to
ligate the low rectosigmoid colon to prevent dissemination of cells within the
lumen of the bowel. There is no evidence that this technique is effective. Some
have advocated early ligation of the mesenteric and lymphatic vessels to prevent proximal dissemination of tumor during manipulation of the rectum.
Again, there is no evidence that this is effective, and evidence suggests that it
makes no difference whether the vessels are ligated. Nonetheless, this is an appropriate time to divide the superior rectal vessels just beneath the takeoff of
the left colic vessels. Again, no advantage has been shown for taking the inferior mesenteric vessels at their origin.

　　The ureters and gonadal vessels are identified and spared. The hypogastric
nerve plexus should be identified and carefully spared unless there is evidence

of fixation or tethering of tumor that would require its resection. It is essential that the left ureter is identified and protected from division with the inferior mesenteric vessels. By drawing the rectum anterosuperiorly, a plane of areolar tissue appears anterior to the sacral promontory. With scissors dissection the retrorectal space can be entered with minimal bleeding. This plane anterior to the presacral nerves is pursued. The nerves bifurcate just below the sacral promontory. This plane is then developed by both blunt and sharp dissection until the rectosacral fascia is encountered. This must be sharply divided; bleeding from the presacral venous plexus is usually caused by attempts to break through this ligament bluntly. After the rectosacral fascia has been incised, the dissection can easily proceed to the coccyx. If bleeding occurs from the presacral veins or the basivertebral veins through the sacral foramina, direct pressure with or without electrocoagulation will usually suffice to restore hemostasis. A titanium thumbtack can be placed directly into the sacrum if required. In patients with a bleeding disorder or who fail to respond to other measures to control bleeding from the presacral tissues, prolonged packing can be used and removed at 2 to 3 days.

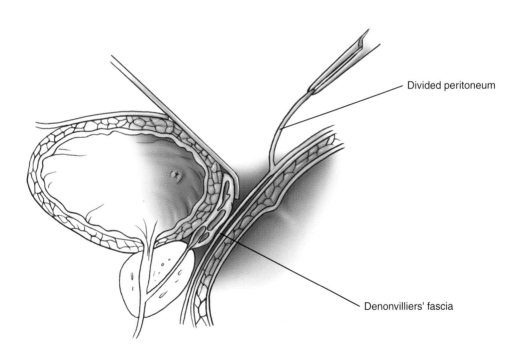

The anterior surface of the rectum is now cleared. In the male, the rectovesical fold is entered, and with traction on the rectum superoposteriorly and on the bladder anteriorly, sharp dissection is continued in the plane between the seminal vesicles anteriorly and Denonvilliers' thin fascia posteriorly. The dissection continues to the base of the seminal vesicles and then over the surface of the prostate gland. Electrocoagulation is helpful to control small bleeding vessels.

In women, the rectovaginal fold is incised and the posterior wall of the vagina cleared to the level at which the pubic bone can be palpated. If there is tethering or fixation, the posterior wall of the vagina can be taken. For adenocarcinoma on the anterior wall of the rectum, the posterior vaginal wall should probably be routinely taken. This does not add to the risk of the procedure or morbidity for the patient.

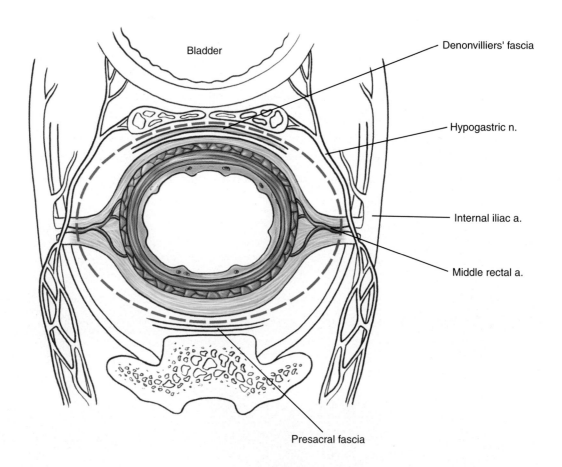

At this point, the hypogastric nerves have been spared and the lateral ligaments are to be taken. At this juncture the anatomy is significant in detail. Heald and Enker both advocate sufficient lateral dissection to clear the mesorectal tissues. Their data suggest that local failure is markedly diminished by such careful wide dissections of the mesorectum. Although attention has been paid to the longitudinal margin on the bowel wall, fairly recent emphasis has been placed on adequate sharp dissection of the lateral margins. The temptation, if clamps and fingers are used laterally, is to cone down through the mesorectum to the distal rectal wall, leaving the distal mesorectal tissues laterally. With the rectum pulled sharply to the left, the ligaments can be divided with an electrocautery or between clamps. A strong, deep pelvic retractor, such as the St. Mark's pelvic retractor, placed anterior to the rectum and lifted forcefully upward, makes it possible to take the lateral stalks under direct vision. In completion of the anterior dissection, a Foley catheter in the trigonal area of the bladder is a useful palpable landmark, just anterosuperior to the prostate and between the seminal vesicles.

A conceptually ideal operation would include Denonvilliers' fascia with the rectum anteriorly, with the plane of dissection being on the outer surface of the fascia, finally divided distally at the prostate. Within the lateral stalks lie the middle rectal vessels, which must be taken along with their associated lymphatics. Also within them lie a condensation of parasympathetic nerve fibers supplying the rectum that must, of necessity, be divided. In addition, there are nerve fibers running longitudinally in the lateral edge of the lateral stalks adjacent to the pelvic sidewall. These may easily be drawn into the dissection and divided, leading to impairment. These partially make up the hypogastric nerves and parasympathetic nerves. The sympathetic or hypogastric nerves, which were followed down from the aortic bifurcation above to the point anterior to the lateral ligaments, can often be visualized and avoided. They course 1 to 2 cm medial to the ureters. If one takes the time to manage the individual vessels in the lateral ligaments, as one would in the superior pole of a thyroid gland, the ligament may be taken between small clips, or with ties, or even with a cautery, minimizing the risk for damage to the truncal parasympathetic nerves and sacral structures, preserving any that are coursing in any direction other than into the bowel wall. There is no evidence that significant innervation lies anteriorly between the rectum and seminal vesicles or prostate. Consequently, one need not be concerned that dissection in this region will contribute to sexual dysfunction. The twin goals in a meticulous dissection of the lateral ligament are preservation of both sympathetic and parasympathetic nerves and the clearance of lymphatics out to those anterior-posterior, and cephalad-caudad running, longitudinal small nerve trunks. This achieves local clearance superior to that achieved with broad clamping and contributes to preservation of function, as demonstrated by the work of both Heald and Enker.

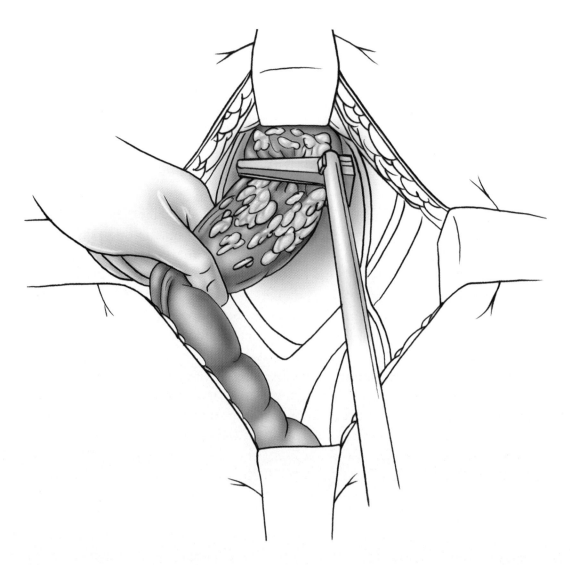

When dissection has progressed to at least 2 cm beneath the inferior margin of the tumor, a right-angle clamp may be gently placed across the bowel wall perpendicularly. The distal rectal stump may then be irrigated with either saline solution or povidone-iodine (Betadine) to eliminate fecal material and possible clumps of tumor cells. This is done for first principles, not for evidence-based considerations. After lateral sutures are placed for support, the distal rectal stump is divided with a scissor or right-angle knife, just beneath the right-angle clamp. Either stapled or open anastomosis may now be performed. Modern circular staple devices allow very low anastomoses with great safety and have virtually eliminated the need for an abdominosacral approach to low tumors. A purse-string suture of 0 or 2-0 monofilament is placed in the rectal stump with bites about 6 mm apart. At an appropriate level, the rectosigmoid colon is divided above and brought down into the pelvis. A purse-string suture is placed, most easily with a crimping instrument. In many illustrations, the stapler has been shown with the distal purse-string tied down and the proximal

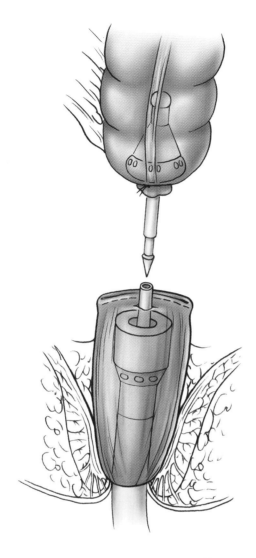

rectosigmoid placed over the anvil. It is dramatically easier to place the stapler through the rectal stump entirely up into the central pelvis and then place the rectosigmoid purse-string suture over the top of the anvil and tie it down. Then the entire instrument is withdrawn through the rectum and the lower purse-string suture tied down. The stapler is closed and twisted to achieve correct approximation and is fired. When it is loosened, the lateral holding sutures on the rectal stump allow the instrument to be easily withdrawn without any traction on the anastomosis. If a right-angle clamp is gently placed above this level in a noncrushing fashion, irrigation of the rectal stump with povidone-iodine with a genitourinary gun or asepto-syringe allows testing the anastomosis to make certain it is watertight. Any suggestion of leak can be sealed with individual sutures. The incision is then closed in the usual fashion. A suction drain may be placed from one lower quadrant into the pelvis to evacuate any hematoma or seroma that might otherwise form adjacent to the anastomosis and is removed by day 3. The anastomosis may also be done with any of the usual freehand techniques.

Coloanal Resection

Coloanal resection is performed after chemotherapy plus radiation therapy for lesions in the low rectum that regress sufficiently that a margin may be obtained above the dentate line. The procedure differs from abdominoperineal resection in that the sphincteric structures, the levator sling, and the lymphatic and blood vessels below the levator muscles are all spared. These must be sterilized with chemotherapy plus radiation therapy, or the surgery will not be successful in controlling tumors at the level of the low rectum. Dissection from above circumscribes the rectum at the level of the levator muscles.

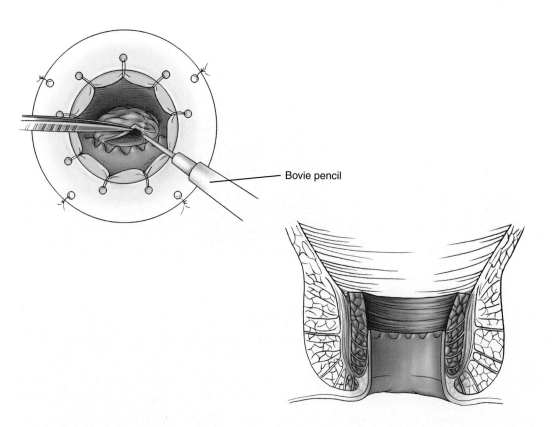

Bovie pencil

From inside, the mucosa is taken from the pectinate line up to the superior margins of the sphincter (submucosal infiltration with epinephrine in saline solution facilitates this dissection); then the entire rectum is circumscribed and excised. A finger placed through the wall of the submucosal rectum guides this division. The splenic flexure must be freed to allow sufficient colonic length into the pelvis, and the left colon must be divided above the level of irradiation so that unirradiated bowel is brought down into the pelvis.

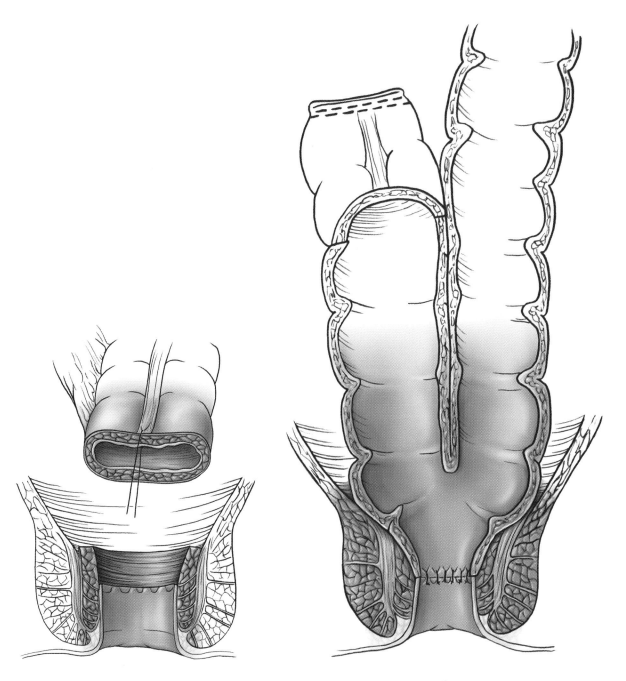

An end-to-end coloanal anastomosis may be made or a J pouch created by stapling the antimesenteric borders together. The pouch has been associated with less stool frequency in the early months after the procedure and appears to engender greater patient satisfaction. It must be again remarked that abdominoperineal resection remains the gold standard for lesions of the low rectum that are not appropriate for treatment by per anal excision and radiation therapy.

Abdominoperineal Resection

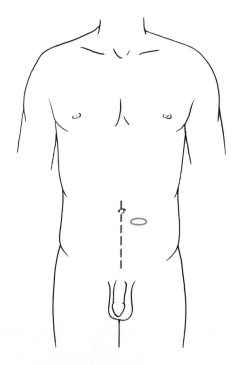

The patient is positioned with legs in Allen or Lloyd-Davies stirrups, and an indwelling Foley catheter is placed. A site for a stoma should be chosen and identified prior to making the skin incision. The best plan is to bring the stoma through the rectus muscle on the left side to minimize the size of the peristomal hernia and place it in an area where there is sufficient flat abdominal wall (i.e., several centimeters from the umbilicus and anterior superior iliac spine) that a stoma disk can lie flat. It must remain in position when the patient is seated and, ideally, not be directly on the beltline but below it. After careful exploration of the abdomen, the rectosigmoid colon is mobilized. Early division of the sigmoid colon facilitates the pelvic dissection. The procedure progresses as described for low anterior resection (see pp. 439 to 445).

To form the stoma, a skin ellipse of appropriate diameter is excised, and the anterior fascia of the rectus muscle is exposed. Either a cruciate incision may be made or a circle excised to allow easy passage of two fingerbreadths. The rectus muscle is spread in the direction of its fibers and the peritoneum incised. When two fingers can very easily pass through, the sigmoid colon is brought out with care to allow it to lie untwisted and without tension. It may be brought out lateral to the peritoneum in a retroperitoneal manner to avoid later herniation, or it may be tacked to the lateral peritoneal wall to avoid this site for internal herniation. There are no convincing data that either of these maneuvers is of any value, but both are widely practiced. It is matured by suturing a single layer of interrupted sutures through the full layer of the bowel wall and full thickness of the skin, once the abdominal incision has been closed.

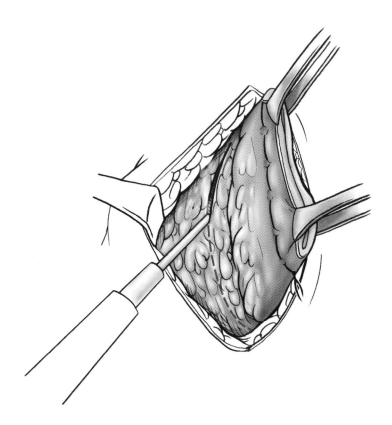

The anus is closed with two purse-string sutures of silk for the comfort of the perineal dissector. In male patients an elliptical incision about the anus is made to remove the pigmented perianal skin. In female patients the posterior vaginal wall may be included in the excision if the tumor lies in the anterior rectal wall. After posterior vaginectomy, the fourchette is reconstituted, and the posterior vaginal wall may be closed or allowed to heal by second intention.

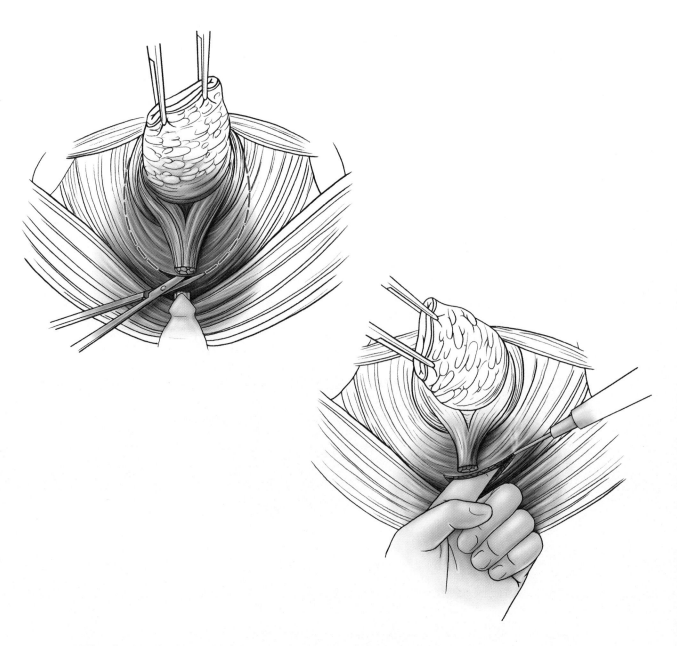

The fatty subcutaneous tissue is taken with an electrocautery. Vascular bundles representing the inferior rectal (hemorrhoidal) vessels are identified both superiorly and inferiorly on the sides in the ischiorectal fat. With a scissors, it is possible to divide the rectococcygeus ligament right at the tip of the coccyx. With a finger placed into the retrorectal space and swept laterally, the levator sling is divided with the electrocautery. This dissection is carried out on both sides, leaving only the area from 11:00 o'clock to 1:00 o'clock intact anteriorly. The rectum should then be passed through from above so that it is only tethered by the puborectalis and rectourethralis muscles anteriorly. These are defined sharply by stripping away the overlying fat with scissors or bluntly with a sponge-covered finger.

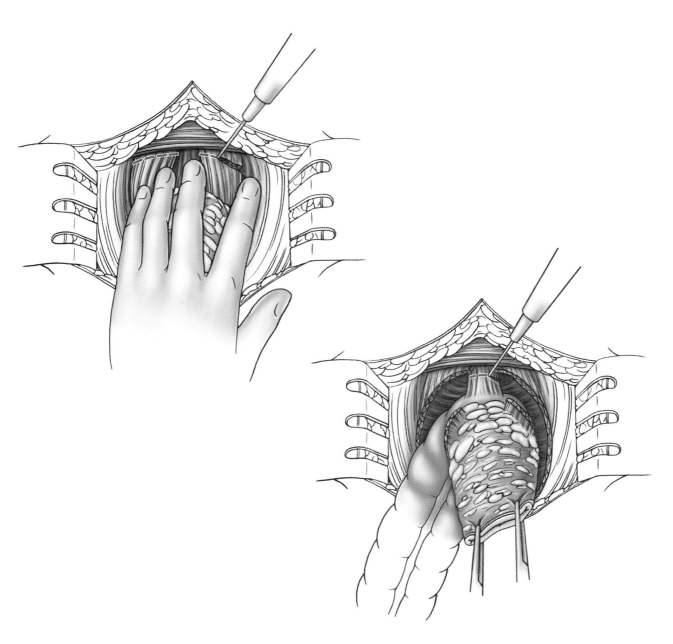

Division of these muscles and the tissue immediately behind them is the most difficult step in the operation. The proper plane is just posterior to the prostate gland and is defined by palpation of the rectum and prostate in the surgeon's noncutting hand. This 2 cm area of division frees the specimen and completes the dissection. Hemostasis is now secured from both above and below. The fatty subcutaneous tissue of the perineum is approximated with at least two, and preferably three, layers of absorbable sutures, followed by skin closure. Suction drains are placed to prevent a pelvic collection. These drains may be brought out through the perineum, but patients are more comfortable when the drains are brought out from above in the lower quadrants of the abdomen. The small bowel is allowed to fall into the pelvis to fill the dead space. There is generally spontaneous reperitonealization with surprisingly little adhesion formation.

Total Pelvic Exenteration

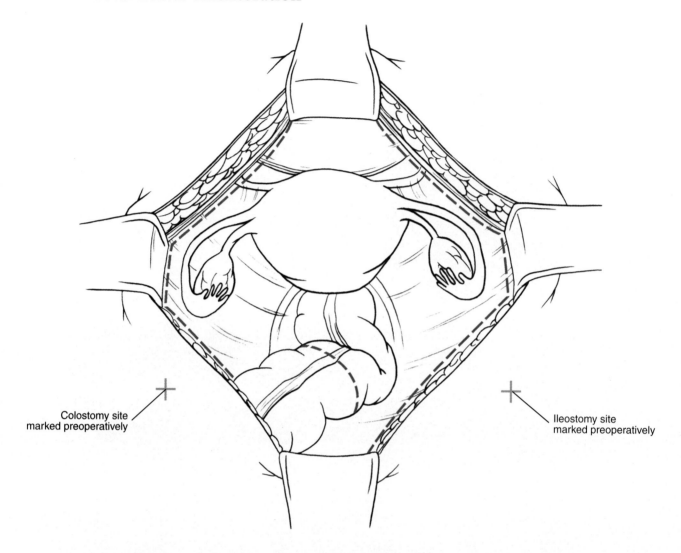

Colostomy site
marked preoperatively

Ileostomy site
marked preoperatively

Rectal cancers invading centrally and free of the pelvic structures peripherally are appropriate for pelvic exenteration. This procedure combines en bloc abdominoperineal resection with cystectomy in male patients and hysterectomy and vaginectomy in female patients if the tumor extends beyond the posterior vagina or uterus. The appropriate chapters should be consulted for more detailed descriptions of the anatomic details that influence these procedures. From below, the ellipse of skin excised includes the vagina and urethra in female patients.

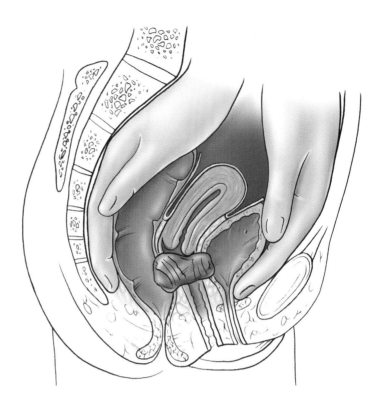

Abdominally from the aortoiliac bifurcation into the sacral hollow and the pelvic sidewalls, all soft tissues are resected. This includes all central branches of the inferior iliac vessels and the obturator vessels, sparing the obturator nerves. The sacral plexus is spared, but all anterior tissues are cleared. The ureters are divided and anastomosed to an ileal conduit.

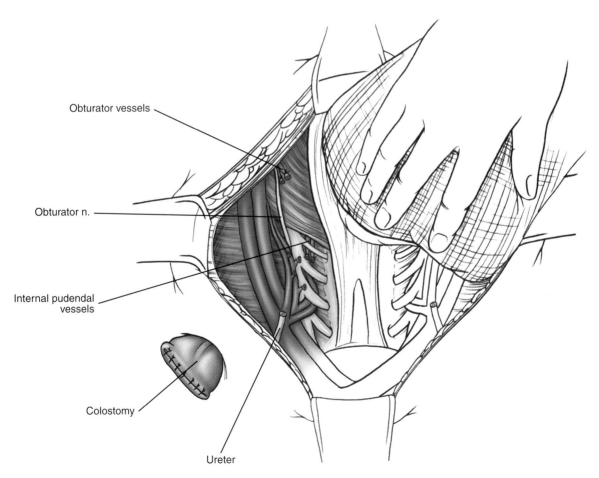

Obturator vessels

Obturator n.

Internal pudendal vessels

Colostomy

Ureter

Per Anal Excision (or Transanal Excision)

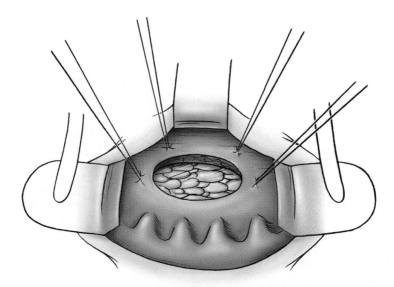

For lesions that are limited to the rectal wall, as seen at ultrasonography, and are exophytic, well differentiated, and mobile, per anal excision followed by radiation therapy provides excellent local tumor control. The lesion can be examined microscopically, and if the tumor was understaged at preoperative evaluation, abdominoperineal resection can still be performed. The patient is positioned in either the lithotomy or Bouie position (prone), depending on the location of the tumor on the rectal wall. The key to effective per anal excision is exposure.

A self-retaining anal retractor or three or four narrow Deaver retractors provide initial visualization of the tumor after the buttocks have been taped apart. Full-thickness stay sutures placed 1.5 to 2 cm from the edge of the tumor permit the tumor to be drawn down and the wall of the bowel to be manipulated. A 1 cm margin is marked on the bowel wall with a Bovie electrocautery. A lateral margin is elevated with a stay suture adjacent to it and another stay suture between the tumor edge and the margin of resection marking. The bowel wall is incised full thickness, so that perirectal fat is encountered. The specimen is excised and oriented with care to prevent fragmentation. Four additional margins of several millimeters of bowel wall provide additional evidence of clear margins, as does a fifth margin deeply off the perirectal fat beneath the tumor. Several small stainless clips in the muscularis propria allow the radiation oncologist to place the boost portion of the radiation dose with precision. If the defect is closed diagonally, minimal narrowing is produced even with specimens as large as 5 or 6 cm in maximal diameter.

Transphincteric Approach

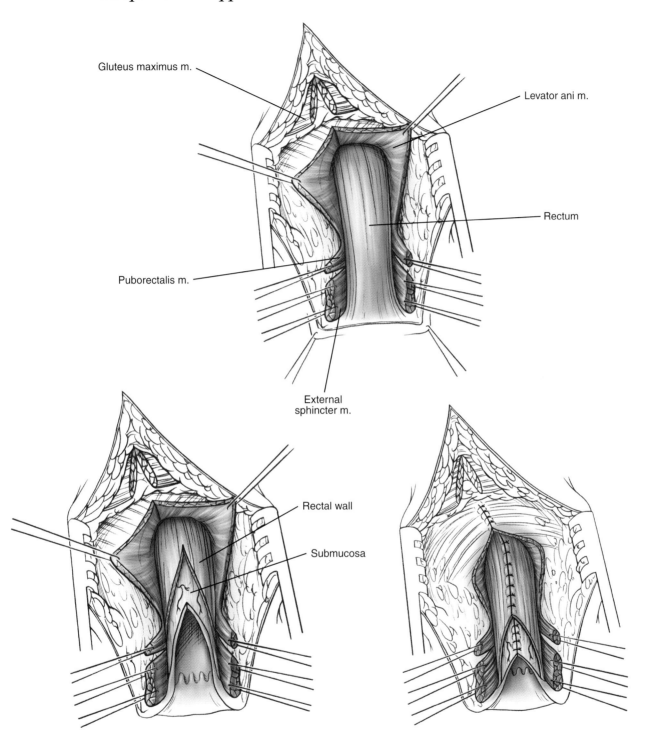

Gluteus maximus m.

Levator ani m.

Rectum

Puborectalis m.

External
sphincter m.

Rectal wall

Submucosa

The sphincter of the rectum may be divided as advocated by York-Mason, the tumor excised as in per anal excision, and the sphincter repaired meticulously in layers. The later morbidity resulting from scarring in some patients makes this approach less appealing than per anal excision. I can see no reason for it presently.

Kraske's Approach

A combination of per anal excision, low anterior resection, and coloanal re-section, this approach has been relegated largely to historical considerations. It is mentioned because it provides a splendid view of the retrorectal anatomy.

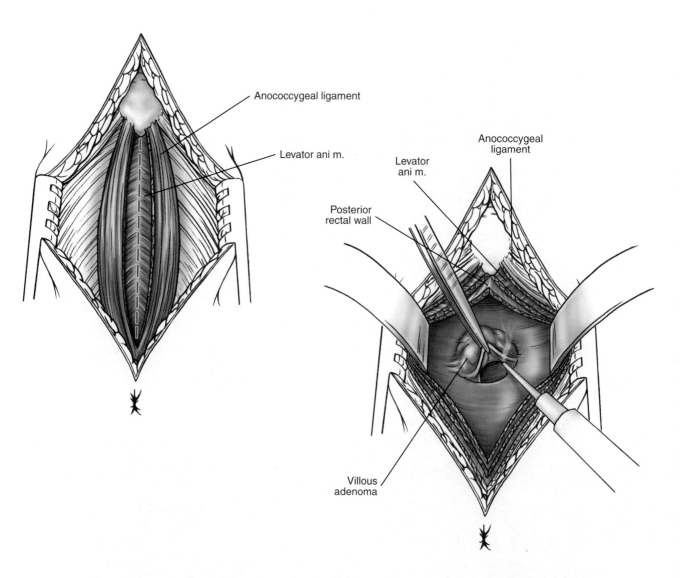

The patient is placed prone with a roll beneath the pelvis. The skin incision extends from the coccyx to just outside the anus. The anococcygeal ligament is incised vertically, and the levator ani deep to that is divided in the midline (vertically). Beneath the perirectal fat lies the posterior wall of the rectum, which can be entered or a sleeve of the rectum can be excised.

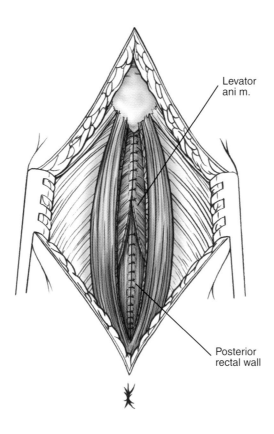

Levator
ani m.

Posterior
rectal wall

After repair of the rectum the tissues divided originally are reapproximated. This procedure has been associated with fecal fistula in approximately 10% of cases.

Anatomic Basis of Complications

- Exact location of the level of rectal tumor and assessment of its mobility allow use of the resection procedure with least morbidity.
- Injury to the hypogastric nerves diminishes sexual function.
- Failure to resect the mesorectum and achieve full radial clearance increases the likelihood of local recurrence of tumor.
- Resection of the presacral fascia increases risk for bleeding from sacral veins.

KEY REFERENCES

Cohen AM, Winawer SJ. Cancer of the Colon, Rectum and Anus. New York: Mc-Graw-Hill, 1995.

This is a superb, comprehensive, multidisciplinary treatise on the subject.

Enker WE. Sphincter-preserving operations for rectal cancer. Oncology 10(11):1673-1684, 1996.

This is a fine review of surgical technique for sphincter-sparing surgery by a superb practitioner of these techniques.

Gordon PH, Nivatvongs S. Principles and Practice of Surgery for the Colon, Rectum, and Anus, 2nd ed. St. Louis: Quality Medical Publishing, 1999.

This beautifully illustrated text focuses on surgical aspects of the management of colon and rectal disease, both benign and malignant.

Heald FJ, Ryall RDH. Recurrence and survival after total mesorectal excision for rectal cancer. Lancet 1:1479-1482, 1986.

The case for careful sharp dissection of the entire mesorectum and the description of the approach are found in this classic paper.

Shafik A. A new concept of the anatomy of the anal sphincter mechanism and the physiology of defecation. IX. Single loop continence: A new theory of the mechanism of anal continence. Dis Colon Rectum 23:37-43, 1980.

This classic paper in surgical anatomy relates the anatomy of the anal sphincter to its function.

Vernava AM III, Moran M, Rotheberger DA, Wong WD. A prospective evaluation of distal margins in carcinoma of the rectum. Surg Gynecol Obstet 175:333-336, 1992.

The paper provides the results of a prospective evaluation of margins. The measurements were based on fixed tissue and must be understood to translate to somewhat larger margins in fresh tissue. A 1 cm margin in the fixed specimen proved adequate distal clearance.

SUGGESTED READINGS

Boxall TA, Griffiths JD, Smart PJG. The blood supply of the distal segment of the rectum in anterior resection. Br J Surg 50:399, 1973.

Goligher JC. Surgery of the Anus, Rectum and Colon, 4th ed. London: Bailliere Tindall, 1980.

Goligher JC. The blood supply to the sigmoid colon and rectum. Br J Surg 37:157-162, 1949.

Lee JF, Maurer VM, Block GE. Anatomic relations of pelvic autonomic nerves to pelvic operations. Arch Surg 107(2):324-328, 1973.

Oh C, Kark AE. The transphinteric approach to mid and low rectal villous adenoma: Anatomic basis of surgical treatment. Ann Surg 176(5):605-612, 1972.

Pearlman NW, Donohue RE, Stiegmann GV, Ahnen DJ, Sedlacek SM, Braun TJ. Pelvic and sacropelvic exenteration for locally advanced or recurrent anorectal cancer. Arch Surg 122(5):537-541, 1987.

Willett CG, Wood WC. Update of the Massachusetts General Hospital experience of combined local excision and radiotherapy for rectal cancer. Surg Oncol Clin North Am 1:131-136, 1992.

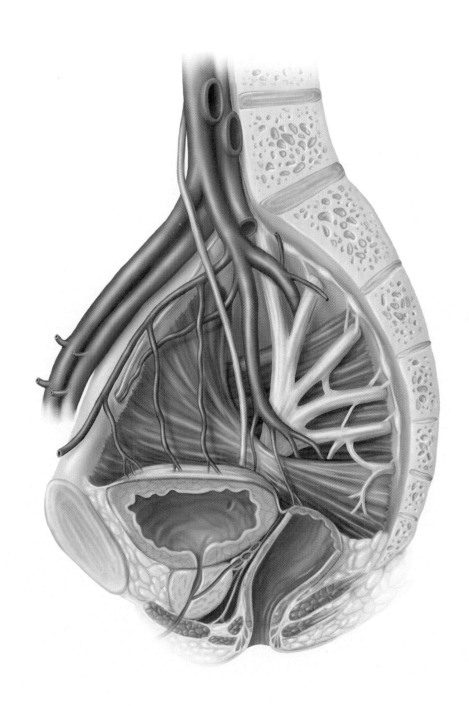

Chapter 11

Pelvis

Albert J. Aboulafia, M.D., and David K. Monson, M.D.

Surgical Applications

Fine-Needle Aspiration Biopsy
Core Needle Biopsy
Open Biopsy
Posterior Flap Hemipelvectomy
Anterior Flap Hemipelvectomy
Partial Pelvic Resection
Internal Hemipelvectomy

*I*t is estimated that approximately 2000 new cases of bone sarcomas and 5700 cases of soft tissue sarcomas are diagnosed annually in the United States. Approximately 5% to 10% of these tumors primarily involve the pelvis. Major advances in our understanding of sarcoma biology have led to advances in chemotherapy and surgical techniques that offer patients with nonmetastatic disease the potential for long-term disease-free survival and cure rates exceeding 50%. This is especially true for the two most common bone sarcomas, osteosarcoma and Ewing's sarcoma. In addition, advances in preoperative imaging studies have allowed surgeons to define the anatomic extent of disease more accurately and thereby plan surgical procedures with curative intent more precisely. Hemipelvectomy was considered the standard surgical procedure for the management of patients with pelvic sarcoma until recently. The procedure, however, is disabling and sacrifices a viable extremity to achieve local tumor control. Predicated on an understanding of sarcoma biology, surgeons have developed limb-sparing procedures that are intended to achieve local tumor control while maximizing function. New reconstructive procedures allow complete or partial resection of the innominate bone, often termed internal hemipelvectomy, with preservation of the extremity.

Sarcomas grow in centrifugal fashion, forming a central core. As they grow they tend to compress normal cells and form a pseudocapsule composed of compressed tumor cells and a fibrovascular zone of reactive tissue. This pseudocapsule gives the appearance of a well-encapsulated tumor. The pseudocapsule is surrounded by grossly normal-appearing tissue that may have tumor cells within it, known as a satellite or micrometastatic lesion. These lesions are believed to be a cause of local recurrence after wide excision. With knowledge of tumor biology and local anatomy, wide surgical excision (i.e., resection beyond the reactive zone) can be planned, with the goal of maximizing function while obtaining local tumor control.

SURGICAL ANATOMY
Topography

The pelvis is the region of the trunk below the abdomen and immediately above the lower extremities. The iliac crest can be felt along its entire length from the anterior superior iliac spine to the posterosuperior iliac spine. The pubic symphysis is in the midline anteriorly, near the distal insertion of the rectus abdominis muscles. The sacral spinous processes are posterior in the midline, within the upper portion of the gluteal cleft, and the coccyx lies in the lower portion of the gluteal cleft behind the anus. The lateral contours of the pelvis are formed by the hip abductor muscles and the greater trochanter of the proximal femur.

Blood Supply

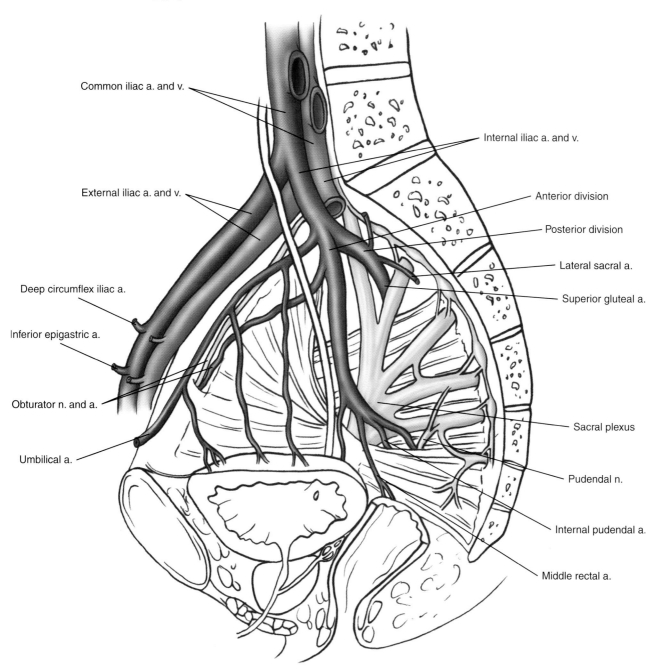

Common iliac a. and v.

External iliac a. and v.

Deep circumflex iliac a.

Inferior epigastric a.

Obturator n. and a.

Umbilical a.

Internal iliac a. and v.

Anterior division

Posterior division

Lateral sacral a.

Superior gluteal a.

Sacral plexus

Pudendal n.

Internal pudendal a.

Middle rectal a.

Each common iliac artery ends at the level of the sacral promontory in front of the sacroiliac joint by dividing into the external and internal iliac arteries. The external iliac artery continues along the medial border of the psoas muscle, giving rise to the deep circumflex iliac and inferior epigastric branches. It then leaves the false pelvis behind the inguinal ligament to become the femoral artery.

The internal iliac artery passes into the true pelvis to the upper margin of the greater sciatic foramen, dividing into anterior and posterior divisions. Branches of these divisions supply the buttocks, pelvic walls, pelvic viscera, and perineum. Branches of the anterior division include the inferior gluteal, obturator, internal pudendal, umbilical, inferior vesical, middle rectal, uterine, and vaginal arteries. Branches of the posterior division include the superior gluteal, iliolumbar, and lateral sacral arteries.

The external iliac vein receives the inferior epigastric and deep circumflex iliac veins. It runs along the medial aspect of the external iliac artery and is joined by the internal iliac vein to form the common iliac vein. The venous tributaries corresponding to the branches of the internal iliac artery join to form the internal iliac vein, which passes upward in front of the sacroiliac joint to join the external iliac vein.

Nerve Supply

The major nerves of the pelvis include the sacral plexus and the sciatic, femoral, pudendal, obturator, genitofemoral, and lateral femoral cutaneous nerves.

The sacral plexus lies on the posterior pelvic wall in front of the piriformis muscle. It is formed from the anterior rami of the fourth and fifth lumbar nerves and the first, second, third, and fourth sacral nerves. The sciatic nerve and other branches to the lower limb leave the pelvis through the greater sciatic foramen.

The pudendal nerve arises from the second, third, and fourth sacral nerves and exits through the greater sciatic foramen deep to the coccygeus muscle and sacrospinous ligament. It then reenters the pelvis through the lesser sciatic foramen and courses in the pudendal canal within the obturator internus fascia to the urogenital diaphragm. Essentially all pelvic resections involving the ischium result in sacrifice of the pudendal nerve, and it is important to inform patients preoperatively of the anticipated sensory losses.

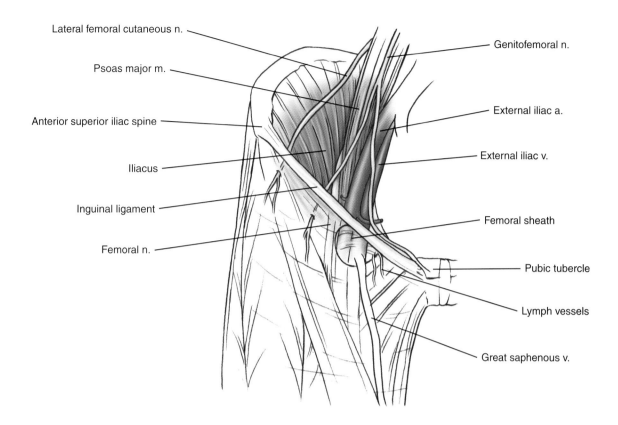

Lateral femoral cutaneous n.

Psoas major m.

Anterior superior iliac spine

Iliacus

Inguinal ligament

Femoral n.

Genitofemoral n.

External iliac a.

External iliac v.

Femoral sheath

Pubic tubercle

Lymph vessels

Great saphenous v.

The femoral nerve is the largest nerve of the lumbar plexus, emerging from the lateral border of the psoas muscle within the abdomen and running between the psoas and iliacus muscles of the false pelvis before exiting the pelvis behind the inguinal ligament to enter the thigh lateral to the femoral vessels and the femoral sheath. The femoral nerve can sometimes be preserved in resection of soft tissue or bone sarcomas arising within the iliac fossa, allowing intact function of the important quadriceps muscle group within the thigh.

The obturator nerve arises from the lumbar plexus along the medial border of the psoas muscle in the abdomen and crosses the front of the sacroiliac joint to enter the pelvis. It continues forward along the pelvic wall in the angle between the internal and external iliac vessels until it reaches the obturator canal and leaves the pelvis to enter the adductor compartment of the thigh. This nerve can often be preserved in resection of soft tissue sarcomas arising within the iliac fossa or bone sarcomas not requiring excision of the obturator ring.

The lateral femoral cutaneous nerve crosses the iliac fossa anterior to the iliac muscle and exits the pelvis behind the lateral end of the inguinal ligament.

Lymphatic Drainage

The external, internal, and common iliac nodes are arranged in a chain along the major blood vessels for which they are named.

Regional lymph node metastases are generally considered uncommon in patients with bone and soft tissue sarcomas. In a review of 2500 cases of soft tissue sarcomas, Weingrad and Rosenberg found a 5% incidence of nodal metastasis during the course of treatment. The incidence of regional node metastasis, however, is much higher in certain histologic subtypes, such as epithelioid sarcomas (20%), synovial sarcomas (17%), malignant fibrous histiocytomas (17%), rhabdomyosarcomas (12%), and clear cell sarcomas. The diagnosis of metastatic melanoma or carcinoma must be excluded in patients with regional node metastasis.

Bony Pelvis

The bony pelvis consists of two innominate bones and the sacrum and coccyx. The innominate bones are divided into three regions: the ilium, the ischium, and the pubis. The two innominate bones are joined anteriorly by the pubic symphysis, and are joined to the sacrum posteriorly at the sacroiliac joints. The pelvic brim is formed by the sacral promontory posteriorly, the iliopectineal line laterally, and the pubic symphysis anteriorly. The false pelvis is above the brim and forms part of the abdominal cavity; the true pelvis lies below.

Ligaments

The sacrotuberous ligament extends from the lateral part of the sacrum and coccyx and the posterior inferior iliac spine to the ischial tuberosity. The sacrospinous ligament lies anterior to the sacrotuberous ligament and extends from the lateral part of the sacrum and coccyx to the ischial spine. These ligaments prevent upward rotation of the lower sacrum and coccyx at the sacroiliac joints and divide the sciatic notch into the greater and lesser sciatic foramina.

The iliolumbar ligament is a posterior structure connecting the tip of the fifth lumbar transverse process to the iliac crest. The posterior sacroiliac ligament and interosseous sacroiliac ligaments stabilize the posterior aspect of the sacroiliac joint; the anterior sacroiliac ligament lies across the anterior aspect of the joint. These structures are important to posterior pelvic stability and must be identified and divided in all resections carried through the sacroiliac articulation.

The inguinal ligament is formed by the inferior margin of the external oblique muscle aponeurosis. It extends from the anterosuperior iliac spine laterally to the pubic tubercle medially and inferiorly.

Musculature

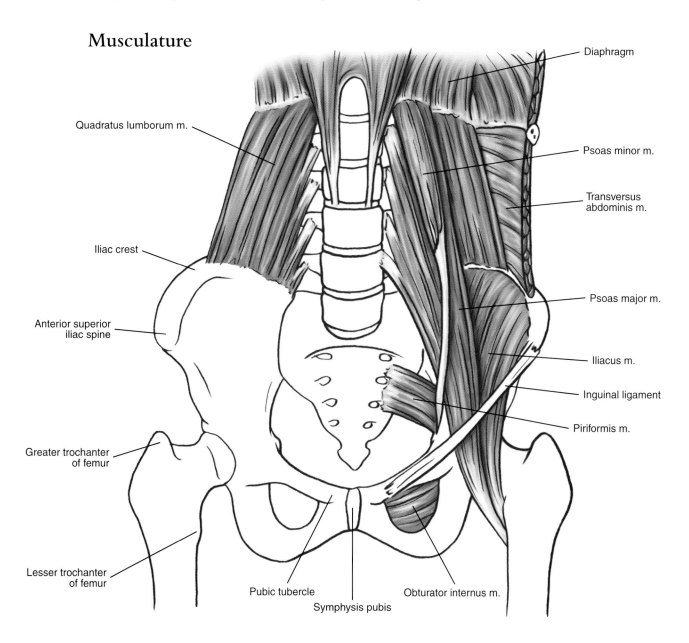

The medial wall of the ilium is covered by the psoas and iliac muscles, which are further separated from the deeper pelvic structures by a distinct fascial plane. The origin of the iliac muscle from the iliac crest serves as a natural barrier to tumor extension, both into the flank superiorly and central pelvic structures medially. The gluteal muscles of the buttocks and the tensor fascia lata muscle cover the lateral wall of the ilium. Their investing fascia and origins from the iliac crest also serve to contain tumor growth external to the ilium. Tumor extension may occur, however, beneath the caudal edge of the gluteus maximus muscle into the proximal portion of the posterior thigh or through the sciatic notch into the pelvis. The muscles arising from or inserting on the ischium and pubis provide poor containment of potential tumor extension and do little to impede tumor growth into the proximal thigh or the ischiorectal fossa, or along the retroperitoneal space.

Within the true pelvis, the pyriformis muscle arises from the front of the sacral lateral masses and passes through the greater sciatic foramen to leave the pelvis. The obturator internus muscle arises from the intrapelvic surface of the obturator membrane and medial wall of the acetabulum to emerge from the pelvis through the lesser sciatic foramen. The parietal pelvic fascia overlies these muscles and assists in tumor containment.

Ureter

The ureter lies in the interval between the peritoneum and the psoas fascia. It enters the pelvis by crossing the bifurcation of the common iliac artery in front of the sacroiliac joint, then lies anterior to the internal iliac artery down toward the ischial spine. It may be displaced by large tumor masses extending medially into the pelvis, but can usually be mobilized away from the medial tumor mass along with the peritoneum, to which it is loosely attached. Direct tumor involvement is rare because of containment of tumor by the psoas fascia.

SURGICAL APPLICATIONS
Biopsy

Complications resulting from poorly planned biopsies adversely affect subsequent surgery and compromise local tumor control. The biopsy site should be chosen such that it can be excised en bloc with the tumor when definitive surgery is performed. In addition, soft tissue compartments not involved with the tumor should not be violated. This requires that the person performing the biopsy be familiar with the various surgical procedures for the management of pelvic sarcomas. The biopsy should be thought of as the first stage of surgery. Therefore, it cannot be overemphasized that the person performing the biopsy should be prepared to do the definitive surgical resection. Even seemingly innocuous procedures such as computed tomography (CT)–directed biopsy contaminate tissue planes and must be performed carefully.

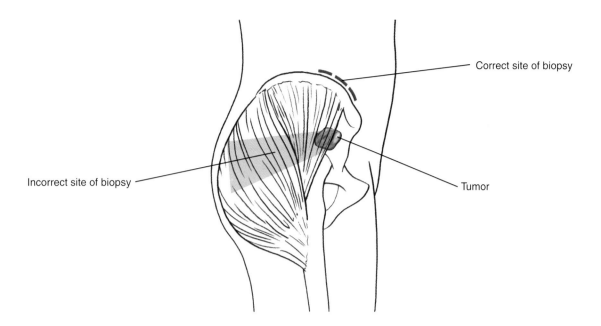

A biopsy performed through the buttock for a pelvic sarcoma can contaminate tissue compartments that would otherwise be preserved and used for wound closure during definitive tumor resection. A patient with a pelvic sarcoma who might be managed with a limb-salvage procedure, such as internal hemipelvectomy, may require an anterior flap hemipelvectomy after contamination of the buttock and gluteal musculature following a poorly planned biopsy.

Such complications resulting from poorly planned biopsy of suspected sarcomas compromising optimum treatment are well documented. This is especially true for pelvic sarcomas because surgeons are less likely to be familiar with the surgical procedures associated with limb sparing than in other extremity sites.

Prior to performing a biopsy, imaging studies such as plain radiographs, CT scans, and magnetic resonance imaging (MRI) studies are obtained to give a three-dimensional representation of the tumor and surrounding anatomy. Performing staging studies prior to biopsy has several distinct advantages. First, characteristics of bone sarcomas evident on plain radiographs or other imaging studies may provide diagnostic clues to the nature of the lesion. Likewise, appropriate imaging of soft tissue lesions may lead to diagnostic considerations of soft tissue masses that mimic sarcoma. Hence, preoperative imaging studies obtained prior to biopsy can alter the prebiopsy differential diagnosis and provide additional information for the pathologist in establishing a diagnosis based on clinical, radiographic, and histologic correlation. In many cases the biopsy serves to confirm what is suspected on the basis of clinical and radiographic information. In such a situation, after intraoperative frozen-section confirmation, definitive surgery can be accomplished in the same operative setting if clinically indicated. Second, preoperative imaging may indicate a soft tissue component of a bone sarcoma, obviating the need to biopsy the bone and allowing biopsy of the soft tissue component of the tumor. By obtaining the biopsy from the soft tissue component of a bone sarcoma, a stress riser in the bone is prevented that potentially can predispose to a pathologic fracture. Third, prebiopsy imaging studies can localize tumor to specific compartments, allowing directed biopsy to be performed without unnecessarily contaminating unaffected compartments. Fourth, after biopsy, imaging studies such as technetium bone scans or MRI studies used to determine the extent of tumor may be different, making accurate assessment of tumor extent more difficult.

While the need for biopsy of suspected pelvic sarcomas prior to initiating treatment is well accepted, the optimal technique for obtaining tissue for diagnosis is not. Once the decision to proceed with biopsy has been made, the surgeon must decide on the most appropriate biopsy technique. Four basic biopsy techniques are described. Factors related to the size, consistency, and location of the tumor, as well as institutional preference and experience, may affect the ultimate choice of biopsy technique.

Fine-Needle Aspiration Biopsy

Fine-needle aspiration biopsy of carcinomas is a widely used and successful diagnostic technique, but its role in the evaluation of pelvic bone and soft tissue sarcomas is controversial. Fine-needle aspiration biopsy was first described in the 1850s. The technique involves use of a fine needle to aspirate cells from a tumor. This is the fundamental difference from other biopsy techniques, which are intended to obtain tissue rather than cells. The procedure offers many advantages over other biopsy techniques: it is simple, with little potential for complications, and can be performed in an office setting with minimal equipment needs. The equipment needed for aspiration of superficial masses includes sterile gloves, alcohol swabs, 10 or 20 ml syringes, an aspiration needle holder, 22- to 25-gauge disposable needles of varying lengths, saline solution, sterile gauze, Coplin jars containing 95% alcohol, nonfrosted slides, and local anesthetic (optional). "Thin" needles (22 gauge or smaller) are used to decrease the amount of obscuring blood obtained; ensure a cytologic, not histologic, specimen; and minimize complications. The work area is prepared with the Coplin jars and saline solution vials opened and ready. Slides are labeled with the patient's name or identifying number, or both. A 10 or 20 ml syringe with attached needle is placed in the aspiration holder. The use of various size needles, from 18 to 25 gauge, has been described for fine-needle aspiration of sarcomas. Once the biopsy site is determined, the skin is prepared and anesthetized. A needle, attached to a syringe, is introduced into the tumor. When the needle is within the tumor the plunger is drawn back, creating negative pressure (suction) in the syringe. With continuous negative pressure, the needle is vigorously moved within the tumor mass using a sawing motion.

When material is noted in the needle hub, negative pressure is released and the needle is removed. Firm pressure is applied over the site to minimize the potential for hematoma formation.

Attention is then directed to preparation of the slides. This step is extremely important to optimize the chances of obtaining an interpretable specimen. The needle is removed from the syringe, a small amount of air is introduced into the syringe, and the needle is reattached. The bevel of the needle is placed directly on the slide surface and a small drop of material is expressed onto the center of the slide. Usually three to six slides can be prepared with each aspiration pass. With a second "spreader" slide gently placed crosswise over the drop of material, the specimen is gently smeared in one smooth motion down the diagnostic slide. The slide is then immediately placed in 95% alcohol fixative. Rapid fixation is extremely important. Several air-dried smears can be made for Romanovsky staining. The needle and syringe are then rinsed with saline solution and collected in a saline solution–filled tube to ensure salvage of all cellular material. Other slides are then made for additional cytologic studies, such as thin smear, cytospin, and cell block. The aspiration procedure can be repeated to ensure optimal sampling of various sites of the mass or to obtain material for flow cytometry and microbiologic cultures. The slides are stained with hematoxylin-eosin, Papanicolaou's stain, or Romanovsky's stain.

The role of fine-needle aspiration biopsy in the evaluation of carcinomas and to document recurrent tumor or metastatic disease involving the pelvis is well accepted. However, the success of obtaining tissue for diagnostic purposes in primary bone and soft tissue sarcomas is less than that achieved with core needle or open biopsy. In addition to its other advantages, fine-needle aspiration biopsy can easily be used to biopsy deep-seated tumors, particularly in the retroperitoneum, with CT assistance. While the diagnostic accuracy for malignancy approaches 90% for fine-needle aspiration biopsy performed at experienced institutions, the accuracy rate is lower for specific tumor type and grade. Establishing the grade and type of tumor is not simply academic but has important implications not only for planning surgical resections but for planning neoadjuvant and adjuvant treatment. For example, a low-grade liposarcoma may be treated with a marginal resection to preserve vital structures, whereas a high-grade liposarcoma requires at least wide margin resection or preoperative irradiation. Similarly, a high-grade osteosarcoma is usually treated with neoadjuvant and adjuvant chemotherapy, whereas a high-grade chondrosarcoma usually is not. Because fine-needle aspiration biopsy is used to obtain cells rather than tissue and does not preserve tissue architecture, many believe it should not have a primary role in the diagnostic evaluation of primary bone and soft tissue sarcomas.

Core Needle Biopsy

Core needle biopsy, like fine-needle aspiration biopsy, is performed percutaneously, usually in an office setting with local anesthesia. Unlike fine-needle aspiration biopsy, with core needle biopsy a core of tissue rather than cells is obtained and tumor architecture is preserved. As a result, diagnostic accuracy of core needle biopsy is superior to that reported for fine-needle aspiration biopsy and is the preferred method for closed biopsy of sarcomas at most centers. Various needles have been used to obtain core specimens from soft tissue or bone. The Tru-cut needle is most useful for biopsy of soft tissue sarcomas or the soft tissue component of bone sarcomas. On occasion, if the cortex of bone has been sufficiently weakened by tumor, a Tru-cut needle can be used to biopsy bone. Use of other core needles, such as the Craig needle, designed to biopsy pathologic bone, generally requires sedation or general anesthesia.

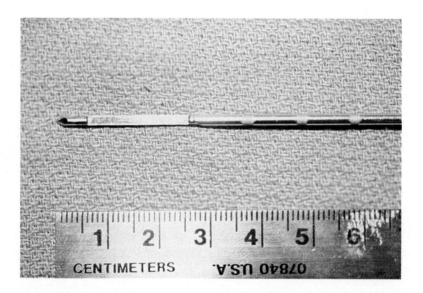

Biopsy with a Tru-cut needle usually is performed in an office setting, with local anesthesia and without radiographic assistance. Compared with open biopsy, which is usually performed in an operating room, closed biopsy is less costly and more convenient. Additional advantages of closed biopsy over open biopsy include (1) less risk for wound complications and infection, and (2) neoadjuvant chemotherapy or radiation therapy, which are an integral part of treatment for pelvic bone and soft tissue sarcomas, can begin immediately, before wound healing. Closed biopsy may be associated with less risk for hematoma formation and local tumor contamination than is open biopsy.

Despite the simplicity of core needle biopsy, the procedure should be performed only by physicians familiar with the surgical procedures involved in managing pelvic sarcomas. Once the decision for closed biopsy of a suspected pelvic sarcoma has been made, the surgeon selects the most appropriate site for biopsy, so that the biopsy site can be excised en bloc with the definitive surgical resection while preventing contamination of compartments not involved with tumor. The individual performing the biopsy should mark the planned skin incision for resection and incorporate the biopsy with the skin markings. If the person planning to perform the biopsy is unable to mark out the skin incision that may be used for future surgery, the biopsy should be deferred and consultation obtained from the surgeon who would likely perform the definitive resection. Additional considerations in selecting the biopsy site include integrity of the skin and averting sampling error. Skin overlying a tumor that is thin and tented should be avoided because it is prone to delayed healing. Similarly, the center of the tumor is likely to be the most necrotic portion, and samples should be obtained from the periphery of the mass, which is more likely to yield viable tissue.

The skin is prepared with povidone-iodine (Betadine) and infiltrated with local anesthetic. With a No. 11 blade, a small puncture wound is made in the skin. This allows the needle to pass freely into and out of soft tissue and creates a small scar marking the biopsy site for later identification so that it can be excised en bloc with the tumor. The needle is then introduced beneath the skin while the trocar is kept closed. The tip of the needle is advanced to the periphery of the tumor. With one hand holding the needle in place, the surgeon uses the other hand to advance the trocar into the tumor, thereby opening the sample tray. Next the cutting sleeve is advanced, closing the sample tray over a piece of tumor. The entire needle is withdrawn and the specimen sterilely retrieved. Several specimens can be retrieved and multiple sites of the tumor can be sampled by repeating the technique and redirecting the needle to other portions of the tumor. Tumor may then be placed in fresh saline solution and given to the pathologist. If adequate tissue is available, frozen sections may be obtained to confirm that diagnostic tissue has been used. Additional portions of tumor may be saved for special studies, such as electron microscopy, cytogenetics, or flow cytometry. Firm pressure is applied to the biopsy site for several minutes to prevent hematoma formation. A single nonabsorbable suture may be used to close the skin and mark the biopsy site.

Despite the high diagnostic yield achieved with closed biopsy, a study that is negative for tumor should not always be interpreted as meaning that no tumor exists. If there is a strong clinical suspicion that tumor exists, open biopsy may be indicated.

Open Biopsy

Open biopsy may be incisional or excisional. Incisional biopsy is performed to obtain a small piece of tumor for diagnostic purposes, whereas excisional biopsy is performed with the intention of removing the entire tumor. Selecting the most appropriate procedure for a suspected pelvic sarcoma may depend on the surgeon's experience and ability in determining preoperatively if a given lesion is malignant. Primary resection for suspected soft tissue sarcomas has been described, but because of the magnitude of this procedure, it would be ill advised for a benign lesion. Similarly, excision along the pseudocapsule of a malignant tumor is likely to result in local recurrence. Given that the optimal surgical procedure for a suspected pelvic sarcoma depends on accurate histologic diagnosis and grade preoperatively, excisional biopsy is generally reserved for selected situations. If open biopsy of a suspected pelvic sarcoma is necessary, incisional biopsy usually is the procedure of choice. Excisional biopsy of pelvic soft tissue tumors should be reserved for small subcutaneous masses with a low probability of malignancy or when MRI studies show the mass to have characteristics of a lipoma. Bone tumors may likewise be managed with excisonal biopsy when the preoperative diagnosis of benign tumor is almost certain, as in the case of an osteochondroma. Excisional biopsy of malignant bone lesions may be performed in selected cases, such as low-grade chondrosarcomas, which are not usually treated with neoadjuvant agents and may have characteristic findings on preoperative imaging studies.

INCISIONAL BIOPSY

Despite the technical ease of incisional biopsy, the procedure requires knowledge and understanding of the complex anatomy of the pelvis and of the surgical procedures used to treat pelvic sarcomas. The hazards of open biopsy of extremity sarcomas are well documented. The incidence of major errors in diagnosis, nonrepresentative or technically poor biopsies, and problems with skin, soft tissue, or bone resulting from open biopsy are alarmingly high. These complications are three to five times more common when the biopsy is performed by someone other than the surgeon who will perform the definitive resection. Complications resulting from biopsy of extremity sarcomas compromise future limb-sparing procedures and adversely affect patient outcome. The complex anatomy of the pelvis and the lack of experience of most surgeons with resections in this area increases the potential for complications.

Prior to selecting the site of biopsy all preoperative imaging studies should be carefully reviewed. The biopsy site should be chosen not necessarily for the shortest route but with the idea that the biopsy should be placed in line with the incision that will be used for the definitive resection. Consequently, the surgeon performing the biopsy must be familiar with the various pelvic resection procedures used for sarcomas. The biopsy should be considered the first part of the surgery, not simply a procedure performed to enable diagnosis. In addition, the site should be selected in an area where skin complications are not likely to result. The temptation to make an incision directly over skin tented from underlying tumor should be avoided.

The imaging studies, such as plain radiographs, CT scans, and MRI studies, are reviewed to select the most appropriate part of the tumor to be biopsied. For bone tumors the least differentiated or mineralized portion of the tumor is most likely to yield diagnostic tissue. Areas of reactive bone should be avoided lest a mistaken diagnosis of osteosarcoma be rendered. For most malignant bone tumors, there is a soft tissue component of the tumor that is frequently best seen with MRI. It is preferable to biopsy the soft tissue component of the bone tumor rather than the bone so that the risk for weakening the bone and resultant pathologic fracture is avoided. In cases of soft tissue sarcomas the MRI studies may reveal areas of necrosis, which are less likely to provide viable tumor when biopsied.

Preoperative antibiotics are usually withheld until after cultures have been obtained if there is any possibility that the diagnosis will be infection rather than neoplasm. The incision should be as small as possible, yet adequate. Vigorous retraction of the skin in an effort to keep the incision small is ill advised and may lead to delayed wound healing, dehiscence, or infection. Similarly, the incision must be adequate to allow visualization so that vital structures are avoided and meticulous hemostasis can be obtained. Following the incision, but prior to reaching the tumor, the surgeon will encounter the pseudocapsule. The pseudocapsule is composed primarily of compressed normal tissue. In muscle it appears salmon colored. Soft tissue sarcomas are usually gray or white. This distinction is important to ensure that the most viable portion of the tumor located at its periphery adjacent to the pseudocapsule-tumor interface is sampled. The specimen is handled carefully to avoid crush artifact. A suture may be placed in the tumor and a wedge cut around the portion secured by the suture to avoid unnecessary handling of the tumor. Tissue is obtained for cultures of aerobic, anaerobic, and fungal organisms, and mycobacteria (tuberculosis) if indicated, and systemic prophylactic antibiotic is administered.

The specimen is given to the pathologist, who performs a touch prep and frozen-section analysis of the tumor to ensure that viable tissue has been obtained before the patient leaves the operating room. If the tissue is nondiagnostic or inadequate, additional material is obtained immediately to obviate the need for repeat surgical procedure and delay in diagnosis. Portions of the tumor are then saved for permanent section analyses and special studies, such as electron microscopy and flow cytometry, if needed. Meticulous hemostasis is obtained to prevent hematoma and thus spread of any viable tumor contained therein. Bone wax, polymethyl methacrylate, or gelatin sponges (Gelfoam) may be used to plug holes created in bone. The wound is closed in layers, with special attention to minimize trauma to the skin. Use of closed suction tubes is recommended, especially after biopsy of deep-seated tumors of the pelvis. The tubes should be brought out through the skin in line with and adjacent to the incision so that the tumor can be excised en bloc with the biopsy material. The diagnostic accuracy of frozen-section analysis is reported to be 90% when performed by a team of experienced surgeons and pathologists. When the frozen-section diagnosis agrees with the clinical and radiographic preoperative diagnosis, immediate surgery may be indicated. If the lesion is confirmed as benign, infectious, or metastatic, definitive surgery may proceed. For many sarcomas, however, it may be preferable to delay surgery until after neoadjuvant chemotherapy or radiation therapy. If there is any doubt as to the definitive diagnosis after frozen-section analysis, definitive surgery should not be performed.

EXCISIONAL BIOPSY

Excisional biopsy may be either marginal or wide. For sarcomas, marginal excision, an excision through the pseudocapsule, requires wide local repeat excision or local recurrence is likely. The surgeon who undertakes wide local repeat excision of a sarcoma that has been inadequately excised will likely need to remove more tissue than would otherwise have been necessary initially. First, the surgeon must excise the biopsy tract and any tissue contaminated by the dissection or subsequent hematoma formation. Second, the tumor margins are no longer apparent clinically or radiographically, so the surgeon must "guess" where the tumor margins are. Consequently, excisional biopsy for suspected sarcomas is rarely indicated except for small (<2 cm) subcutaneous lesions that can be widely excised without more morbidity than with marginal excision.

Hemipelvectomy

Classic hemipelvectomy involves disarticulation through the sacroiliac joint posteriorly and the symphysis pubis anteriorly. Modified hemipelvectomy refers to amputation through the pelvis in which the plane of bony resection posteriorly is anterior and lateral to the sacroiliac joint, thereby preserving a variable portion of the ilium. Extended hemipelvectomy involves resection of the pelvis in which the posterior bony resection is medial to the sacroiliac joint and through the sacral neural foramina; consequently, the sacroiliac joint is included in the resection. Internal hemipelvectomy refers to limb-sparing resection of the pelvis with partial or complete resection of the innominate bone.

Various surgical techniques have been described for hemipelvectomy. In many cases the surgical technique chosen will depend on the location and extent of the tumor rather than simply surgical preference. Tumors extending into the buttock involving the gluteal muscles are not amenable to posterior flap hemipelvectomy and may require management with an anterior flap hemipelvectomy.

Early descriptions of hemipelvectomy (during the first half of this century) reported a mortality of 60%. The major complication from surgery was shock secondary to blood loss. More recent reports have shown that hemipelvectomy can now be performed safely with an operative mortality of approximately 1%. In some cases, especially in patients who refuse blood products because of religious reasons, it may be possible to perform the procedure without the need for blood transfusion.

The physical and psychological effects of hemipelvectomy are substantial. Some patients may benefit from the opportunity to visit with other patients who have undergone similar surgery. The procedure and potential consequences, including bowel, bladder, and sexual dysfunction, should be thoroughly discussed with the patient so that informed consent can be obtained. Psychological support should be offered by appropriate persons, including family, clergy, social workers, and other patients. Preoperatively, the patient's metabolic and hematologic status should be optimized. Bowel preparation is done to decrease bacterial count. A diet of clear liquids only, for 24 hours, is used, and enemas are administered prior to the procedure to decrease the chances of fecal contamination of the wound during surgery. Although the operative blood loss is usually less than 1500 ml, packed red blood cells should always be available. In obese patients or in technically difficult hemipelvectomies, when operative blood loss is expected to be high, it is advisable to have fresh-frozen plasma and platelets available as well. Techniques to minimize transfusion requirements are advised, such as hemodilution and hypotensive anesthesia. If time permits, patients may give blood for autotransfusion.

Posterior Flap Hemipelvectomy

The primary indications for posterior flap hemipelvectomy include primary malignant neoplasms of the innominate bone or femur that have invaded the hip joint and sarcomas involving the upper thigh and extending through the obturator foramen to invade the pelvic wall and those that involve the pelvic wall primarily. A general anesthetic is administered, and a Foley catheter is inserted into the bladder. An arterial catheter is inserted for continuous hemodynamic monitoring, and a central venous catheter is advisable. One or more large-bore peripheral venous catheters are secured in place. A rectal tube is inserted and sutured in place to avoid fecal contamination of the wound. A nasogastic or orogastric tube is inserted and attached to suction to decompress the gastrointestinal tract.

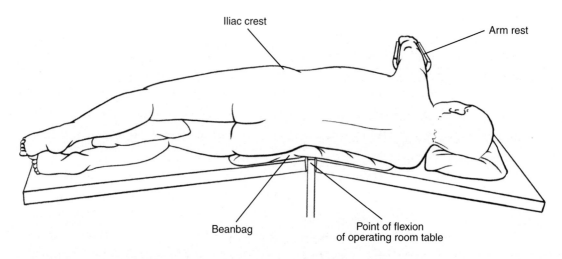

We prefer the patient in a semilateral position, which allows more accurate orientation for division of the sacroiliac joint by allowing access to the anterior and posterior portions of the joint. The patient is placed in the lateral position with the affected side up and the contralateral iliac crest centered over the point of flexion of the operating room table. Care is taken to protect the axilla and bony prominances of the contralateral side, and the ipsilateral upper extremity is placed on a Krasky arm rest or pillow. The operating room table is then extended beneath the iliac crest to allow greater access between the iliac crest and vertebral column on the involved side. A beanbag is placed beneath the patient and kept well below the midline posteriorly and anteriorly to help secure the patient in position. By keeping the beanbag well below the midline posteriorly and anteriorly, the patient can easily be rolled slightly forward during the posterior dissection and backward during the anterior dissection.

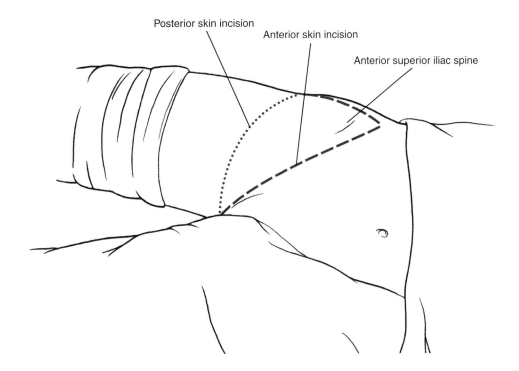

A U drape is used to isolate the perineum, genitalia, and anus from the operative field. The skin is prepared from the distal aspect of the great toe to the level of the xiphoid proximally and beyond the midline anteriorly and posteriorly. The extremity must be included in the preparation so that it can be manipulated during the procedure, permitting tissues to be divided under tension. The involved extremity is exsanguinated using an Esmarch bandage from proximal to distal for "autotransfusion" in the extremity to be sacrificed. The Esmarch bandage should remain distal to the tumor.

ANTERIOR DISSECTION

Anteriorly the incision begins approximately 5 cm proximal to the anterosuperior iliac spine and 2 cm medially. The incision curves gently distally and medially, paralleling the inguinal ligament to the symphysis pubis. The lateral incision is made beginning at the proximal portion of the incision and continuing distally and laterally to the anterosuperior iliac spine, over the anterior portion of the greater trochanter, and continuing posteriorly distal and parallel to the gluteal groove, to the perineum, and around the proximal thigh to meet the anterior incision at the superior border of the symphysis pubis.

Previous biopsy sites are incorporated with the incision and widely excised en bloc with the tumor. Attention is directed first to the anterior portion of the dissection. While the surgeon is positioned anterior to the patient, the patient is rolled back into a semilateral position, giving greater exposure anteriorly and facilitating medial retraction of the abdominal contents. Recall that by keeping the beanbag below the midline anteriorly and posteriorly the patient can be logrolled forward or backward as needed. The incision is deepened through subcutaneous tissue, Scarpa's fascia, and the external oblique aponeurosis. The internal oblique and transversus muscles are cut under tension, and the deep epigastric artery and vein are ligated. The spermatic cord in male patients or the round ligament in female patients is identified, and a Penrose drain is placed around it and retracted medially.

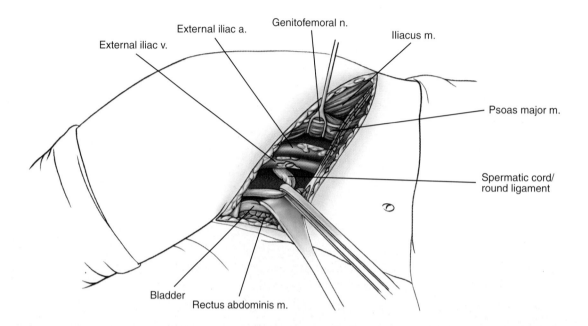

The ipsilateral rectus abdominis muscle is freed from its insertion on the pubic symphysis. The inguinal ligament is released from its medial and lateral pelvic attachments along the pubis and anterosuperior iliac spine, respectively. The anterior abdominal wall is thereby freed from its attachments to the pelvis, forming the anterior flap. The iliac fossa is exposed by bluntly dissecting the extraperitoneal fat from the fascia over the iliac and psoas muscles, and the urinary bladder is retracted medially and downward.

The external iliac artery and vein are identified and traced proximally to the common iliac artery and vein. The ureter is identified as it crosses the external iliac artery at the common iliac bifurcation and is retracted medially with the peritoneum. The common iliac vessels are then ligated and divided. The bladder and rectum are gently retracted medially while lateral traction is applied to the internal iliac artery and vein, and its branches to the pelvic side wall, rectum, and bladder are identified under tension, ligated, and transected. Then the iliolumbar and lateral sacral vessels and the superior and inferior gluteal vessels, and the internal pudendal, and middle hemorrhoidal and inferior and superior vesicular arteries are divided. The bladder and rectum are now free from the pelvic sidewall, and the sacral nerve roots to the bladder and rectum are visualized and preserved, if possible, to minimize the risks for bowel, bladder, and sexual dysfunction. The anterior wound is then packed with moist sponges, and attention is directed to the posterior incision.

POSTERIOR DISSECTION

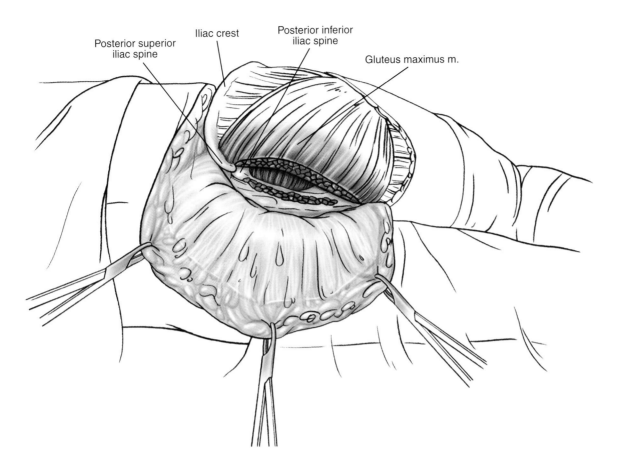

The surgeon moves to the posterior side of the patient, and the posterior incision is carried deep to the gluteal fascia. The skin incision is extended between the perineum and the thigh to join the anterior incision. The hip is flexed and adducted, placing tension on the gluteal muscles, and the incision is deepened through the gluteal fascia. The attachments of the gluteal fascia to the iliotibial tract and the tensor fascia lata are released, and a fasciocutaneous flap with the gluteal fascia is created. While placing traction on the posterior flap, it is elevated proximal to the iliac crest, and dissection proceeds until the posterosuperior and posteroinferior iliac spines are visualized.

A variable amount of the gluteus maximus muscle may be preserved with the flap if tumor margins permit. The muscular attachment along the ilium, namely, the external oblique aponeurosis and the erector spinae, latissimus dorsi, and quadratus lumborum muscles, are released. Transection of these muscles as close to bone as possible using an electrocautery minimizes blood loss. The inferior margin of the gluteus maximus muscle is identified, and a gloved digit is placed deep to the muscle and superficial to the sacrum. While maintaining tension on the muscle, it is released from its attachments on the sacrum, coccyx, and sacrotuberous ligament. The hip is then placed in neutral position and the psoas muscle is isolated. The genitofemoral nerve is identified on the anterior surface of the muscle and transected. While keeping tension on the muscle it is transected, and muscular vessels are cauterized as they are encountered. The proximal cut ends of the psoas muscle are ligated using a 0-silk suture. Deep to the psoas muscle the obturator and femoral nerves are transected, as is the lumbosacral nerve trunk.

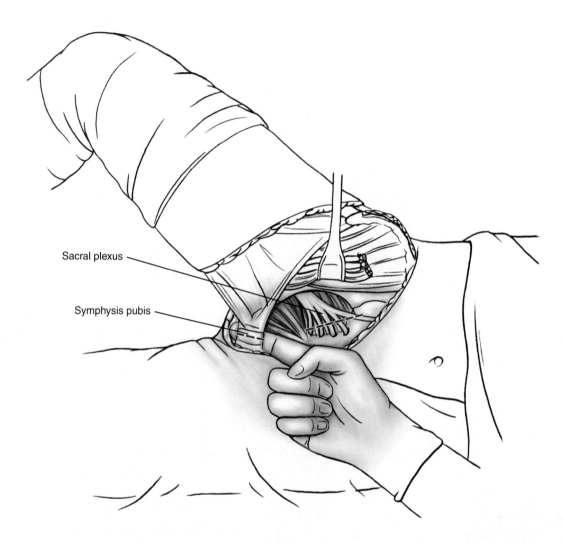

Sacral plexus

Symphysis pubis

The hip is flexed and abducted and externally rotated, placing tension on the ligaments of the symphysis pubis. The retropubic space is identified, and a gloved digit or a narrow ribbon retractor is placed beneath the symphysis to protect the urethra, prostate gland, and bladder. The symphysis is divided using a Gigli wire saw or osteotome. The sacral nerve roots are transected approximately 2 cm distal to the sacral foramina while preserving the nervi erigentes.

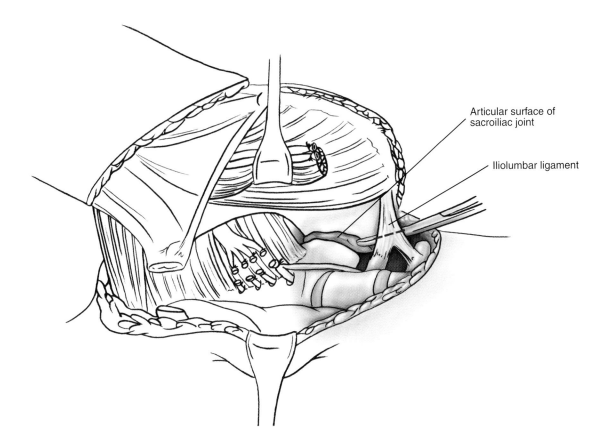

The iliac muscle is reflected laterally, and downward pressure is applied to the anterosuperior iliac spine to expose the anterior portion of the sacroiliac joint. The capsule of the sacroiliac joint is then opened. An osteotome may be needed to enter the sacroiliac joint if a synostosis exists between the sacrum and ilium, which is not uncommon, especially in older patients. The iliolumbar ligament is identified as it courses from the transverse process of the fifth lumbar vertebra to the ilium, a clamp is passed beneath the ligament, and the ligament is transected.

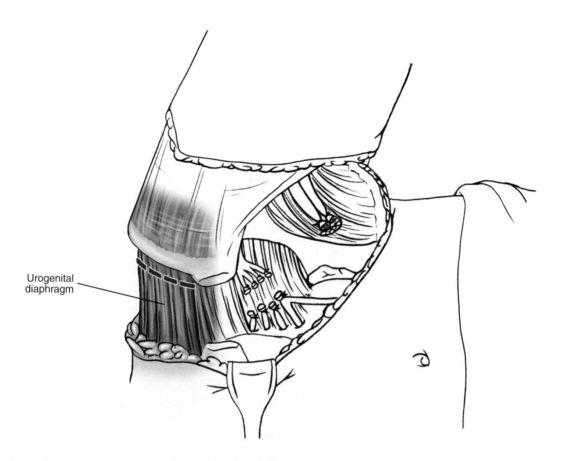

Urogenital
diaphragm

All that remains to complete the amputation is transection of the pelvic diaphragm. This is facilitated by the assistant constantly pulling upward on the extremity while the patient's hip is maximally flexed, placing the structures of the
urogenital diaphragm and levator ani muscles under tension.

Starting at the symphysis and continuing toward the ischial tuberosity, the
muscles of the urogenital diaphragm and the pubococcygeus muscles are divided at their origins along the inferior pubic ramus. A gloved digit is placed
in the ischiorectal fossa to prevent inadvertent injury to the rectum. The remaining muscular and ligamentous structures are transected, namely, the is-
chiococcygeus, iliococcygeus, and piriformis muscles and the sacrotuberous and
sacrospinalis ligaments.

The hip is then flexed and adducted to expose the posterior portion of the
sacroiliac joint, which is divided with an osteotome, thereby completing the
amputation.

The wound is irrigated with copious quantities of solution, and bleeding
sites are cauterized or ligated as needed. Sharp bony prominences, if present,
are removed with a rongeur or file. Avitene powder or other hemostatic agents
may be spread in the wound, and bone wax is applied to cut surfaces of bone
to minimize postoperative bleeding.

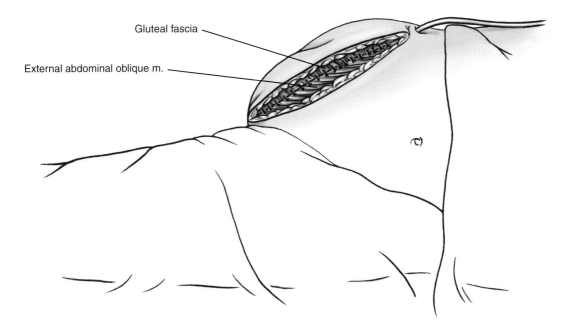

Gluteal fascia

External abdominal oblique m.

Closed-suction catheters are placed deep within the wound and are brought out through the skin without violating the posterior skin flap. The gluteal fascia is sutured to the fascia of the abdominal wall with interrupted sutures.

The skin is closed in layers with minimal handling of the posterior skin. A bulky sterile dressing is applied and covered with a circular woven elastic wrap (Ace bandage), providing a well-padded compression dressing. The patient is transferred to a well-padded bed or one with an air mattress, with an overhead trapeze to minimize excessive pressure on the posterior flap and to encourage mobility and facilitate positioning.

Anterior Flap Hemipelvectomy

Anterior flap hemipelvectomy in patients with sarcoma is indicated when tumor involves the upper thigh or buttock and cannot be managed by local excision. This situation is commonly encountered when tumor recurs after prior buttockectomy or previously irradiated posterior skin. The anterior flap hemipelvectomy utilizes a myocutaneous flap based on the preserved external iliac and superficial femoral artery.

The patient is prepared for surgery and placed on the operating table as previously described and illustrated for posterior flap hemipelvectomy (see p. 478). If an Esmarch bandage is used, it should not extend proximal to the knee joint. The skin incision is marked to ensure an adequate skin flap is obtained anteriorly for wound closure and that surgical margins are free of tumor. The skin incision in the thigh is along the posteromedial and posterolateral aspects of the thigh and joined by a transverse incision proximal to the patella. Anteriorly the incision begins 2 cm proximal and posterior to the anterosuperior iliac spine and parallels the inguinal ligament to the pubic tubercle approximately 1 to 2 cm proximal to the inguinal ligament. Laterally the incision parallels the iliac wing, passing medial and distal to the anterosuperior iliac spine, and then is directed distally along the lateral aspect of the thigh to the level of the tendinous portion of the quadriceps muscle, just proximal to the superior pole of the patella. Beginning at the origin of the anterior incision near the anterosuperior iliac spine, the incision is continued posteriorly along the proximal edge of the posterior iliac wing beyond the posteroinferior iliac spine. The incision continues distally and medially toward the midline of the sacrum, passes just lateral to the anus, and stops in the perineal region just distal to the gluteal crease.

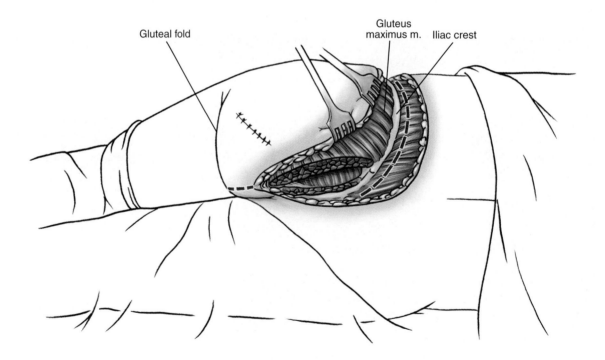

The iliac crest and sacrum are skeletonized by releasing the muscular attachments of the external oblique, latissimus dorsi, quadratus lumborum, erector spinae, and gluteus maximus muscles.

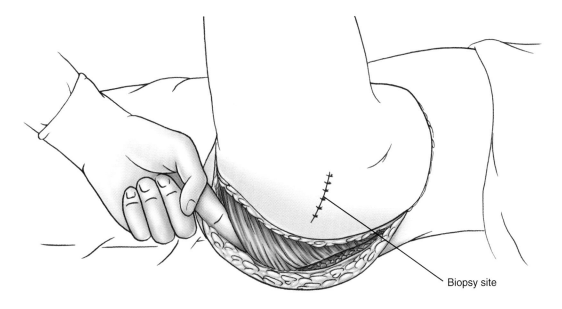

Biopsy site

A gloved digit is placed deep to the remaining fibers of the distal origin of the gluteus maximus muscle, along the coccyx and sacrotuberous ligament, to identify the ischiorectal fossa. These structures are placed under tension by the assistant, flexing the patient's hip while applying gentle internal rotation. The remaining fibers of the gluteus maximus muscle are then transected using an electrocautery, and the rectum is protected by a gloved digit in the ischiorectal fossa.

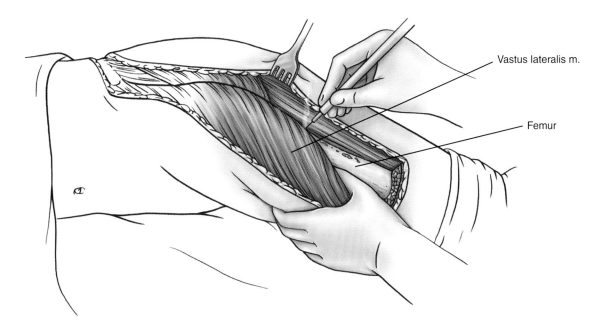

Vastus lateralis m.

Femur

The surgeon moves to the opposite side of the table to stand anterior to the patient. The transverse skin incision distally is carried through skin, subcutaneous tissue, fat, and the entire quadriceps muscle to expose the anterior surface of the distal femur. The incision is then continued proximally along the lateral thigh toward the greater trochanter, terminating at the medial portion of the anterior skin incision just medial and distal to the anterosuperior iliac spine. The iliotibial band is incised in line with the skin incision, and the tensor fascia lata is separated from investing fascia and retracted posteriorly to be resected en bloc with the specimen. The lateral edge of the vastus lateralis muscle is identified by placing traction on the muscle medially. While maintaining medial traction on the muscle the plane between the vastus lateralis and the biceps femoris muscles posteriorly is identified, and the fascial covering of the vastus lateralis muscle is freed to its origin on the greater trochanter.

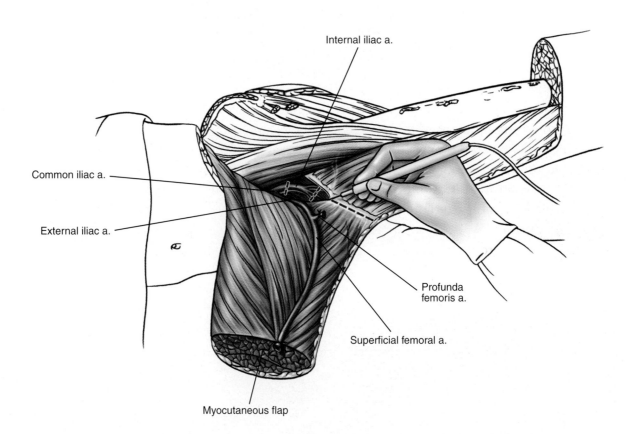

The vastus lateralis muscle is then released from its insertion along the linea aspera on the posterior surface of the femur. The vastus lateralis muscle is kept in continuity with full-thickness skin, subcutaneous tissue, and fascia overlying it on the anterior thigh. Attention is then directed to the distal medial aspect of the thigh where the anterior transverse incision joining the medial and lateral thigh incision has been created. The medial incision is extended proximally to the pubic crest. The sartorius muscle is identified, and the vastus medialis muscle is retracted anteriorly and medially to expose the subsartorial canal. The femoral artery and vein are traced proximally to the adductor hiatus, where they are ligated and divided. Proximal traction is placed on the anterior flap, and the origins of the vastus medialis and intermedius muscles are released from their attachments along the shaft of the femur. The dissection remains anterior and medial to the adductor magnus and adductor longus muscles, which ultimately are sacrificed with the specimen.

As the dissection continues proximally, the profunda femoris artery is encountered as it passes behind the femoral artery and adductor longus muscle, approximately 4 cm distal to the inguinal ligament. The vessels are ligated and divided just distal to the common femoral artery and vein. After the quadriceps muscles are released from the femur, attention is directed to release of the anterior myocutaneous flap from its attachments to the pelvis. The flap is continually retracted proximally and inverted so that the superficial femoral artery can be visualized and protected while maintaining continuity with the flap. The abdominal muscles are released from their attachments along the iliac crest, then the sartorius muscle is released from its origin on the anterosuperior iliac spine, and the rectus femoris from its origin on the anteroinferior iliac spine. The femoral canal is identified and the femoral sheath divided. Dissection is continued proximally, and the remaining origin of the rectus femoris muscle on the pubis is identified and transected. Blunt dissection is continued proximally along the femoral nerve to enter the pelvis. The symphysis is divided as previously illustrated (see p. 482) while protecting the bladder and urethra. With the hip flexed, abducted, and externally rotated, medial traction on the pelvic viscera is applied, allowing exposure of the internal iliac artery. The internal iliac artery and vein are traced proximally to the common iliac vessels, where the ureter is identified and protected. The internal iliac vessels are then ligated and transected near their origin from the common iliac vessels. As in posterior flap hemipelvectomy, branches of the internal iliac vessels are ligated and divided.

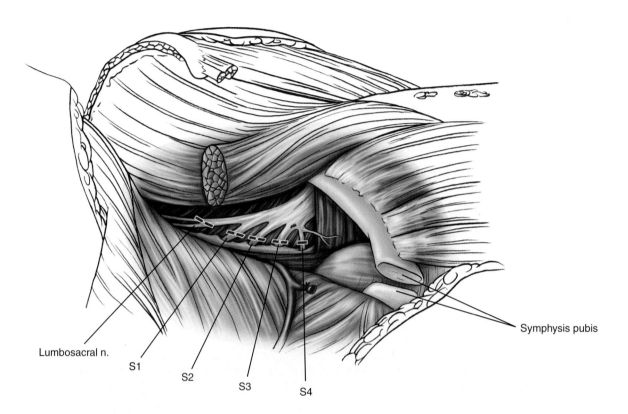

Lumbosacral n.

S1

S2

S3

S4

Symphysis pubis

The lumbosacral nerve and sacral nerves 1 through 4 are visualized on the anterior surface of the levator ani muscle. The femoral nerve is retracted with the
myocutaneous flap, and the psoas muscle is identified and divided under tension. Muscular bleeds are cauterized as they are encountered, or the cut ends
of the psoas muscle may be ligated with 0-silk suture. The lumbosacral nerve
and sacral nerve roots S1 to S4 are transected near the sacral foramina.

The hip is flexed and abducted to place the medial structures of the pelvic
diaphragm under tension. The urethra, bladder, and rectum are protected with
one hand, applying medial and proximal traction on the intrapelvic structures
while the urogenital diaphragm, pubococcygeus, and piriformis muscles are
divided near their pelvic attachments. Attention is then directed posteriorly in
preparation for division of the sacrum. The surgeon moves now to stand posterior to the patient.

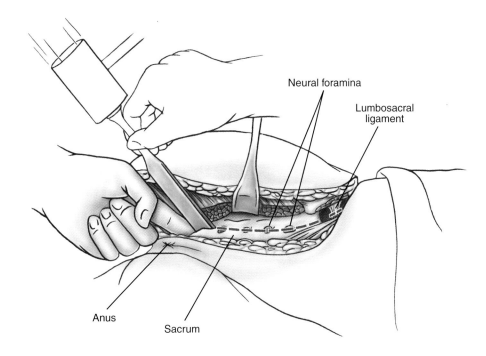

While reaching around the coccyx, the surgeon palpates the S5 neural foramina along the anterior sacrum. An osteotome is used to divide the coccyx and sacrum through the sacral foramina. The lumbosacral ligament extending from the transverse process of L5 to the sacrum is transected, completing the amputation.

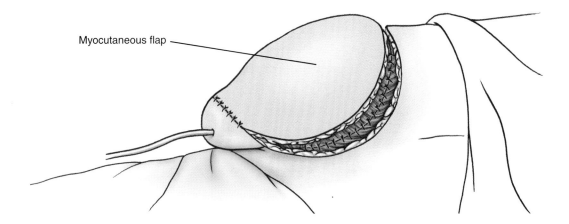

Hemostasis is obtained, and rough or pointed bony prominences are smoothed in preparation for wound closure. Suction drains are placed deep within the wound and brought out through the skin, avoiding the flap. The anterior flap is folded posteriorly with the most distal end oriented toward the most posterior aspect of the defect. The fascia of the quadriceps muscle is reapproximated to the fascia of the anterior abdominal wall, to the quadratus lumborum muscle, the sacrum, and the muscles of the levator ani. The skin and subcutaneous tissue are closed with interrupted sutures.

Partial Pelvic Resection

Partial pelvic resection involves removal of a portion of the innominate bone, with preservation of the lower extremity.

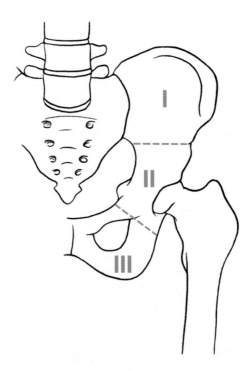

The surgical goal is to obtain a wide surgical margin to control local tumor. Depending on the extent of the soft tissue portion of the tumor, a variable amount of soft tissue is resected with a portion of the resected bone. Based on anatomic, surgical, and functional considerations, the innominate bone can be divided into three parts.

The first part is the iliac wing, extending from the sacroiliac joint to the neck of the ilium just proximal to the acetabulum. The second portion of the innominate bone is the periacetabular portion, which extends from the neck of the ilium to the lateral portion of the pubic rami and includes the ischium. The third portion of the innominate bone extends from the lateral margin of the obturator foramen to the symphysis pubis. Various portions of the innominate bone can be removed singly or in combination. Removal of the first part of the innominate bone is classified as a type I pelvic resection; removal of the second part of the innominate bone a type II pelvic resection; and removal of the third part of the innominate bone a type III pelvic resection. When two portions of the pelvis are resected in combination (e.g., first and second parts of the innominate bone), the resection is classified as a type I/II resection. When all three parts of the innominate bone are resected (type I/II/III) with limb preservation, the procedure is called internal hemipelvectomy. Partial pelvic resections that do not involve the acetabulum (type I and type III) do not usually require any bony reconstruction. When the acetabulum is resected either singly (type II) or in combination with the ilium (type I/II) or pubis (type II/III), reconstruction can be accomplished using a variety of techniques.

Patient positioning and surgical incision depend on the portion of pelvis and soft tissue to be resected. For access to the entire innominate bone, the patient is positioned supine with a sandbag or 3 L fluid bag beneath the lower thoracic spine and the proximal buttock on the affected side to help roll the patient anteriorly during posterior dissection. This "floppy lateral" position allows the patient to be rolled back into a supine position during anterior dissection and forward during posterior dissection. The skin is prepared from the distal aspect of the great toe on the involved side to the level of the xiphoid proximally, and beyond the midline anteriorly and posteriorly. For type III pelvic resections the patient is placed in the supine position.

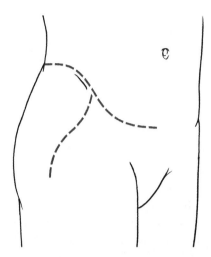

A utilitarian incision that provides access to the inner and outer aspects of the innominate bone and the lower part of the abdomen and hip joint can be used for partial pelvic resection involving the acetabulum and for internal hemipelvectomy. The incision begins at the posteroinferior iliac spine and follows the crest of the ilium to the anterosuperior iliac spine, where it curves to parallel the inguinal ligament to the symphysis pubis. The second arm of the incision begins just anterior to the anterosuperior inferior iliac spine and extends distally with a gentle curve directed posterior to the greater trochanter.

For type I pelvic resection, only the first portion of the incision is needed. Anteriorly the lateral attachment of the inguinal ligament is released, as are Scarpa's fascia, the external oblique aponeurosis, and the internal oblique and transversus abdominis muscles. The femoral vessels are identified distal to the inguinal ligament and protected. The parietal peritoneum is elevated, the inferior epigastic vessels ligated, and the retroperitonem exposed. The femoral nerve is identified and protected, and retracted medially with the abdominal contents. The iliac muscle is identified and transected to expose the inner portion of the iliac wing. The origins of the sartorius, tensor fascia lata, and rectus femoris muscles are divided near their respective origins along the anterosuperior iliac spine, anterior outer lip of the iliac crest, and anteroinferior iliac spine to allow access to the supra–acetabular portion of the iliac wing. Blunt dissection from lateral to medial along the inner table of the iliac wing enables identification of the greater sciatic notch. Attention is directed posteriorly where the origins of the gluteus maximus, medius, and minimus muscles are released from their attachments on the outer surface of the ilium, exposing the greater sciatic notch and the sacroiliac joint posteriorly. The neck of the ilium is transected with a Gigli wire saw. The Gigli wire saw is passed anteriorly to posteriorly around the greater sciatic notch under direct visualization to prevent injury to the superior gluteal nerve. By directing the line of transection from the greater sciatic notch to the anterosuperior iliac spine, the resection will be across the supra–acetabular portion of the pelvis, thereby preserving the hip joint.

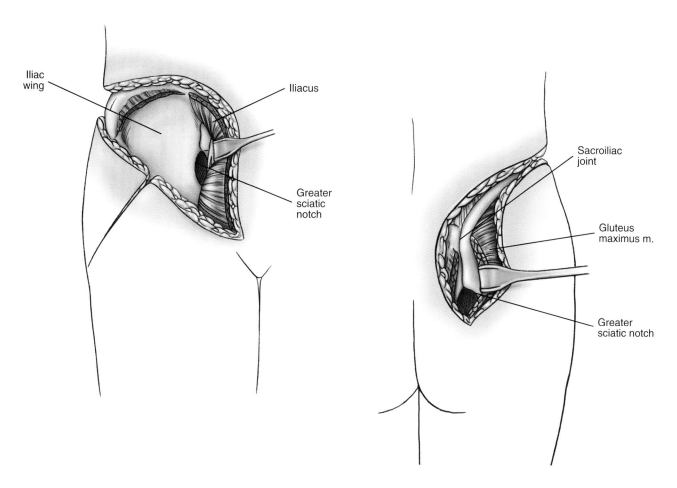

The sacroiliac joint is transected with an osteotome directed from posterior to anterior, with the lumbosacral trunk and sacral roots visualized and protected. The sacrotuberous and sacrospinous ligaments are transected, thereby completely releasing the ilium, which is then removed.

Internal Hemipelvectomy

The utilitarian incision described for partial pelvic resection involving the acetabulum is used for internal hemipelvectomy. In contrast to iliac resection, internal hemipelvectomy involves romoval of the entire innominate bone, from the sacroiliac joint to the symphysis pubis, with limb preservation. The utilitarian incision allows exposure of the entire innominate bone as well as the major motor nerves (femoral and sciatic nerves). The incision begins along the posteroinferior iliac spine and extends to the anterosuperior iliac spine, then continues along the inguinal ligament to the symphysis pubis (as described for type I pelvic resection). To visualize and remove the portion of innominate bone extending from the neck of the ilium to the symphysis pubis, while preserving the femoral and sciatic nerves, a second incision is made. This incision begins just anterior to the anterosuperior inferior iliac spine and extends distally with a gentle curve directed posterior to the greater trochanter. The anterior incision is deepened through skin and subcutaneous tissue, Scarpa's fascia, and the external oblique aponeurosis. The origins of internal oblique and transversus abdominis muscles are cut under tension, and the deep epigastric artery and vein are ligated. The rectus abdominis muscle is released from its insertion, as is the inguinal ligament from its medial and lateral attachments to the pelvis. The round ligament in female patients or the spermatic cord in male patients is identified and protected, and retracted medially. Blunt dissection behind the retroperitoneal fat allows medial retraction of the abdominal contents with the round ligament or spermatic cord and the identification of the iliac vessels and femoral nerve. A large vessel loop is placed around the common iliac vessels to assist with their mobilization.

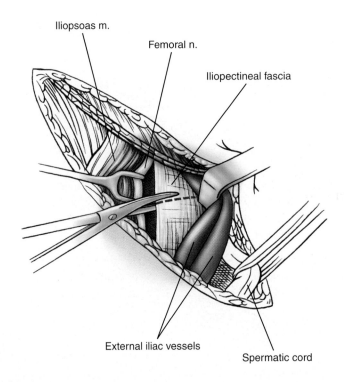

Arising from the medial and lateral aspects of the common femoral artery are the external pudendal and superficial circumflex iliac arteries, which are ligated and divided to allow mobilization of the femoral vessels. The iliopectineal fascia separating the vessels from the iliopsoas muscle and nerve is identified. The vessels are bluntly dissected from the medial aspect of the iliopectineal fascia, thereby preserving the lymphatic vessels. The femoral nerve and iliopsoas muscle are retracted laterally and the iliopectineal fascia incised to the pectineal eminence, thereby further mobilizing the femoral vessels.

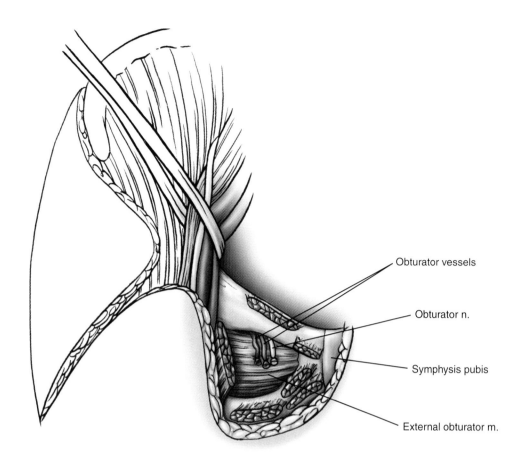

Obturator vessels

Obturator n.

Symphysis pubis

External obturator m.

In some patients an anastomosis between the femoral and obturator vessels exists and should be identified and ligated. The femoral nerve is traced proximally in the groove between the psoas and iliacus. A Penrose drain is repositioned around the psoas muscle along with the neurovascular bundle if the psoas muscle is to be preserved. The neurovascular bundle is retracted laterally, and dissection is continued to expose the adductor muscle origins along the pubic symphysis, pectineal line, pubic tubercle, and outer surface of the inferior pubic ramus. The gracilis, adductor longus, pectineus, adductor brevis, and adductor magnus muscles are released from their insertions on the pelvis. The obturator vessels and nerve, which divide into anterior and posterior branches that run along the anterior and posterior surfaces of the adductor brevis muscle, are transected. The dissection along the anterior and inferior pubic rami continues distally to expose the origin of the obturator externus muscle on the medial margin of the obturator foramen, which is left intact and removed with the specimen. The most posterior fibers of the origin of the adductor magnus muscle arising from the ischial tuberosity cannot be visualized from the anterior incision and are released later in the procedure after the lateral arm of the incision is fully developed.

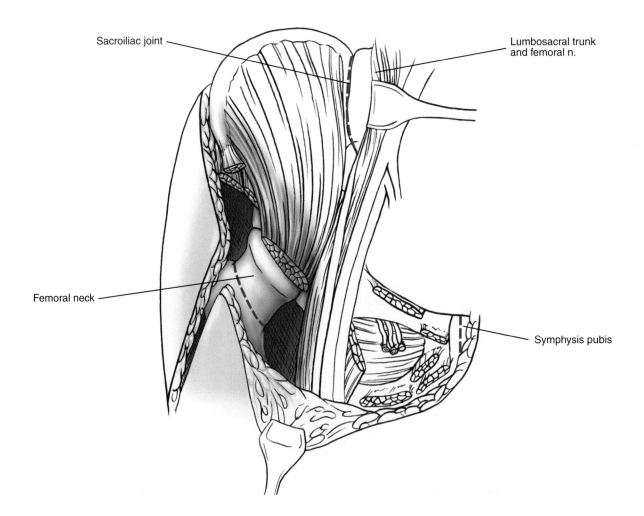

Sacroiliac joint

Lumbosacral trunk
and femoral n.

Femoral neck

Symphysis pubis

The lateral arm of the incision is developed through skin and subcutaneous
tissue. The tensor fascia lata and sartorius muscles along with the straight head
of the rectus femoris muscle are released from their insertions on the anterior
part of the outer lip of the iliac crest and anterosuperior iliac spine, respectively.
The reflected head of the rectus femoris muscle is released from its insertion
on the groove on the upper brim of the acetabulum, exposing the anterior hip
capsule. The capsule is incised to expose the femoral neck. If tumor extends
into the hip joint, the femur is transected at a level distal to the intertrochanteric
line to ensure that the hip joint, is not opened, risking tumor contamination
into the operative field. Alternatively, if tumor does not extend into the hip
joint, an intra-articular resection is carried out either by transecting the femoral
neck or cutting the ligamentum teres. Exposure of the ligamentum teres is facilitated by placing longitudinal traction on the extremity while maintaining
the hip in extension and external rotation. Posteriorly the dissection continues
on top of the surface of the fascia lata and gluteus minimus and medius mus-

cles. The origin of the gluteus maximus muscle from the posterior gluteal line near the sacroiliac joint is divided, exposing the sacroiliac joint. The gluteus maximus muscle is retracted in continuity with the posterior flap. The iliotibial tract is incised, as is the tendinous insertion of the gluteus maximus muscle. The sciatic nerve is identified and retracted posteriorly and medially. The piriformis muscle is divided near its insertion on the upper border of the greater trochanter of the femur, as are the insertions of the gluteus minimus and medius, obturator internus and externus, inferior and superior gemillus, and quadratus femoris muscles from their respective insertions in the proximal femur. The ischial tuberosity is exposed to release the biceps femoris, semitendinosus and semimembranosus muscles, the remaining fibers of the adductor magnus muscle, and the attachment of the sacrotuberous ligament. The bladder and rectum are retracted medially away from the obturator internus muscle. The anterior aspect of the sacroiliac joint is identified along its most proximal portion. The L5 nerve root is identified and retracted medially along with the lumbosacral trunk.

The sacroiliac joint is divided with an osteotome under direct vision with a hand on the opposite side of the joint to ensure proper orientation of the line of transection. The remaining sacrospinous ligament is then transected. The pubic symphysis is divided after identifying the retropubic space of Retzius and protecting the bladder and urethra with either a gloved digit or ribbon retractor. The pelvis is thereby released and the specimen removed. The skin and subcutaneous tissue along with any remaining fascia are closed in layers over drains. Postoperatively the patient is placed in skeletal traction to allow wound healing.

RECONSTRUCTION FOLLOWING INTERNAL HEMIPELVECTOMY

Reconstruction procedures following complete or partial internal hemipelvectomy are designed to maximize function. Generally for partial internal hemipelvectomy in which the acetabulum and hip joint are preserved (types I and III), no reconstructive procedures are needed to maintain reasonable function. For pelvic resection in which the acetabulum is removed (type II), a variety of reconstructive procedures have been described in an attempt to maximize function. Reconstructive options for type II pelvic resections include simple soft tissue closure, pelvic allograft, autoclaved allograft, composite allograft, custom and noncustom endoprosthetic replacement, and iliofemoral and ischiofemoral arthrodesis. In cases where the ischium is sacrificed with the acetabulum but a portion of the ilium can be preserved (types II and III resection), the saddle prosthesis may be a reconstructive option.

Anatomic Basis of Complications

- A high rate of posterior flap necrosis was noted in early reports of hemipelvectomy. Ligation of the external iliac artery, rather than the common iliac artery, was recommended in an effort to preserve blood supply to the posterior flap. We and Karakousis have had no problems with posterior flap necrosis with ligation of the common iliac artery when the gluteal fascia is preserved with the gluteus maximus muscle (see p. 481).

- Postoperative bleeding from the cut edges of bone and muscle may occur. This can be prevented by cutting muscles close to their tendinous origins and insertions whenever possible. When the psoas muscle is transected, Kelly clamps can be placed around the muscle, which is placed under tension, and bleeds are cauterized as they are encountered. The cut ends of the muscle are then ligated with a 0-silk suture (see p. 482). Bone wax is applied to the cut surfaces of bone to minimize bleeding from exposed cut bone surfaces.

- Skin flap necrosis is decidedly rare with anterior flap hemipelvectomy. Viability of the flap is ensured with meticulous attention to maintaining the overlying skin and fascia in continuity with the muscle mass of the quadriceps mechanism.

- Transient sciatic and femoral nerve palsy may result from vigorous traction on the nerve during the procedure. Permanent nerve injury may result from injury to the lumbosacral trunk of the sciatic nerve during division of the sacroiliac joint as the nerve courses over the sacral ala.

- Postoperative extremity swelling may occur as a result of disruption of lymphatic drainage during dissection in the region of the common femoral vessels. This can be minimized by bluntly dissecting the common femoral vessels, along with their lymphatic vessels, from the medial portion of the iliopectineal fascia.

KEY REFERENCES

Chretien PA, Sugarbaker PH. Surgical technique of hemipelvectomy in the lateral position. Surgery 90:900-909, 1981.

The authors describe in detail an orderly sequence of steps used to perform hemipelvectomy. Each portion of the procedure is described in detail with excellent accompanying diagrammatic illustrations. Throughout the article the authors emphasize two important surgical principles: maintaining tissues to be divided under tension and dividing muscles as close to their origin or insertion as possible to minimize blood loss.

Enneking WF, Dunham WK. Resection and reconstruction for primary neoplasms involving the innominate bone. J Bone Joint Surg 60A:731-746, 1978.

The article describes the authors' criteria used to select patients for hemipelvectomy vs. resection (partial or complete internal hemipelvectomy). The types of resection and methods of reconstruction are described, as are the functional outcomes and incidence of local recurrence for the two procedures.

Huth JF, Eckardt JJ, Pignatti G, et al. Resection of malignant bone tumors of the pelvic girdle without extremity amputation. Arch Surg 123:1121-1124, 1988.

The authors review their experience with 53 patients who were evaluated for nonamputative surgery during a 12-year period. Three patients were considered to have unresectable tumor, 17 underwent wide local excision, 27 underwent internal hemipelvectomy, and six underwent classic hemipelvectomy with amputation. The incidence of local recurrence was 11.8% for wide local excision, 7.4% for internal hemipelvectomy, and 33% for classic hemipelvectomy. The authors conclude that internal hemipelvectomy has the advantage of preserving a functional lower extremity, with acceptable hip stability and function.

Mankin HJ, Mankin CJ, Simon MA. The Hazards of Biopsy: The Biopsy, Revisited. For the Members of the Musculoskeletal Tumor Society. J Bone Joint Surg 78A:656-663, 1992.

In a 1982 study the hazards of biopsy in 329 patients with primary malignant musculoskeletal sarcomas showed alarmingly high rates of complications when the biopsy was performed outside the treating institution. Ten years later, in the present study of 597 patients, the authors found that complications, errors, and changes in the patient course and outcome were significantly greater when the biopsy was performed outside of the treating institution. The authors emphasize the importance of planning the biopsy, and recommend that surgeons who are not prepared to proceed with definitive treatment should refer patients with suspected sarcomas to a treating center prior to biopsy.

Simon MA, Biermann JS. Biopsy of bone and soft-tissue lesions. In Schafer M, ed. Instructional Course Lectures: American Academy of Orthopaedic Surgeons, 1994, pp 521-526.

The authors outline the appropriate management of patients with musculoskeletal tumors as it relates to biopsy. Prebiopsy strategy, tissue handling, biopsy site, and techniques are discussed.

SUGGESTED READINGS

Aboulafia AJ, Buch R, Mathews J, et al. Reconstruction using the saddle prosthesis following excision of primary and metastatic periacetabular tumors. CORR 314:203-213, 1995.

Aboulafia AJ, Malawer M. Surgical management of pelvic and extremity osteosarcoma. Cancer 71:3358-3366, 1993.

Ball ABS, Fisher C, Watkins RM, et al. Diagnosis of soft tissue tumors of Tru-cut biopsy. Br J Surg 77:756-758, 1990.

Barth RJ, Merino MJ, Solomon D, et al. A prospective study of the value of core needle biopsy and fine needle aspiration in the diagnosis of soft tissue masses. Surgery 112:536-543, 1992.

deSantos LA, Lukeman JM, Wallace S, et al. Percutaneous needle biopsy of bone in the cancer patient. Am J Roentgenol 130:641-649, 1978.

Dollahite HA, Tatum L, Moinuddin SM, et al. Aspiration biopsy of primary neoplasms of bone. J Bone Joint Surg 71A:1166-1169, 1989.

Eilber FR, Grant TT, Sakai D, et al. Internal hemipelvectomy—Excision of the hemipelvis with limb preservation. An alternative to hemipelvectomy. Cancer 43:806-809, 1979.

Enneking WF, Menendez LR. Functional evaluation of various reconstructions after periacetabular resection of iliac lesions. In Enneking WF, ed. Limb Salvage in Musculoskeletal Oncology. New York: Churchill Livingstone, 1987, pp 117-135.

Harrington KD. The use of hemipelvic allografts or autoclaved grafts for reconstruction after wide resections of malignant tumors of the pelvis. J Bone Joint Surg 74A:331-341, 1992.

Johnson JTH. Reconstruction of the pelvic ring following tumor resection. J Bone Joint Surg 60A:747-751, 1978.

Karakousis CP. The abdominoinguinal incision in limb salvage and resection of pelvic tumors. Cancer 54:2543-2548, 1984.

Karakousis CP, Emrich LJ, Driscoll DL. Variants of hemipelvectomy and their complications. Am J Surg 158:404-408, 1989.

Kearney MM, Soule EH, Ivins JC. Malignant fibrous histiocytoma: A retrospective study of 167 cases. Cancer 45:167, 1980.

Knelson M, Haaga J, Lazarus H, et al. Computed tomography–guided retroperitoneal biopsies. J Clin Oncol 7:1169-1173, 1989.

Kreicbergs A, Bauer HCF, Brosjo O, et al. Cytological diagnosis of bone tumours. J Bone Joint Surg 78B:258-263, 1996.

Lotze MT, Sugarbaker PH. Femoral artery based myocutaneous flap for hemipelvectomy closure: Amputation after failed limb-sparing surgery and radiotherapy. Am J Surg 150:625-629, 1985.

Mazeron JJ, Suit HD. Lymph nodes as sites of metastases from sarcomas of soft tissue. Cancer 60:1800-1808, 1997.

Mink J. Percutaneous bone biopsy in the patient with known or suspected osseous metastases. Radiology 161:141-194, 1986.

Simon MA, Biermann JS. Biopsy of bone and soft-tissue lesions. J Bone Joint Surg 75A:616-621, 1993.

Steel HH. Partial or complete resection of the hemipelvis. An alternate to hindquarter amputation for periacetabular chondrosarcoma of the pelvis. J Bone Joint Surg 60A:719-730, 1978.

Sugarbaker PH, Chreitien PA. Hemipelvectomy for buttock tumors utilizing an anterior myocutaneous flap of quadriceps femoris muscle. Ann Surg 197:106-115, 1983.

Sundaram M, McGuire MH, Herbold DR. Magnetic resonance imaging of osteosarcoma. Skeletal Radiol 16:23-29, 1987.

Walaas L, Kindblom LG. Light and electron microscopic examination of fine-needle aspirates in the preoperative diagnosis of osteogenic tumors: A study of 21 osteosarcomas and two osteoblastomas. Diagn Cytopathol 6:27-38, 1990.

Weingrad DW, Rosenberg SA. Early lymphatic spread of osteogenic and soft-tissue sarcomas. Surgery 84:231-240, 1978.

Zimmer WD, Berquist TH, McLeod RA, et al. Bone tumors: Magnetic resonance imaging versus computed tomography. Radiology 155:709-718, 1985.

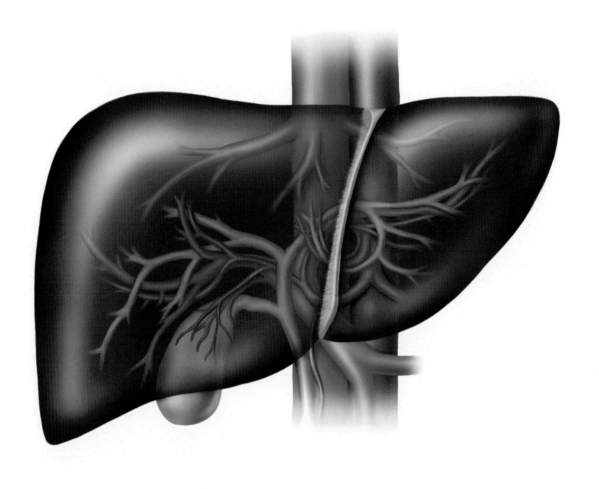

Chapter 12

Liver

George W. Daneker, Jr., M.D.

Surgical Applications

Complete operative resection remains the principal curative treatment of liver metastasis from colorectal carcinomas and of hepatocellular carcinomas with adequate hepatic reserve. The successful emergence of operative therapy has resulted from improvements in imaging and tumor staging, in surgical technique due to better understanding of hepatic anatomy, and in ability to assess hepatic tolerance and maximize hepatic reserve. At present, the 5-year survival rate following successful resection of metastatic colorectal cancer and hepatocellular carcinoma is 25% to 35%, and the operative mortality after resection is less than 5%.

Surgical interventions are also helpful in treating liver metastasis not amenable to resection. Chemotherapeutic agents delivered through the surgically implanted hepatic arterial infusion pump have been used effectively for palliation while preserving quality of life.

Selection of the appropriate therapy in each clinical situation is based on understanding of the biologic behavior of the primary tumor, familiarity with the indications and limitations of each therapeutic modality, and a thorough knowledge of hepatobiliary anatomy and its variations. Although challenging, major hepatic surgery may be performed safely with a well-planned, careful, respectful operative approach. This chapter reviews the surgical management of liver tumors from an anatomic orientation, and includes the clinically relevant anatomy of the liver and hepatobiliary tree, preoperative evaluation of liver malignancies, indications and technical details of anatomic and nonanatomic liver resections, indications and technical details of hepatic arterial infusion pump insertion, and an overview of potential complications.

SURGICAL ANATOMY
Topography

The liver, which is the largest glandular organ in the body, principally occupies the right subcostal and epigastric regions and extends into the left subcostal region and downward into the right lumbar region. It lies directly beneath the diaphragm and is covered by ribs over the majority of its lateral surface. A small part of the liver's anterior surface is in contact with the anterior abdominal wall; the remainder normally lies hidden.

The anterosuperior surface of the liver is convex and molded to the diaphragm but is accessible within the free abdominal cavity. Similarly, the visceral or inferior surface of the liver conforms to the surrounding intra-abdominal organs. The inferior surface is covered by a continuation of the peritoneal lining of the lesser omentum. The interface between abdominal cavity and liver is susceptible to surface implantation of free intra-abdominal tumor, and this must be kept in mind when assessing "superficial" hepatic metastasis.

The right lateral surface of the liver lies beneath the costal margin in the midaxillary line. It rests against the diaphragm and is adjacent to the costodiaphragmatic pleural recess and a portion of the thoracic wall composed of the seventh to eleventh ribs.

The posterior surface of the liver, in contrast to other surfaces, is only partially covered by peritoneum. The peritoneal covering of the anterosuperior, inferior, and lateral surfaces of the liver reflect onto the diaphragm, leaving most of the right lobe's posterior surface and a strip of the left lobe's posterior surface in direct contact with the diaphragm. This "bare area" of the liver is contained within these peritoneal reflections, called the coronary ligaments, and the lateral fusion of the coronary ligaments, called the triangular ligaments. Of surgical significance, the inferior vena cava (IVC) and hepatic veins are fully contained within the liver's bare area.

Functional Hepatic Anatomy

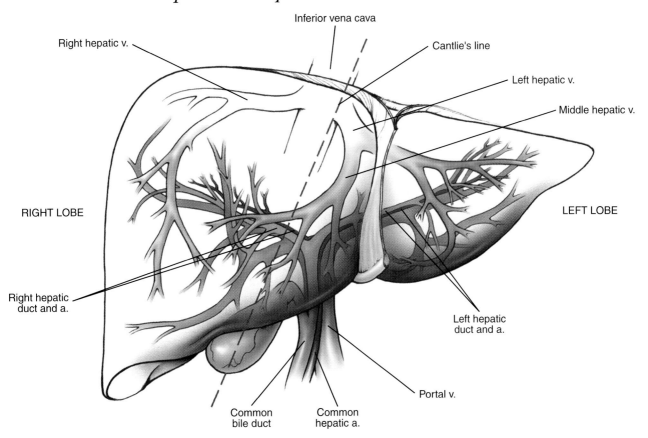

The liver is functionally divided into lobes and segments based on its hepatic arterial blood supply, portal venous blood supply, biliary drainage, and hepatic venous drainage. The major divisions of the liver are the right and left lobe. Each lobe, or more accurately, hemiliver, is defined by the branching of the proper hepatic artery, portal vein, and common bile duct into major right and left subdivisions. The topographic division between these lobes follows a plane (Cantlie's line) that runs vertically through the liver and connects the gallbladder fossa anteriorly to the left side of the IVC posteriorly.

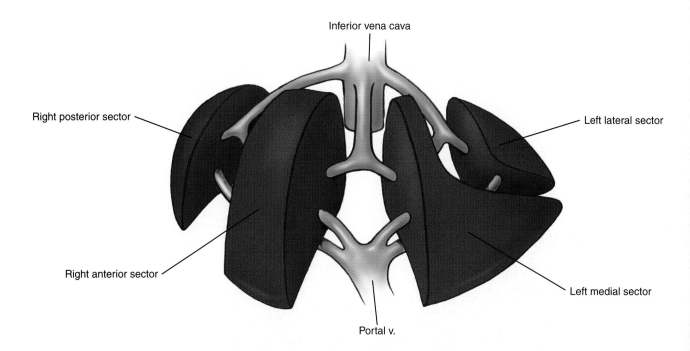

Inferior vena cava

Right posterior sector

Left lateral sector

Right anterior sector

Left medial sector

Portal v.

The right and left lobes can be further subdivided into sectors based on the distribution of the portal pedicles and hepatic veins. The planes of division along each of the three main hepatic veins are called scissura. These scissura are used to divide the liver into four sectors, known as the right anterior, right posterior, left medial, and left lateral sectors, each supplied by a portal pedicle comprised of a major lobar hepatic artery branch, portal vein branch, and bile duct branch. The configuration of right-sided liver sectors is dependent on their surroundings. When the liver is in its normal location in the body, the anterior sector is directly in front of the posterior sector. In contrast, when the liver is splayed out on the dissecting table, the posterior sector is directly lateral to the more medial anterior sector. No clear topographic features or morphologic boundaries exist between the sectors in the right lobe. Within the left lobe, the umbilical fissure and falciform ligament are used to define the plane of division between the medial and lateral sectors. Although this plane of division has been commonly adopted, it is not completely correct.

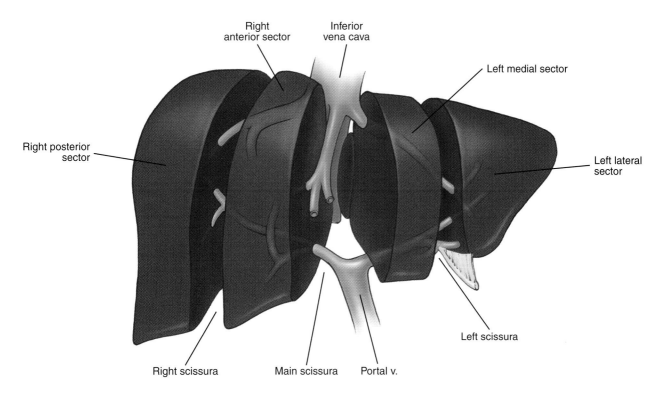

The portal pedicle contents are the main structures within this plane, not the left hepatic vein.

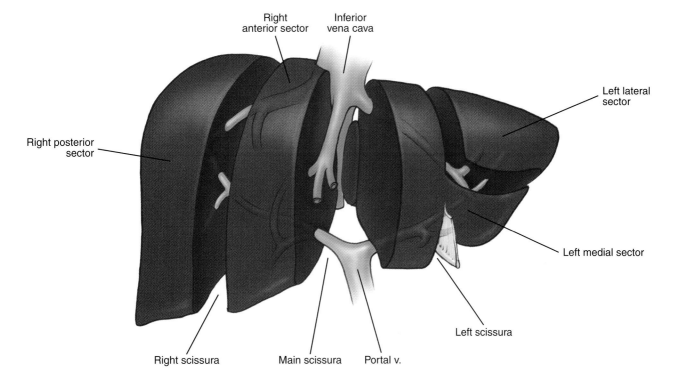

By properly using the scissura, the left lobe is divided into the medial sector that contains segments III and IV and the lateral sector that contains segment II.

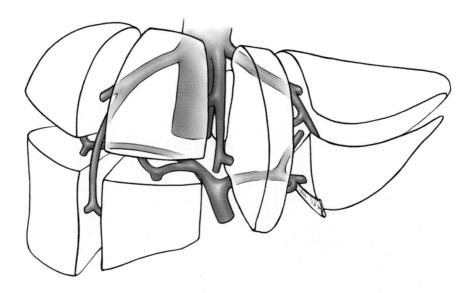

Each hepatic sector can be further subdivided into numbered segments, as described by Couinaud. There are eight liver segments, including the caudate lobe, segment I, which is a separate entity. This segmentation is one step beyond division of the liver into lobes and sectors and is based on the major bifurcation of each portal pedicle within the sectors. The logic of remembering the liver's segmental anatomy is as follows. Clockwise from the vena cava, the first segment encountered is the superiolaterally situated segment II. The more inferiorly situated segment III, together with segment II, comprise the liver to the left of the falciform ligament. Segment IV is the portion of the liver between the falciform ligament and Cantlie's line. Segment IV is often divided into a superior half (segment IV-A) and an inferior half (segment IV-B). Segments V, VI, VII, and VIII make up the right lobe and are labeled according to this clockwise system. Segments V and VIII comprise the right anterior sector, and segments VI and VII comprise the right posterior sector.

Segment I, or the caudate lobe, is considered an autonomous segment from the viewpoint of functional anatomy. This segment receives branches from both hepatic arteries and portal veins, although the majority of the blood supply comes from the left-sided branches. Venous drainage is not through the hepatic veins but through a variable number of branches that drain directly into the IVC.

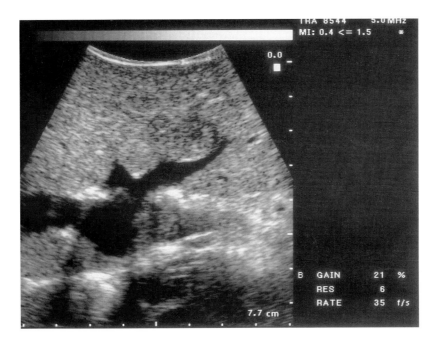

Again, the point must be made that no hepatic topographic features or morphologic boundaries delineate the majority of sectors or segments. The sectoral-segmental anatomy of the liver has practical significance because it can be determined in the operating room with intraoperative ultrasonography. With ultrasound, the surgeon not only can see and mark the exact anatomy but can also examine the hepatic parenchyma for lesions.

Portal Anatomy

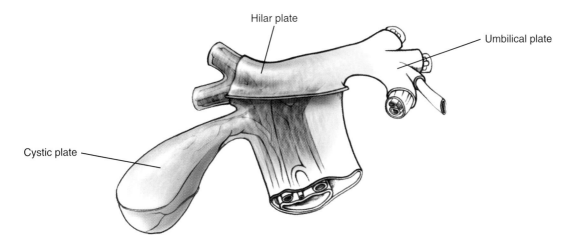

The liver is covered by a thin layer of connective tissue known as Glisson's capsule. This capsule surrounds the parenchyma and extends into the porta hepatis, where it forms sheaths that envelop the bile duct, hepatic artery, and portal vein. At the level of the liver hilum, the capsule and vasobiliary sheaths coalesce and thicken to form a series of fibrous plates that surround the portal structures. Division of these plates is required to gain access for mobilization, control, and division of the portal pedicles during liver resection. The vasobiliary sheaths then continue to invest the intrahepatic portal components up to the level of the sinusoid. This continuation of Glisson's capsule produces a hyperechoic ring around each portal component when visualized with intraoperative ultrasonography. These rings are clinically important because they can be used to differentiate intrahepatic portal structures from the hepatic veins, which have no capsule or fascial covering.

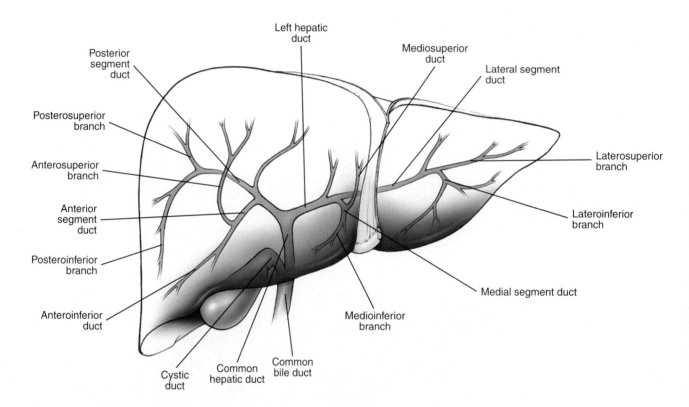

The common hepatic duct branches into the main right and left hepatic ducts at the right side of the liver hilum, anterior to the portal vein bifurcation and overlying the origin of the right main portal trunk. The bifurcation is usually at or above the level of the hilar plate; thus dissection of the hepatic ducts often requires division of the plate and may require intraparenchymal dissection. The right hepatic duct is short and rapidly ascends into the parenchyma after the bifurcation. In 28% of cases, one of the right segmental ducts crosses Cantlie's line to join the main left hepatic duct. Because of its length and orientation, and the variable anatomy of the biliary tree, the right ductal system is more vulnerable to injury during portal dissection. In contrast, the left hepatic duct is longer, with a more horizontal course through the hilum. These features generally contribute to easier dissection with less surgical risk to the left duct.

Blood Supply

The liver receives its blood from two sources: the hepatic artery and the portal vein. The hepatic artery provides 25% of the hepatic blood and half of the oxygen supply, and the portal vein contributes about 75% of the blood and the other half of the oxygen supply. Of all the portal components, the hepatic arterial blood supply is the most variable, with 10 different vascular patterns identified. The most modern description of the blood supply is that of VanDamme and Bonte.

Hepatic Artery Variations

Type I	The right hepatic, midhepatic, and left hepatic arteries are from the celiac artery (55%).
Type II	The right hepatic and the midhepatic are from the celiac artery, replaced left hepatic from the left gastric artery (10%).
Type III	The midhepatic and left hepatic are from the celiac artery, replaced right hepatic from the superior mesenteric artery (11%).
Type IV	The midhepatic is from the celiac artery, replaced right hepatic from the superior mesenteric artery and replaced left hepatic from the left gastric artery (1%).
Type V	The right hepatic, midhepatic, and left hepatic are from the celiac artery, and an accessory left hepatic is from the left gastric artery (8%).
Type VI	The right hepatic, midhepatic, and left hepatic are from the celiac artery, and an accessory right hepatic is from the superior mesenteric artery (7%).
Type VII	The right hepatic, midhepatic, and left hepatic are from the celiac artery, an accessory right hepatic is from the superior mesenteric artery, and an accessory left hepatic is from the left gastric artery (1%).
Type VIII	Patterns are combined. A replaced right hepatic and an accessory left hepatic, and an accessory right hepatic and a replaced left hepatic (2%).
Type IX	Absent celiac hepatic artery. The entire hepatic trunk is from the superior mesenteric artery (4.5%).
Type X	Absent celiac hepatic artery. The entire hepatic trunk is from the left gastric artery (0.5%).
Type X (variant)	Double celiac hepatic arteries (no common hepatic artery). The right hepatic is from the proximal celiac artery, the left hepatic is from the distal end of the celiac artery.

From Michels NA. Newer anatomy of the liver and its variant blood supply and collateral circulation. Am J Surg 112:337-347, 1966, with permission from Excerpta Medica, Inc.

The frequency of arterial variability mandates the need for celiac artery and superior mesenteric artery (SMA) arteriograms prior to liver resection or intra-arterial pump insertion. Typically, the proper hepatic artery divides into the main right and left lobar branches within the porta hepatis outside the liver parenchyma. Usually the proper hepatic artery branches lower in the porta than does the bile duct or portal vein. A middle hepatic branch usually arises from the proximal left hepatic artery.

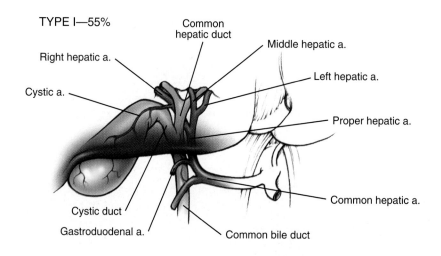

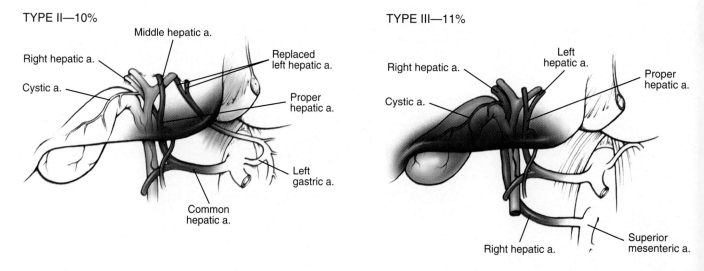

This variation of arterial anatomy, known as type I, is the most common and occurs in 55% of patients. Two other common variations are type III (11%), in which the main right hepatic artery arises from the SMA and is situated in the posterolateral porta, and type II (10%), in which the main left hepatic artery arises from the left gastric artery and travels into the liver in the proximal gastrohepatic ligament, and the middle hepatic artery arises from the proximal right hepatic artery. Within the liver, arteries follow the course of the bile ducts, dividing into anterior and posterior branches within the right lobe and into medial and lateral branches within the left lobe.

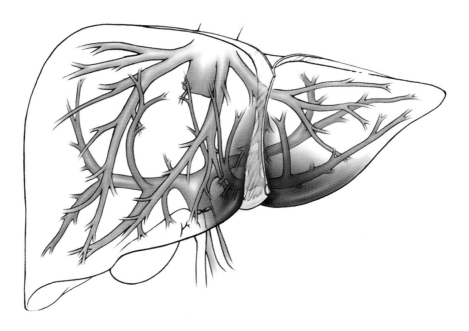

Portal Vein

The portal vein and its branches are the least variable components of the porta hepatis. The portal vein is the most posterior portal structure, situated beneath the bile ducts and hepatic artery. Like the right hepatic duct, the main right portal vein is short and branches soon after it ascends into the parenchyma. The left main portal branch, also like the left duct, is relatively long and has a predictable horizontal course through the liver.

Hepatic Veins

The hepatic veins arise from the IVC as it emerges from the liver immediately below the diaphragm. These veins have a short extrahepatic course before they enter the scissura, dividing the liver into sectors. The right hepatic vein is usually single and drains the anterior and posterior sectors of the right lobe. In 61% of patients the right hepatic vein has no branches for a distance of 1 cm from its origin on the vena cava. In these patients, extrahepatic division of the vein prior to transection of the liver may be contemplated. In 61% of patients there is an additional one or two large veins draining from the posterior or posteroinferior right lobe directly into the infrahepatic vena cava. These branches must be ligated during mobilization of the right lobe from the infrahepatic cava. The middle hepatic vein runs along Cantlie's line and drains the right anterior and left medial sectors. The left hepatic vein drains the left lateral sector and a small portion of the left medial sector. In 84% of patients the left and middle hepatic veins arise from a common trunk. The bifurcation of the common trunk into the left and middle veins usually occurs within 1 cm of its origin from the vena cava. With the frequency of the common trunk and difficulty with proximal control, ligation of the left and middle hepatic veins prior to transection of the liver generally should be avoided.

SURGICAL APPLICATIONS

When metastasis from colorectal carcinoma or a hepatoma has been diagnosed, treatment decisions are made following sequential evaluation for the presence of extrahepatic tumor and the extent of intrahepatic tumor. The initial evaluation consists of a thorough history, physical examination, and laboratory studies including liver transaminases, alkaline phosphatase, and albumin levels, and prothrombin and partial thromboplastin times. This evaluation is designed to screen for the presence and severity of liver diseases such as chronic hepatitis and liver dysfunction from coexisting diseases or tumor burden. Tumor markers such as carcinoembryonic antigen (CEA) and alpha-fetoprotein are checked as an indirect reflection of tumor volume and as a baseline to follow after therapy. A chest x-ray film is obtained to look for pulmonary disease, including metastasis. The most definitive initial liver studies are computed tomography (CT) scans of the abdomen. While the current generation of scanners provides as sensitive and specific a routine study as possible, there remain weaknesses, especially with detection of peritoneal and regional nodal metastasis. Following this battery of studies, patients with a good performance status, good hepatic function, well-controlled comorbid diseases, no evidence of extrahepatic tumor, four or fewer metastases, and metastasis or hepatoma without prohibitive vascular encroachment or invasion are further considered as candidates for resection. These patients then undergo celiac and SMA angiography, followed by CT arteriography and portography. Standard arteriography provides a road map for resection as well as a guide for placement of a hepatic arterial infusion catheter when resection is not feasible. CT angioportography is used because it is more sensitive than routine CT for detection of intrahepatic tumors and provides more information about the relationship of tumor to intrahepatic vascular structures. The usefulness of CT angioportography in patients with cirrhosis can be limited by the heterogeneous liver perfusion patterns resulting from fibrosis. Magnetic resonance imaging (MRI) with or without vascular contrast medium can be used in these patients; the general role of MRI for staging the liver continues to expand with recent technological improvements. If after these studies the patient continues to meet criteria as mentioned for liver resection, the procedure is scheduled.

Lateral "segmentectomy"

"Trisegmentectomy"
(including segment IV)

Left lobectomy

Right lobectomy

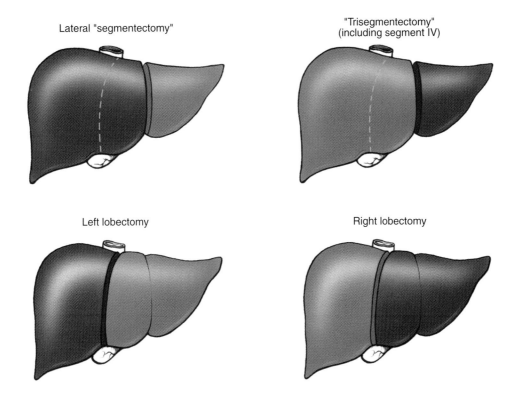

Liver resection can be classified as either anatomic or nonanatomic. Anatomic resections follow defined anatomic features and involve removal of a lobe, sector, or segment. The four major types of anatomic resections, in addition to segmental resections, are the right lobectomy, left lobectomy, resection of the right lobe and the medial segment (segment IV) of the left lobe (trisegmentectomy), and resection of the lateral segments (segments II and III) of the left lobe. Nonanatomic resections are based on tumor location and can cross anatomic boundaries. The determination of segmental anatomy is important prior to nonanatomic resection, but tumors are rarely confined solely within a single segment (other than segment I), nor is formal segmental resection often required to obtain the desired 1 to 2 cm margin. In general, anatomic resections have not been associated with superior survival rates, compared with nonanatomic resections. Thus we currently use the resection technique that will permit complete removal of the tumor or tumors with a 1 to 2 cm margin of normal liver.

Some colorectal cancer metastases strictly limited to the liver are not resectable. When the preoperative studies, particularly CT angioportography, clearly show more than four metastases or metastasis encroaching on both right and left main portal trunks, hepatic arterial infusion chemotherapy is an optimal palliative alternative. At present, hepatic arterial infusion therapy has up to a 75% response rate, which is significantly better than the response rates from systemic chemotherapy. The improvement in patient survival with hepatic arterial infusion therapy, compared with systemic chemotherapy, trends toward significance when data from randomized trials are reviewed by meta-analysis. This trend is present despite problems in trial design where treatment crossover from systemic chemotherapy to hepatic arterial infusion therapy arms was allowed.

Right Hepatic Lobectomy

Right hepatic lobectomy involves removal of liver segments V, VI, VII, and VIII, which comprise the right hemiliver. Indications are four or fewer lesions within the right lobe where (1) resection requires sacrifice of major portal structures or major portal structures and hepatic vein, or (2) metastases are scattered within the lobe and cannot be fully encompassed with a nonanatomic or segmental resection.

Incision and Exposure

The patient is supine on the operating table with the arms extended. For larger patients, a folded sheet is placed transversely across the back at the level of the lower ribs. The full abdomen and chest up to the sternal notch is prepared and draped into the field. During the initial exploration, an incision is made two fingerbreadths below the right costal margin. Through this limited incision a thorough exploration of the abdomen, including close examination of the liver and portal structures, is conducted. An enlarged lymph node in the porta adjacent to the duodenum and posterior to the common bile duct is often found. This node is routinely sent for frozen-section analysis, and the procedure is terminated if it contains metastatic cancer. If no extrahepatic tumor or more extensive intrahepatic tumor is detected, a generous bilateral subcostal (chevron) incision is made. The right arm of the incision is extended toward the flank to the lateral peritoneal reflection. The left arm of the incision is extended as far beyond the left lateral rectus sheath as will allow easy access to the left upper quadrant structures. For large, bulky tumors a paraxiphoid midline extension (the Mercedes-Benz incision) is helpful for gaining access to the suprahepatic vena cava and hepatic veins. A thoracoabdominal incision may be contemplated for large posterior right lobe tumors, but in our experience this incision has been rarely needed.

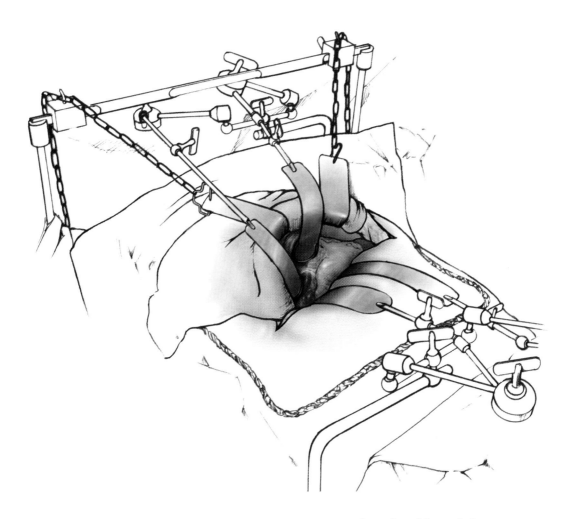

After the incision is made, exposure is secured with self-retaining retractors. Goligher-type or chain retractors provide constant upward and lateral retraction of the costal margin, giving excellent access to all surfaces of the liver. These retractors are suspended from a frame anchored to the operating table at the level of the patient's chin. Two double-jointed octopus-type self-retaining retractors are also used. One retractor is anchored at the level of the Goligher frame so that it can provide upward traction on the liver, and a second is positioned at the level of the patient's hips to provide downward traction on the intra-abdominal viscera.

Mobilization and Assessment of Resectability

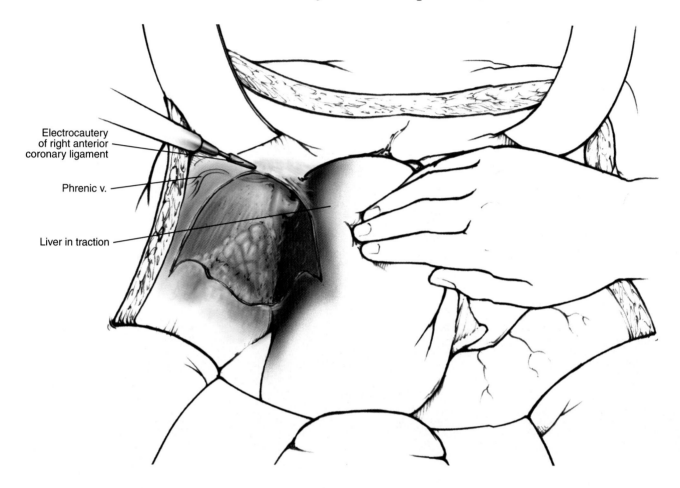

Electrocautery of right anterior coronary ligament

Phrenic v.

Liver in traction

The falciform ligament is divided halfway between the abdominal wall and the liver so that it can be reapproximated at the completion of the resection. While the first assistant exerts gentle clockwise traction on the liver, the right triangular, right anterior, and right posterior coronary ligaments are divided medially to the level of the IVC. As these ligaments are divided the liver can be carefully rotated anteriorly and to the left, exposing the right adrenal gland, the bare area, and the retrohepatic IVC. If the diaphragm is adherent to the liver in the vicinity of the tumor, it should be resected en bloc with the right lobe. If necessary, the left triangular and coronary ligaments are divided, taking care to prevent injury to the phrenic vein. Transverse division of the peritoneum over the suprahepatic IVC is completed and the hepatic veins are identified. There usually are no vessels contained within the ligaments and bare area of the liver, so the preceding dissection is relatively bloodless. Following mobilization of the liver, thorough inspection and bimanual palpation more clearly shows the relationship of the tumor or tumors to the adjacent landmarks and key structures. The liver is now examined with intraoperative ultrasound for number, size, and location of tumors and for vascular anatomy.

Venous Dissection

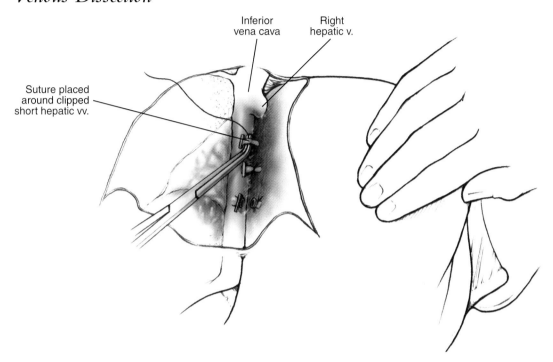

Mobilizing the liver from the IVC commences with the veins at the inferior surface of the liver. While the liver is retracted anteriorly and to the left, two to 12 pairs of short hepatic veins extending from the anterior surface of the IVC are encountered. These veins are fragile and can result in troublesome bleeding if not ligated carefully. Our preferred method is ligature in continuity with 3-0 silk sutures, followed by placement of a small hemoclip on the caval side prior to scalpel transection. Occasionally a large inferior hepatic vein, often near the main right hepatic vein, is encountered. Care should be taken to avoid confusing the inferior hepatic vein with the main hepatic vein. This vein is divided between vascular clamps and oversewn with a running 4-0 Prolene suture. The suture is placed in two layers, with a deeper horizontal mattress suture run in one direction and an over-and-over stitch incorporating the cut edge of the vein in the other direction. Access to the short hepatic veins on the left side of the midline is improved by division of the gastrohepatic ligament and mobilization of the caudate lobe from the IVC by division of its peritoneal attachments.

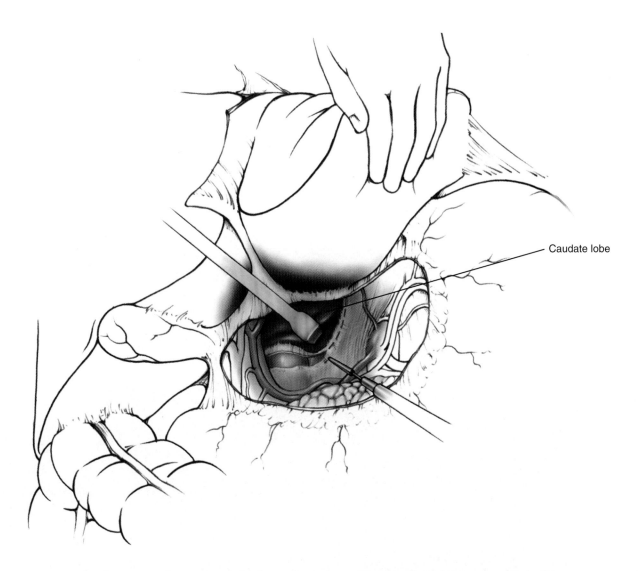

Caudate lobe

Just inferior to the main right hepatic vein, a fibrotic ligament extending from the caudate lobe to segment VII is encountered. Careful division of this structure is necessary to adequately visualize the main right hepatic vein.

Extrahepatic division of the hepatic veins prior to parenchymal transection remains controversial. In general, we believe that hemostasis is better and resection of posterior tumor near the hepatic veins is safer if the right hepatic vein is divided prior to parenchymal transection. These advantages are not compelling enough to warrant a risky and potentially fatal maneuver if the circumstances are not ideal. Ideal circumstances are clear visualization of at least 1 cm of the superior and inferior border of the right hepatic vein as it enters the liver parenchyma.

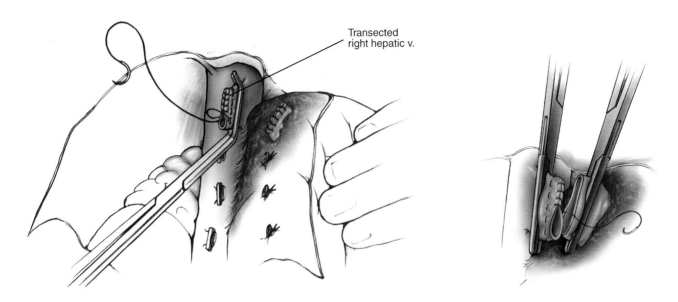

Once this extent of visualization has been achieved by careful dissection with a large blunt right-angled clamp, the vein is divided between vascular clamps and the ends oversewn, as described above, with a running 3-0 Prolene suture. If extrahepatic division of the vein is not possible, careful blunt dissection above and behind the liver usually allows encirclement and control of the vein with a Rommel tourniquet. In this situation and when the vein is not controlled outside the liver, the main right hepatic vein is divided within the parenchyma near the last step in the transection.

Portal Dissection

With the preoperative mesenteric angiogram on hand, the portal peritoneum is divided longitudinally over the anteriorly placed hepatic artery. The proper hepatic artery is dissected up to and slightly beyond the bifurcation where the cystic artery is identified, ligated, and divided as it courses to the right. Dissection of the lateral leaf of portal peritoneum proceeds laterally to where the common bile duct and cystic duct are identified. The cystic duct is divided and the gallbladder dissected from its bed in either an antegrade or retrograde fashion. Although cholecystectomy is not mandatory, it usually greatly improves access to the portal structures, especially the bile ducts. The medial leaf of portal peritoneum is then dissected, giving clear access to the common hepatic and proper hepatic arteries. Attention is turned to the common bile duct, which is dissected up to the liver. Division of the hepatic plate is usually necessary to visualize the bifurcation and the proximal right and left hepatic ducts. Dissection on the distal common duct is kept predominantly to the right side of this structure so that injury to the proximal left duct and crossing segmental ducts may be prevented. Dissection of the bile ducts is usually the most tedious and technically difficult step of portal dissection. For this reason, extrahepatic division of the bile ducts may be readily abandoned and these structures controlled during parenchymal transection. If division of the main right hepatic duct is possible, care is taken to identify segmental ducts passing from right to left, which are individually ligated and divided. The proximal right hepatic duct is doubly ligated with 2-0 Vicryl ties, then divided clearly away from the bifurcation.

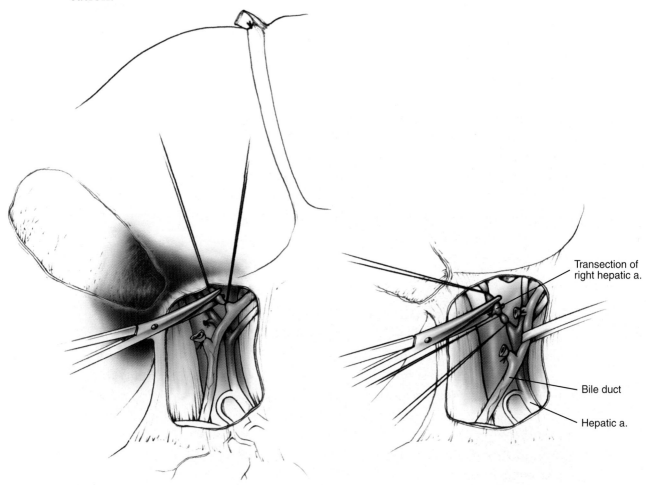

After accurate identification of the arterial anatomy, the proximal right hepatic artery is triply ligated with ties and a proximal suture ligature of 2-0 silk, then divided. In the type III variant of arterial anatomy, the right hepatic artery is identified and divided in the right posterolateral porta as it courses up from the SMA. The common duct is then retracted to the right, and the hepatic artery retracted to the left, giving access to the posteriorly placed portal vein.

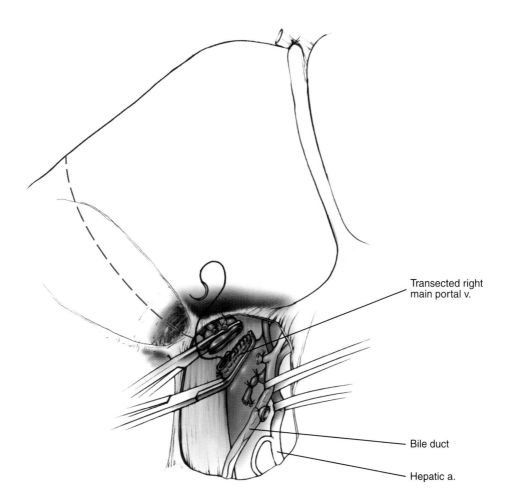

Transected right
main portal v.

Bile duct

Hepatic a.

The right main portal vein is dissected proximally to the bifurcation and distally to the anterior segment branch. At least 1 cm of main right portal vein is dissected free before it is divided between vascular clamps clearly away from the bifurcation. Both ends of the divided vein are oversewn with a running 3-0 Prolene suture as described above. After division of the portal vein a clear line of demarcation should be seen between the devitalized right lobe and perfused left lobe. The portal structures, exclusive of the common duct, are then encircled with a Rommel tourniquet to provide vascular isolation should it be needed during the parechymal transection.

Parenchymal Transection

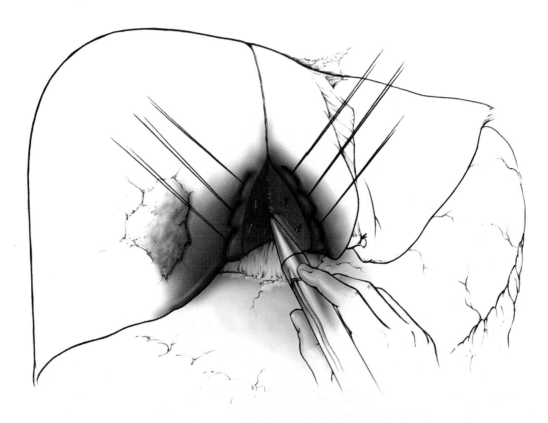

The capsule of the liver is scored with an electrocautery at the line of demarcation between the lobes. No. 1 chromic horizontal mattress sutures on a blunt liver needle, incorporating 2 to 3 cm of liver parenchyma per suture, are placed extending inward from the anterior edge 4 to 6 cm for traction and exposure. The liver parenchyma is then divided using short "brush strokes" of the ultrasonic dissector, leaving the intraparenchymal vascular structures intact. Structures smaller than 0.5 mm are controlled with electrocautery, those 0.5 to 1.5 mm with hemoclips, and structures larger than 1.5 mm with ties or suture ligatures. Division of the parenchyma should proceed at a steady, controlled pace to prevent unnecessary blood loss. The parenchyma should be transected over a broad front, with the surgeon ever cognizant of the location of the tumor or tumors and major structures, especially the left portal pedicle. As work proceeds toward the dome of the liver, the middle hepatic vein or its larger branches will be encountered in or to the left of the plane of transection. Care should be taken to preserve this structure.

Vascular isolation via portal occlusion is commonly, albeit not invariably, used during parenchymal transection. If troublesome bleeding occurs, especially from arterial collaterals, vascular isolation allows dissection in a relatively bloodless field. Although the normal liver will tolerate continuous occlusion for up to 90 minutes, we routinely occlude inflow for 15 to 20 minutes followed by a 2- to 3-minute "rest" period. In patients with parenchymal disease we attempt to avoid vascular isolation if possible. If vascular isolation is necessary, we strictly adhere to 15-minute occlusion and 5-minute rest cycles.

Once the parenchyma has been transected and the specimen removed, additional hemostasis is achieved with the argon beam coagulator. Major vascular structures, especially biliary, along the line of transection are carefully examined and additional sutures placed as needed. The specimen is then hand carried to the pathology suite and oriented for examination of the gross and microscopic margins. The resected surface is drained with one large sump drain placed above and a second large sump drain below the edge of the liver. If mobile, the omentum is draped over and tacked to the resected edge of the liver. The falciform ligament is then reconstructed to avoid portal torsion. The abdomen is closed in two layers with a No. 1 monofilament suture.

Left Hepatic Lobectomy

Left hepatic lobectomy involves removal of liver segments II, III, and IV, which comprise the left hemiliver. Indications are four or fewer lesions within the left lobe where (1) resection requires sacrifice of major portal structures or major portal structures and hepatic veins, or (2) metastases are scattered within the lobe and cannot be fully encompassed with a nonanatomic or segmental resection.

Incision and Exposure

Incision and exposure are identical as for right hepatic lobectomy (see pp. 518 and 519).

Mobilization and Assessment of Resectability

The falciform ligament is divided so that it can be reapproximated at the completion of the resection. With the operating surgeon exerting gentle anterior and clockwise traction on the left lobe, the left triangular and the commonly

fused left coronary ligaments are divided medially to the level of the suprahepatic IVC. If the diaphragm is adherent to the liver in the vicinity of the
tumor it should be resected en bloc with the left lobe. As the dissection approaches the IVC, care should be taken to prevent injury to the phrenic vein,
particularly as it empties into the left hepatic vein. Division of the peritoneum
over the suprahepatic IVC is completed and the left and middle hepatic veins
are identified. At this point, mobilization of the right lobe is begun if necessary. The most common indication for mobilization of both lobes is a posteriorly located tumor or tumors lying close to the hepatic veins or IVC.

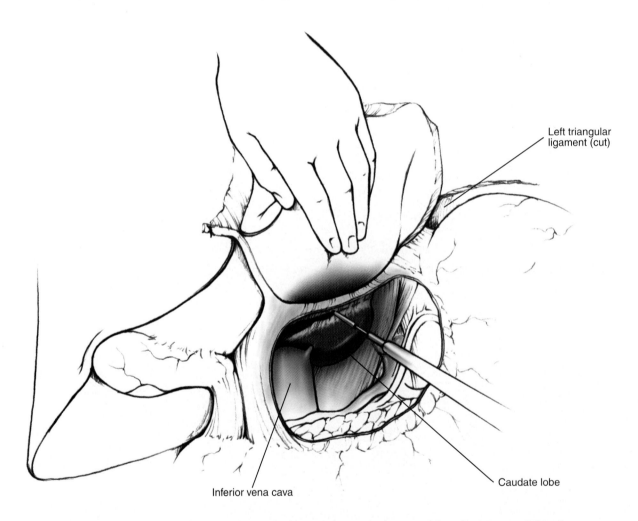

Left triangular
ligament (cut)

Inferior vena cava

Caudate lobe

Access to the line of parenchymal transection is improved by division of the fibrous attachments between the caudate lobe and segments II and III. After mobilization of the liver, thorough inspection and bimanual palpation will more
clearly show the relationship of the tumor to the adjacent key structures. The
liver is then examined with intraoperative ultrasound.

Venous Dissection

Access to the infrahepatic IVC and medial porta is obtained by division of the gastrohepatic ligament. Exposure of the vena cava is not routinely necessary but can be achieved as described for right hepatic lobectomy. Although extrahepatic division of the right hepatic vein is frequently attempted, we discourage extrahepatic division of the left hepatic vein prior to parenchymal transection. Reasons for this recommendation are the complexity of obtaining safe control of a short common trunk with a major venous bifurcation, and control of two closely approximated major venous trunks.

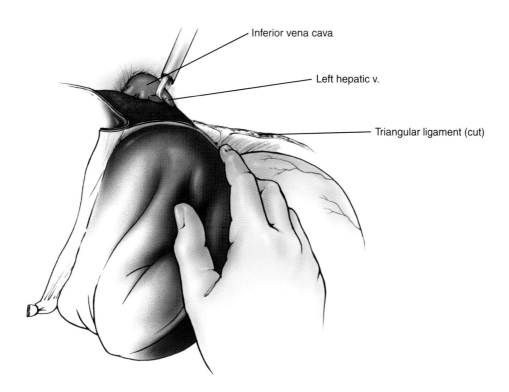

Very careful blunt dissection above and behind the liver can allow encirclement and control of the vein with a Rommel tourniquet; however, this move should be abandoned at the slightest indication of difficulty. The most common method of venous control is intraparenchymal division of the left hepatic vein at the completion of the resection. Not only is this method safer and easier, but it reduces the chance of major damage to the middle hepatic vein. Preservation of the middle hepatic vein is desirable but not critical for survival of the right lobe. Ligation of the divided left hepatic vein stump with a running 3-0 Prolene suture is as described for the right hepatic vein.

Portal Dissection

With the preoperative mesenteric angiogram on hand, the portal peritoneum is divided longitudinally over the anteriorly placed hepatic artery. The proper hepatic artery is dissected up to and slightly beyond the bifurcation where the cystic artery is identified and divided. Dissection of the lateral leaf of portal peritoneum then proceeds laterally to where the common bile duct is identified and the cystic duct is divided. The gallbladder is dissected from its bed in either an antegrade or retrograde fashion. The medial leaf of the portal peritoneum is dissected to the left, giving clear access to the common hepatic and proper hepatic arteries. Attention is turned to the common bile duct, which is dissected up to the liver. Dissection on the distal common duct is kept predominantly to the left side of this structure so that injury to the proximal right duct may be prevented. Dissection of the bile ducts is usually the most technically difficult step of the portal dissection; however, a long segment of the left hepatic duct passes horizontally within the hepatic plate, making it more amenable to safe extrahepatic division than the right duct.

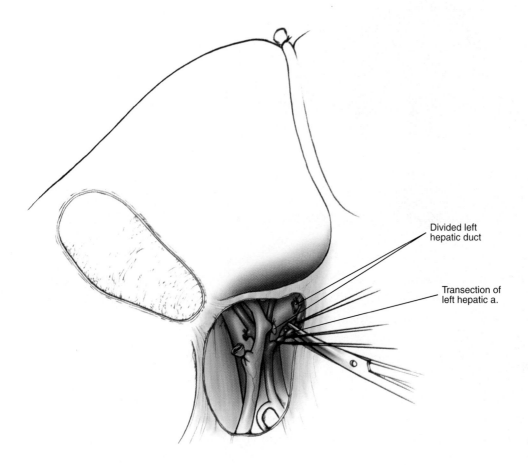

Divided left
hepatic duct

Transection of
left hepatic a.

If division of the left duct is possible, care is taken to identify segmental ducts passing from right to left and the duct is divided distal to these branches. The proximal left hepatic duct is doubly ligated with 2-0 Vicryl ties, then divided clearly away from the bifurcation. After accurate conformation of the arterial anatomy, the proximal left hepatic artery is triply ligated with ties and a proximal 2-0 silk suture ligature, then divided. In the type II variant of arterial anatomy, the main left hepatic artery is identified and divided within the proximal gastroduodenal ligament. The common duct and the hepatic artery are retracted to the right, giving access to the posteriorly placed portal vein.

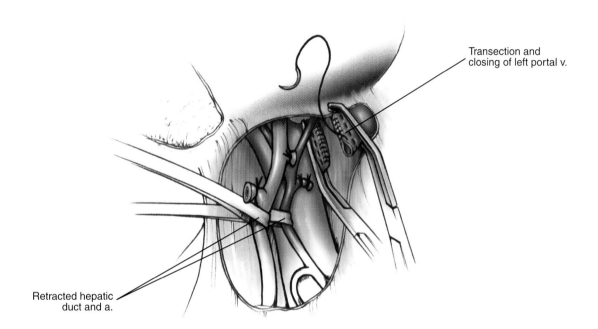

Transection and
closing of left portal v.

Retracted hepatic
duct and a.

The left portal vein is dissected proximally to the bifurcation of the main right and left trunks and distally so that at least 1 cm of the main left portal vein is free. The vein is then divided between vascular clamps clearly away from the bifurcation. Both ends of the divided vein are oversewn with a running 3-0 Prolene suture as described above. Following division of the portal vein a clear line of demarcation between the devitalized left lobe and perfused right lobe should be seen. The portal structures, exclusive of the common duct, are then encircled with a Rommel tourniquet.

Parenchymal Transection

The liver parenchyma is divided using the ultrasonic aspirator, as described for right hepatic lobectomy. Care should be taken to preserve the middle hepatic vein by creating the line of transection lateral to it. The course of the middle vein has no topographic features but can be delineated by the use of intraoperative ultrasound.

Resection of Right Hepatic Lobe Plus Medial Segment (IV) of Left Lobe (Trisegmentectomy)

Trisegmentectomy involves removal of liver segments IV, V, VI, VII, and VIII. The major indications are four or fewer lesions within the right lobe and segment IV where (1) resection requires sacrifice of the major right portal structures or major portal structures and hepatic veins, or (2) metastases are scattered within the right lobe and segment IV and cannot be fully encompassed in with a nonanatomic or segmental resection. Trisegmentectomy involves removal of 75% of the liver parenchyma and should be reserved for patients with normal livers and excellent overall liver function. Over time, the parenchymal mass will be reconstituted by hepatocytes in the remaining segments II and III.

Incision and Exposure

Incision and exposure are as described for right hepatic lobectomy (see pp. 518 and 519).

Mobilization and Assessment of Resectability

The liver is mobilized and assessed as described for right hepatic lobectomy (see pp. 520 and 521).

Venous Dissection

Venous dissection in left hepatic lobectomy is similar to that in right hepatic lobectomy. Dissection of the entire retrohepatic IVC from the caudate lobe is necessary. This dissection is aided by approaching the IVC both laterally, rotating the liver anteriorly and to the left, and medially, through the gastrohepatic omentum, rotating the liver anteriorly and to the right. Attempts are made at extraparenchymal division of the right hepatic vein. Very cautious attempts are made at encirclement and control of the middle and left hepatic veins; however, a safer approach is to identify these vessels and divide the middle hepatic vein within the parenchyma at the completion of the transection. Prevention of injury to the left hepatic vein is absolutely critical to the viability of the remaining left lobe.

Portal Dissection

Portal dissection in left hepatic lobectomy is as described for right hepatic lobectomy (see pp. 523 to 525).

Parenchymal Transection

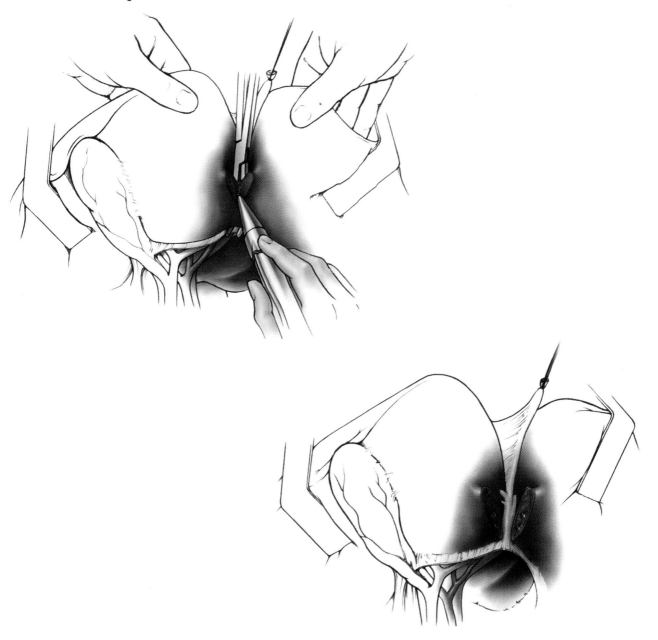

The parenchyma is transected 0.5 to 1.0 cm to the right of the falciform ligament with the ultrasonic aspirator. Transection is begun by dividing the tissue
bridge joining the left lateral sector to segment IV at the lower end of the umbilical fissure. With this bridge divided it is possible to identify and divide vessels passing to segment IV in the umbilical fissure. Because the line of transection passes through the perfused left lobe, vascular isolation is normally used.
Other technical details are as described for right hepatic lobectomy.

Resection of Lateral Segments II and III of Left Lobe

Left lateral segmentectomy involves removal of liver segments II and III. The indications are four or fewer lesions within the left lateral sector (1) where resection requires sacrifice of the sectoral portal pedicle or left hepatic vein, or (2) metastases are scattered within the sector and cannot be fully encompassed in a nonanatomic or segmental resection.

Incision and Exposure

Incision and exposure are as described for right hepatic lobectomy (see pp. 518 and 519).

Mobilization and Assessment of Resectability

The liver is mobilized and assessed as described for right hepatic lobectomy (see pp. 520 and 521). The gastrohepatic omentum is fully divided. The right lobe is not mobilized.

Venous Dissection

The phrenic vein, left hepatic vein, and junction of the left hepatic vein with the IVC are identified. No attempt at extrahepatic control of the left hepatic vein is needed. The IVC is not mobilized from the liver.

Portal Dissection

The common bile duct is dissected free from the remaining portal structures. A Rommel tourniquet is placed around the portal structures, excluding the common duct. Vascular isolation is usually necessary during parenchymal transection.

Parenchymal Transection

The bridge of tissue at the lower end of the umbilical fissure is divided. A line of transection 0.5 to 1.0 cm to the left of the falciform ligament is scored on the liver. No. 1 chromic horizontal mattress sutures on a blunt liver needle are placed 1 cm lateral to the line of transection as far posteriorly as can be done with ease. This move should control the portal pedicles to segments II and III. Transection is then performed with the ultrasonic aspirator. At the superior border of the transection the main left hepatic vein is identified and divided. Other technical details are as described for lobectomy.

Nonanatomic Resections

Nonanatomic resections were originally designed to optimally preserve functioning hepatic parenchyma in the cirrhotic patient with a hepatoma. Such resections have subsequently been shown to diminish morbidity and mortality, without affecting survival, in patients with normal livers undergoing resection of metastasis. The indications for nonanatomic resections are (1) four or fewer lesions where resection does not require sacrifice of a major portal branch or major portal branch and hepatic vein; (2) a confined distribution of four or fewer lesions that can be fully resected in a nonanatomic or segmental resection; or (3) a bilobar distribution of four or fewer lesions that can be fully resected in a nonanatomic or segmental resection.

Incision and Exposure

Incision and exposure are as described for right hepatic lobectomy (see pp. 518 and 519).

Mobilization and Assessment of Resectability

The need for mobilization of the hepatic lobes is dictated by the size and location of the tumor. In general, we err on the side of more mobilization, because lack of mobility may jeopardize recovery from technical problems, particularly bleeding. The technical details of liver mobilization are as described for the right and left hepatic lobectomies. Assessment of resectability is based on both bimanual palpation and intraoperative ultrasonography.

Venous Dissection

Dissection of the IVC and hepatic veins is rarely needed. Division of the peritoneum over the suprahepatic IVC with identification of the hepatic veins is helpful when resecting posterior tumors. Identification and ligation of hepatic vein branches is completed during parenchymal division.

Portal Dissection

No formal dissection or division of the portal structures is necessary. A Rommel tourniquet is placed around the porta, excluding the common bile duct. Identification and ligation of portal pedicles is completed during parenchymal division.

Parenchymal Transection

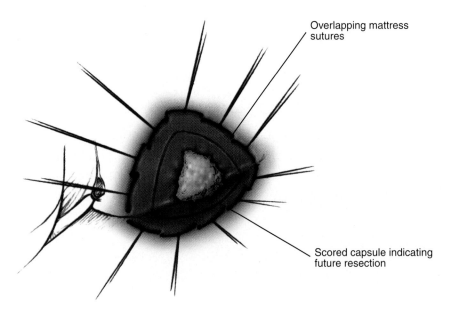

Overlapping mattress sutures

Scored capsule indicating future resection

Lesions at the periphery of the liver are amenable to wedge resection. A wedge that encompasses the tumor and an additional 1.5 to 2 cm of normal liver is scored on the capsule. For small superficial tumors, No. 1 chromic horizontal mattress sutures are placed 1 cm lateral to the scored line of resection from the base to the apex of the wedge. An electrocautery is then used for parenchymal division. For larger, deeper lesions, horizontal mattress sutures are placed 1 cm away from the line of resection as far posterior as can be done with ease. The parenchyma is then divided with the ultrasonic aspirator. Larger vessels and bile ducts are clipped or ligated, and divided. Vascular isolation is often not necessary during wedge resection.

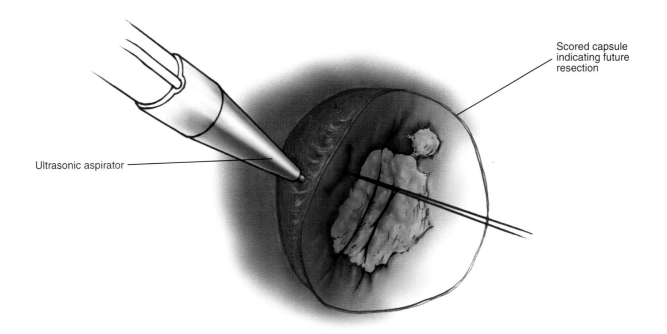

Chromic sutures are not used for more centrally located lesions. The capsule is scored with electrocautery, leaving a 1.5 to 2 cm margin of normal liver. The parenchyma is then divided with the ultrasonic aspirator. Parenchymal division progresses over a broad front, with identification and division of larger vessels and bile ducts. An exact determination of the edge of the tumor by palpation can be difficult. The surgeon should regularly palpate the liver to assure there is at least 1 cm of normal liver between the tumor and the resection margin. Bleeding during resection can be troublesome, and vascular isolation is often necessary.

Once the parenchyma is transected and the specimen removed, additional hemostasis is achieved with the argon beam coagulator. Vascular structures, especially biliary vessels, along the line of transection are carefully examined and additional sutures placed as needed. The specimen is then hand carried to the pathology suite and oriented for examination of the gross and microscopic margins. The resected surface is drained with one large sump drain placed in the resection defect. If mobile, the omentum is draped over and tacked to the defect in the liver. The falciform ligament is reconstructed. The abdomen is closed in two layers with a No. 1 monofilament suture.

Insertion of Hepatic Artery Infusion Pump

Hepatic arterial infusion therapy is used in patients without extrahepatic tumor but with more than four metastases or metastasis encroaching on both main right and left portal trunks. In general, patients with 50% or more of the liver replaced by tumor or with significant liver dysfunction are not candidates for hepatic arterial infusion therapy. The technique described is used in patients with type I ("normal") anatomy. Techniques used in patients with other anatomic variants are not described in detail, although in general the catheter is placed in the dominant lobar hepatic artery and the nondominant artery is ligated after test clamping to ensure cross-perfusion.

Incision and Exposure

The patient is positioned supine with the arms extended. A limited right subcostal incision is made. Through this incision a thorough exploration of the liver, abdomen, and portal structures is conducted. An enlarged lymph node in the porta adjacent to the duodenum and posterior to the common bile duct is routinely sent for frozen-section analysis, and the procedure is terminated if the node contains metastatic cancer. If no extrahepatic tumor is detected the incision is extended laterally two thirds the distance to the flank and medially to the midline. Exposure is then maintained with a Goligher retractor and one Octopus-type retractor anchored to the operating table at the level of the patient's chin.

Portal Dissection

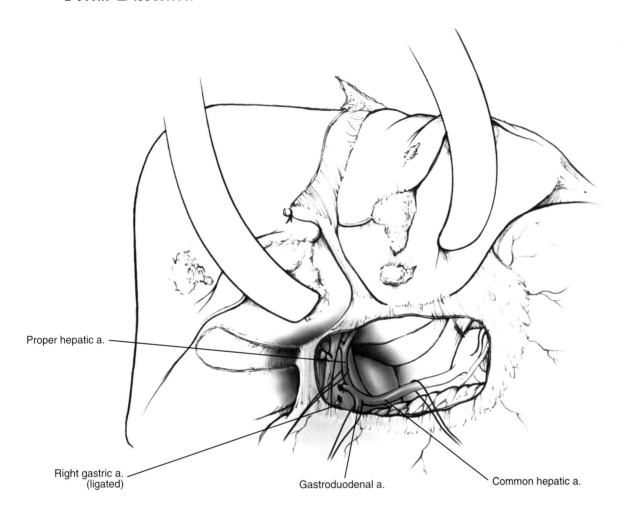

Proper hepatic a.

Right gastric a.
(ligated)

Gastroduodenal a.

Common hepatic a.

With the preoperative mesenteric angiogram on hand, the portal peritoneum is divided longitudinally over the anteriorly placed hepatic artery. The proper hepatic artery is dissected up to and beyond the bifurcation. The cystic artery is then identified, ligated, and divided as it courses to the right. Dissection of the lateral leaf of portal peritoneum then proceeds laterally with identification of the common bile duct and cystic duct. This cystic duct is divided, and the gallbladder is dissected from its bed in either antegrade or retrograde fashion.

(Cholecystectomy is performed to prevent the development of chemical chole-cystitis.) The medial leaf of the portal peritoneum is dissected to the left, giving clear access to the common hepatic and proper hepatic arteries. The gastro-duodenal artery is identified as it originates from the common hepatic artery. The common hepatic artery is then dissected proximally for at least 4 cm. The supraduodenal and right gastric arteries are commonly encountered during this dissection. These vessels are doubly ligated with 3-0 silk ties, then divided. The common hepatic artery is then encircled with a vessel loop. Using retraction on the common hepatic artery, the proper hepatic artery is dissected circum-ferentially for at least 2 cm beyond the bifurcation, then encircled with a vessel loop. Care is taken that small vessels originating from the proper hepatic artery are ligated and divided. Using vessel loops for retraction, the gastroduodenal artery is dissected distally to where it passes under the duodenum. It is impor-tant that all branches of the common hepatic artery, proper hepatic artery, and gastroduodenal artery are divided within the confines of the dissection de-scribed, to prevent perfusion of chemotherapy into the stomach, duodenum, and common bile duct. If meticulous attention is not paid to the dissection, difficult chemical gastritis and duodenitis can result when chemotherapy is in-fused. When the arterial dissection is complete, attention is turned to the ab-dominal wall. Assistants are given instructions to begin filling the pump with heparinized saline solution during the portal dissection.

Placement of Infusion Pump in Abdominal Wall Pocket

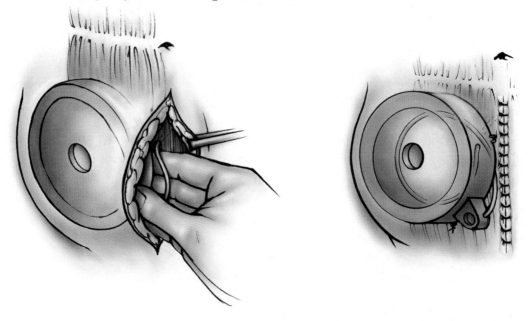

Six centimeters below the midpoint of the subcostal incision, a second inci-sion is made in the midline of the abdomen. This incision is deepened down into the subcutaneous fat to a thickness of 5 mm in normal and obese patients or to the rectus fascia in thin patients. With an electrocautery, a pump pocket is then created to the left of the midline incision. Thickness of the overlying pocket is crucial. The pocket should be thin enough that both the reservoir and bolus infusion ports are easily palpable, but not so thin that there is danger of the pump eroding through the pocket. When the pocket has been tailored to the exact size of the pump, the catheter is passed through the abdominal wall. Special care is taken to prevent injury to abdominal contents, especially the intestine.

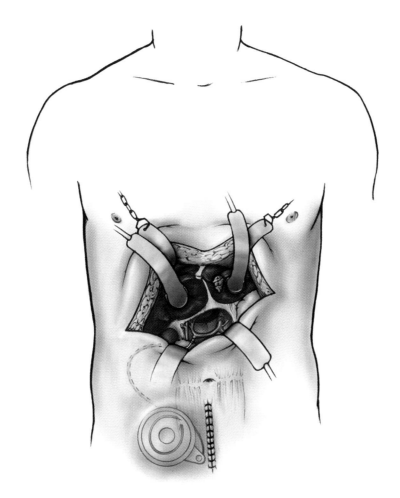

The catheter is passed through the abdominal wall posterior to the pump so that it is out of the way of errant needles. The catheter is routed up the right colic gutter and over the right kidney so that it approaches the porta lateral to the duodenum. The length of the catheter is adjusted so that it forms gentle curves, with no tension at the site of the arterial insertion. The extra catheter is retrieved into the pocket and coiled under the pump. The pump is then fixed into the pocket at three points with tie-down loops on the pump secured to the fascia with No. 1 Prolene sutures. The pump pocket may be closed at this point or after arterial insertion of the catheter. The pocket is closed with deep subcutaneous interrupted 2-0 Vicryl sutures and a 2-0 nylon running vertical mattress skin suture.

Catheter Insertion

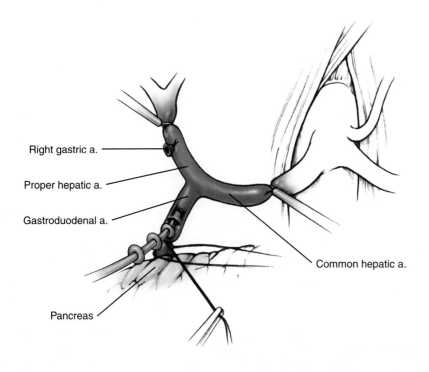

Right gastric a.

Proper hepatic a.

Gastroduodenal a.

Common hepatic a.

Pancreas

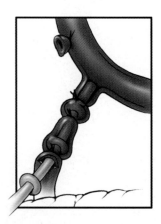

The gastroduodenal artery is ligated distally with a 2-0 silk ligature, which is then used for traction. An arteriotomy site is chosen on the gastroduodenal artery. Using the distance from the arteriotomy to the gastroduodenal orifice as a guide, the catheter is cut to length so that the end is flush with the orifice, the proximal bead is well contained within the artery, and the distal bead is just beyond the arteriotomy. The common and hepatic arteries are occluded with vessel loops, and a 2 mm arteriotomy is made with a No. 11 blade and Pott's scissors. The catheter is then threaded into the artery and secured with 3-0 silk ligatures proximal and distal to the proximal bead and distal to the distal bead. The bolus infusion port of the pump is then accessed with a noncoring needle, and 10 ml of a fluorscein solution is slowly injected. The right upper abdomen is then observed under Wood's lamp to assure that there is homogeneous perfusion of the liver without extrahepatic perfusion. The abdomen is then thoroughly irrigated and closed in two layers with a No. 1 monofilament suture.

Anatomic Basis of Complications

- The most serious and life-threatening intraoperative complication of liver resection is intraoperative bleeding from the hepatic veins. These veins can be damaged during their dissection or by excessive torquing of the liver during mobilization. Injury to the hepatic veins can also produce a hemodynamically significant air embolus. Attempts may be made at direct control and repair, but the surgeon should be readily prepared for insertion of an intracaval shunt if bleeding persists.

- Postoperative complications of liver resection can be broken down into the phases of the operation. Diaphragmatic injury and paresis can result during mobilization of the liver. Budd–Chiari syndrome can result from thrombosis of the hepatic veins secondary to operative injury during venous dissection or during parenchymal transection. Hepatic ischemia can develop from arterial or portal vein thrombosis due to injury during portal dissection. Biliary fistulas can arise from ductal damage during portal dissection or from inadequate ligation of ducts during parenchymal transection. Hepatic insufficiency can result from ischemia and inadequate hepatic reserve remaining after parenchyma transection. Intra–abdominal infection and abscesses can develop from enteric and skin contamination and inadequate hemostasis.

- Intraoperative complications from hepatic arterial infusion pump placement are mostly vascular. The most serious problems are occlusion of the hepatic artery or its major branches from thrombosis or dissection of an intimal flap. These problems require urgent exploration and repair of the artery.

- Postoperative complications from hepatic arterial infusion pump placement include infection, particularly within the pump pocket, heterogeneous perfusion of chemotherapy solution in the liver, and misperfusion of chemotherapy into the stomach or duodenum. Heterogeneous perfusion of chemotherapy can result in undertreated areas within the liver, and misperfusion can result in gastritis or duodenitis.

KEY REFERENCES

Bismuth H, Chiche L. Surgical anatomy and anatomical surgery of the liver. In Blumgart LH, ed. Surgery of the Liver and Biliary Tract. Edinburgh: Churchill Livingstone, 1994, pp 3-9.

This book offers an excellent description of the functional anatomy of the liver, with a clear explanation of the anatomic basis of the sectoral and segmental divisions of the liver.

Blumgart LH, Fong Y. Surgical options in the treatment of hepatic metastasis from colorectal cancer (review). Curr Probl Surg 32:346-355, 1995.

This thorough, detailed, comprehensive monograph reviews all aspects, including anatomic and procedural, of surgical treatment for hepatic metastasis. This work is an extremely valuable current review and contains a lengthy list of important references.

Broelsch CE. Atlas of Liver Surgery. New York: Churchill Livingstone, 1993, pp 1-118.

This beautifully illustrated and comprehensively written atlas includes in-depth details of liver resection techniques. The completeness and accuracy of the illustrations and accompanying text add greatly to the practical usefulness of this work by inclusion of information not found in other atlases.

Cameron JL, ed. Atlas of Surgery, vol 1. Philadelphia: BC Decker, 1990, pp 152-205.

This is a beautifully illustrated and clearly written atlas that includes the techniques of liver resection and hepatic arterial infusion pump insertion used by the Johns Hopkins surgical faculty. The detail and accuracy of the illustrations add greatly to the realism and practical usefulness of this work.

Nagorney DM. Hepatic resections. In Chassin JL, ed. Operative Strategy in General Surgery. New York: Springer-Verlag, 1994, pp 585-598.

This concise and clearly written chapter contains detailed sequential step-by-step descriptions of hepatic resections. The chapter is structured so that the novice surgeon can be comfortable with the steps involved in anatomic and nonanatomic resections. The illustrations are closely associated with the text and provide important anatomic details.

Roh MS. Liver resection. In Roh MS, Ames FC, ed. Advanced Oncologic Surgery. London: Wolfe, 1994, pp 5.2-5.17.

This chapter provides a thorough review of indications for liver resection, radiologic assessment, and technique of anatomic (lobar and segmental) liver resections. The technical details and illustrations for critical steps in the operation are detailed and extremely helpful. Overall, the chapter is written for the more experienced surgeon who is beginning to undertake liver resections or is trying to improve operative technique.

SUGGESTED READINGS

Anson BJ, McVay CB. Surgical Anatomy. Philadelphia: WB Saunders, 1984, pp 616-629.

Farmer DG, Rosove MH, Shaked A, et al. Current treatment modalities for hepatocellular carcinoma. Ann Surg 219:236-247, 1994.

Kemeny N. Review of regional therapy of liver metastasis in colorectal cancer. Semin Oncol 19(Suppl 3):155-162, 1992.

Kemeny NE, Seiter K, Conti JA. Hepatic arterial floxuridine and leucovorin for unresectable liver metastasis from colorectal cancer. Cancer 73:1134-1142, 1994.

Makucchi M, Yamamoto J, Takayama T, et al. Extrahepatic division of the right hepatic vein in hepatectomy. Hepatogastroenterol 38:176-179, 1991.

Meta-Analysis Group in Cancer. Reappraisal of hepatic arterial infusion in the treatment of non-resectable liver metastasis from colorectal cancer. J Natl Cancer Inst 88:252-257, 1996.

Meyers WC. Segmental hepatic resection. In Sabiston DC, ed. Atlas of General Surgery. Philadelphia, WB Saunders, 1994, pp 534-544.

Michels NA. Newer anatomy of the liver and its variant blood supply and collateral circulation. Am J Surg 112:337-347, 1966.

Mizumoto R, Suzuki H. Surgical anatomy of the hepatic hilum with special reference to the caudate lobe. World J Surg 12:2-10, 1988.

Nakamura S, Toshiharu T. Surgical anatomy of the hepatic veins and the inferior vena cava. Surg Gynecol Obstet 152: 43-50, 1981.

Rosen CB, Donohue JH, Nagorney DM. Liver resection for metastatic colonic and rectal carcinoma. In Cohen AM, Winawer SJ, eds. Cancer of the Colon, Rectum and Anus. New York: McGraw-Hill, 1995, pp 805-821.

Skandalakis JE, Skandalakis PN, Skandalakis LJ. Surgical Anatomy and Technique: A Pocket Manual. New York: Springer-Verlag, 1995, p 471.

Smadja C, Blumgart LH. The biliary tract and the anatomy of biliary exposure. In Blumgart LH, ed. Surgery of the Liver and Biliary Tract. Edinburgh: Churchill Livingstone, 1994, pp 11-24.

VanDamme JP, Bonte J. Vascular Anatomy in Abdominal Surgery. New York: Thieme Medical Publishers, 1990.

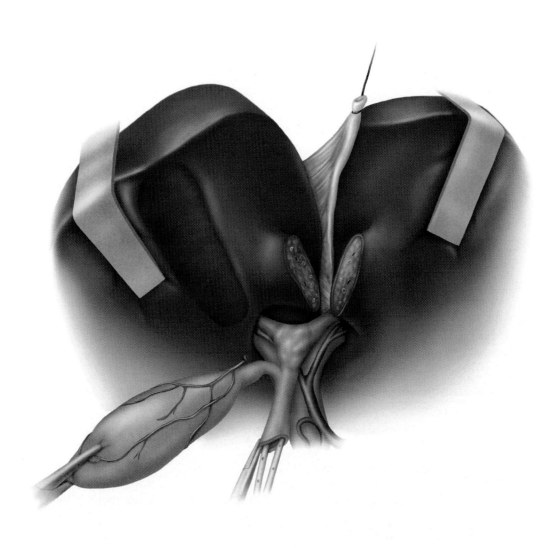

Chapter 13

Biliary Tree and Gallbladder

John R. Galloway, M.D., and George W. Daneker, Jr., M.D.

Surgical Applications

Cancers arising within the biliary tree and gallbladder are relatively rare, with a yearly incidence in the United States of 3 to 4 per 100,000 persons. Due to differences in their presentation, clinical features, and biologic behavior, these malignancies may be conveniently separated into cholangiocarcinoma (biliary tree) and gallbladder carcinomas.

Cholangiocarcinoma is a disease of older persons (50 to 70 years), without proclivity for gender. Although cholangiocarcinoma can arise anywhere in the intrahepatic or extrahepatic biliary tree, 60% to 80% of tumors arise in the peri-hilar region, particularly at the common hepatic duct bifurcation. Cholangio-carcinomas that arise within the liver are the second most common primary hepatic malignancy, after hepatocellular carcinoma. The development of chol-angiocarcinoma is associated with preexisting diseases, including biliary cir-rhosis, sclerosing cholangitis (often related to coexisting ulcerative colitis), choledochal cysts, and hepatolithiasis. Common features in these diseases in-clude chronic inflammation and chronic exposure of the biliary tree to stag-nant or infected bile. More than 90% of patients with cholangiocarcinoma have obstructive jaundice. A radiologic evaluation for jaundice usually shows a di-lated proximal biliary tree, irregular strictured biliary segment, collapsed distal biliary tree, and normal pancreas. The finding of a mass related to the stricture is an exception rather than the rule.

Management of cholangiocarcinoma follows two principles: curative re-section, when possible, and relief of biliary obstruction. At present, surgical in-tervention is the treatment of choice for potentially curable disease. The usual surgical procedure is resection of the malignant stricture with a biliary-enteric reconstruction augmented by long-term endoluminal stenting. Current 5-year survival rates after curative surgery are 10% to 20%. Surgical palliation with a similar procedure is desirable if the tumor is deemed unresectable at the time of exploration. Lesions determined to be unresectable during the preoperative evaluation are managed with endoluminal stenting and drainage. Stents are placed via a percutaneous transhepatic approach for proximal (infrahepatic) bil-iary lesions and via endoscopic retrograde cholangiopancreatography (ERCP) for more distal lesions. Median survival after palliative interventions is 5 to 30 months, with no long-term survivors. The addition of adjuvant therapy to surgery has not resulted in improved survival and is currently not routinely rec-ommended.

Carcinoma of the gallbladder is predominantly a disease of older women. Review of the literature shows that at least 75% of patients are women, with an average age of 69 years at presentation and a peak disease incidence after age 70. The few men who develop the disease are also older, with an average age of 67 years. The most common associated disease, implicated as a risk factor, is cholelithiasis. Gallstones are found in 68% to 98% of patients, and carcinoma is associated with larger stones. The majority of patients have symptoms, including abdominal pain, nausea, vomiting, and weight loss. These symptoms can easily be mistaken for symptoms of benign cholelithiasis. This mistaken identity is further perpetuated by the low diagnostic accuracy of ultrasonography and computed tomography (CT). These imaging studies enable identification of cancer in fewer than 50% of patients.

In patients with early disease, whose tumors are confined to the mucosa or invade superficially into the muscularis propria, simple cholecystectomy is adequate treatment, with a survival rate of 60% to 90%. Patients with invasion of the deep muscularis, invasion into the serosa, or invasion breaching the serosa should undergo resection of the gallbladder bed with a 3 to 4 cm margin (segments IV-B and V) and complete portal lymphadenectomy; 5-year survival rate in this group of patients is 25% to 40%. Transmural extension of the tumor into other organs (including liver) and regional lymphadenopathy may occasionally be cured with radical surgery (<10%), but given the age and associated medical problems of the average patient, conservative management is usually recommended. The use of adjuvant radiation therapy has shown promise in small retrospective reports, but a general recommendation awaits confirmation of these results in larger prospective trials. Radiation therapy or systemic chemotherapy has had little effect in the treatment of advanced disease.

Selection of the appropriate therapy in each clinical situation is based on understanding of the biologic behavior of the primary tumor, familiarity with the indications and limitations of each therapeutic modality, and a thorough knowledge of hepatobiliary anatomy and its variations. This chapter reviews the surgical management of biliary tree and gallbladder malignancies from an anatomic orientation. Topics included are the clinically relevant anatomy of the liver, biliary tree, and its accessory structures; the preoperative evaluation and patient selection in the management of biliary malignancies; the technical details of bile duct resections and radical cholecystectomy with portal lymphadenectomy; and an overview of potential complications.

SURGICAL ANATOMY
Topography

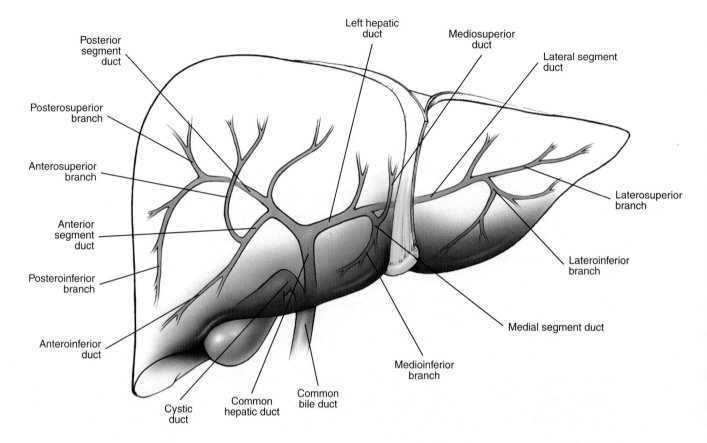

The main extrahepatic biliary system begins as the right and left lobar ducts, which join to form the common hepatic duct. As the hepatic duct passes through the porta hepatis it is joined by the cystic duct to form the common bile duct. The common bile duct passes through the lower porta and pancreatic head to empty into the duodenum. The main extrahepatic biliary system is joined by the accessory biliary structures, which consist of the gallbladder and its associated cystic duct.

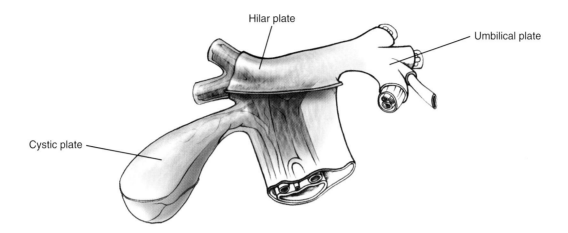

The common hepatic duct arises from the junction of the lobar ducts in the right half of the liver hilum, anterior to the portal venous bifurcation and overlying the right branch of the portal vein. The origin of the common hepatic duct is usually contained within a series of fibrous "plates," the hepatic plates, which surround the portal structures. The plate system is formed at the level of the liver hilum by coalescence and thickening of the liver capsule and vasobiliary sheaths. Dissection of the lobar ducts and the proximal common hepatic duct often requires division of these plates. The common hepatic duct runs downward and anterior to the portal vein for approximately 4 cm before it is joined by the cystic duct. The common hepatic duct is usually in close association with the proper hepatic artery, which lies to its left. The right hepatic branch of the proper hepatic artery crosses either the common hepatic or common bile duct. This crossing is usually anterior to the biliary structures, although crossing of the artery posterior to the ducts is also common.

The common bile duct, properly considered to be the union of the cystic and common hepatic ducts, is more conveniently thought of as the continuation of the common hepatic duct. The duct, which is approximately 9 cm long, begins in the porta hepatis and descends in the free margin of the lesser omentum (supraduodenal portion). It continues behind the first portion of the duodenum (retroduodenal portion) and enters a groove in or behind the superior lateral part of the head of the pancreas (pancreatic portion). The duct then descends obliquely and to the right, to enter below the middle of the second portion of the duodenum on its posteromedial surface (intraduodenal portion). The intraduodenal portion of the duct is usually joined on its left side by the main pancreatic duct. Once united, the ducts form a reservoir within the duodenal wall, known as the ampulla of Vater. The distal constricted end of the ampulla opens into the duodenum on the summit of the major duodenal papilla.

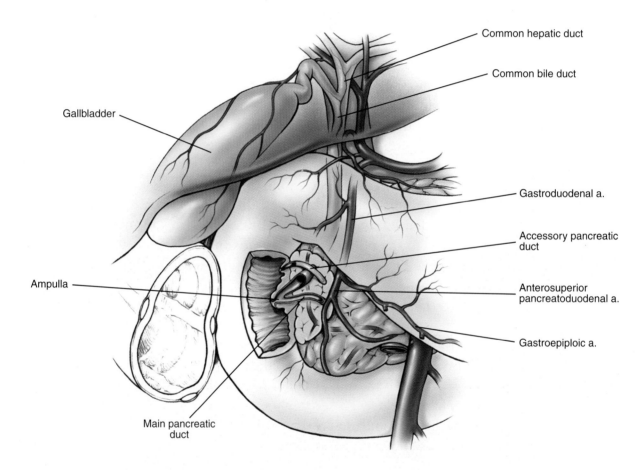

Relations of major vascular structures to the common bile duct include the following:

1. The infrahepatic supraduodenal portion of the duct usually descends adjacent and to the right of the hepatic artery. The artery often passes obliquely toward the midline, away from the duct, toward the distal end of this portion. The anterior surface of the portal vein is directly posterior or posteromedial to the supraduodenal portion of the duct.

2. The retroduodenal portion of the duct is situated to the lateral or right side of the gastroduodenal artery and is anterior to the right edge of the portal vein.
3. The pancreatic portion of the duct is accompanied by the gastroduodenal artery, which at a variable distance along its course gives off a superior pancreaticoduodenal branch that crosses the duct anteriorly or posteriorly. In addition, this portion of the duct is contained within a cage of vessels formed by the vasa recti of arcades from superior and inferior pancreaticoduodenal arteries. The significant venous relation of the pancreatic portion is the right edge of inferior vena cava, which is separated from the duct by a thin layer of connective tissue or pancreas. The duct has no relationship with the portal vein, which approaches it obliquely from below and from the left.

The gallbladder is a thin-walled pear-shaped sac approximately 8 to 10 cm in length capable of holding 50 ml of bile. It lies in a fossa on the inferior surface of the liver along a line (Cantlie's line) dividing the right and left lobes. The gallbladder is usually surrounded on its inferior and lateral surfaces by loose connective tissue and peritoneum, which attach it to the liver. Although the gallbladder is usually suspended from the gallbladder fossa, it may also be enveloped by parenchyma so that only a portion of the inferior surface is visible. The fundus of the gallbladder is its large bulbous cap, which commonly protrudes approximately 1 cm beyond the liver margin. When the gallbladder is full, the fundus comes in contact with the anterior abdominal wall opposite the ninth costal cartilage in an angle formed between the right rectus muscle and the costal margin. The body is the main part of the gallbladder and lies within the gallbladder fossa. The superior surface of the body is usually in direct contact with the liver without intervening peritoneum. Small vessels and bile ducts can pass directly from the liver into the body through the fossa. The lateral and inferior surfaces, which are covered with peritoneum, are in close proximity to the second portion of the duodenum and the transverse colon. The neck of the gallbladder, which results from tapering of the body, is folded into a S curve that terminates in the cystic duct. The neck is contained in the deepest part of the gallbladder fossa and lies in the uppermost free portion of the lesser omentum. The mucosa of the neck is ridged, forming the spiral valve (of Heister). Pathologic dilation of the gallbladder results in formation of a bulge or pouch in the neck, called the infundibulum. The infundibulum may overhang and obscure the cystic or bile ducts. Division of the right edge of the lesser omentum and mobilization of the infundibulum from the duodenum and biliary structures are necessary to prevent misidentification and accidental injury.

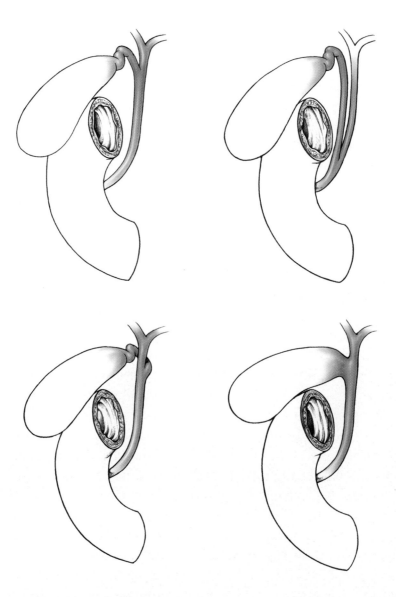

The cystic duct is approximately 4 cm long and extends from the gallbladder neck to the porta hepatis, where it runs beside, then joins, the common hepatic duct to form the common bile duct. Although the cystic duct is relatively long, it is usually folded on itself so that its union with the common hepatic duct is close to the neck of the gallbladder. The tortuosity of the duct is attributable to the spiral valves, which continue into the cystic duct from the gallbladder neck. The anatomy described is the usual arrangement, but variations of the cystic duct are common and should be kept under consideration.

Blood Supply

Of all the porta hepatis components, the hepatic arterial blood supply is the most variable, with 10 different vascular patterns identified. Typically, the proper hepatic artery divides into the main right and left lobar branches within the porta hepatis and outside the liver parenchyma. Usually the proper hepatic artery branches lower in the porta hepatis than does the bile duct or portal vein. A middle hepatic branch usually arises from the proximal left hepatic artery.

Hepatic Artery Variations

Type I	The right hepatic, midhepatic, and left hepatic arteries are from the celiac artery (55%).
Type II	The right hepatic and the midhepatic are from the celiac artery, replaced left hepatic from the left gastric artery (10%).
Type III	The midhepatic and left hepatic are from the celiac artery, replaced right hepatic from the superior mesenteric artery (11%).
Type IV	The midhepatic is from the celiac artery, replaced right hepatic from the superior mesenteric artery and replaced left hepatic from the left gastric artery (1%).
Type V	The right hepatic, midhepatic, and left hepatic are from the celiac artery, and an accessory left hepatic is from the left gastric artery (8%).
Type VI	The right hepatic, midhepatic, and left hepatic are from the celiac artery, and an accessory right hepatic is from the superior mesenteric artery (7%).
Type VII	The right hepatic, midhepatic, and left hepatic are from the celiac artery, an accessory right hepatic is from the superior mesenteric artery, and an accessory left hepatic is from the left gastric artery (1%).
Type VIII	Patterns are combined. A replaced right hepatic and an accessory left hepatic, and an accessory right hepatic and a replaced left hepatic (2%).
Type IX	Absent celiac hepatic artery. The entire hepatic trunk is from the superior mesenteric artery (4.5%).
Type X	Absent celiac hepatic artery. The entire hepatic trunk is from the left gastric artery (0.5%).
Type X (variant)	Double celiac hepatic arteries (no common hepatic artery). The right hepatic is from the proximal celiac artery, the left hepatic is from the distal end of the celiac artery.

From Michels NA. Newer anatomy of the liver and its variant blood supply and collateral circulation. Am J Surg 112:337-347, 1966, with permission from Excerpta Medica, Inc.

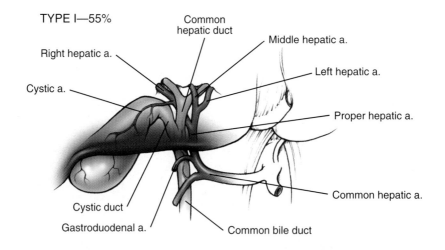

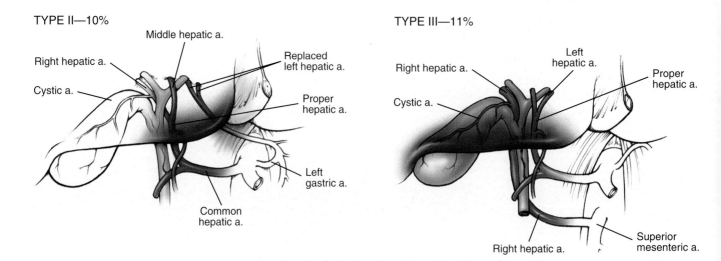

This variation of arterial anatomy, type I, is the most common and occurs in 55% of patients. Two other common variations are type III (11%), in which the main right hepatic artery arises from the superior mesenteric artery (SMA) and is situated in the posterior lateral porta hepatis, and type II (10%), in which the main left hepatic artery arises from the left gastric artery and travels into the liver in the proximal gastrohepatic ligament, while the middle hepatic artery arises from the proximal right hepatic artery.

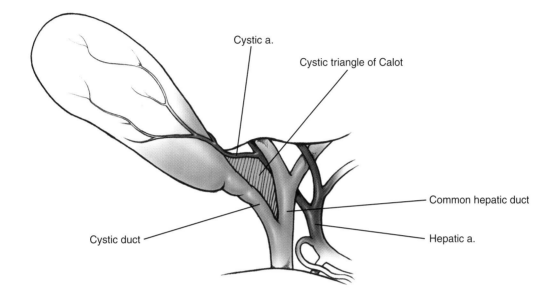

Cystic a.

Cystic triangle of Calot

Common hepatic duct

Cystic duct

Hepatic a.

The cystic artery supplies the gallbladder and is one of the most anomalous structures in the body. In the most common anatomic variant, found in 60% of patients, the cystic artery arises as a branch of the right hepatic artery. In this arrangement the cystic artery runs laterally through the porta hepatis, passing anteriorly or posteriorly to the common hepatic duct to supply the gallbladder. When this anatomic variant is present, the cystic triangle of Calot is formed. The superior base of this triangle is formed by the cystic artery, the medial border by the common hepatic duct, and the inferolateral border by the cystic duct. Important structures contained within Calot's triangle can include anomalous cystic arteries, the right hepatic artery, anomalous hepatic arteries, and bile ducts. Overall, 12 variants of cystic arterial anatomy have been described.

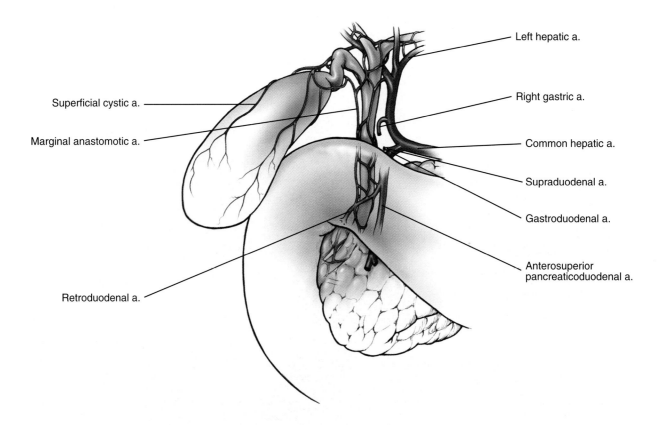

Left hepatic a.

Superficial cystic a.

Right gastric a.

Marginal anastomotic a.

Common hepatic a.

Supraduodenal a.

Gastroduodenal a.

Anterosuperior
pancreaticoduodenal a.

Retroduodenal a.

The blood supply of the bile duct is deserving of special emphasis. Despite an apparent rich arterial supply, segmental devascularization of the duct with resulting ischemia and stricture is a well-recognized and serious complication of hepatobiliary surgery. The blood supply of the bile duct is based on division of the bile duct into hilar, supraduodenal, and retropancreatic segments. The blood supply to the supraduodenal duct is axial, with most of the vessels arising from the retroduodenal artery, the gastroduodenal artery, the right hepatic artery, the cystic artery, and the retroportal artery. On average, eight 0.3 mm diameter arteries supply the supraduodenal duct. The most significant of these vessels run along the lateral borders of the duct at the 3- and 9-o'clock positions. Of the blood supply to the supraduodenal duct, 60% ascends from inferior vessels and 38% descends from superior vessels; the additional 2% comes from the direct contribution of small proper hepatic artery branches. The hilar ducts receive a rich blood supply from the plexus of vessels in continuity with the plexus surrounding the supraduodenal duct. The retropancreatic bile duct is supplied by a plexus of vessels derived from the retroduodenal artery.

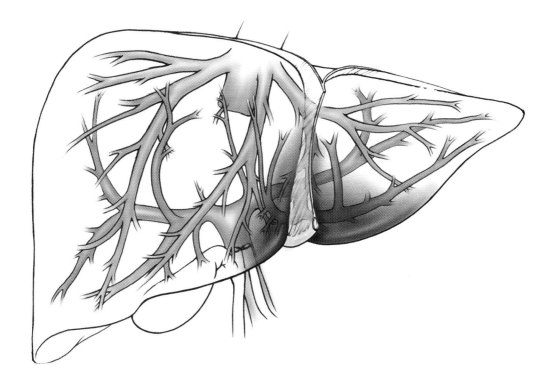

The portal vein and its branches are the least variable components of the porta hepatis. The portal vein is the most posterior portal structure, situated beneath the bile ducts and hepatic artery. Like the right hepatic duct, the main right portal vein is short and branches soon after it ascends into the parenchyma. The left main portal branch, like the left duct, is relatively long with a predictable horizontal course through the liver.

The venous drainage of the bile ducts and gallbladder is in the form of a continuous venous plexus. The veins draining the bile ducts accompany the small axial arteries and empty into larger veins along the lateral borders of the duct at the 3- and 9-o'clock positions. The venous drainage of the lower bile duct eventually enters the portal vein. Veins draining the gallbladder empty into this system, as well as into the liver parenchyma at the gallbladder fossa. The venous drainage of the gallbladder into the liver does not enter the portal circulation.

Lymphatic Drainage

The lymphatic vessels of the gallbladder and biliary tree drain medially into vessels and nodes along the common hepatic and common bile ducts, as well as directly into the liver parenchyma at the gallbladder fossa.

SURGICAL APPLICATIONS
Preoperative Evaluation of Cholangiocarcinomas and Carcinoma of Gallbladder

Preoperative evaluation of cholangiocarcinoma or carcinoma of the gallbladder is complex, and multiple modalities are used to define histologic features, anatomy, underlying liver function, and the presence of metastatic disease. While a great deal of nonoperative information can be obtained, many patients with cholangiocarcinoma have obstructive jaundice without a definable associated mass. This makes the successful preoperative histologic diagnosis of cholangiocarcinoma often difficult. Therefore, the preoperative diagnosis of cholangiocarcinoma is frequently made on the basis of clinical and radiographic findings. Nevertheless, an attempt at histologic confirmation of cholangiocarcinoma should be attempted preoperatively, if possible, particularly if there is a dominant mass or enlarged lymph node readily accessible to percutaneous biopsy. Liver function is important in determining whether a patient with cholangiocarcinoma is a candidate for surgical resection. A routine biochemical profile, which includes levels of total bilirubin, the hepatocellular enzymes aspartate transaminase and alanine transaminase, and the ductal enzymes alkaline phosphatase and γ-glutamyl transpeptidase, indicates biliary obstruction and identifies underlying hepatocellular damage, which may result from ongoing obstruction of the biliary tree. Serum albumin and prothrombin time are important measures of underlying hepatic function. Studies such as galactose elimination capacity, although not widely available, can serve to quantify hepatocellular reserve and are particularly important in patients who may require liver resection. Finally, marked elevation of the biochemical marker CA 19-9 correlates well with the presence of malignancy, although it can be elevated to a lesser degree in benign biliary obstruction.

Transabdominal ultrasonography is important in the screening for suspected obstructive jaundice, but it is not often so successful in delineating the level of obstruction. It can identify the presence of multiple hepatic metastases that would preclude surgical intervention. Endoscopic ultrasound is becoming more widely available and, as further experience is gained with this modality, it will become particularly useful in assessing the size and invasion of distal cholangiocarcinomas. Abdominal and pelvic CT is the diagnostic study of choice. CT scans provide a great deal of information regarding the presence of liver metastases, lymphadenopathy, and remote peritoneal metastases. If a mass 2 cm or larger is found in the porta hepatis or within the liver, percutaneous CT-directed biopsy has a good chance of confirming the diagnosis of cholangiocarcinoma. Ascites, as seen on ultrasonograms or CT scans, should be aspirated and subjected to cytologic evaluation to rule out malignancy. Malignant extraportal lymphadenopathy and malignant ascites are contraindications to a curative surgical intervention. The CT scan is also potentially valuable in identifying tumor encasement of the portal vein and hepatic arteries, as well as ruling in the presence of portal hypertension by demonstration of splenomegaly and significant intra-abdominal collateral venous development. Finally, CT also identifies the presence of lobar atrophy from long-standing unilateral biliary obstruction, which is important if an en bloc hepatic resection is anticipated. In our experience, magnetic resonance imaging (MRI) does not yield additional information beyond that obtained with CT, but this may change with improvements in MRI technology, especially in the area of MRI cholangiography. A routine chest x-ray film is important to rule out the occasional pulmonary metastases. Finally, any patient with significant bone pain should be examined with plain radiography of the painful area and bone scans as indicated. We have occasionally seen patients with skeletal metastasis from cholangiocarcinomas.

Visualization of the obstructing cancer is within the realm of the endoscopist or interventional radiologist. ERCP can be used to define the level of the lesion, as well as to rule out other potentially obstructing cancers in the upper gastrointestinal tract. Endoscopic biliary stent placement can also be used to palliate obstructive jaundice. It is our experience, however, that ERCP is more valuable for middle to distal common bile duct lesions, and often does not define the level of involvement of proximal bile duct lesions. Endoscopic stenting of a proximal cholangiocarcinoma can also be very technically challenging. For these reasons, percutaneous transhepatic cholangiography (PTC) is the diagnostic study of choice when the obstruction is in the region of the hepatic duct bifurcation or more proximally in either the right or left hepatic lobes. Bilateral PTC is often necessary when both right and left hepatic ducts are obstructed. Once again, this modality is useful as both a diagnostic and therapeutic tool to relieve obstructive jaundice. Because of the risk of cholangitis from instrumentation, some authors do not recommend preoperative intubation of the biliary tree. To the contrary, we believe that preoperative stenting, usually by transhepatic means, not only assists in defining important anatomy but also helps with the intraoperative dissection and resection. It should be noted that ERCP and PTC are not necessarily competing tests but complementary studies utilized to define the level of obstruction and assist in the preoperative relief of jaundice. Both ERCP and PTC can also serve as a port of entry to obtain cytologic brushings from the biliary tree. Because of the scant amount of tissue obtained and the significant amount of inflammation usually present, the success rate in obtaining a diagnosis of cholangiocarcinoma with brushings is approximately 30%. Transhepatic choledochoscopy may allow more accurate visualization and biopsy of suspect lesions; however, we have had inadequate experience with this technique at the present time.

If the patient remains a candidate for resection after these studies, preoperative visceral angiography is scheduled. Selective arterial injections are made into the celiac axis and superior mesenteric artery and visualization is followed through until the superior mesenteric vein, splenic vein, and portal veins are defined. Although not absolutely necessary, we believe angiography yields important information regarding the variations in hepatic arterial anatomy. This is particularly true for type III anatomy, in which replaced right hepatic artery courses through the posterior lateral porta and must be preserved during the portal dissection. Arterial encasement may also be noted on visceral angiograms and is a contraindication to resection. Although portomesenteric venous anatomy is more constant, occlusion or encasement of the portal vein or its major branches by tumor is critical preoperative information. Venous encasement may preclude surgical exploration if extensive, or predict the need for resection and reconstruction if localized.

The role of diagnostic laparoscopy should be mentioned. Unlike the case in pancreatic carcinoma, we do not routinely perform laparoscopy prior to formal exploration, because of the relatively low incidence of metastatic disease, which would preclude exploration. It is not clear whether the cost of routine laparoscopy to those patients with equivocal preoperative radiographic studies for metastatic disease is warranted.

Potential Contraindications to Surgical Resection

The extensive preoperative evaluation should determine those instances in which the tumor is not resectable, and obviate the need for surgical exploration, unless palliation by endoscopic or transhepatic stenting is unsuccessful. In our opinion, the following are contraindications to surgical resection of suspected cholangiocarcinoma:

1. Significant comorbid medical conditions such as chronic obstructive pulmonary disease (COPD), coronary atherosclerotic heart disease, or morbid obesity.
2. Poor underlying liver function, especially in the patient who may require liver resection.
3. Malignant ascites.
4. Evidence of diffuse hepatic metastases.
5. Evidence of extensive progression of the tumor into the secondary or tertiary bile ducts. This is more a biologic consideration than technical. Several groups have reported large central hepatic resections with multiple biliary enteric reconstructions to the secondary and tertiary bile ducts. We do not believe this is biologically appropriate in patients for whom significant palliation can be obtained with less extensive nonsurgical means.
6. Evidence of systemic metastases.
7. Small volume or atrophic hepatic lobe with very proximal invasion of the tumor into the secondary or tertiary bile ducts of the contralateral lobe, thereby requiring resection of that contralateral lobe.
8. Angiographic evidence of vascular encasement of the portal vessels. Although some groups have described en bloc resections of portal vein and hepatic arteries, we do not think this is biologically appropriate.

Resection of Proximal Cholangiocarcinoma Without Hepatic Lobectomy

Cholangiocarcinomas can develop from the very distal common bile duct as it courses through the head of the pancreas all the way into the hepatic duct bifurcation, with extension into the liver. Very distal cholangiocarcinomas often require pancreatoduodenectomy (see Chapter 14). The technique for resection of a lesion in the mid–common bile duct or located more proximally at the level of the common hepatic duct bifurcation is described.

Incision and Exposure

The patient is positioned on the operating table supine with the arms extended. Exposure is improved, particularly in obese patients, by placing a folded sheet transversely across the back at the level of the lower ribs or by "breaking" the table and extending the patient's back 10 to 15 degrees. Sequential compression stockings are used to decrease the risk of deep venous thrombosis. The full abdomen and lower chest, including the transhepatic biliary stents, are prepared and draped into the field. A limited incision is made two fingerbreadths below the right costal margin, and the abdomen is explored to assess for the presence of liver metastases or peritoneal implants.

Two lymph node groups are assessed. An enlarged lymph node in the porta, adjacent to the C loop of the duodenum and posterior to the common bile duct, is usually found. This node and several other posterior portal lymph nodes are often enlarged secondary to the desmoplastic processes associated with cholangiocarcinoma. The nodes are sent for frozen-section analysis, although they are rarely positive for metastatic disease. If these nodes prove to be positive for tumor, the decision to resect is made as follows:

1. For small cancers when resection of only the common bile duct is necessary, all nodes are resected en bloc with the extrahepatic biliary tree.
2. If the portal nodes are positive and the resection is to be more extensive, including possible hepatic resection, the procedure is terminated.

The celiac lymph nodes are examined after the gastrohepatic ligament is opened. Care is taken to preserve a replaced left hepatic artery (type III anatomy), which may be encountered within the proximal gastrohepatic ligament. The celiac nodes are often enlarged and are usually also negative for tumor. Suspicious nodes are sent for frozen-section analysis, and if they prove to be positive for tumor, the procedure is terminated. Regardless of the other intraoperative findings, the presence of tumor within these lymph nodes usually reflects the likelihood of additional distant metastases.

At the initial exploration the portal structures are carefully examined; however, the tumor frequently cannot be visualized. In addition, the gallbladder and extrahepatic biliary tree often appear normal in the case of more proximal tumors. Despite its seemingly occult nature, with palpation up into the hilum of the liver, the tumor and its surrounding inflammatory response may be recognized.

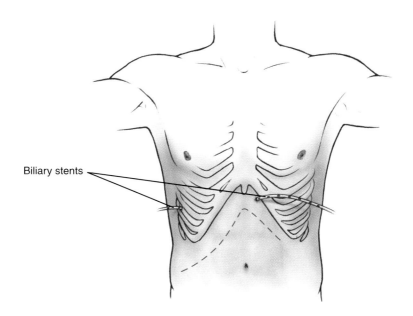

Biliary stents

If no extrahepatic tumor, vascular invasion, or more extensive intrahepatic tumor is detected, the right subcostal incision is extended into a generous bilateral subcostal, or chevron, incision. The right arm of the incision is extended toward the flank to the lateral peritoneal reflection. The left arm of the incision is extended as far beyond the left lateral rectus sheath as will allow easy access to the left upper quadrant structures. In cases when hepatic lobectomy is anticipated, a paraxiphoid midline extension, also known as the Mercedes-Benz incision, is helpful for gaining access to the suprahepatic vena cava and hepatic veins. After the incision is made, exposure is obtained with use of several types of self-retaining retractors. The Roshad retractor or the Goligher-type chain retractor is used to provide upward and lateral retraction of the costal margin, giving excellent access to the portal structures and the liver. These retractors are suspended from a frame anchored to the operating table at the level of the patient's chin. Two double-jointed octopus-type self-retaining retractors, attached to the bed frame, are also utilized. One retractor is anchored just below the level of the Roshad or Goligher retractor so that it can provide upper traction on the liver. A second double-jointed octopus retractor is placed at the level of the patient's hip to provide downward traction on the abdominal viscera.

Mobilization and Assessment of Resectability

The ligamentum teres is ligated and divided, and the falciform ligament is taken down with the cautery halfway between the abdominal wall and liver. Two Dever-type retractor blades are attached to the upper double-jointed octopus arms and placed beneath the liver to elevate it superiorly and expose the portal structures.

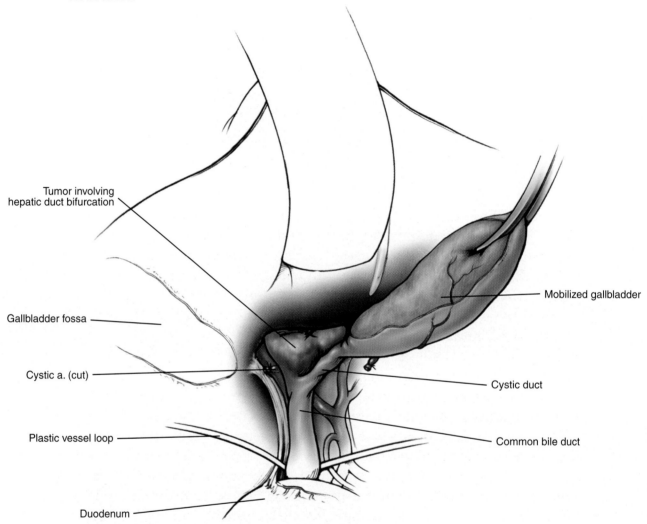

Two maneuvers, described by Cameron et al., greatly aid in exposure and dissection of the portal bifurcation. The first is mobilization of the gallbladder out of the gallbladder fossa. If the gallbladder is present, the cystic artery is identified, doubly clamped, ligated, and divided. The gallbladder is then mobilized out of the liver bed, and the cystic duct is mobilized to where it enters into the common hepatic duct. This maneuver greatly improves access to the portal bifurcation and, in particular, to the right hepatic duct. The second maneuver is dissection and encirclement of the distal common bile duct, just above the duodenum, early in the dissection of the porta hepatis.

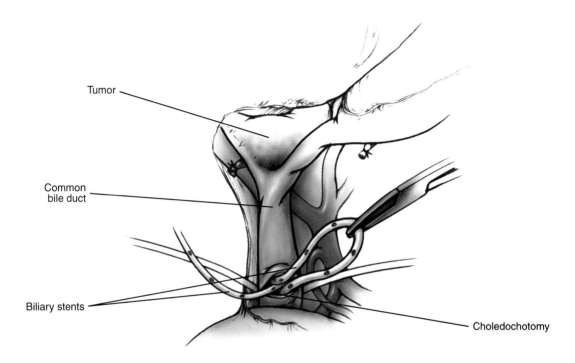

Identification and dissection of the common bile duct is facilitated by preoperative placement of transhepatic biliary stents. The common bile duct is surrounded by a vessel loop, the anterior wall of the distal bile duct is opened, and the transhepatic stents are extracted from the distal bile duct and duodenum. The distal bile duct is completely transected and a frozen section from the distalmost margin is sent for analysis. If this margin contains tumor a pancreatoduodenectomy will be necessary, and the anticipated additional morbidity and mortality must be assessed before proceeding. However, if this margin is negative for tumor, the transected distal bile duct can be either doubly ligated with 2-0 silk sutures or closed with interrupted 3-0 Vicryl vertical mattress sutures. These two maneuvers, mobilization of the gallbladder and early division of the distal common bile duct, greatly facilitate dissection of the extrahepatic biliary tree.

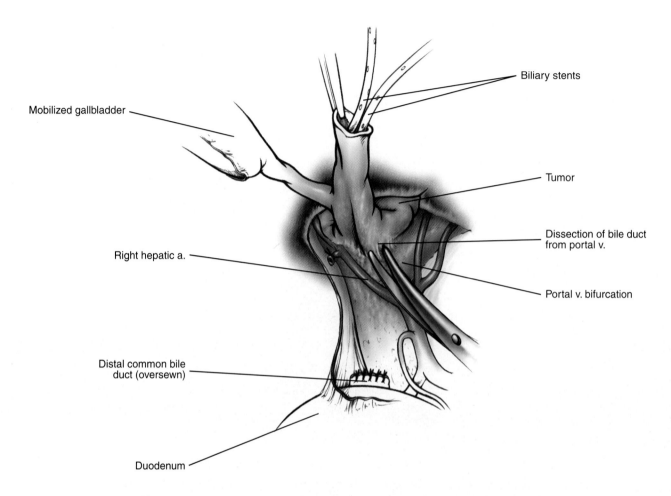

Biliary stents

Mobilized gallbladder

Tumor

Dissection of bile duct from portal v.

Right hepatic a.

Portal v. bifurcation

Distal common bile duct (oversewn)

Duodenum

Further dissection can be accomplished by traction on the biliary stents anteriorly and superiorly, exposing the plane between the posterior aspect of the common bile duct and the anterior surface of the portal vein. Dissection usually proceeds, either sharply or bluntly, distal to proximal. If at any point tumor involvement of the anterior surface of the portal vein becomes apparent, it may be necessary to abandon the procedure or consider portal vein resection and reconstruction. In most cases, if the preoperative imaging studies were normal, the dissection proceeds without incident. Associated nerves and lymphatic channels surrounding the bile duct are dissected away from the hepatic arterial structures medially and are resected en bloc with the specimen.

Further Proximal Portal Dissection

As dissection proceeds proximally, eventually the tumor and its associated desmoplastic process are reached. At this point, dissection at the bile duct off the portal structures, and in particular the portal vein, becomes more difficult. Nevertheless, careful sharp dissection, combined with gentle traction anteriorly and superiorly on the biliary stents, will aid in elevation of the posterior surface of the bile duct, tumor, and associated inflammatory reaction off the portal vein. Attempts at this maneuver without early division of the bile duct can result in a poorly accessible injury to the portal vein.

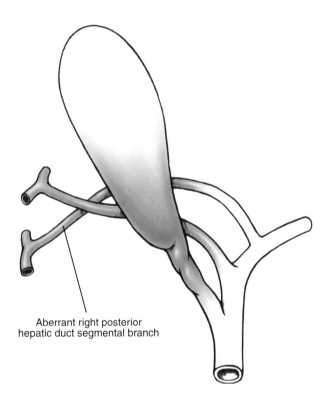

Aberrant right posterior hepatic duct segmental branch

After the bifurcation has been separated from the anterior surface of the portal vein, the dissection is carried out as far proximally as possible along the posterior aspects of the right and left hepatic ducts. At this point in the dissection, the surgeon can find an aberrant hepatic duct from the right anterior or posterior segment crossing the midline to enter the medioposterior aspect of the left hepatic duct. This structure, if present, should be identified and preserved.

Once the posterior dissection has been completed, it is usually possible to see the portal vein bifurcation. Care must be taken to prevent injury to the right hepatic artery, which usually courses posteriorly to the common bile duct but may cross anteriorly anywhere along this line of dissection. If the right hepatic artery courses anteriorly, it must be fully mobilized, encircled, and displaced beneath the bile duct during the dissection.

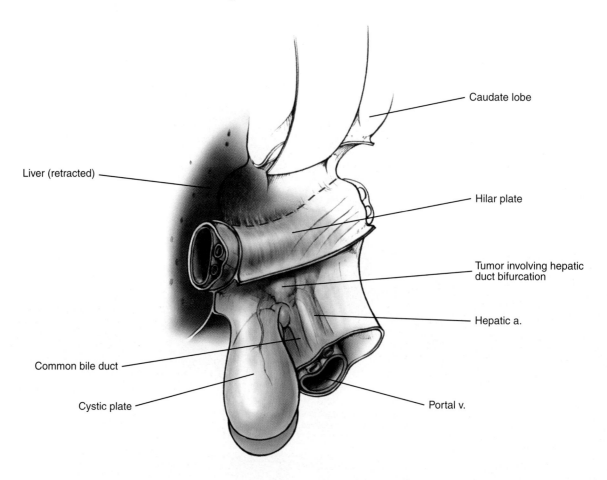

Attention is then turned to the hepatic bifurcation. Octopus-mounted Dever retractors are replaced at the bottom of segment IV-B and the bottom of segment V. Traction is then applied in an anterior and superior direction to expose the hilar plate, which is entered anteriorly.

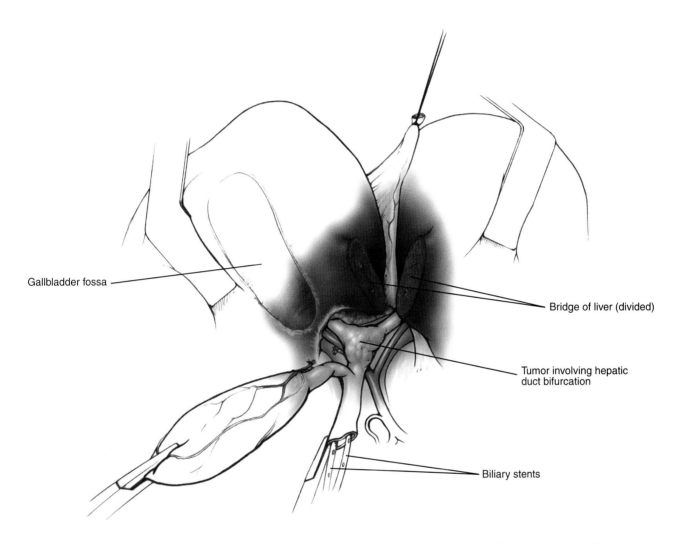

Gallbladder fossa

Bridge of liver (divided)

Tumor involving hepatic duct bifurcation

Biliary stents

If the tumor is small, dissection continues in this relatively bloodless plane until the superior aspect of the bifurcation can be identified. If the tumor is more invasive, parenchymal division (segment IV-B plus segment V) must be carried out anterior to the tumor to obtain an adequate margin.

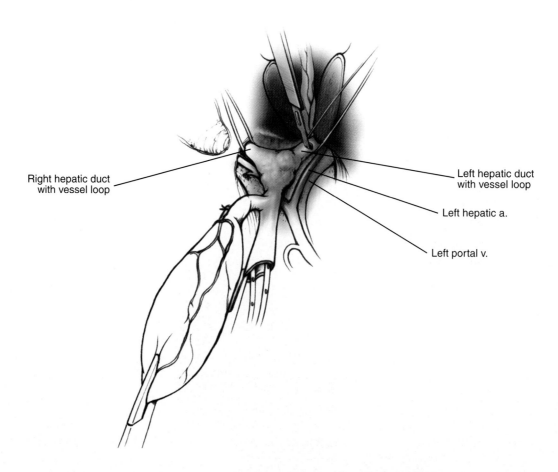

Right hepatic duct
with vessel loop

Left hepatic duct
with vessel loop

Left hepatic a.

Left portal v.

At this point the right and left hepatic ducts can be fully palpated, particularly with the intrahepatic biliary stents in place. Both bile ducts are individually encircled with vessel loops. Care is taken not to injure the portal vein, which lies posteriorly, as well as any aberrant right hepatic ducts that cross the midline to enter the left hepatic duct. The right and left hepatic ducts are divided just beyond the tumor, and the specimen is removed en bloc with the gallbladder. Occasionally when an aberrant right hepatic duct enters the left duct just proximal to the bifurcation, all three ducts of this "trifurcation" are divided during the resection. The distal common bile duct margin and the right and left hepatic ducts are tagged to aid the pathologist with orientation of the specimen. Frozen-section examination of the proximal right and left hepatic duct margin is controversial because these margins have proved difficult to accurately interpret. Some authors have noted that delineation of tumor extent is difficult even after careful examination of the entire specimen after permanent sectioning. This problem is due to the scirrhous nature of cholangiocarcinomas, which can spread discontinuously within the wall of the bile ducts. Despite these arguments, we usually send margins for frozen-section analysis so that if tumor is found the proximal bile ducts can be further resected in the hope of obtaining a negative margin.

Biliary Enteric Reconstruction

After the specimen has been removed, the biliary enteric reconstruction, over silicone (Silastic) transhepatic biliary stents placed in both right and left hepatic ducts, is performed. Although stenting is not absolutely necessary, we believe it aids in performing the anastomosis and also makes available the opportunity for postoperative brachytherapy radiation. If the bile ducts are of large caliber, Jackson-Pratt drain tubing, with the drain portion removed and with multiple side holes cut tangentially into the catheter for a distance of 10 cm, makes an excellent and readily available stent. Any transhepatic catheters placed preoperatively are brought in through the chest or abdominal wall into the abdominal cavity. If these catheters are at least 12 to 14 Fr, they are secured directly to the Silastic tubing by placing the stent into the tubing and anchoring it with a 0 silk transfixion suture. The Silastic stent, which is now attached to the transhepatic biliary catheter, is pulled through the hepatic duct and out through the surface of the liver, using the pathway created by the catheter as a guide. The Silastic stents are positioned so that the side holes begin within the intrahepatic bile duct and extend out of the distal lobar ducts or remaining common duct. This portion of the catheter is placed within the jejunal limb brought up to create the anastomosis. To prevent reflux of bile and leakage into the suprahepatic space, it is important to make certain that no side holes are outside the surface of the liver. For this purpose a No. 1 chromic horizontal mattress suture is placed around the stent as it emerges from the capsule of the liver.

If the preoperatively placed biliary catheters are 10 Fr or smaller, it is usually necessary to dilate the intrahepatic tract with a 12 Fr Coudé catheter, as described by Cameron. In order not to lose the tract if one of the catheters should break or become dislodged, guidewires are placed through the catheters. A 12 Fr Coudé catheter with the tip excised is passed over the guidewire and sutured to the biliary catheter. The biliary catheters are withdrawn, leaving the right and left hepatic ducts intubated with the Coudé catheters.

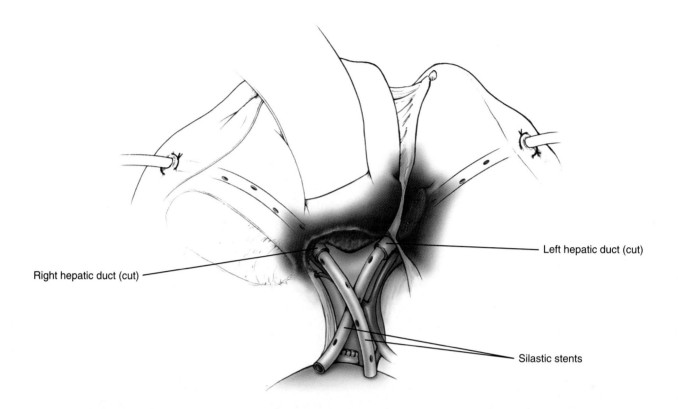

Right hepatic duct (cut)

Left hepatic duct (cut)

Silastic stents

The Silastic stents (Jackson-Pratt drains) are placed over the guidewires into the flanged end of the Coudé catheters and anchored to the catheters with 0 silk transfixion sutures. By withdrawing the Coudé catheters, the silicone stents are appropriately positioned. The stents are secured as described above.

After placement of the stents, a biliary enteric anastomosis to a 60 cm Roux-en-Y loop is constructed. A proximal loop of jejunum, just distal to the ligament of Treitz, is divided using a gastrointestinal stapling device (GIA) at a convenient arcade. The associated jejunal mesentery is then divided to its base, giving excellent bowel mobility. The Roux-en-Y loop is brought into the right upper quadrant via a retrocolic route over the second and third portions of the duodenum.

Enteric continuity is reestablished with an end-to-side jejunojejunostomy 60 cm distal to the end of the Roux-en-Y loop. The anastomosis is carried out in usual two-layer fashion, utilizing an outer interrupted layer of 3-0 silk and an inner continuous layer of 3-0 Vicryl sutures. The mesenteric defect is closed with interrupted 3-0 silk sutures.

At the appropriate site on the antemesenteric border, two enterotomies are made for anastomoses to the right and left ducts. Care must be taken to match the length of the enterotomies with the width of the bile ducts. If there is adequate length of the right and left hepatic ducts and if they are in close proximity to each other, the sidewalls of the ducts are sutured together medially to form a single, common orifice for the anastomosis.

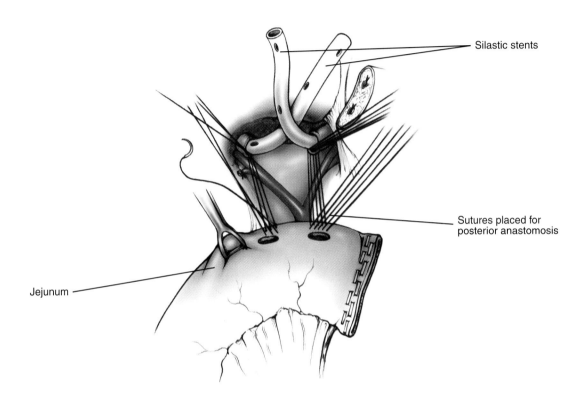

Silastic stents

Sutures placed for
posterior anastomosis

Jejunum

After enterotomies are made on the jejunum, we tack the mucosa to the serosa circumferentially with interrupted 4-0 Vicryl sutures. This ensures eversion of the mucosa and mucosal-to-mucosal apposition during the anastomosis. The hepaticojejunostomy is constructed using one layer of interrupted 3-0 Vicryl or PDS sutures. Corner stitches are placed first, outside to inside, so that the knot is on the outside. The subsequent entire back row of sutures is then placed before any of the sutures are tied. Each suture passes through the full thickness of the jejunal wall, inside to outside, and then through the full thickness of the bile duct, outside to inside. Thus the knots of the posterior row will be inside the lumen. Since synthetic absorbable material is being used, these knots are not long-term niduses for stone formation. When both posterior rows have been placed, the sutures are tied. Prior to placement of the anterior row of sutures, the silicone biliary stents are inserted through the jejunal enterotomies.

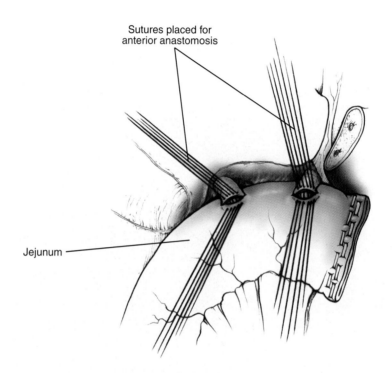

The anterior layer is then completed with interrupted 4-0 sutures. The sutures are not tied until all have been placed for both right and left hepaticojejunostomies. These sutures are placed through the full thickness of the jejunum, outside to inside, then through the bile duct, inside to outside, so that all knots for the anterior row are on the outside.

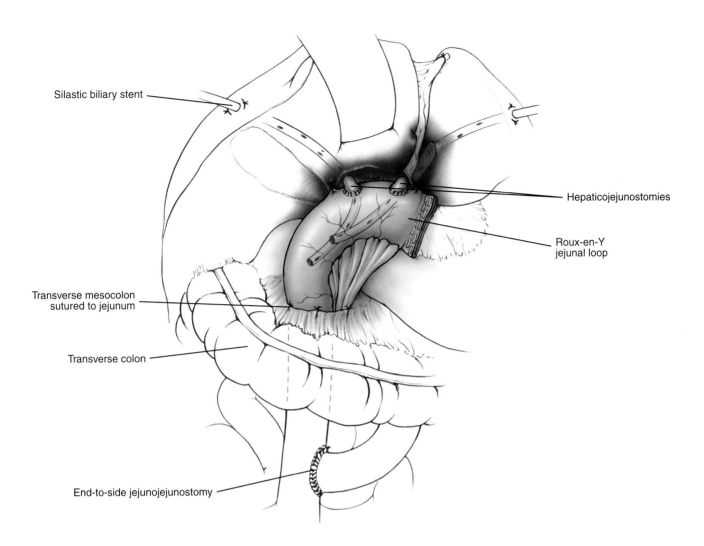

Silastic biliary stent

Hepaticojejunostomies

Roux-en-Y
jejunal loop

Transverse mesocolon
sutured to jejunum

Transverse colon

End-to-side jejunojejunostomy

The Roux-en-Y loop is then tacked to the undersurface of the liver using interrupted 3-0 silk sutures to ensure there is no tension on the anastomosis. The Roux-en-Y loop is then sutured to the opening in the transverse mesocolon with interrupted 3-0 silk sutures to prevent herniation of small bowel. Each Silastic stent is then brought out through a stab wound in the right or left upper quadrant and anchored to the skin with a 2-0 nylon suture. Three 10 mm Jackson-Pratt drains are placed through separate abdominal stab wounds. One drain is used at each stent exit site on the superior surface of the liver. The hepaticojejunostomy is drained with a Jackson-Pratt drain placed posterior to the anastomoses, with part of the drain extending into Morrison's pouch and brought out through a separate lateral stab wound. The abdomen is then closed in two layers with a No. 1 monofilament suture.

Resection of Proximal Cholangiocarcinoma At or Above the Common Hepatic Duct Bifurcation With En Bloc Liver Resection

Cholangiocarcinomas located at the common hepatic duct bifurcation or proximally within the right or left hepatic ducts often require resection of the extrahepatic biliary tree with en bloc resection of a hepatic lobe, followed by biliary enteric anastomosis to the remaining lobar bile duct. Preoperative evaluation, within the limitations previously outlined, is extremely important in determining the extent of proximal hepatic duct invasion and the potential need for hepatic lobectomy. Also, preoperative evaluation of liver volume and function is important for determining the extent of hepatic resection possible without producing hepatic insufficiency. Finally, it is not infrequent for one or both lobar branches of the portal vein or hepatic artery to be encased or occluded by tumor extension. These tumors may still be resectable if en bloc hepatic lobectomy is performed along with resection of the bifurcation and extrahepatic biliary tree. The technique for resection of a cholangiocarcinoma located at or above the hepatic bifurcation with en bloc resection of the left hepatic lobe is described. Resection of the extrahepatic biliary tree with en bloc resection of the right hepatic lobe can also be accomplished with similar techniques, utilizing the principles for right hepatic lobe resection described in Chapter 12.

Incision and Exposure

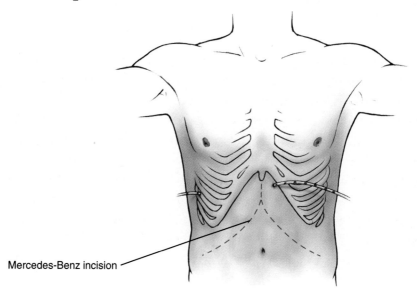

Mercedes-Benz incision

The incision and exposure are similar to that for resection of proximal cholangiocarcinomas at or below the bifurcation of the common hepatic duct (see p. 565). A limited right subcostal incision is made, and the abdomen is explored to assess for the presence of more extensive liver involvement by tumor or peritoneal implants. Assessment of the portal and celiac lymph nodes, as previously described, is performed with removal of several of these nodes for frozen-section evaluation. Metastatic disease in one or both of these nodal groups precludes resection of the bile duct with en bloc liver resection, and, if present, the procedure is terminated.

If there is no extrahepatic tumor, extensive vascular invasion, or more extensive intrahepatic tumor, the right subcostal incision is extended into a generous bilateral subcostal, or chevron, incision. Since in this case hepatic lobectomy is anticipated, a paraxiphoid midline extension (Mercedes-Benz incision) is helpful for gaining access to the suprahepatic inferior vena cava and hepatic veins. Exposure is obtained by use of self-retaining retractors, as described for proximal cholangiocarcinoma.

Mobilization and Assessment of Resectability

After the abdominal cavity is entered and the retractors are placed, the ligamentum teres is divided and ligated and the falciform ligament is taken down with a cautery halfway between the abdominal wall and liver. At this point, two Dever-type retractor blades are attached to the upper double-jointed octopus arms and placed beneath the liver to elevate it superiorly and expose the portal structures. The initial operative strategy for this part of the procedure is similar to that described for resection of proximal cholangiocarcinoma without hepatic lobectomy. Two maneuvers that greatly aid in the exposure and dissection of the portal bifurcation, as described by Cameron et al., are now performed: mobilization of the gallbladder, and dissection with division of the distal common bile duct just above the duodenum. Mobilization of the gallbladder improves exposure to the bifurcation, and division of the distal common bile duct facilitates dissection of the bifurcation off the portal vascular structures. A frozen-section of the distal common bile duct is obtained for analysis. If positive for tumor, the procedure is abandoned and a Roux-en-Y hepaticojejunostomy below the level of obstruction is constructed. The remainder of the biliary dissection is as described for the resection of proximal cholangiocarcinoma without hepatic lobectomy.

Further Proximal Portal Dissection and Left Hepatic Lobectomy

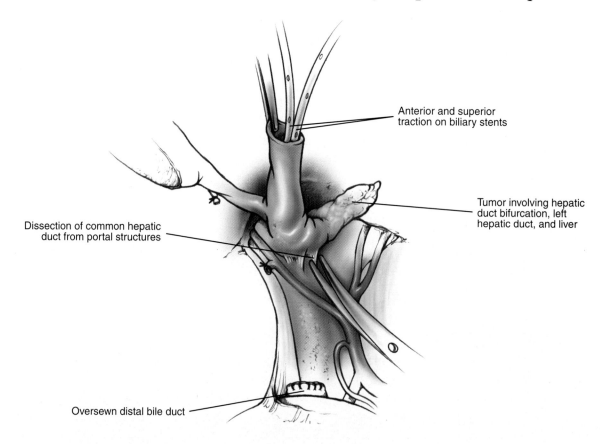

Anterior and superior traction on biliary stents

Tumor involving hepatic duct bifurcation, left hepatic duct, and liver

Dissection of common hepatic duct from portal structures

Oversewn distal bile duct

As the dissection proceeds proximally within the porta, the tumor and its associated inflammatory process are encountered. Dissection of the portal structures, and in particular the portal vein, becomes more difficult. Nevertheless, careful sharp dissection combined with gentle anterior and superior traction on the biliary stents will aid in mobilization of the posterior surface of the bile duct, tumor, and associated inflammatory reaction off the portal vein. Once the bifurcation has been separated from the anterior surface of the portal vein, the dissection is carried out along the right hepatic duct as far as possible. At this point, the tumor usually extends well up into the left lobe and may also involve the left hepatic artery and the portal vein. When this becomes obvious, no attempts at dissecting the tumor from the left hepatic artery or portal vein are made, because serious bleeding may occur. Care must also be taken not to injure the right hepatic artery, which may cross anteriorly or posteriorly to the common bile duct anywhere along this line of dissection. The surgeon must attempt to gain access to the proximal right hepatic duct above the tumor. This duct is usually normal and can be identified by palpating the biliary catheter, within the duct, above the tumor. This maneuver may necessitate division of the hilar hepatic plate at the level of the gallbladder bed (segment V).

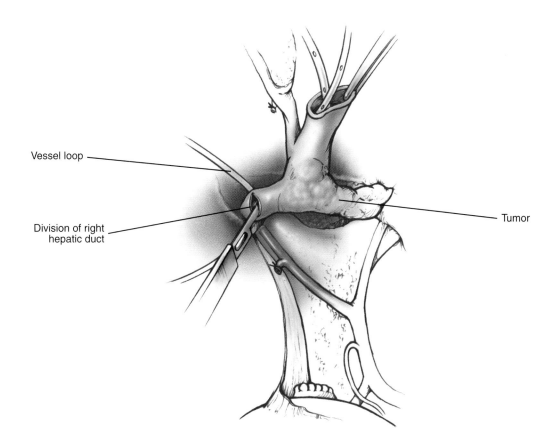

Vessel loop

Division of right hepatic duct

Tumor

By dissecting in this relatively bloodless plane, it is possible to encircle the right hepatic duct completely. The right hepatic duct is then divided and the biliary catheter exposed. Attention is now turned to identification and division of vascular inflow to the left lobe of the liver. Preoperative hepatic and mesenteric arteriograms greatly assist in clear delineation of hepatic arterial and portal venous anatomy. The peritoneum of the hepatoduodenal ligament is divided longitudinally over the common hepatic artery. Dissection along the proper hepatic artery up to and slightly beyond its bifurcation into the left and right hepatic arteries is performed. The cystic artery is identified and ligated, if not done during mobilization of the gallbladder.

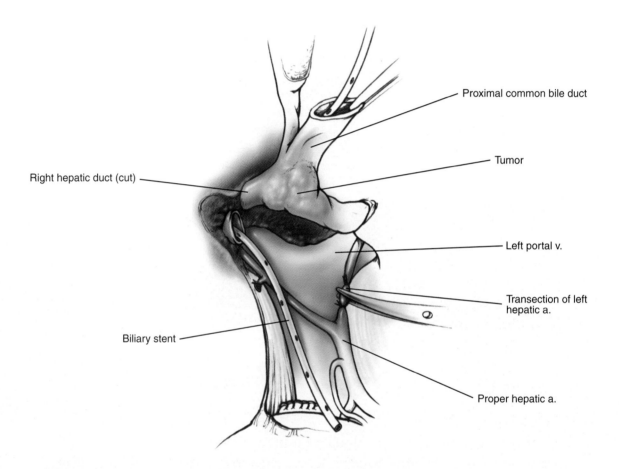

After accurate confirmation of the arterial anatomy, the proximal left hepatic artery is divided between double ligatures of 2-0 silk. Any replaced or accessory left hepatic arteries are divided as well. The common hepatic artery and its branch to the right lobe are retracted laterally, giving access to the posteriorly situated portal vein.

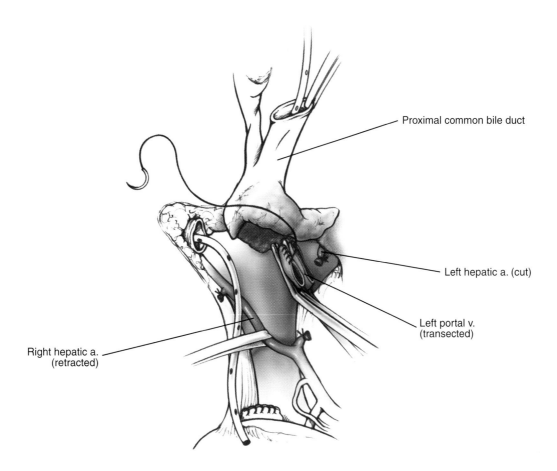

Proximal common bile duct

Left hepatic a. (cut)

Left portal v.
(transected)

Right hepatic a.
(retracted)

Dissection of the main portal vein proximally to its bifurcation into the right and left branches is completed, and at least 2 cm of left portal vein is cleared free. The left portal vein is then divided between Cooley vascular clamps, clearly away from the bifurcation. The proximal end of the left portal vein is then over-sewn with a continuous 4-0 or 5-0 Prolene suture. The distal end of the vein can also be oversewn with a similar suture, or suture ligated with 2-0 silk if length permits.

If at this point in the portal dissection it becomes obvious that the tumor is encroaching on the portal bifurcation, resection of some or all of the portal vein bifurcation en bloc with the tumor as it extends into the left hepatic lobe may be necessary. Prior to any attempt at resection, proximal venous control of the main portal vein below the bifurcation and distal venous control of the right branch of the portal vein above the level of the bifurcation must be ob-tained. After partial excision of the bifurcation, lateral venorrhaphy using running 5-0 Prolene sutures may be used to repair the vein if the caliber of remaining portal vein is adequate. If the caliber of remaining portal vein is too small (<50%), a vein patch, utilizing a piece of harvested internal iliac or saphenous vein sewn into the defect with 5-0 Prolene suture, is usually sufficient. If the entire bifurcation has been excised, an end-to-end anastomosis between the main trunk of the portal vein and the right portal vein is needed. Two 5-0 Prolene corner sutures are placed so that the knots are on the two ends of the portal vein. The first corner suture is brought inside, and the posterior row is sewn in a continuous fashion inside the vein to the opposite corner suture, where it is brought outside and tied. The other half of the first corner suture is used to complete the anterior row of the anastomoses in a continuous fashion on the outside of the vein, to the opposite corner. These two ends of the front suture are then tied, leaving a small "air knot" (called a "growth stitch" by transplant surgeons) to allow for expansion of the anastomosis.

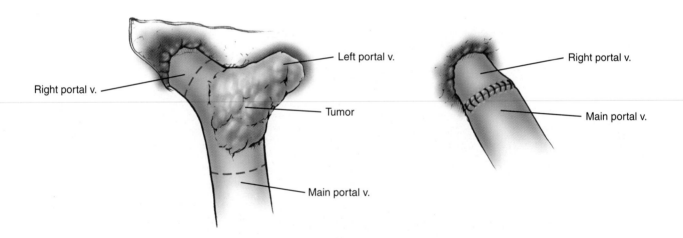

This end-to-end anastomosis can be accomplished without difficulty if less than 2 cm of vein has been resected. However, if more than 2 cm of vein has been removed, a small vein graft is usually necessary. In this case, we prefer to use a small section of internal jugular vein because it is a perfect size match for the portal vein. If we anticipate the possibility of a venous reconstruction based on preoperative angiography, the left side of the patient's neck is prepared and draped in anticipation of harvesting the left internal jugular vein.

After division of the portal vein, a clear line of demarcation between the devitalized left lobe and the perfused right lobe should be seen. The hepatic artery and portal vein supplying the right lobe are encircled with a Rommel tourniquet. Further mobilization of the left lobe is now performed.

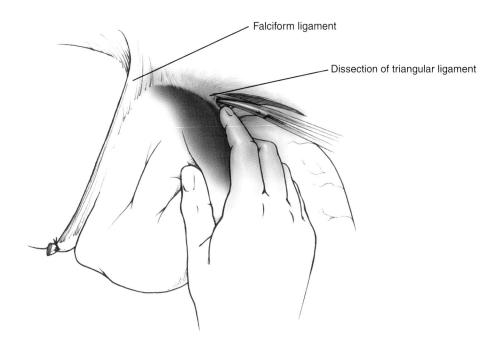

Falciform ligament

Dissection of triangular ligament

With the assisting surgeon exerting gentle anterior and counterclockwise retraction on the left lobe, the left triangular and commonly fused left coronary ligaments are divided medially to the level of the suprahepatic inferior vena cava. As the dissection approaches the inferior vena cava, care should be taken to prevent injury to the left phrenic vein, particularly as it empties into the left hepatic vein.

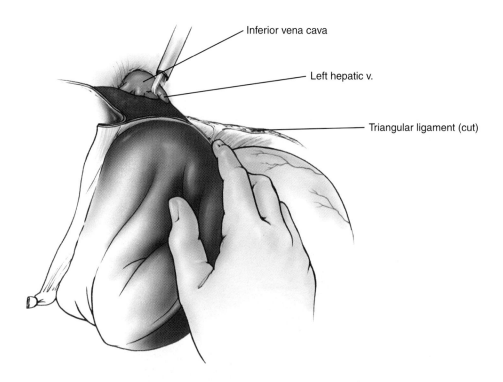

Division of the peritoneum over the suprahepatic inferior vena cava is completed and the left and middle hepatic veins are identified. At this point mobilization of the right lobe may be necessary. The most common indication for mobilization of both lobes is the posterior extension of a large cholangiocarcinoma into the caudate lobe with close proximity to the hepatic veins, or the retrohepatic inferior vena cava. Mobilization of the right lobe of the liver allows access to the plane between the caudate lobe and the anterior surface of the retrohepatic inferior vena cava. In this region of the cava multiple paired veins pass directly into the caudate lobe. By rotating the liver from lateral to medial, one can sequentially divide these small veins beginning inferiorly and working superiorly. Division of these veins is facilitated by division of the gastrohepatic omentum, which allows exposure of the medial side of the retrohepatic inferior vena cava. This step allows full mobilization of the liver off of the retrohepatic inferior vena cava and aids in en bloc resection of the caudate lobe. Again, exposure of the retrohepatic inferior vena cava is not routinely necessary, but is helpful in resecting a large tumor invading posteriorly into the caudate lobe.

Although extrahepatic division of the right hepatic vein is frequently attempted, extrahepatic division of the left hepatic vein prior to parenchyma transection is discouraged because the difficulty in obtaining safe control of a short, common trunk with a major venous bifurcation, or control of two closely approximated major venous trunks (e.g., middle hepatic vein and left hepatic vein together). It is possible to selectively encircle the left and middle hepatic veins with very careful blunt dissection around these veins at their junction with the inferior vena cava, but this maneuver should be abandoned at the slightest sign of difficulty. The most common method of venous control is intraparenchymal division of the left hepatic vein. Not only is this method safer and easier, it also reduces the chance of damage to the middle hepatic vein. Preservation of the middle hepatic vein is desirable but not critical for the survival of the right lobe. The left hepatic vein is doubly clamped with sharply curved Cooley clamps and divided. The parenchymal portion of the hepatic vein can be over-sewn with a continuous 4-0 Prolene suture if it is divided early in the removal of the left lobe. The proximal stump of the left hepatic vein, as it enters the vena cava, is oversewn with a continuous 4-0 Prolene suture.

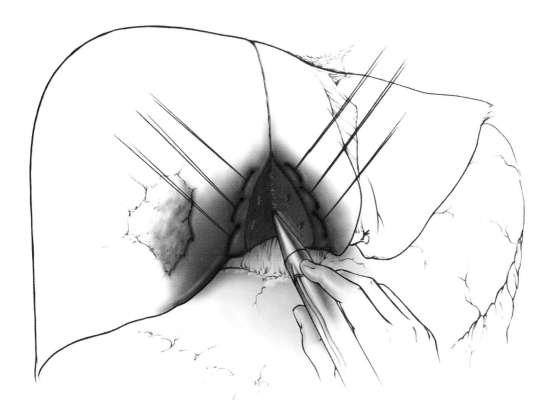

With division of hepatic vascular inflow and control of hepatic vascular out-flow, the parenchyma can be transected. The capsule of the liver is scored with a cautery along the line of demarcation between the right and left lobes of the liver. This line extends from the gallbladder fossa to the hepatic veins as they enter the inferior vena cava. Parallel rows of No. 1 chromic sutures, incorpo-rating approximately 2 cm of liver, are placed in a horizontal mattress fashion approximately 1 cm on either side of the plane of division between the lobes. The liver parenchyma is then divided with a combination of cautery and finger fracture technique. We have found use of the ultrasonic dissector (Cavitron ul-trasonic surgical aspirator [CUSA]) in the chronically obstructed liver secondary to cholangiocarcinoma difficult, because the parenchyma tends to become firmer and more fibrous and is less yielding to the ultrasound dissector. Therefore we tend to use a combination of finger fracture technique and cautery, being careful to leave the intraparenchymal vascular structures intact. Structures smaller than 5 mm are controlled with cautery, those 0.5 to 1.5 mm with hemoclips, and structures larger than 1.5 mm with ties or suture ligatures. Division of the parenchyma should proceed at a steady, controlled pace, averting unnecessary blood loss. The parenchyma should be transected over a broad front, with the surgeon ever aware of the location of the tumor and major vascular structures, especially the right portal pedicle. As work proceeds toward the dome of the liver, the middle hepatic vein and its larger branches will be encountered in or to the left of the plane of transection. Care should be taken to preserve the middle hepatic vein, if possible, without jeopardizing complete removal of the tumor.

Vascular isolation, via portal occlusion with a Rommel tourniquet, is commonly used during parenchymal transection for other types of tumors. We have found, however, that vascular inflow occlusion in the patient with obstructive cholangiopathy is not as well tolerated and can lead to an increased incidence of postoperative liver dysfunction, particularly of a cholestatic nature. If inflow occlusion is to be used, we routinely occlude for only 15 to 20 minutes at a time, followed by a 5-minute "rest" period.

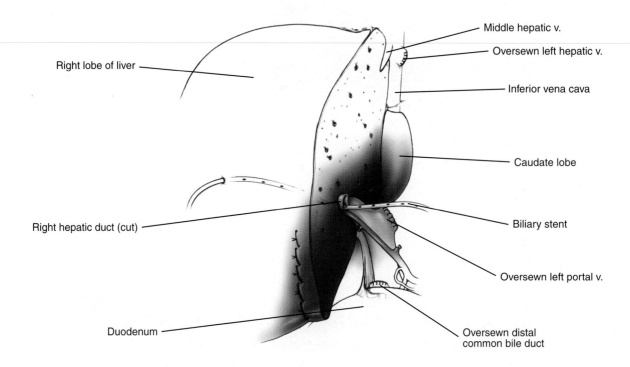

The resected specimen, which includes the entire extrahepatic biliary tree along with the gallbladder and the bifurcation and the left lobe of the liver, is taken to the pathology suite and oriented for the pathologists. Frozen sections are used to evaluate any questionable margins. Additional hemostasis is achieved with the argon beam coagulator. Major vascular structures, especially biliary, along the line of transection are carefully examined, and additional sutures are placed as needed.

Biliary Enteric Reconstruction

The biliary enteric reconstruction to the transected right lobe duct is essentially performed as described for resection of proximal cholangiocarcinoma without hepatic lobectomy (see p. 574 to 577).

Palliation of Proximal Cholangiocarcinoma by Transhepatic Stenting and Hepaticojejunostomy

Proximal cholangiocarcinomas are staged preoperatively and explored when they are thought to be curable based on cholangiographic and angiographic criteria. In patients who do not meet the criteria for resection, biliary obstruction is palliated by radiographically placed transhepatic biliary catheters, and exploratory surgery is not performed. Of those tumors thought to be curable at the time of exploration, only half will be resectable; the other half will be unresectable because of unrecognized tumor extension into both lobes or involvement of the common hepatic artery or main portal vein, which is often not apparent until after division of the distal common bile duct. If this is the case, we believe that it is appropriate to replace the radiographically placed catheters with silicone transhepatic biliary stents and to drain the biliary tree by constructing an end-to-side jejunal choledochojejunostomy. The larger Silastic stents provide better palliation than do the smaller percutaneous catheters alone in that they are better tolerated by patients and less frequently associated with complications. An hepaticojejunostomy is necessary, not only for placement of the larger catheters, but also because the distal common bile duct below the level of the tumor has already been divided during assessment of resectability.

Incision and Exposure

Positioning, preparation, and draping of the patient are as described above. The abdominal cavity is explored though an incision two fingerbreadths below the right costal margin. If tumor extends into both lobes, the diagnosis is confirmed by frozen-section analysis (if not confirmed preoperatively). It may be difficult to diagnose cholangiocarcinoma on frozen-section examination, but it is important to persist so that appropriate palliative therapy can be delivered postoperatively.

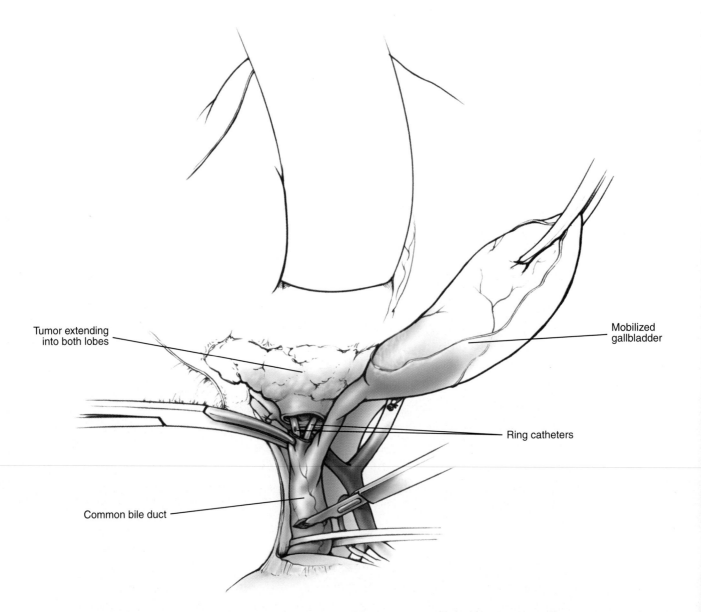

Tumor extending
into both lobes

Mobilized
gallbladder

Ring catheters

Common bile duct

Once the determination of unresectability has been made, the gallbladder should be removed and the common duct mobilized and looped with a vessel loop. The cystic artery is identified, doubly clamped, ligated, and divided. The gallbladder is mobilized out of the gallbladder fossa, and the common hepatic duct is divided distal to the common hepatic duct bifurcation. The distal common bile duct is divided below the cystic duct, and the gallbladder with a segment of extrahepatic tree is removed. The distal common bile duct, below the level of transection, is then either ligated or oversewn with interrupted 3-0 silk sutures. In many cases it is not clear that the tumor is unresectable until after the distal common bile duct has been divided and the tumor extension into the portal vein bifurcation or into the contralateral branches of the portal vein is noted. Even then, it is still necessary to remove the gallbladder, because the large Silastic stents may lead to obstruction of the cystic duct and to the development of acute cholecystitis.

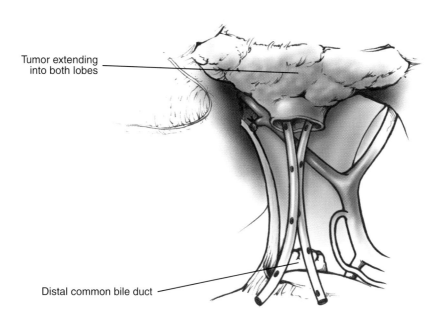

Tumor extending into both lobes

Distal common bile duct

After the gallbladder and segment of extrahepatic biliary tree have been removed, there remains a short segment of common hepatic duct extending below the tumor. The biliary stents placed preoperatively into both right and left hepatic ducts exit through the lumen of this short segment of common hepatic duct.

Biliary Enteric Reconstruction

Biliary enteric reconstruction is performed as described for resection of proximal cholangiocarcinoma at or above the common hepatic duct bifuraction without hepatic lobectomy (see pp. 574 to 577).

Resection of Gallbladder Fossa With Portal Lymphadenectomy

In most patients with carcinoma of the gallbladder the tumor extends into the liver, extrahepatic biliary tree, or regional lymph glands, making cure difficult if not impossible. Occasional patients have symptoms of gallstone disease and undergo elective cholecystectomy, only to find at pathologic examination of the gallbladder that an incidental adenocarcinoma is present. These patients with incidentally discovered superficially invasive gallbladder carcinoma have an excellent opportunity for cure by simple cholecystectomy. In rare patients the tumor is still confined primarily to the gallbladder and the surrounding liver parenchyma, and wedge resection of the liver and regional lymphadenotomy will yield at least significant palliative benefit and an occasional cure.

Incision and Exposure

Many patients are seen after a cholecystectomy via laparoscopic or open technique, during which carcinoma of the gallbladder was discovered. Nevertheless, all patients undergo exploratory surgery through a right subcostal incision. In obese patients the incision may be extended to the lateral peritoneal reflection on the right and to the lateral border of the rectus sheath on the left, for additional exposure. If the gallbladder has already been removed, the adhesions between the omentum, right hepatic flexure of the colon, or duodenum, to the gallbladder bed are gently taken down to expose the gallbladder bed and porta hepatis. If the gallbladder has not been removed at prior surgery, the part or all of the gallbladder wall may contain a thickened, whitish mass that is firmer than the typical chronic cholecystitis. In this case, wedge biopsy of the gallbladder wall with frozen-section examination is performed. If frozen-section analysis confirms carcinoma of the gallbladder, or if the surgeon's index of suspicion remains high despite a negative biopsy, the operative procedure is extended to wedge resection of the gallbladder fossa and regional lymphadenectomy.

Wedge Resection of Gallbladder Fossa

Resection of the gallbladder bed includes resection of a portion of liver segments IV-B, and V. If the tumor is confined to the muscularis of the gallbladder, the line of resection should be approximately 2 cm lateral and medial to the gallbladder fossae and extend at least 2 cm deep into the hepatic parenchyma. If there is invasion through the gallbladder wall into the hepatic parenchyma, the excision should extend at least 2 cm beyond the deepest portion of tumor. Preoperative CT scans are helpful, but intraoperative ultrasonograms are ultimately more useful in determining the depth of invasion.

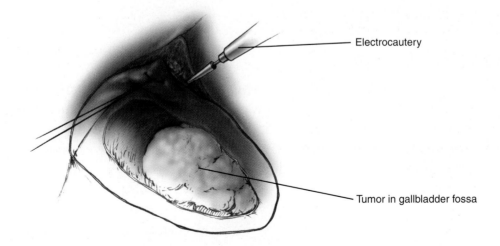

Electrocautery

Tumor in gallbladder fossa

The margins of the wedge resection are scored on the liver with an electrocautery. Overlapping No. 1 chromic mattress sutures are then placed circumferentially around the line of resection and secured to compress the surrounding hepatic parenchyma. After this has been accomplished, the wedge resection can be performed, utilizing a variety of techniques. For nonanatomic resection, use of the ultrasonic dissector is preferable because it clearly delineates vascular and biliary structures while removing the surrounding hepatic parenchyma. Structures smaller than 0.5 mm are controlled with electrocautery, those 0.5 to 1.5 mm with hemoclips, and structures larger than 1.5 mm with ties or suture ligatures. Vascular control using portal occlusion assists in controlling blood loss, which sometimes exceeds that seen in formal hepatic lobectomies. Formal portal dissection with control of specific lobar vessels is not needed for this procedure. Once the specimen has been removed, small bleeding points or small bile ducts are further controlled with suture ligatures.

Regional Portal Lymphadenectomy

Following the wedge liver resection, regional portal lymph node dissection is performed. All of the tissues surrounding the biliary and major vascular structures, extending from the bifurcation of the common hepatic duct to the distal common bile duct as it enters the pancreas behind the duodenum, are removed en bloc. The majority of the lymph nodes within this tissue are posterior to the common bile duct and adjacent to the portal vein. Care must be taken in removing these nodes to prevent injury to the portal vein or to a replaced right hepatic artery, which originates from the superior mesenteric artery and travels through the lateral posterior aspect of the hepatoduodenal ligament (type III anatomy). Palpation of the posterior lateral aspect of the porta prior to dissection usually identifies the replaced right hepatic artery if preoperative angiograms are not available.

Sometimes a Kocher maneuver will assist in removal of the lymph nodes posterior to the common bile duct, which extend behind the C loop of the duodenum. The dissection must also include the nodes extending medially along the common hepatic artery as it arises from the celiac axis. These lymph nodes travel in a groove between the common hepatic artery and the superior border of the pancreas. When the porta hepatis and the hepatic artery down to the celiac axis have been skeletonized, the dissection is complete. The liver resection and the periportal areas are drained with two closed suction drainage catheters (Jackson-Pratt drains). All laparoscopic port sites are then excised to prevent an abdominal wall recurrence. The port sites are closed primarily. The abdomen is then closed with two layers of running nonabsorbable monofilament suture.

Anatomic Basis of Complications

- Surgery for biliary tract tumors, particularly those of the proximal third, remains difficult and is associated with potential for significant mortality and high early morbidity. The main complications include bleeding, anastomotic leakage, abscess formation, portal vein or hepatic artery thrombosis, cholangitis, and liver abscess.

- Bleeding usually occurs during the operation, but also can occur in the early postoperative period. Contributing to this problem is coagulopathy secondary to vitamin K deficiency in patients with prolonged obstructive jaundice. This coagulopathy should be anticipated during the preoperative preparation of the patient and corrected by administration of vitamin K, fibrinogen, and fresh-frozen plasma.

  Intraoperative bleeding from the portal vein and the hepatic artery tends to occur during dissection of the tumor off these individual structures. Injury to the portal vein can be prevented by early mobilization, division, and elevation of the distal common bile duct, in an effort to expose the portal vein trunk and bifurcation. Injury to the hepatic artery can occur during dissection of the tumor mass. Special attention must be paid to prevent injury to a right hepatic artery originating from the superior mesenteric artery (type III anatomy) during lymphatic clearance of the hepatoduodenal ligament. Blind dissection is to be avoided at all times. Injury to the common hepatic artery or its branches can be prevented by identification of the artery in the distal hepatoduodenal ligament early in the dissection, followed by complete mobilization and retraction of the artery and its branches laterally and away from the bile duct and associated tumor. Again, early division and mobilization of the distal common bile duct tumor lessens the chance for injury to the arterial blood supply to the liver.

  Life-threatening intraoperative bleeding may also occur from the vena cava or the hepatic veins, if a combined liver resection is also performed. These veins can be damaged during dissection or by excessive torquing of the liver during mobilization. An adequate incision, with careful dissection under visual control, is mandatory to prevent such injuries. Careful dissection and division of the veins bridging the vena cava and posterior caudate lobe allow complete elevation of the liver off the vena cava and a more accessible dissection with control of the hepatic veins at their entrance into the inferior vena cava.

Anatomic Basis of Complications—cont'd

Prevention of postoperative bleeding starts at the time of the initial surgery, with meticulous hemostasis and careful inspection of the operative field before closing the abdominal cavity. Bleeding from the hepaticojejunostomy or jejunojejunostomy can be difficult to diagnose, but usually occurs later than bleeding into the intra-abdominal cavity. This complication almost always requires repeat exploration and takedown of the anastomosis with control of specific bleeding points.

- Anastomotic dehiscence with leakage can occur in either the early or late postoperative period. If it occurs in the early postoperative course, it will usually heal spontaneously if the leak is small. A late postoperative leak, however, may be due to bile duct ischemia and may require repeat operation. Abscess formation may also occur secondary to contaminated collections of bile or blood accumulated after the operation. Preventive measures are paramount, including good hemostatis, careful fashioning of the hepaticojejunostomies, and adequate drainage of the abdominal cavity. In most cases, CT-directed drainage of the abscess and intravenously administered antibiotics successfully control anastomotic leakage.
- Thrombosis of either the portal vein or the hepatic artery may also occur in the postoperative period. Portal vein thrombosis may be occult and not recognized until symptoms of portal hypertension develop later in the postoperative period. Acute hepatic artery thrombosis, however, may be recognized by elevation in hepatocellular enzyme levels, and may be associated with acute liver failure or a late anastomotic leak or stricture.
- Cholangitis is often seen in the early postoperative period, and is usually the result of surgical manipulation of the colonized stented biliary tree. Management with intravenously administered antibiotics, assurance of the patency of any transhepatic biliary stents, and a search for any remaining obstructed biliary segments are the hallmarks of therapy.
- Liver abscess may develop due to failure to establish adequate biliary drainage during surgery. Management of liver abscesses, in the majority of the patients, can be achieved by percutaneous drainage under ultrasound or CT guidance. On occasion, however, formal laparotomy with debridement and evacuation of the abscess cavity, followed by drainage, is necessary.

KEY REFERENCES

Ahrendt SA, Cameron JL, Pitt HA. Current management of patients with perihilar cholangiocarcinoma. Adv Surg 30:427-452.

This is a thorough, detailed, and comprehensive review of all aspects of cholangiocarcinoma management. Included in this chapter are sections on preoperative evaluation, surgical decision making, surgical technique, palliative therapy, and treatment results. This work is an extremely valuable current review and contains a lengthy list of important references.

Broelsch CE. Atlas of Liver Surgery. New York: Churchill Livingstone, 1993, pp 176-195.

This beautifully illustrated and comprehensively written atlas includes in-depth details of biliary and liver resection techniques. The completeness and accuracy of the illustrations and accompanying text add greatly to the practical usefulness of this work by inclusion of information not found in other atlases.

Cameron JL, ed. Atlas of Surgery, vol 1. Philadelphia: BC Decker, 1990, pp 58-198.

Beautifully illustrated and clearly written, this atlas includes the techniques of biliary and liver resection used by the Johns Hopkins surgical faculty. The detail and accuracy of the illustrations add greatly to the realism and practical usefulness of this work.

Chassin JL. Operations for carcinoma of hepatic duct bifurcation. In Operative Strategy in General Surgery. New York: Springer-Verlag, 1994, pp 585-598.

This concise, clearly written chapter contains a detailed sequential step-by-step description of bile duct resection for cholangiocarcinoma. This chapter is structured so that the novice surgeon can be comfortable with the steps involved in curative resection. The illustrations are closely associated with the text and provide important anatomic details.

Pitt HA, Dooley WC, Yeo CJ, et al. Malignancies of the biliary tree. Curr Probl Surg 32:1-100, 1995.

Although slightly dated, this is an excellent overview of biliary tree malignancies, including cholangiocarcinoma and gallbladder cancer. This valuable review article is comprehensive and contains a lengthy list of references.

Smadja C, Blumgart LH. The biliary tract and the anatomy of biliary exposure. In Blumgart LH, ed. Surgery of the Liver and Biliary Tract. Edinburgh: Churchill Livingstone, 1994, pp 11-24.

This is an excellent in-depth description of biliary tree anatomy from a surgical prospective. All important variations of anatomy have been included in the thorough work, which also includes a section describing techniques of biliary exposure with emphasis on anatomic detail.

SUGGESTED READINGS

Abi-Rached B, Neugut AL. Diagnosis and management issues in gallbladder carcinoma. Oncology 9:19-30, 1995.

Anson BJ, McVay CB. Surgical Anatomy. Philadelphia: WB Saunders, 1984, pp 616-629.

Bismuth H, Chiche L. Surgical anatomy and anatomical surgery of the liver. In Blumgart LH, ed. Surgery of the Liver and Biliary Tract. Edinburgh: Churchill Livingstone, 1994, pp 3-9.

Bismuth H, Nakache R, Diamond T. Management strategies in resection for hilar cholangiocarcinoma. Ann Surg 215:31-38, 1992.

Boema EJ. Research into the results of resection of hilar bile duct cancer. Surgery 108:572-580, 1990.

Cameron JL, Pitt HA, Zinner MJ, et al. Management of proximal cholangiocarcinoma by surgical resection and radiotherapy. Am J Surg 159:91-98, 1990.

Cubertafond P, Gainant A, Clucchairo G. Surgical treatment of 724 carcinomas of the gallbladder: Results of the French Surgical Association survey. Ann Surg 219:275-280, 1994.

Donohue JH, Nagorney DM, Grant CS, et al. Carcinoma of the gallbladder. Arch Surg 125:237-241, 1990.

Gall FP, Kockerling F, Scheele J, et al. Radical operations for carcinoma of the gallbladder: Present status in Germany. World J Surg 15:328-336, 1991.

Nordback IH, Pitt HA, Coleman JA, et al. Unresectable hilar cholangiocarcinoma: Percutaneous versus operative palliation. Surgery 115:597-603, 1992.

Piehler JM, Crichlow RW. Primary carcinoma of the gallbladder. Surg Gynecol Obstet 147:929-942, 1978.

Sugiura Y, Nakamura S, Iida S, et al. Extensive resection of the bile ducts combined with liver resection for cancer of the main hepatic duct junction: A cooperative study of the Keio Bile Duct Cancer Study Group. Surgery 115:445-451, 1994.

Thorek P. Anatomy in Surgery. New York: Springer-Verlag, 1985, pp 534-545.

Wanebo HJ, Vezeridis MP. Carcinoma of the gallbladder. J Surg Oncol (Suppl 3):134-139, 1993.

Warwick R, Williams PL, Dyson M, et al. Gray's Anatomy. Philadelphia: WB Saunders, 1989, pp 1393-1396.

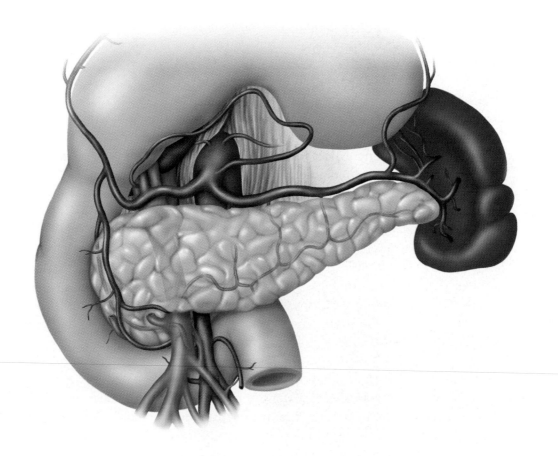

Chapter 14

Pancreas and Duodenum

Gene Branum, M.D., and Lee J. Skandalakis, M.D.

Surgical Applications

Transduodenal Biopsy of Pancreas
Whipple Operation With Hemigastrectomy
Whipple Operation With Pylorus Preservation
Distal Pancreatectomy With Splenectomy
Enucleation of Insulinoma
Local Excision of Ampullary Tumor
Excision of Duodenal Tumor
Duodenal Resection
Resection of Third or Fourth Portion of Duodenum

P ancreatic exocrine neoplasms are common. The early signs and symptoms of pancreatic exocrine tumors are vague and nonspecific (e.g.,
anorexia, malaise, weight loss), making delayed diagnosis the rule, not
the exception. Pancreatic endocrine tumors may cause vague symptoms as well, but are often associated with recognizable clinical syndromes that
lead to the diagnosis. Duodenal tumors are more unusual and are characterized
by the same difficulties in diagnosis. Despite the vagaries of diagnosis, pancreatic resection remains an important tool in the treatment of pancreatic neoplasms and is challenging for even the most experienced surgeon.

Preoperative evaluation of pancreatic and duodenal tumors is improving
with the development of spiral computed tomography (CT) and endoscopic
ultrasonography. These two modalities are increasingly accurate for diagnosis
of vascular invasion, a notoriously difficult task in the past. Moreover, preoperative laparoscopy is useful to rule out peritoneal and hepatic metastases and
allows peritoneal washing for cytologic analysis.

Trials are ongoing to evaluate preoperative treatment with chemotherapy
and radiation, and fine-needle aspiration biopsy is crucial to confirm the diagnosis in patients for whom this treatment is chosen. After induction chemoradiation therapy and prior to resection, repeat laparoscopy may be performed
to exclude peritoneal or hepatic spread. Adjuvant chemoradiation therapy
shows promise in improving survival after resection in some trials and is routinely offered to patients after resection.

SURGICAL ANATOMY
Topography
Duodenum

The first portion of the duodenum is approximately 5 cm long. The proximal
half is mobile; the distal half is fixed. The first duodenum passes upward from
the pylorus to the neck of the gallbladder. It is related posteriorly to the common bile duct, portal vein, inferior vena cava, and gastroduodenal artery; anteriorly to the quadrate lobe of the liver; superiorly to the epiploic foramen;
and inferiorly to the head of the pancreas. The first 2.5 cm is covered by the
same two layers of peritoneum that invest the stomach. The hepatoduodenal
portion of the lesser omentum attaches to the superior border of the duodenum; the greater omentum attaches to its inferior border. The distal 2.5 cm
is covered with peritoneum only on the anterior surface; thus the posterior
surface is in intimate contact with the bile duct, portal vein, and gastroduodenal artery. The duodenum is separated from the inferior vena cava by a small
amount of connective tissue.

The second (descending) portion is approximately 7.5 cm long. It extends
from the neck of the gallbladder to the upper border of L4. The second duodenum is crossed by the transverse colon and mesocolon and consists of a supra-

mesocolic segment and an inframesocolic segment. The segments above and below the attachment of the transverse colon are covered with visceral peritoneum. The first and second portions of the duodenum join behind the costal margin slightly above and medial to the tip of the ninth costal cartilage and on the right side of L1. The second portion of the duodenum forms an acute angle with the first portion and descends from the neck of the gallbladder anterior to the hilum of the right kidney, the right ureter, the right renal vessels, the psoas major muscle, and the edge of the inferior vena cava. The second portion of the duodenum is related anteriorly to the right lobe of the liver, the transverse colon, and the jejunum. At about the midpoint of the second part of the duodenum, the pancreaticobiliary tract opens into its concave posteromedial side. The right side is related to the ascending colon and the right colic flexure.

The third portion of the duodenum (horizontal or inferior) is approximately 10 cm long. It extends from the right side of L3 or L4 to the left side of the aorta. The third portion of the duodenum begins about 5 cm from the midline, to the right of the lower end of L3 at about the level of the subcostal plane. It passes in a transverse pathway to the left, anterior to the ureter, right gonadal vessels, psoas muscle, inferior vena cava, lumbar vertebral column, and aorta and ends to the left of L3.

The inframesocolic portion of the duodenum is covered anteriorly by the peritoneum. It is crossed anteriorly by the superior mesenteric vessels. Near its termination it is crossed by the root of the mesentery of the small intestine. The third portion is related superiorly to the head and uncinate process of the pancreas. The inferior pancreaticoduodenal artery lies in a groove at the interface of the pancreas and duodenum. Anteriorly and inferiorly this part of the duodenum is related to the small bowel, primarily to the jejunum.

The second and third portions are overlapped by the head of the pancreas, so there is a pancreatic bare area of the duodenum not covered by peritoneum. A second bare area exists on the anterior surface of the second part of the duodenum, where the transverse colon is attached. With pancreatic cancer or pancreatitis, the pancreas and mesocolon with its middle colic artery become firmly fixed. The anatomic entities responsible for duodenal fixation are the pylorus, the superior mesenteric vessels, the ligament of Treitz, and the peritoneum.

The fourth portion of the duodenum (ascending) is approximately 2.5 cm long. It extends from the left side of the aorta to the left upper border of L2 and is directed obliquely upward, slightly to the left. It ends at the duodenojejunal junction (flexure) at the level of L2 at the root of the transverse mesocolon. This junction occurs approximately 4 cm below and medial to the tip of the ninth costal cartilage. The fourth portion is related posteriorly to the left sympathetic trunk, the psoas muscle, and the left renal and gonadal vessels. Its termination is very close to the terminal part of the inferior mesenteric vein, the left ureter, and the left kidney. The upper end of the root of the mesentery attaches here also. The duodenojejunal junction is suspended by the ligament of Treitz, a remnant of the dorsal mesentery, which extends from the duodenojejunal flexure to the right crus of the diaphragm.

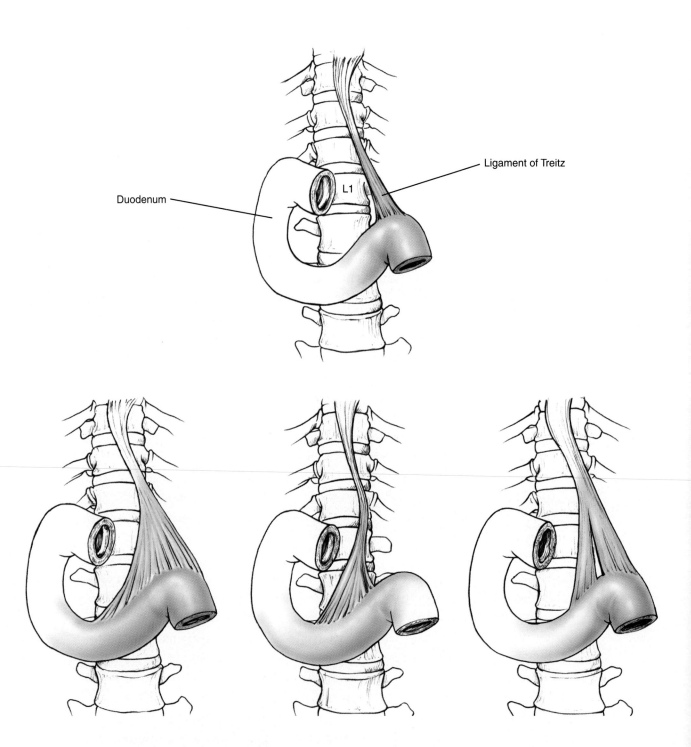

The suspensory ligament usually inserts on the duodenal flexure and the third and fourth portions of the duodenum. It may insert on the flexure only, or on the third and fourth portions only. There may also be multiple attachments. In almost one fifth of cadavers, the ligament is absent.

Pancreas

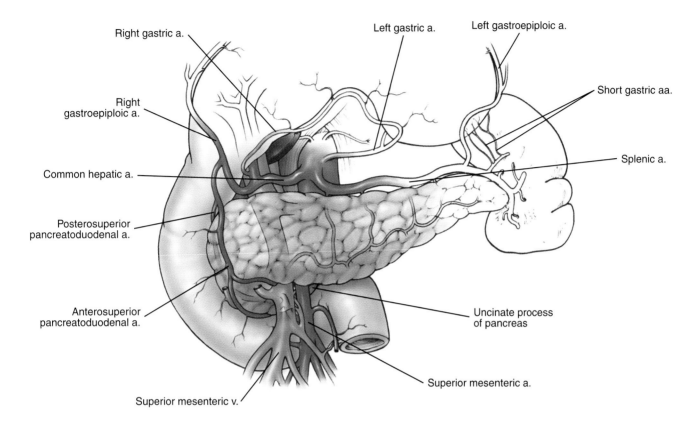

The pancreas is an elongated organ with a lobular surface extending from the C loop of the duodenum to the hilum of the spleen. The gland is retroperitoneal and is divided topographically into the uncinate, head, neck, body, and tail. The head lies to the right of the second lumbar vertebra in apposition to the duodenum. The uncinate process lies posterior to the head, extends medially to lie beneath the superior mesenteric vessels, and contacts the vena cava posteriorly.

The neck is a narrowed 2.0 to 2.5 cm portion of the gland that lies directly over the superior mesenteric vein and beneath the first duodenum. Only rarely are there vascular attachments between the neck and the superior mesenteric vein. Development of the plane between these structures is a critical step in performing pancreatic resection.

The body extends across the second lumbar vertebral body anterior to the left kidney and tapers slightly cephalad into the tail, terminating in or near the splenic hilum.

The anterior surface of the pancreas is covered by the parietal peritoneum, which separates the gland from the stomach. The inferior surface abuts the transverse mesocolon and is closely associated with the duodenojejunal junction. The splenic vein is imbedded by varying degrees in the posterior surface of the pancreas, occasionally completely encased by pancreatic tissue. The splenic artery runs along the superior edge of the gland.

Pancreatic Ducts

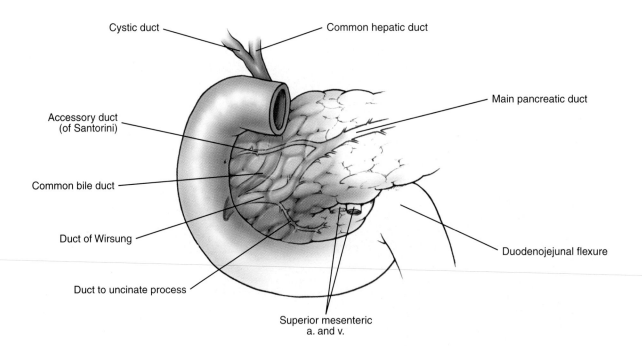

The pancreatic ductal system is formed by the fusion of two embryologic ductal systems. The main pancreatic duct originates in the tail and travels longitudinally through the gland to the head, where in most cases it turns slightly caudally and posterior to its termination in the duodenal papilla. At the point of deviation of the duct, an accessory duct travels more directly through the head to the duodenum, terminating in the minor or lesser papilla. In a minority (10%) of patients the ductal systems fail to fuse, and the accessory duct serves as the major drainage system for the gland. This anatomic variant constitutes pancreas divisum. Tributaries to the main duct are generally at right angles to it, an arrangement upheld in the secondary and tertiary ducts as well.

Ampulla of Vater

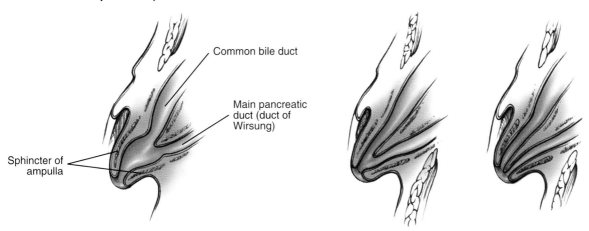

The pancreatic duct and the bile duct terminate in the duodenum at the ampulla (papilla) of Vater. The major papilla is an elevation of the duodenal mucosa at the point where the common bile duct and the pancreatic duct enter the duodenum. It is usually 7 to 10 cm from the pylorus, but may be as close as 1.5 cm or as distant as 12 cm. The bile duct and the pancreatic duct typically join to form a common channel of varying length (the ampulla) within the papilla. In a minority of cases the two ducts enter the duodenum separately through the papilla, in which case the ampulla is said to be absent. In rare instances the ducts may enter the duodenum via separate papillae. The minor papilla is present in approximately 70% of patients and lies slightly anterior and 2 cm cephalad to the major papilla.

The following classification seems the most useful:

Type 1   The pancreatic duct opens into the common bile duct at a variable distance from the opening in the major duodenal papilla. The common channel may or may not be dilated (85%).

Type 2   The pancreatic and bile ducts open close to one another but separately on the major duodenal papilla (5%).

Type 3   The pancreatic and bile ducts open into the duodenum at separate points (9%).

The variations in the distance between the pancreaticobiliary junction and the duodenal lumen result from developmental processes. In the embryo the main pancreatic duct arises as a branch of the common bile duct, which in turn arises from the duodenum. Growth of the duodenum absorbs the proximal bile duct up to its junction with the pancreatic duct. When resorption is minimal there is a long ampulla and the junction of the ducts is high in the duodenal wall (type 1), or even extramural. With increased resorption of the terminal bile duct the junction lies closer to the duodenal orifice and the ampulla is shortened. Maximum resorption results in separate orifices for the main pancreatic duct and the common bile duct (type 3).

MAJOR DUODENAL PAPILLA

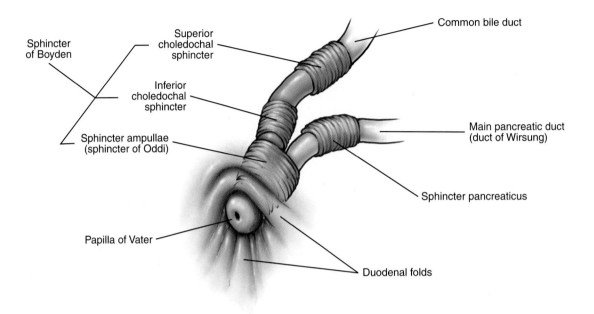

Endoscopically, the major papilla may be recognized at the junction of a transverse and a longitudinal fold of duodenum mucosa (plica longitudinalis), which forms a T configuration. The orifice of the papilla is often filled with villus-like projections called valvulae.

Like the papilla of Vater, the sphincter of Oddi at the duodenal end of the pancreatic and common bile ducts is misnamed. By priority of description, it should have been named for Francis Gilsson (1654), who described annular fibers around the entire intramural portion of the bile duct and believed they guarded the opening against reflux of duodenal contents.

The sphincter lies within the ampulla and is a complex series of muscular valves that work in conjunction with hormonal and neural signals to control secretion from the pancreatic and bile ducts. This sphincteric mechanism constitutes the narrowest portion of both the bilary and pancreatic ductal systems and is the most common site of stone-related obstruction of these ducts.

MINOR DUODENAL PAPILLA

The minor papilla is about 2 cm cranial and slightly anterior to the major papilla. The accessory pancreatic duct (of Santorini) opens through the minor papilla, which is smaller and less easily identified than the major papilla. The most useful landmark is the gastroduodenal artery, behind which lies the accessory duct and the minor papilla. Duodenal dissection for gastrectomy should end proximal to the artery.

The minor papilla may contain no duct or only a microscopic, tortuous channel. A true sphincter (of Helly) is rarely present. In about 10% of patients, the duct of Santorini is the only duct draining most of the pancreas. Accidental ligation of this duct, together with the gastroduodenal artery, would result in catastrophic pancreatitis.

Blood Supply
Arteries

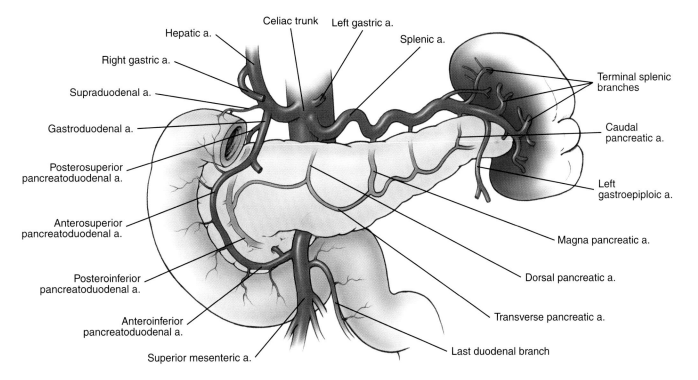

The blood supply of the duodenum is confusing because of the diverse possibilities of origin, distribution, and individual variations. This is especially true of the blood supply of the first portion of the duodenum.

The first part of the duodenum is supplied by the supraduodenal artery and the posterosuperior pancreaticoduodenal branch of the gastroduodenal artery (retroduodenal artery of Edwards, Michel, and Wilkie), which is a branch of the common hepatic artery. In many patients the upper part of the first 1 cm is also supplied by branches of the right gastric artery. In some patients there may be separate small branches to the superior and posterior aspects of the first part of the duodenum. These can be properly called supraduodenal and retroduodenal, respectively. Each may arise separately or in various combinations. It is preferred, therefore, that the term retroduodenal not be used as a synonym for the posterosuperior pancreaticoduodenal artery, the principal role of which is to supply the second part of the duodenum and the pancreatic head.

After giving origin to the supraduodenal, retroduodenal, and posterosuperior pancreatoduodenal branches, the gastroduodenal artery descends between the first part of the duodenum and the head of the pancreas. It terminates by dividing into the right gastroepiploic and anterosuperior pancreatoduodenal arteries, both supplying twigs to this part of the duodenum.

The remaining three parts of the duodenum are supplied by an anterior and a posterior arcade. From the arcades spring pancreatic and duodenal branches. Those supplying the duodenum are called arteriae rectae, and they may be embedded in the substance of the pancreas.

The pancreas has an extremely rich blood supply from varied sources, the most major of which comes from branches of the gastroduodenal, superior mesenteric, and splenic or celiac arteries. Numerous smaller tributaries arise from the splenic, hepatic, and gastroduodenal arteries.

The gastroduodenal artery is critical to any discussion of pancreatic arterial anatomy. It arises from the hepatic artery approximately 2 cm from its origin and passes medially and inferiorly to the common bile duct, where it passes beneath the first portion of the duodenum and across the anterior surface of the head of the pancreas. The anterosuperior pancreatoduodenal artery is a continuation of the gastroduodenal artery and passes downward and through the sulcus between the duodenum and the pancreas. It continues and anastomoses with the inferior pancreatoduodenal artery along the medial surface of the duodenum. The posterosuperior pancreatoduodenal artery branches from the gastroduodenal artery at the superior border of the pancreas and traverses posteriorly behind the pancreas, traversing medially to anastomose with the posteroinferior pancreatoduodenal artery.

Two other major arterial branches supplying the body and tail of the pancreas are the inferoanterior and inferoposterior pancreatoduodenal arteries. These two arteries arise from the superior mesenteric artery, or one of its primary branches, and form an arcade that supplies the duodenojejunal junction and portions of the neck of the pancreas.

The superior dorsal pancreatic artery is somewhat inconstant, but when present arises from either the celiac or splenic artery and courses along the superior border of the body and tail of the pancreas. The inferior transverse pancreatic artery is fairly constant and arises from either the superior mesenteric artery, the superoanterior pancreatoduodenal artery, or the superior dorsal pancreatic artery and passes through the body of the pancreas along the inferior margin of the gland.

The body and tail of the gland receive numerous branches from the splenic artery, which leave the artery intermittently as it courses along the superior border of the gland.

There are surgically significant arterial anomalies. The most common major anomaly is the origin of the right hepatic artery from the superior mesenteric artery. When this occurs the artery passes through the head of the pancreas or posterior to the head in intimate contact and enters the porta hepatis posterior and lateral to the common bile duct. More rarely the common hepatic artery may arise from the superior mesenteric artery and travel anterior, posterior, or through the pancreatic substance to the porta hepatis. Recognition of these anomalies is critical to the safe performance of pancreatoduodenal resection and certain hepatobiliary procedures. When either artery travels posterior to the head of the gland, it can usually be dissected free and preserved. When an anomalous artery passes through the substance of the gland, it will be sacrificed and may need to be reconstructed via reimplantation in the common hepatic artery or the gastroduodenal artery, or grafted into the aorta.

Veins

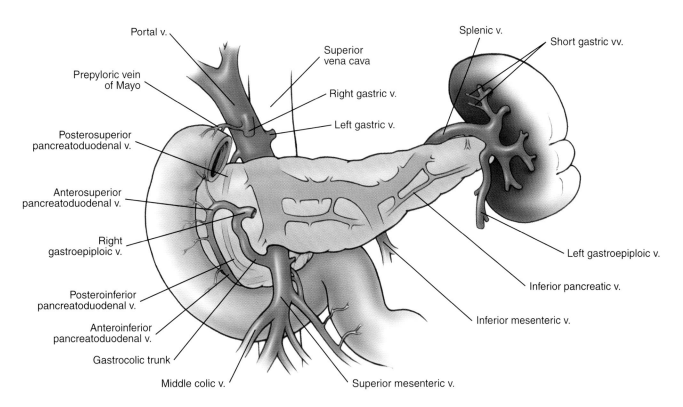

Veins of the lower first part of the duodenum and the pylorus usually open into the right gastroepiploic veins; they are the subpyloric veins. The upper first part of the duodenum is drained by suprapyloric veins, which open into the portal vein or the posterosuperior pancreatoduodenal vein. Anastomoses between subpyloric and suprapyloric veins pass around the duodenum. One of these has been said to mark the site of the pylorus (prepyloric vein of Mayo). It is not a constant indicator of the location of the pylorus.

The venous arcades draining the duodenum follow the arterial arcades and tend to lie superficial to them. The anterosuperior vein drains into the right gastroepiploic vein. The posterosuperior vein usually passes behind the common bile duct to enter the portal vein. The inferior veins can enter the superior or the inferior mesenteric vein, the splenic vein, or the first jejunal branch of the superior mesenteric vein. The veins may terminate separately or by a common stem.

The superior mesenteric vein, the splenic vein, and the portal vein are intimately associated with the pancreas. The anterior surface of the superior mesenteric vein passes directly beneath the neck of the gland and only rarely receives branches. The splenic vein receives numerous branches from the body and tail of the pancreas along its course to its junction with the superior mesenteric vein beneath the neck of the gland. The inferior mesenteric vein is constant in its course, but variable in its drainage into either the splenic vein or superior mesenteric vein. The left gastric (coronary) vein is constant in its course along the lesser curve of the stomach, but terminates at the splenoportal junction or along the portal vein some distance from the splenoportal junction.

This trunk is ligated for exposure of the anterior surface of the pancreas. The head of the gland is drained via an arcade of venous structures forming the anterosuperior pancreaticoduodenal vein and the anteroinferior pancreatoduodenal veins. The former receives numerous duodenal tributaries and passes upward and medially from the duodenojejunal junction to enter the gastrocolic trunk. The latter passes medially through the substance of the pancreas, joining a jejunal tributary of the superior mesenteric vein. The posterior aspect of the head is drained by two significant veins, the posterosuperior and posteroinferior pancreatoduodenal veins. The superior vein courses behind the bile duct and wraps medially to drain directly into the portal vein, and the inferior vein passes around the superior mesenteric vein and drains into that vein's first duodenojejunal tributary.

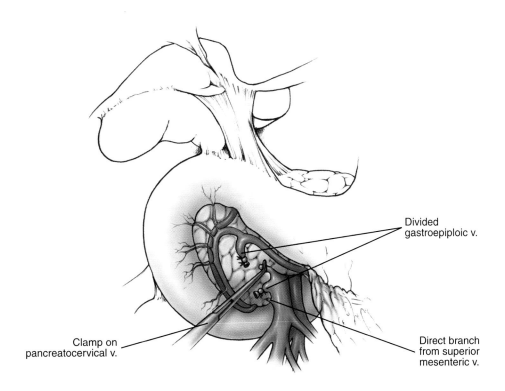

The right gastroepiploic vein courses along the greater curvature of the stomach between the two leaves of the gastrocolic ligament and curves downward where it joins the superior mesenteric vein just below the neck of the pancreas. The right gastroepiploic vein is significant because it is joined near its insertion into the superior mesenteric vein by the inferosuperior duodenal vein and one or more colic veins. This short but relatively broad attachment is called the gastrocolic trunk.

The superior portion of the neck and body of the pancreas is drained through multiple short tributaries into the splenic vein. The inferior portion of the neck and body of the pancreas are drained by a relatively constant inferior pancreatic vein, which courses along the inferior border of the body of the gland and commonly empties into either side of the superior mesenteric vein.

Major anomalies of the pancreatoduodenal venous drainage are unusual. Particular care must be paid, however, to rare but anomalous connections of the neck of the pancreas to the portal vein via short tributaries. In addition, when mobilizing the pancreas from the anterior surface of the superior mesenteric vein short but relatively wide tributaries directly into the vein from the uncinate process are often encountered and must be ligated and evaluated with care to prevent their being torn from the superior mesenteric or portal vein.

Lymphatic Drainage

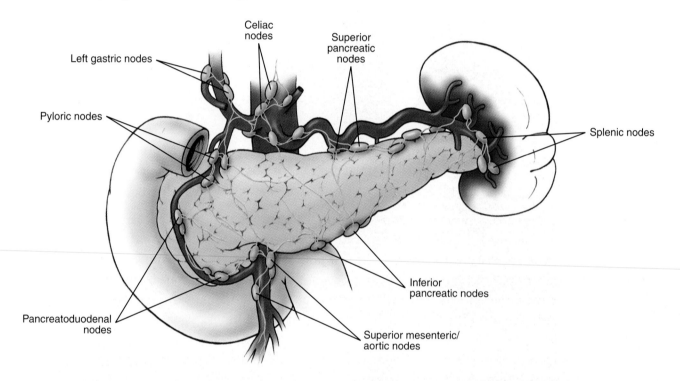

The duodenum is richly supplied with lymphatic vessels. They originate as blind-ending vessels (lacteals) in each villus of the mucosa. These vessels form a plexus in the lamina propria and, piercing the muscularis mucosae, form a second submucosal plexus. Still another lymphatic plexus lies between the circular and longitudinal layers of the muscularis. Collecting trunks pass over the anterior and posterior duodenal wall toward the lesser curvature to enter the anterior and posterior pancreaticoduodenal lymph nodes.

The anterior extramural collecting ducts drain to nodes anterior to the pancreas. The posterior ducts pass to nodes posterior to the head of the pancreas. The ducts follow the veins and arteries to nodes related to the superior mesenteric artery.

Nerve Supply

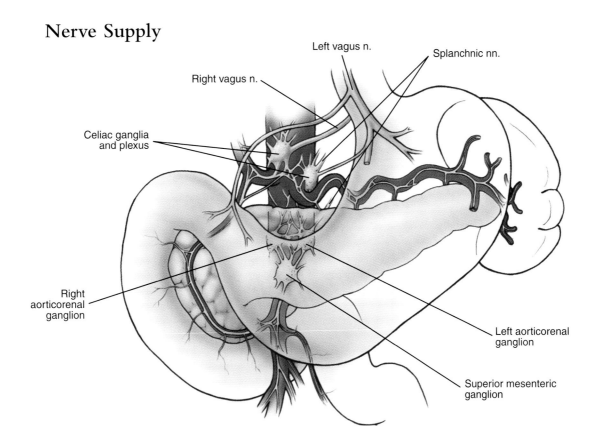

Within the duodenal wall are the two well-known neural plexuses of the gastrointestinal tract, each of which is composed of groups of neurons interconnected by networks of fibers. One plexus (of Meissner) is in the submucosa; another plexus (of Auerbach) is in the connective tissue between circular and longitudinal layers of muscularis externa. Some of the neuronal cells bodies and processes in the plexuses are assumed to be postganglionic parasympathetic fibers. However, recent studies indicate that many are related to circuitry for processing information received from various types of sensory receptors, synaptic complexes for directing neural outflow, and interconnecting neurons.

The preganglionic parasympathetic fibers in the plexuses are carried initially by the vagus nerves. The postganglionic sympathetic fibers arise from cell bodies located in the celiac and superior mesenteric plexuses, and perhaps the upper thoracic sympathetic chain ganglia also. The extrinsic nerve supply to the duodenum probably includes contributions that leave the anterior hepatic plexus close to the origin of the right gastric artery. In unusual cases, nerves from the hepatic division of the anterior vagal trunk give rise to one or more branches that innervated the first part of the duodenum. In most specimens, some branches can be traced upward to the gastric incisura.

Innervation of the pancreas largely accompanies the vascular structures. Sympathetic fibers travel via the celiac ganglion, where preganglionic efferent fibers pass before reaching the pancreas. The sympathetic efferent fibers are located in the dorsal root ganglia T10 through T12, an important concept in consideration of operations to relieve pain from chronic pancreatitis or pancreas exocrine cancer. The parasympathetic fibers invade the pancreas via the vagus nerve and have their cell bodies in the brain.

SURGICAL APPLICATIONS
Incisions

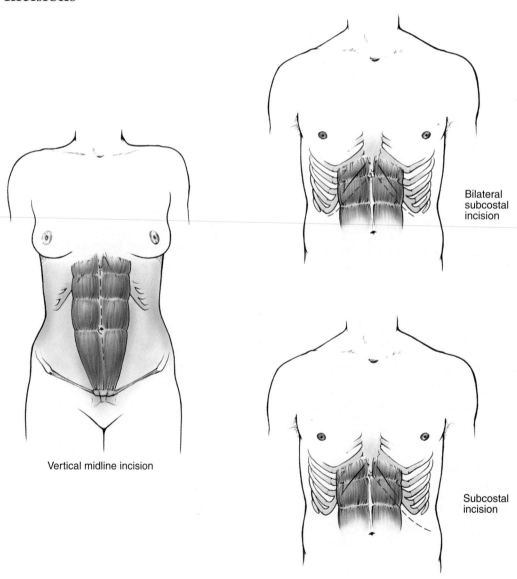

Bilateral subcostal incision

Vertical midline incision

Subcostal incision

Several incisions can be used to expose the pancreas. A vertical midline incision provides adequate exposure to the entire pancreas in most patients. The bilateral subcostal ("bucket handle") incision may be extended along the left or right subcostal margin to provide better exposure for either the head, or tail and spleen. For more limited exposure of the head and duodenum for procedures such as ampullary resection, a right subcostal incision may be adequate. Likewise, for distal pancreatectomy with or without splenectomy, a left subcostal incision may suffice.

Exposure of Pancreas

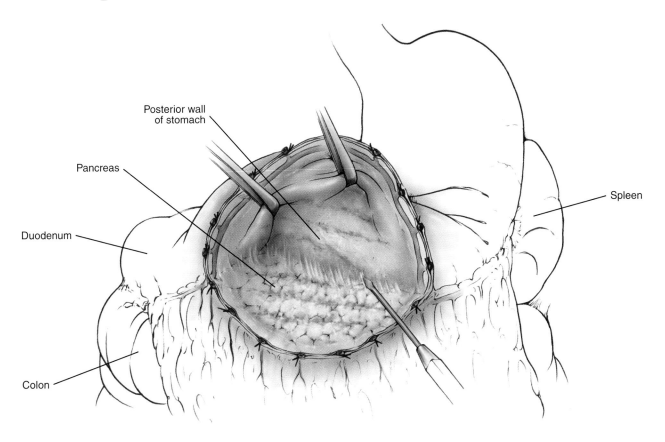

The pancreas may be exposed via several approaches, tailored to the procedure. The most commonly used exposure is via the gastrocolic approach. The gastrocolic omentum is divided between clamps, preserving, if possible, the gastroepiploic arteries. Progressing laterally to the right, the superior and lateral peritoneal reflections of the right colon are divided either between clamps or with an electrocautery, and the colon is retracted inferiorly for the remainder of the operation.

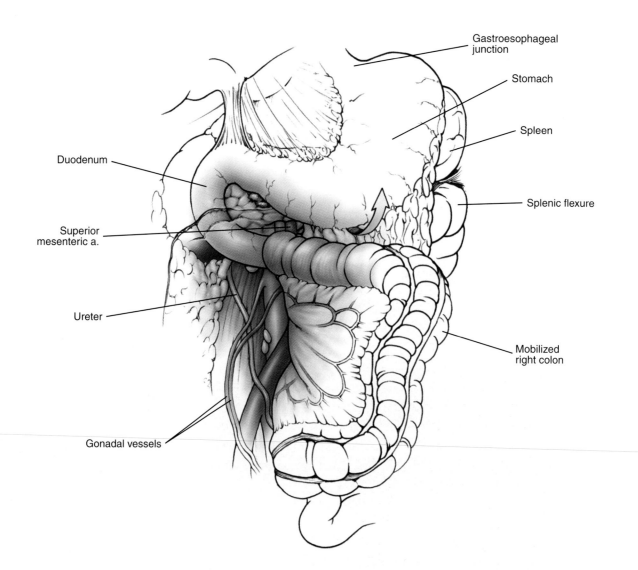

The Cattell maneuver may be performed to allow increased exposure of the superior mesenteric vein, vena cava, and pancreatic tissues. The lateral reflection of the right colon and hepatic flexure are mobilized, and the entire right colon retracted inferomedially. For procedures involving the tail of the gland, and especially if splenectomy is to be performed, the short gastric vessels should be divided between clamps and tied. When this exposure has been obtained, the stomach can be retracted superiorly for the remainder of the operation. Retrogastric adhesions between the stomach and pancreas can be divided sharply or with an electrocautery for complete exposure of the surface of the gland.

Kocher Maneuver

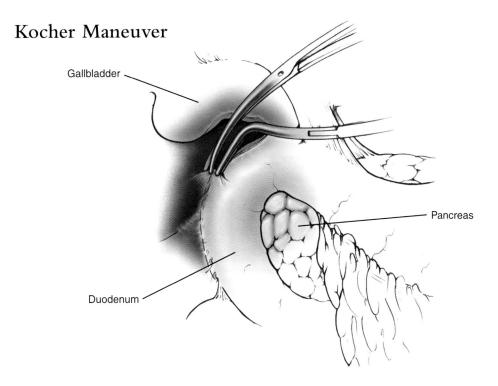

All procedures performed on the head of the pancreas require elevation of the duodenum and head of the pancreas from the retroperitoneum, with the Kocher maneuver. Under direct vision and with sharp dissection or electrocautery, the lateral peritoneal reflection of the duodenum is divided from the level of the common duct around the second, third, and fourth portions of the duodenum. The maneuver is facilitated by aggressive medial retraction of the duodenum and head of the pancreas by the assistant, whose fingers bluntly elevate the peritoneal layers to be divided. When the Kocher maneuver is complete and the pancreas is rolled medially, the vena cava will form the base of the wound and the entire duodenum and head of the pancreas can be grasped within the operator's hand. Care must be taken in performing this maneuver to prevent injury to the structures of the porta hepatis and vena cava.

Exposure of the third portion of the duodenum, proximal to the superior mesenteric vessels, can be obtained by an incision through the transverse mesocolon, an incision through the gastrocolic omentum, or reflection of the right half of the colon.

Exposure of the duodenum distal to the superior mesenteric vessels can be accomplished by incision through the gastrocolic omentum and further reflection of the right colon. In addition, division of the parietal fold just inferior to the paraduodenal fossa will permit visualization of the distal duodenum. Further mobilization of the duodenum can be obtained by transection of the suspensory muscle. In dividing the mesocolon, the surgeon must watch for the right colic, middle colic, and marginal vessels. The gastroepiploic arteries lie near the greater curvature of the stomach, within the gastrocolic ligament, and should be handled appropriately.

Transduodenal Biopsy of Pancreas

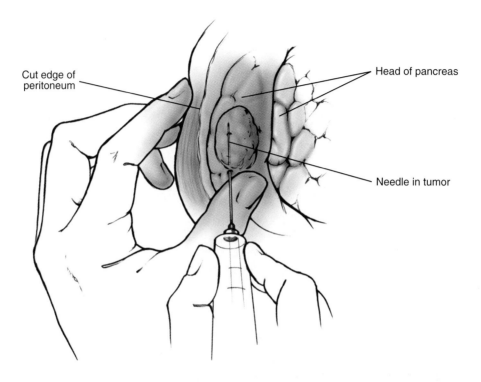

Transduodenal biopsy of the pancreas is accomplished through either a midline or subcostal incision. The hepatic flexure of the colon is mobilized as previously described, and the Kocher maneuver performed. When the Kocher maneuver is complete, the duodenum and pancreas are elevated from the retroperitoneum. The lesion may be imaged ultrasonographically, or the operator's hand is used to palpate the abnormal area within the head. When the location of the lesion is determined, a Tru-cut or fine needle is introduced through the duodenal wall and into the lesion. The Kocher maneuver should be adequate to allow the needle to be directed away from the superior mesenteric vein and the needle should not be allowed to penetrate the anterior or posterior surface of the gland. For fine-needle aspiration, the needle is directed into the area in question, and multiple forceful aspirations are performed. This technique may have little value in a scirrhous lesion or in a gland that has had recurrent bouts of pancreatitis. If a Tru-cut needle is used, the incision site along the duodenal wall is oversewn with a Lembert suture to prevent leakage of duodenal contents.

Neither biopsy method is 100% accurate. Preoperative planning and discussion, as well as intraoperative findings such as lymph nodes metastases and invasion of the superior mesenteric artery or vein, should determine whether resection should proceed without a tissue diagnosis. Most surgeons who perform the Whipple operation to treat cancer proceed without a positive biopsy if the evidence for malignancy is strong.

Whipple Operation With Hemigastrectomy

Pancreatoduodenectomy taken as a whole seems complex. However, when condensed to an orderly series of steps, it can be performed safely and with elegance.

After a midline ("bucket handle") incision is made, extensive exploration of the abdomen is performed to rule out metastatic disease and confirm preoperative staging. Intraoperative staging is performed by excluding gross metastases from the peritoneal surfaces, the liver, the omentum, and direct extension into the transverse mesocolon. The gastrohepatic ligament is divided between clamps, and the Kocher maneuver performed.

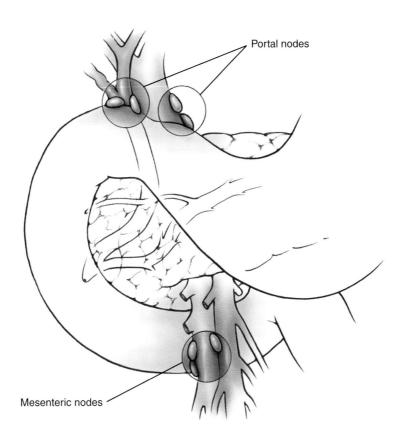

Lymph nodes should be sought posterior to the common bile duct near the junction of the bile duct to the duodenum. Other common places for adenopathy include along the superior border of the porta hepatis near the duodenum and along the lesser curvature of the stomach. Lymph nodes along the hepatic artery and at the celiac origin should also be sought. Lymph nodes at the base of the transverse mesocolon are also common, but less so than the others. It is important to continually progress through the operation. If lymph nodes are papalated and sent for frozen-section analysis, the operation should proceed with further mobilization and cholecystectomy.

Resectability is based not only on the absence of metastatic disease but lack of invasion of the tumor into vital structures such as the superior mesenteric vessels. The next step should be identification of the superior mesenteric vein. This is best accomplished along the inferior border of the pancreas. As the Kocher maneuver proceeds through the third portion of the duodenum, the superior mesenteric vein is encountered. The vein is covered by a thin layer of adventitial tissue, and this is incised sharply or with an electrocautery. With gentle dissection with a finger or Kidner dissector, a plane is developed between the vein and the posterior surface of the pancreas. There is often a short wide venous tributary from the uncinate process to the superior mesenteric vein in this area that is conveniently ligated to prevent its tearing and bothersome bleeding.

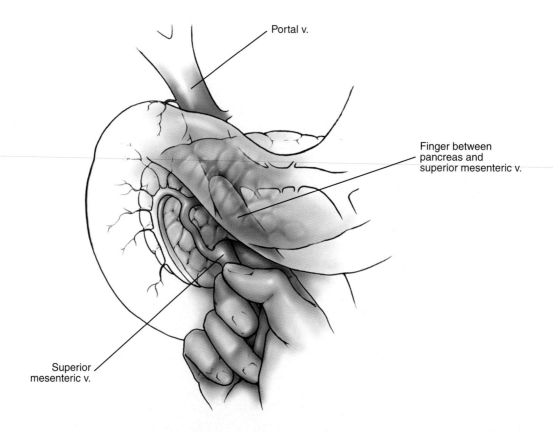

Portal v.

Finger between
pancreas and
superior mesenteric v.

Superior
mesenteric v.

The space anterior to the superior mesenteric vein can be developed beyond the neck of the pancreas, then connected to the equivalent space from above the duodenum. If the pancreas is inseparable from the portal vein because of tumor invasion, most surgeons consider the tumor to be unresectable. Some groups do resect involved portal vein, reconstructing it with vein patches or synthetic material (see p. 624). If this plane is clear and frozen sections are negative for metastatic disease, the first portion of the duodenum should be mobilized.

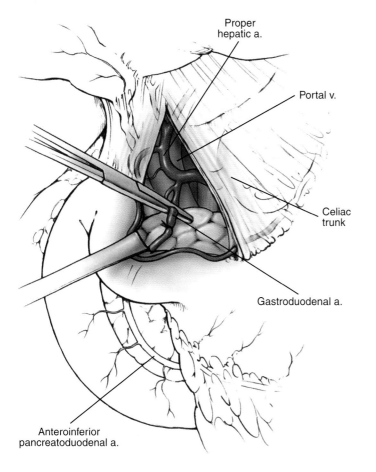

Proper hepatic a.

Portal v.

Celiac trunk

Gastroduodenal a.

Anteroinferior pancreatoduodenal a.

The hepatic artery is identified in the gastrohepatic ligament and followed to the branch of the gastroduodenal artery. The gastroduodenal artery is dissected free from the surrounding tissues and doubly clamped and divided. Attention is turned to the common bile duct. The adventitial tissue overlying the porta hepatis is incised and the duct identified by palpation of the indwelling stent or by aspiration with a needle. Periportal tissues are divided between clamps and tied to prevent leakage of lymphatic fluid, and any nodal tissue encountered and the gallbladder are taken en bloc with the specimen. The common bile duct is divided, a suture is placed at the 6-o'clock position, and the duct is retracted superiorly to prevent ongoing leakage of bile into the operative field.

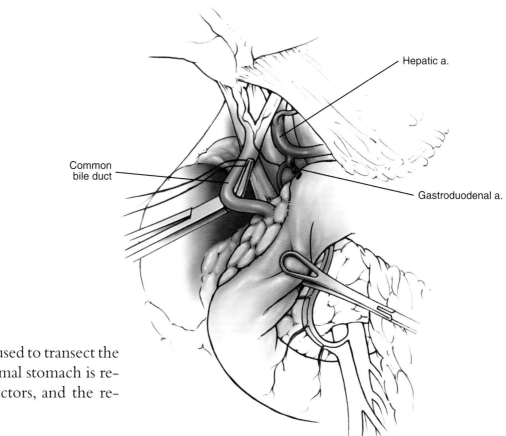

Hepatic a.

Common bile duct

Gastroduodenal a.

A stapling device is used to transect the stomach. The proximal stomach is replaced behind retractors, and the resection proceeds.

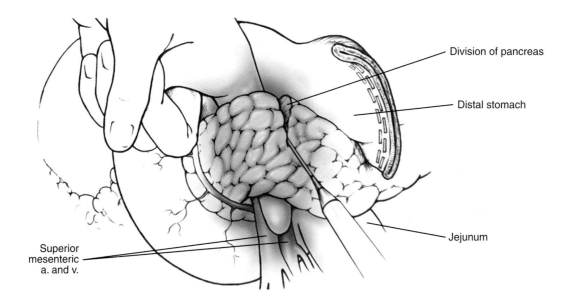

The pancreas is now transected with a knife or cautery, taking care to protect the superior mesenteric vein. Bleeding points are immediately noted near the superior and inferior margins of the gland and are controlled with interrupted sutures. Alternatively, a linear stapler may be passed and fired on the specimen side of the pancreas to control bleeding.

Small vessels that drain directly from the uncinate process to the superior mesenteric vein are now meticulously dissected and ligated between clips or sutures. A larger venous branch is typically encountered at the superior edge of the uncinate process and must be carefully ligated.

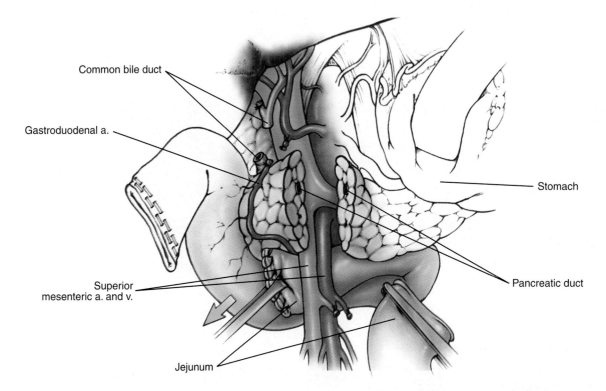

Attention is turned to mobilization and removal of the third and fourth portions of duodenum. This mobilization allows the jejunum to be rotated beneath the superior mesenteric artery. The ligament may be broad or narrow, encompasses approximately 270 degrees of the circumference of the duodenal wall, and attaches superiorly to the right crus of the diaphragm. This may occasionally be accomplished from above the transverse mesocolon, but usually requires its elevation with division of the ligament under direct vision. The duodenojejunal junction is divided with a linear stapler, and the short duodenal mesentery is divided between fine clamps and secured with silk ligatures.

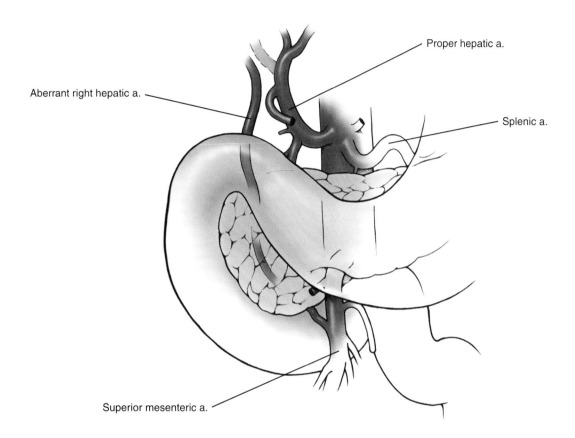

The specimen is now anchored only by the retroperitoneal attachments of the medial uncinate process. These may be transected using multiple clamps and ligatures. Alternatively, a linear stapler may be passed across the retroperitoneal attachments on the uncinate process and fired. Care is taken not to impinge on the superior mesenteric artery or the portal vein when placing the stapling device. Any residual bleeding points are controlled with silk sutures.

The most commonly encountered arterial anomaly that affects performance of the Whipple operation is the right hepatic artery arising from the superior mesenteric artery. The artery usually courses along the posterior surface of the pancreas and can be dissected free, or is completely posterior to the gland and does not interfere with the dissection. When the artery courses through the pancreatic head, it may be ligated superior to the pancreas and either reimplanted, grafted using vein, or simply left.

The extended nodal dissection has been championed by some surgeons as leading to a lower local recurrence rate, although no prospective randomized studies have been performed. The R2 resection is carried out by adding regional nodal dissection to the Whipple operation. During the course of the Kocher maneuver, the node-bearing tissue adjacent to the vena cava and aorta are dissected free and remain with the specimen. In addition, the portal, celiac, and renal nodes are cleared.

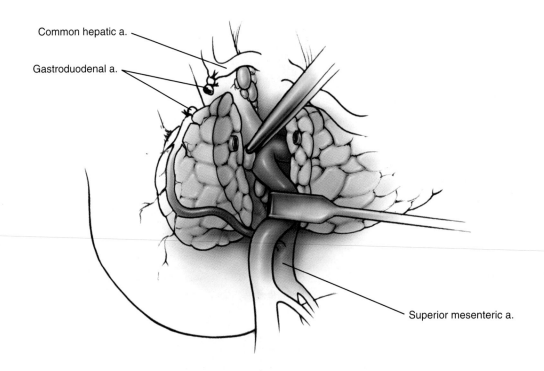

Common hepatic a.

Gastroduodenal a.

Superior mesenteric a.

Small tumors may sometimes involve the superior mesenteric vein, typically on the right lateral side of the vein, and are not discovered until after division of the gland. The superior mesenteric vein is mobilized at the inferior border of the pancreas, and dissection of the gland from the anterior surface of the vein proceeds in the usual fashion. The gland is divided as usual, and the site of invasion is noted when dissection of the uncinate process begins. When venous resection is deemed necessary, the splenic vein is divided and oversewn. The entire and retroperitoneal dissections are completed, and the specimen is attached by the superior mesenteric and pancreatic veins only. Proximal and distal control are obtained with Rommell tourniquets, and vascular clamps or a Rommell tourniquet is applied to the superior mesenteric artery to prevent mesenteric engorgement. The specimen is then removed and end-to-end reanastomosis performed. In rare cases, end-to-end reconstruction is not possible and internal jugular vein or 10 to 12 mm reinforced polytetrafluoroethylene (PTFE) graft may be used.

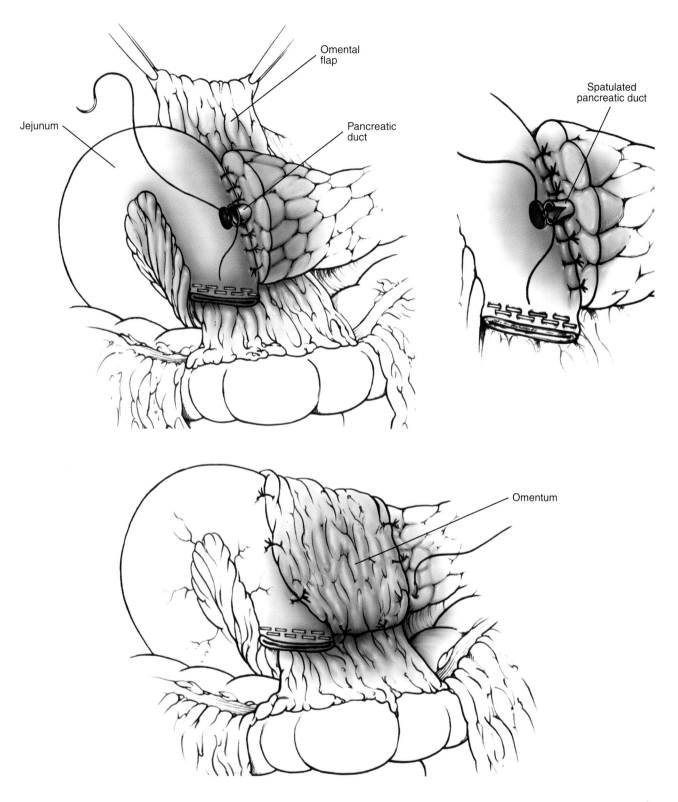

Once hemostatis is assured, reconstruction of pancreatic, gastrointestinal, and biliary continuity may proceed. Reconstruction is typically begun with the pancreatic duct, affording the best visualization for the most critical portion of the operation. Multiple techniques have been used for construction of a pancreaticojejunostomy. Two techniques are described here. A vascularized pedicle of greater omentum is mobilized between clamps and rotated superiorly. The jejunum and pancreas are placed above this omental tongue, and the capsule of the pancreas is approximated to the serosa of the jejunum using interrupted silk or absorbable sutures. The pancreatic duct, if dilated, is anastomosed mucosa-to-mucosa with interrupted absorbable sutures. Alternatively, if the pancreatic duct is normal in size, the duct is spatulated using a needle-tip cautery or scissors, and a mucosal anastomosis is performed. The anterior pancreatic capsule is then approximated to the jejunal serosa, and the entire anastomosis is wrapped with the omental flap.

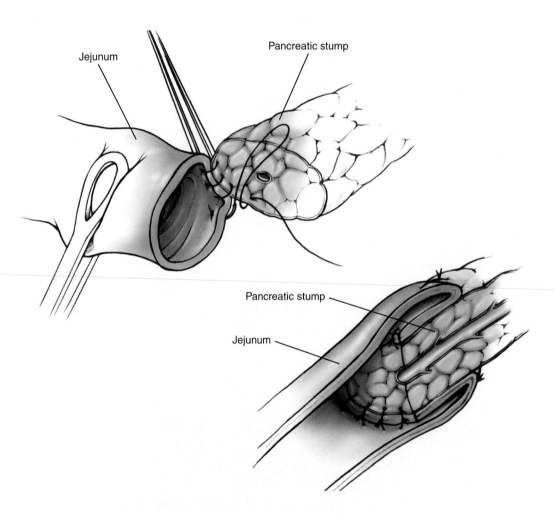

Alternatively, the pancreatic stump may be dunked into the transected end of the jejunum. An outer capsule to the seromuscular layer of silk sutures is placed posteriorly, followed by a second inner layer of pancreaticojejunal sutures. The anterior row of pancreaticojejunal sutures is then placed and the pancreatic stump rotated into the jejunum. A second anterior layer of serocapsular sutures is then placed, completing the invagination. The invagination process is often difficult because of edema of the gland or jejunum by this point in the operation and may be facilitated with intravenous administration of glucagon to relax the intestine prior to anastomosis. A small (6 to 8 Fr) stent may be placed in the pancreaticojejunostomy and secured with an absorbable stitch, allowing the tube to pass spontaneously in a few weeks.

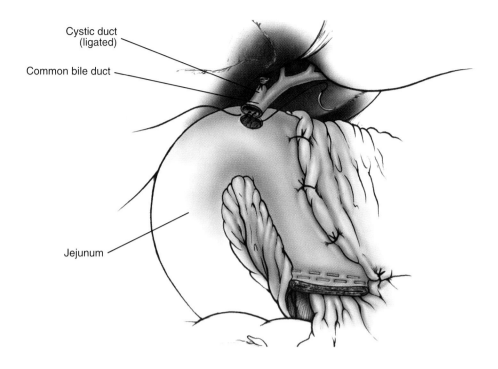

Cystic duct (ligated)

Common bile duct

Jejunum

Attention is then turned to the choledochojejunostomy. A jejunotomy is made at an appropriate distance from the pancreaticojejunostomy, and reapproximation of the bile duct to the jejunum is performed with interrupted absorbable sutures. For ease of construction, the posterior row of sutures is placed with the knots on the interior of the anastomosis and the anterior row with the knots on the exterior. A running stitch may also be used for either layer. If a transhepatic stent has been placed preoperatively, it may be left in place, although the bile duct is typically dilated and stenting is not necessary.

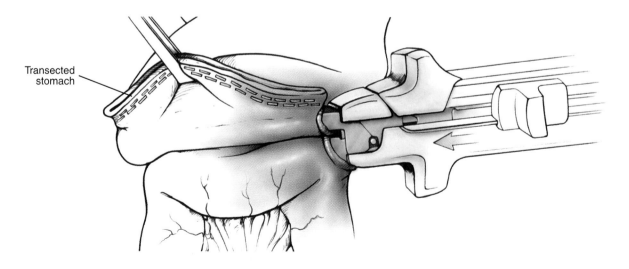

Transected stomach

An antecolic posterior gastrojejunostomy is then constructed using a linear stapling device or by sewn anastomosis. Closed suction drains are placed posterior to the biliary and pancreatic anastomoses, and a feeding jejunostomy tube is placed 20 to 30 cm downstream from the gastrojejunostomy.

Whipple Operation With Pylorus Preservation

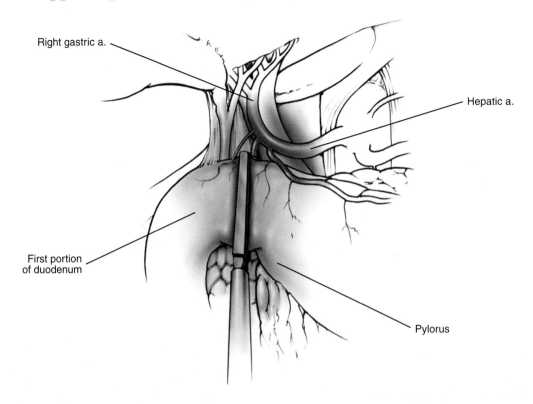

A common alternative to the classic Whipple operation includes preservation of the pylorus in an attempt to maintain more normal physiology of gastric emptying. In applying this technique, mobilization of the duodenum, proximal jejunum, pancreas, and biliary tree is performed as described for the Whipple operation. Mobilization of the stomach, however, is modified. The blood supply coursing through the gastrohepatic ligament is left intact. Moreover, when the gastrocolic attachments are divided between clamps, it is done inferior to the gastroepiploic arteries, leaving these intact with their supply of the greater curvature. The first portion of the duodenum is mobilized to a distance of 2 cm beyond the pylorus. This leaves an adequate cuff of duodenum for subsequent duodenojejunostomy. It is preferable in performing this dissection to identify the gastroduodenal artery prior to transaction of the duodenum. If an arteriogram has been obtained and it is clear that the anatomy is classic, the gastroduodenal artery may be ligated. The right gastric artery typically arises off the proximal hepatic artery, yielding an adequate blood supply to the pylorus and proximal duodenum. This artery often is preserved when in its normal position, but its preservation is not critical. The duodenum is now transected 2 cm beyond the pylorus with a linear stapler.

At this point variations in the hepatic arterial anatomy should be sought. The most common variation is the right hepatic artery originating from the superior mesenteric artery. In this case, the right hepatic artery typically passes along the posterior surface or directly through the head of the pancreas. Its course may be similar to that of the gastroduodenal artery at the superior border of the pancreas. The gastroduodenal, hepatic, and replaced right hepatic arteries may be differentiated by temporary exclusion of the right hepatic artery. If a pulse remains on the pancreatic side of this exclusion, the structure is likely to be a replaced right hepatic artery rather than the hepatic artery. On the other hand, if a pulse remains superior to the exclusion, the structure is likely to be the gastroduodenal artery. Once this differentiation is made, the gastroduodenal artery is ligated and transected, and the right hepatic is left intact.

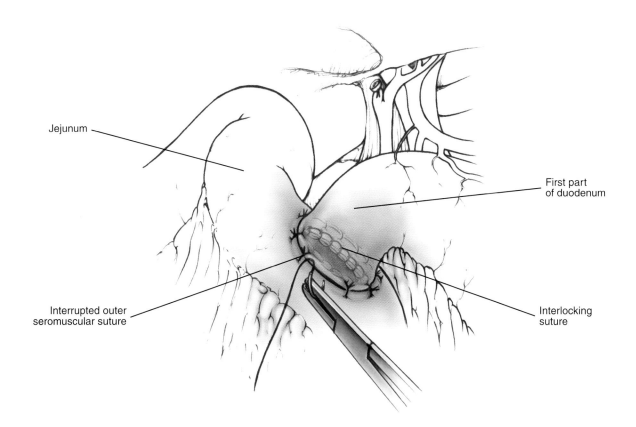

Jejunum

First part of duodenum

Interrupted outer seromuscular suture

Interlocking suture

The procedure then continues as previously described. Reconstruction of enteric continuity in the pylorus-preserving Whipple operation is accomplished after pancreaticojejunostomy and hepaticojejunostomy, with an end-to-side duodenojejunostomy. The anastomosis may be performed to the loop of jejunum that has been rotated beneath the superior mesenteric vessels or more distally in the same loop bought antecolic or transmesocolic. A two-layer anastomosis is made using interrupted seromuscular silk sutures and a running absorbable inner layer. This inner layer is made hemostatic and watertight using over-and-over locking sutures for the posterior row and Connell sutures for the anterior row. The anastomosis is completed with an anterior layer of seromuscular silk sutures.

Distal Pancreatectomy With Splenectomy

Adenocarcinoma of the body and tail of the pancreas typically presents late in the course of the disease, with vague or nonspecific symptoms. The tumors are often large and exhibit local invasion or metastases by the time the patient is evaluated. Distal pancreatectomy is also used for extirpation of cystic neoplasms and neuroendocrine tumors, which are often located in body and tail of the pancreas.

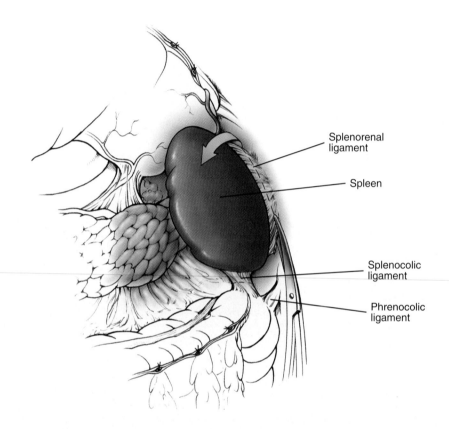

Splenorenal
ligament

Spleen

Splenocolic
ligament

Phrenocolic
ligament

A left subcostal incision with extension across the midline is preferred for the distal pancreatectomy and splenectomy. Exploration is begun with a search for metastatic disease in the liver and throughout the abdomen. The gastrocolic omentum is divided between clamps, and the stomach is retracted superiorly. The vasa brevia are likewise divided between clamps, exposing the entire anterior surface of the pancreas and spleen. The splenophrenic and splenocolic attachments are likewise divided and splenic flexure of the colon retracted inferiorly. When performed early in the operation these maneuvers remove the stomach and colon from consideration for the remainder of the procedure and allow excellent exposure.

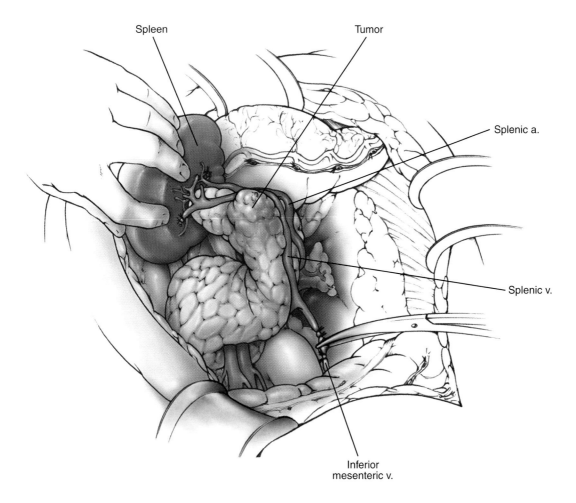

Spleen

Tumor

Splenic a.

Splenic v.

Inferior
mesenteric v.

The peritoneum at the inferior border of the pancreas is incised sharply or with an electrocautery, taking care not to injure the superior or inferior mesenteric veins. The inferior mesenteric vein is identified, cleared of surrounding tissues, doubly clamped, and ligated. This allows mobilization of the inferior border of the pancreas through an avascular plane. The spleen has been mobilized from the diaphragm by the division of its lateral peritoneal attachments, allowing medial rotation of the spleen and the tail of the pancreas. The body of the pancreas is then bluntly dissected from the retroperitoneum and gerotas fascia through avascular tissue.

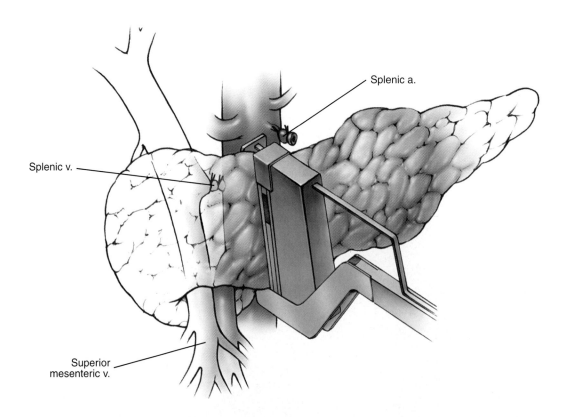

With the pancreas and spleen rolled medially, the splenic artery is easily identified at the superior border of the gland. The artery is isolated from surrounding tissues near its origin from the celiac axis, clamped, and suture ligated. A site 2 cm proximal to the tumor is identified where the pancreas is to be transected. The splenic vein is isolated from the pancreas at this point and suture ligated. Alternatively, the vein may be stapled along with the pancreas in the next step. Care is taken not to impinge on the superior mesenteric vein.

If the site for transection of the pancreas is soft, a linear stapling device may be used. If the gland has become fibrotic from chronic pancreatitis, the gland is divided with an electrocautery. Bleeding points are controlled with figure-of-eight nonabsorbable sutures. Whether transected with a stapler or electrocautery, the end of the gland is secured with interrupted interlocking mattress sutures. Particular attention is paid to the region of the main pancreatic duct, which if readily apparent is separately ligated. Once the end of the gland is secured, the resection bed is inspected for bleeding points and hemostatis assured. A closed suction drain is placed in the pancreatic bed near the stump of the pancreas and brought out through the left abdomen.

Enucleation of Insulinoma

Recent advances in imaging techniques have made the preoperative diagnosis of insulinoma more secure. Fine-cut spiral CT scans and arteriograms depict the location of insulinoma in up to 80% of cases. Endoscopic ultrasonography is a relatively new technique that is highly sensitive for mass lesions of the pancreatic head and uncinate process as small as 5 mm, but somewhat less sensitive for body and tail lesions. In some cases the exact location of an insulinoma is not known prior to exploratory surgery. Intraoperative ultrasonography is useful in such cases.

The abdomen is explored through a midline (bucket-handle) incision. An extensive Kocher maneuver is performed, the gastrocolic omentum is divided, and the stomach is retracted superiorly. The inferior border of the pancreas is identified and the overlying peritoneum divided with an electrocautery or sharp dissection. The pancreas is then elevated from the retroperitoneum in the avascular plane between its posterior surface and Gerota's fascia. Palpation of body and tail is then undertaken. Palpation of the head and neck is performed, although the pancreas is thickest in this area and palpation of small tumors is difficult.

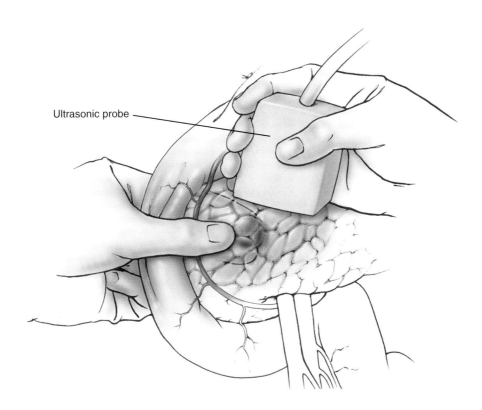

Intraoperative ultrasonography is performed to search for the primary tumor and for multifocal disease. Insulinomas are reddish brown and typically 1 to 2.5 cm in diameter. If the tumor is located in the body or tail and exhibits local invasion, or is buried in the pancreatic substance, distal pancreatectomy should be performed. Likewise, if the lesion is buried in the head or uncinate process and is not accessible for enucleation, pancreaticoduodenectomy should be performed. Most insulinomas, however, are on the surface of the gland and can be enucleated.

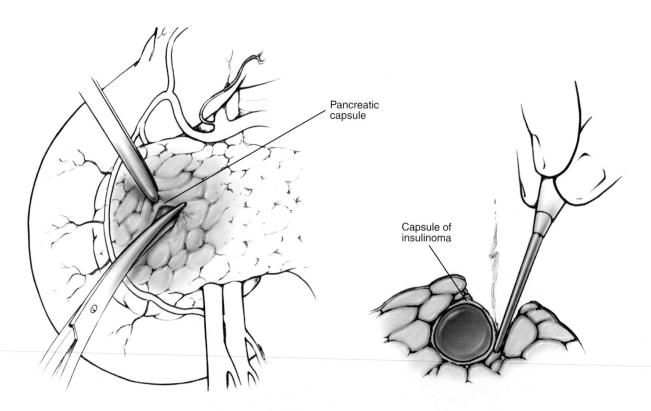

Pancreatic capsule

Capsule of insulinoma

Enucleation is accomplished by sharply incising the pancreatic capsule around the evident portion of the tumor. The pancreatic substance is then dissected free from the wall of the tumor, and small clips or sutures are placed on bleeding points in the pancreatic substance. Electrocautery is applied to the wall of the lesion, allowing rapid and bloodless excision of the tumor. There is no ductal communication with these tumors; however, small ducts may be injured during the dissection, and these should be searched for and suture ligated. When hemostasis is assured, a closed suction drain is placed in the lesser sac near the site of the tumor excision and brought out through the abdominal wall.

Local Excision of Ampullary Tumor

Tumors of the ampulla of Vater represent a small percentage of pancreatic and periampullary tumors. Most such lesions are carcinomas and should be treated with pancreaticoduodenectomy. However, adenomas and neuroendocrine tumors are being found more frequently in an era of increased use of endoscopic retrograde cholangiopancreatography. Ampullary adenomas are premalignant lesions that are cured by resection. Neuroendocrine tumors of the ampulla are typically benign and can be cured with local excision. Although the Whipple operation is the treatment of choice for ampullary carcinoma or adenomas with dysplasia or carcinoma in situ, some patients are too frail for or refuse the operation, and palliation can be achieved with ampullary resection.

Abdominal exploration is performed through a right subcostal or midline incision, and extensive Kocher maneuver of the duodenum is performed. If an endoscopic stent is in place, the stent and mass are usually easily palpable through the duodenal wall. A small duodenotomy is performed over the lesion to ensure its position. This duodenotomy is then extended proximally and distally until sufficient room is obtained for resection of the tumor. Six silk stay sutures are then placed circumferentially in the duodenal wall, and the ampulla is visualized.

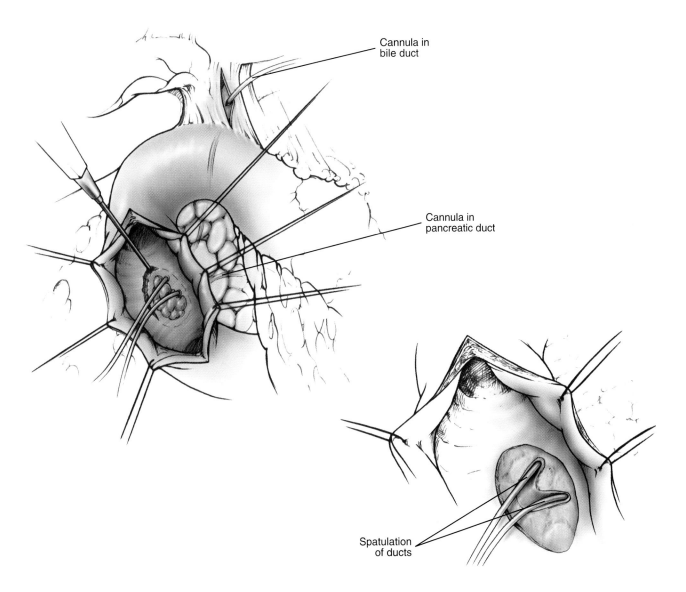

Cannula in bile duct

Cannula in pancreatic duct

Spatulation of ducts

Lacrimal duct probes are placed in the bile duct and pancreatic ducts as soon as possible to ensure their locations. The bile duct is in the 11-o'clock position, coursing cephalad through the pancreatic substance. If a biliary stent has been placed, the duct is identified by this method. It may be necessary to resect a portion of the tumor or enter the duodenal wall directly to identify the exact position of the pancreatic duct. Intravenous secretin may also be used to increase the flow of pancreatic juice and aid in the identification of the pancreatic duct. Once identification has been accomplished, circumferential resection of the duodenal mucosa to a depth necessary to excise the tumor is undertaken with needle electrocautery. If abnormal tissue lies along the surface of the bile duct, the duct may be spatulated to ensure removal of all neoplastic tissue. Frozen-section analysis should be performed to ensure negative margins and benignity of lesion. If negative margins cannot be obtained or if in the process of local excision it becomes obvious that the entire tumor cannot be removed, consideration is given to pancreaticoduodenectomy.

The bile and pancreatic ducts will have been transected or spatulated at variable distances from the duodenal mucosa. The reconstruction is critical to ensure adequate biliary and pancreatic drainage and to repair the transduodenal defect. Loupe magnification is useful for accurate reconstruction.

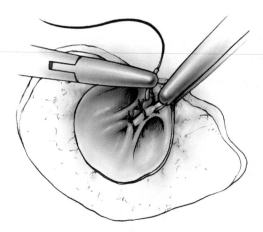

Reconstruction is accomplished by approximating the common walls of the pancreatic and bile ducts. After approximation of the common wall of the ducts, circumferential reapproximation of the duodenal mucosa to the pancreatic bile duct mucosae is undertaken, with absorbable monofilament sutures.

After this reapproximation, the ducts should be probed with biliary dilators to ensure appropriate size. A diameter of 6 to 8 mm for the bile duct and 4 to 5 mm for the pancreatic duct should be obtained.

Once adequate patency has been ensured, the duodenotomy is closed transversely with sutures or a linear stapler.

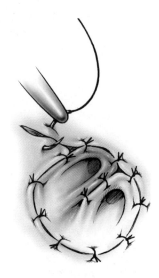

Excision of Duodenal Tumor

Duodenal tumors, whether benign or malignant, primary or metastatic, epithelial or nonepithelial, are all "unusual." Forty percent of adenocarcinomas of the small bowel develop in the duodenum. (Bear in mind that the duodenum is 22 cm long, compared with 258 cm for the jejunoileum.)

The overall distribution of benign and malignant duodenal tumors, which also includes jejunoileal tumors, as well as the classification of tumors of the jejunum and ileum, is shown in Tables 14-1 and 14-2.

The most common benign tumor is the leiomyoma; the most common (but rare) duodenal malignant tumor is adenocarcinoma.

Table 14-1 *Distribution of Benign Tumors of the Small Bowel by Site in 13 Series*

Tumor Type	Duodenum	Jejunum	Ileum	Total (%)
Leiomyoma	24	64	47	135 (37)
Polyp/adenoma	34	17	17	68 (19)
Lipoma	11	13	30	54 (15)
Hemangioma	1	10	26	37 (10)
Fibroma	4	7	12	23 (6)
Other	27	8	13	48 (13)
Total (%)	101 (27)	119 (33)	145 (40)	365 (100)

From Coit DC. Cancer of the small intestine. In DeVita VT Jr, Hellman S, Rosenberg SA, eds. Cancer: Principles and Practice of Oncology, 5th ed. Philadelphia: Lippincott-Raven, 1997.

Table 14-2 *Distribution of Malignant Tumors of the Small Bowel by Site in 27 Series*

Tumor Type	Duodenum	Jejunum	Ileum	Total (%)
Adenocarcinoma	634	454	301	1389 (44)
Carcinoid	60	92	781	933 (29)
Lymphoma	34	183	276	493 (15)
Sarcoma	61	159	148	368 (12)
Total (%)	789 (25)	888 (28)	1506 (47)	3183 (100)

From Coit DC. Cancer of the small intestine. In DeVita VT Jr, Hellman S, Rosenberg SA, eds. Cancer: Principles and Practice of Oncology, 5th ed. Philadelphia: Lippincott-Raven, 1997.

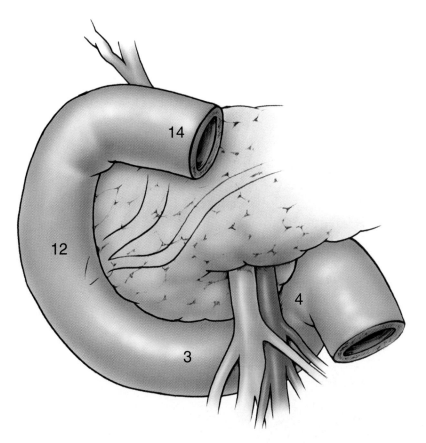

Leiomyomas are found in the first or second portions of the duodenum. The majority of leiomyosarcomas are found in the second and third portions.

Malignant smooth muscle tumors of the duodenum metastasize to other organs at varying rates.

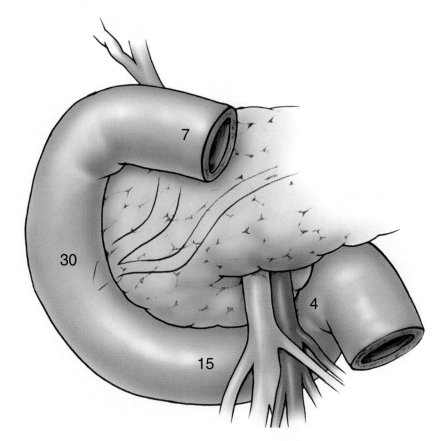

Surgical treatment of these tumors ranges from simple excision to radical procedures such as pancreatoduodenectomy. The procedure used in any patient is governed by the answers to the following questions:

1. Is the tumor benign or malignant?
2. How large is it, and where is it?
3. Is it endogastric, exogastric, or intramural?
4. Is it fixed to neighboring structures?
5. Are any lymph nodes involved?
6. Is there evidence of metastasis?

The answers to these questions must be evaluated against the known natural history of the specific tumor and the age and general condition of the patient. In addition, the surgeon must be familiar with the anatomic basis of duodenal surgery, the physiology that may be changed by the operation, and the pathologic changes that may take place as a result of surgical treatment in its absence.

Benign Tumors

If the tumor is benign and small, excisional biopsy is the proper procedure, not enucleation or simple biopsy. For enucleation or excisional biopsy the duodenum is mobilized with the Kocher maneuver and elevated. The tumor is identified, and if it encompasses less than half the circumference of the duodenum, proximal and distal stay sutures are placed and the tumor is excised with a surrounding border of normal duodenal wall. The defect is then closed in two layers with a running absorbable transmural layer of sutures and serial muscular sutures. For a benign leiomyoma in the submucosal plane, this same procedure is followed, but the serial muscular layers are incised directly over the tumor and it is enucleated. Hemostasis is assured, and the serial muscular layers are reapproximated with interrupted silk sutures.

Enucleation should be considered if the tumor lies close to the papilla of Vater of if the age and condition of the patient do not permit a more radical operation.

At the other extreme is the giant ulcerated leiomyoma, which even though benign dictates proximal or distal subtotal gastrectomy.

Malignant Tumors

The surgeon must differentiate adenocarcinoma of the duodenum from peri-ampullary malignancies. The 5-year survival rate after resection of peri-ampullary lesions is approximately 40%.

Another peculiar tumor of the duodenum is the extrapancreatic gastrinoma, which produces Zollinger-Ellison syndrome. Extrapancreatic gastrinoma may be located in the duodenal wall and is a cause of persistent disease if not found during exploration.

When the diagnosis of malignant tumor of the duodenum is established, and if the age and general condition of the patient permit, the procedure of choice is pancreatoduodenectomy. If the lesion is small and proximal to the ampulla of Vater, however, segmental resection with antrectomy is advisable. For a lesion close to the ampulla, pancreatoduodenectomy should be performed. For a lesion distal to the ampulla, segmental resection will suffice. Palliative bypass procedures may be used for huge unresectable tumor of the duodenum.

The surgeon should remember the blood supply of the duodenum and head of the pancreas and must not ligate the superior and inferior pancreaticoduodenal arteries. Such ligation will produce both duodenal ischemia and necrosis. The surgeon should remember that in 10% of instances the patient has only one pancreatic duct, the accessory duct (of Santorini). Ligation of this duct would be catastrophic. The duct of Santorini is always located just beneath the gastroduodenal artery.

Duodenal Resection

The first portion of the duodenum is surgically treated by resection (see Chapter 7). Pancreatoduodenectomy is used in the second and third portions of the duodenum.

Resection of Third or Fourth Portion of Duodenum

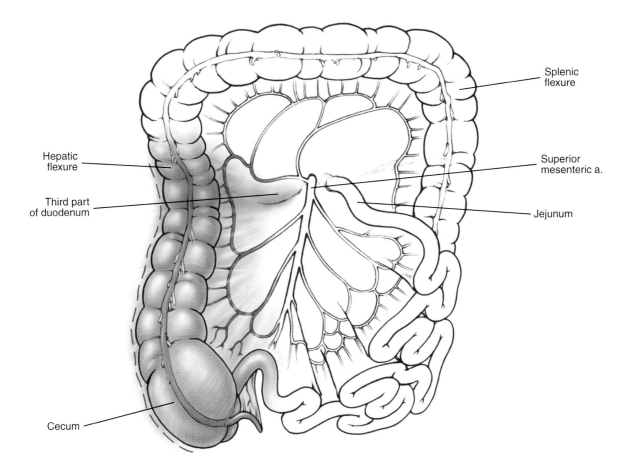

After a long midline or chevron incision is made, total mobilization of the right colon is achieved with the Cattell maneuver. The separation should extend from the hepatic flexure to the cecum to separate the renal covering from the cecum. It includes a segment of the terminal ileum.

The mesentery of the small bowel is elevated from the posterior abdominal wall in such a way that the small bowel in toto will be free and mobile. The right colon and small bowel are now mobile. The second, third, and fourth parts of the duodenum may be visualized by medial and upward rotation of the right colon and small bowel. After this maneuver the superior mesenteric vessels no longer overlay the third portion of the duodenum. The tumor is evaluated. If it is fixed to the pancreas, pancreatoduodenectomy or total pancreatectomy is required. If the tumor and the duodenal wall are free, individual ligation of small mesenteric vessels should be done with fine clamps, effecting duodenal resection. Continuity is reestablished with end-to-end or side-to-side duodenojejunostomy, after closure of the duodenal stump. The small bowel and right colon are carefully replaced in the normal position.

Anatomic Basis of Complications of the Whipple Operation

MAJOR

- Anastomosis of the pancreatic surface to a limb of jejunum is prone to leakage (in 25% to 30% of patients) because of ongoing pancreatic secretion and inability of the normal pancreas to hold stitches well.
- Bleeding can occur at any of the anastomotic sites, but bleeding at the pancreaticojejunostomy is most dangerous. Ongoing pancreatic secretion and inflammation can lead to erosion of a jejunal vessel, causing bleeding that is difficult to diagnose and requires exploration of the pancreatic anastomosis.
- Leakage from the pancreatic or biliary anastomosis may lead to abscess formation in the subhepatic, subhernia, or retrogastric space.
- Removal of the pancreatic head and uncinate process will lead to diabetes in patients with marginal endocrine function prior to the resection. Pancreatic exocrine insufficiency may also result if the residual gland has been damaged by ongoing or recurrent pancreatitis.

MINOR

- Delayed gastric emptying occurs secondary to edema at the gastrojejunostomy or duodenojejunostomy, loss of the duodenal pacemaker, or vagal interruption.
- Splenectomy creates the slight but real possibility of postsplenectomy sepsis.

KEY REFERENCE

Berger HB, Warshaw AL, Büchler MW, Carr-Locke DL, Neoptolemos JP, Russell C, Sarr MG, eds. The Pancreas. Oxford: Blackwell Science, 1998.
This two-volume opus is the "alpha and omega" of information about the pancreas. It presents the newest findings in the fields of pancreatic anatomy, pathology, and surgery.

SELECTED READINGS

DiGiuseppe JA, Hruban RH. Pathobiology of cancer of the pancreas. Semin Surg Oncol 11:87, 1995.

Norton JA. Neuroendocrine tumors of the pancreas and duodenum. Curr Probl Surg 31:79, 1994.

Wilson JM, Melvin DB, Gray G, et al. Benign small bowel tumors. Ann Surg 181:247, 1975.

Yeo CJ, Cameron JL, Lillemore KD, et al. Periampullary adenocarcinoma: Analysis of 5-year survivors. Ann Surg 227:821-831, 1998.

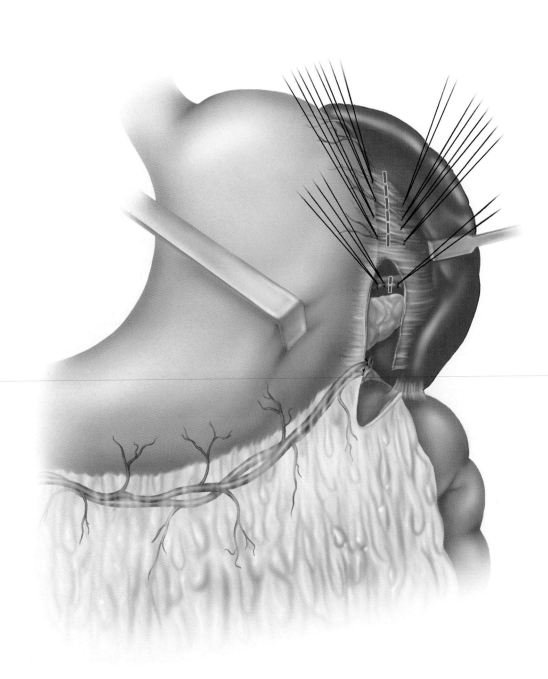

Chapter 15

Spleen

John E. Skandalakis, M.D., Ph.D., Lee J. Skandalakis, M.D.,
Panajiotis N. Skandalakis, M.D., M.S., and C. Daniel Smith, M.D.

Surgical Applications

*P*rimary tumors of the spleen are rare (Morgenstern et al.). Although lymphoma can arise primarily in the spleen, it is not treated surgically. Splenectomy is sometimes required because of isolated metastases of epithelial tumors, such as melanoma. In this chapter, open approaches to splenectomy are discussed, with specific note of the staging procedures for Hodgkin's disease. Also included is a discussion of laparoscopic splenectomy, a procedure that is being performed with increasing frequency.

SURGICAL ANATOMY
John E. Skandalakis, M.D., Ph.D.

Topography

The spleen is located in the left upper quadrant of the abdomen, in a niche formed by the diaphragm above (posterolateral), the stomach medially (anteromedial), the left kidney and left adrenal gland posteriorly (posteromedial), the phrenocolic ligament below, and the chest wall (ninth to eleventh left ribs) laterally. The spleen is concealed at the left hypochondrium and cannot be palpated under normal conditions.

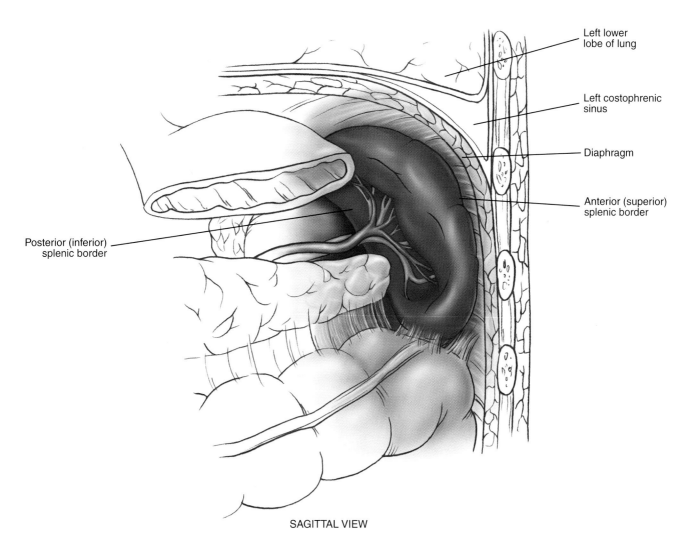

Left lower
lobe of lung

Left costophrenic
sinus

Diaphragm

Anterior (superior)
splenic border

Posterior (inferior)
splenic border

SAGITTAL VIEW

The spleen is associated with the posterior portions of the left ninth, tenth, and eleventh ribs. It is separated from them by the diaphragm and the costodi-aphragmatic recess. The patient with fractures of the left ninth to eleventh ribs is a prime candidate for underlying splenic rupture and should be closely monitored.

The spleen is oriented obliquely; its upper end is about 5 cm from the dorsal midline and approximates the level of the spinous processes of the tenth and eleventh thoracic vertebrae. The lower end lies just behind the midaxillary line. The average spleen is 5 cm wide and 14 cm long, as seen on radiographs. The organ descends about 2 to 5 cm at deep inspiration.

The spleen is always located in front of the splenic flexure in splenomegaly, and vascular adhesions almost always are present. An enlarged spleen is often fixed heavily with the colon. If splenomegaly is present, intestinal preparation is essential for elective splenectomy.

The upper third of the spleen relates to the lower lobe of the left lung, the middle third to the left costophrenic sinus, and the lower third to the left pleura and costal origin of the diaphragm. The lower splenic pole in most persons is related to the upper half of the first lumbar vertebra or to the upper half of the fifth lumbar vertebra. Most frequently the lower splenic pole is related to the upper third of the third lumbar vertebra.

Spleens vary in weight. Extremes of 1 ounce to 20 pounds, including both healthy and diseased organs, have been reported. The spleen responds readily to stimuli, increasing in volume with a rise in blood pressure and after meals. It decreases in volume after exercise or immediately postmortem. Like lymphoid tissue elsewhere in the body, the lymphoid tissue of the spleen undergoes diminution after the age of 10 years. After age 60, there is some involution of the spleen as a whole.

Shape, Surfaces, and Borders

Knowledge of the surfaces, borders, and topographic anatomy of the spleen permits the radiologist to view and read the spleen correctly. The shape, surfaces, and borders of the spleen should also be carefully noted by the surgeon to alert him or her to possible trouble that may arise during splenectomy. The careful surgeon will proceed with deliberation to prevent bleeding from the spleen, the greater curvature of the stomach, and perhaps from the capsule of the left kidney.

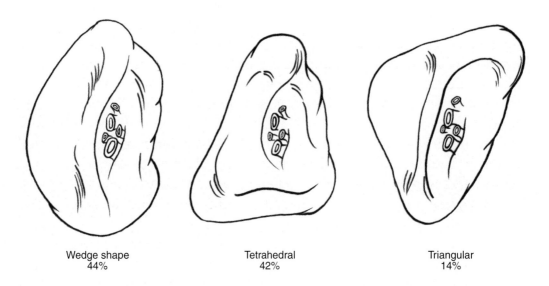

Wedge shape
44%

Tetrahedral
42%

Triangular
14%

Michels described three basic spleen shapes: wedge, in 44% of specimens; tetrahedral, in 42%; and triangular, in 14%.

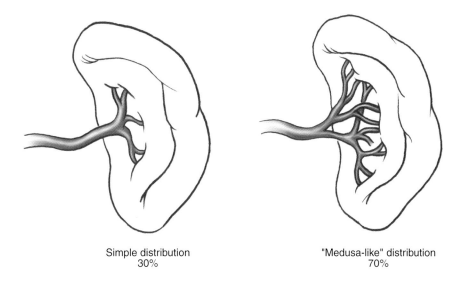

Simple distribution
30%

"Medusa-like" distribution
70%

Michels' alternate description of spleen shape according to arterial distribution, however, may have greater surgical relevance. Two types are compact or simple distribution, in 30% of specimens; and "Medusa-like" distribution, in 70%. The compact type has almost even borders and a narrow hilus in which the arterial branches are few and large; the distributed type has notched borders and a large hilus in which the arterial branches are small and numerous.

If a notched anterior border is present in an enlarged spleen, it may still be palpated. Michels furthermore advises surgeons that a notched anterior border warns of a difficult splenectomy. Spleens with notched borders have multiple arteries (more than two) entering the medial surface of the spleen, and polar arteries are common.

We have also observed these types of vascular distribution in notched and unnotched spleens in laboratory dissections and operating room splenectomies. A notched spleen has multiple arteries that should be ligated carefully, one by one, close to the splenic portas.

The spleen can be said to have two surfaces: parietal and visceral. The relations of the convex parietal surface are with the diaphragm; the relations of the concave visceral surface are with the stomach, kidney, colon, and tail of the pancreas (gastric, renal, colonic, and pancreatic). The tail of the pancreas must be separated cautiously from the spleen to prevent pancreatic injury. The pancreatosplenic ligament should be ligated when present. Although the convex parietal surface related to the diaphragm is in most cases avascular, it is wise to ligate the short or long splenophrenic ligament.

The spleen has two borders: superior (anterior) and inferior (posterior). The superior border separates the gastric and diaphragmatic areas; the inferior border separates the renal and diaphragmatic areas. Since the posterior splenic border is related to the renal and diaphragmatic areas, separation should be toward the diaphragm to prevent injury of the renal capsule.

Peritoneum and Ligaments

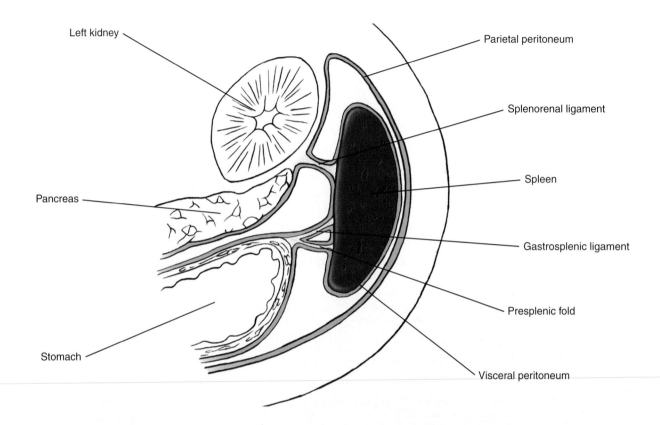

The peritoneum covers the entire spleen in a double layer, except for the hilus. The gastrosplenic and splenorenal ligaments are the two chief ligaments of the spleen. These ligaments comprise part of the embryonic dorsal mesentery, the mesogastrium, whose leaves separate to surround the spleen.

The visceral peritoneum joins the right layer of the greater omentum at the hilus to form the gastrosplenic and splenorenal ligaments, which in turn form the splenic pedicle. The visceral peritoneum also forms the capsule itself, which is as friable and easily injured as the spleen.

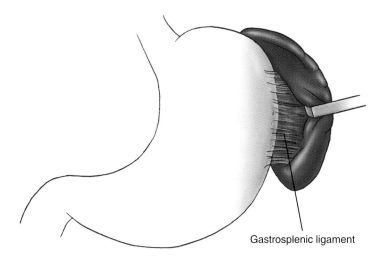

Gastrosplenic ligament

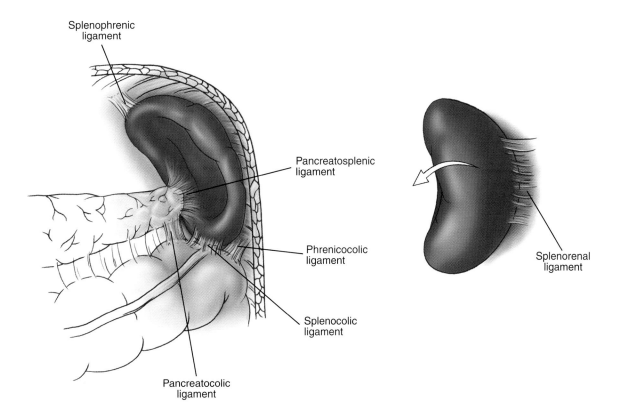

Splenophrenic
ligament

Pancreatosplenic
ligament

Phrenicocolic
ligament

Splenocolic
ligament

Pancreatocolic
ligament

Splenorenal
ligament

There are several minor splenic ligaments in addition to the two chief ligaments. The names of these ligaments indicate their connections: the splenophrenic ligament, splenocolic ligament, pancreatosplenic ligament, presplenic fold, phrenocolic ligament, and pancreatocolic ligament.

The mobility of the spleen depends on the degree of laxity of the splenic ligaments and the splenic blood vessels. In our opinion, only four ligaments can affect the position of the spleen: the gastrosplenic, splenocolic, phrenocolic, and splenorenal ligaments.

GASTROSPLENIC LIGAMENT

The gastrosplenic ligament is the portion of the dorsal mesentery between the stomach and the spleen. Whitesell conceived of the ligament as a triangle. Two sides form the upper portion of the greater curvature of the stomach and the medial border of the spleen. At its apex, the superior pole of the spleen lies close to the stomach and may be fixed to it. Also at the apex of this triangle, the leaves of the mesentery are reflected to the posterior body wall and to the inferior surface of the diaphragm, the splenophrenic ligament. At its base, the inferior pole lies 5 to 7 cm from the stomach. The gastrosplenic ligament contains the short gastric arteries above and the left gastroepiploic vessels below. During splenectomy care must be taken to ligate the short gastric vessels and the left gastroepiploic vessels separately and to incise the gastrosplenic ligament between clamps.

SPLENORENAL LIGAMENT

Curiously, the existence of the splenorenal ligament is often overlooked. This almost avascular ligament is the posterior portion of the primitive dorsal mesogastrium. The splenorenal ligament envelops the splenic vessels and the tail of the pancreas. Therefore incisions and finger excavation to mobilize the organ must be done with care. In addition, no more traction than usual should be applied to a short splenophrenic ligament, to prevent tearing the capsule, which may produce bleeding. Incision of its peritoneal layer, together with mobilization of the tail of the pancreas, reestablishes the primitive condition.

The posterior layer of the gastrosplenic ligament forms the outer layer of the splenorenal ligament. Careless division may injure the short gastric vessels.

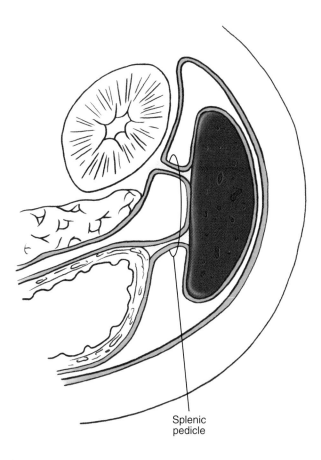

Splenic
pedicle

The extent to which the primitive dorsal mesogastrium was absorbed into the body wall determines whether the splenic pedicle is narrow or wide. The length of the splenic vessels after incision of the ligament is a greater factor than the splenorenal ligament in controlling the degree of effective mobilization of the spleen. A short splenic artery may make it impossible to deliver the spleen out of the abdomen. Splenic mobility may be increased by gently pushing the tail of the pancreas away from the hilus of the spleen.

Rosen et al. reported that the length of the splenorenal ligament ranges from 2.5 to 5.5 cm. The relations between the pancreatic tail and the splenic porta (hilum splenicum) are as follows: tail not penetrating the ligament, 24%; tail within the ligament without reaching the porta, 32%; tail reaching the porta, 27.9%; and tail penetrating the gastrosplenic ligament, 13%.

MINOR LIGAMENTS

SPLENOPHRENIC LIGAMENT. The splenophrenic ligament is the reflection of the leaves of the mesentery to the posterior body wall and to the inferior surface of the diaphragm at the area of the upper pole of the spleen close to the stomach. It is an extension of the splenorenal ligament to the diaphragm. Although usually avascular, it should be checked for possible bleeding after division.

SPLENOCOLIC LIGAMENT. The splenocolic ligament is a remnant of the extreme left end of the transverse mesocolon, which develops a secondary attachment to the spleen during embryonic fixation of the colon to the body wall. As a secondary attachment, it might not be expected to contain large blood vessels. However, massive bleeding may result from careless incision of the ligament; tortuous or aberrant inferior polar vessels, or a left gastroepiploic artery, may lie close enough to be injured. Because of its close relation to the lower polar and left gastroepiploic vessels, the splenocolic ligament should be incised between clamps.

PANCREATOSPLENIC LIGAMENT. The pancreatosplenic ligament can be found when the tail of the pancreas does not touch the spleen. The pancreatosplenic ligament, if present and long enough, should be incised between clamps. If absent or short, careful separation of the pancreatic tail from the spleen is necessary to prevent pancreatic or splenic injury.

PRESPLENIC FOLD. A peritoneal fold lies anterior to the gastrosplenic ligament. The fold is usually free on its lateral border, but in a large diseased spleen it may be attached. This fold may be derived from the anterior limb of the inverted-Y arrangement of some hili.

The left gastroepiploic vessels are often contained in the presplenic fold. Excessive traction during upper abdominal operations can result in a tear in the splenic capsule. Conservative procedures are then mandatory for splenic salvage. Excessive traction on the presplenic fold may produce bleeding because of its proximity to the left gastroepiploic vessels.

PHRENOCOLIC LIGAMENT. The phrenocolic ligament extends between the splenic flexure and the diaphragm. It is not really a splenic ligament, but the spleen rests on it. It is the "splenic floor," but is unconnected to the spleen. The phrenocolic ligament acts as a barricade at the left gutter and is responsible in most instances for prohibiting downward travel of blood from a ruptured splenic artery or from the spleen. Instead, the blood collects at the anterior pararenal space retroperitoneally or around the spleen at the left upper quadrant by displacing the colon laterally. If the phrenocolic ligament is short or fused, injury to the lower pole or the splenic flexure of the colon is remote but possible.

It is a mistake to describe the phrenocolic ligament as the left phrenocolic ligament, because there is no corresponding right ligament; there is only one phrenocolic ligament, and it is on the left side.

PANCREATOCOLIC LIGAMENT. The pancreatocolic ligament is the upper extension of the transverse mesocolon. Careless traction of a short or fused pancreatocolic ligament may lead to colonic or pancreatic injury.

Blood Supply
Segmental Anatomy

A number of studies have reported the separation of the spleen into lobes and segments by its arterial supply (Redmond et al.). Few mention the fact that the same segmental pattern can be observed based on venous drainage. This reflects the embryologic development of the organ, which is formed by the fusion of vascularized, isolated mesenchymal aggregates.

Gupta et al. made corrosion casts of human splenic arterial trees. In 84%, there were two splenic segments (superior and inferior); in 16% there were three segments (superior, middle, and inferior). The arterial segments were separated by avascular planes.

After studying 127 human spleens, Redmond et al. stated that the spleen is composed of anywhere from three to seven segments. Each segment has its own independent blood supply, separated by avascular planes. Segmental anatomy is not useful in tumor surgery involving the spleen.

Splenic Artery

In most people, the splenic artery is a branch of the celiac trunk, together with the hepatic and left gastric arteries. The common tripodal form of the celiac trunk (82%, according to Michels) may be replaced by a dipodal or tetrapodal pattern of branching when any of these or other upper abdominal arteries arise from atypical sources (VanDamme and Bonte). The normal course of the splenic artery is as follows.

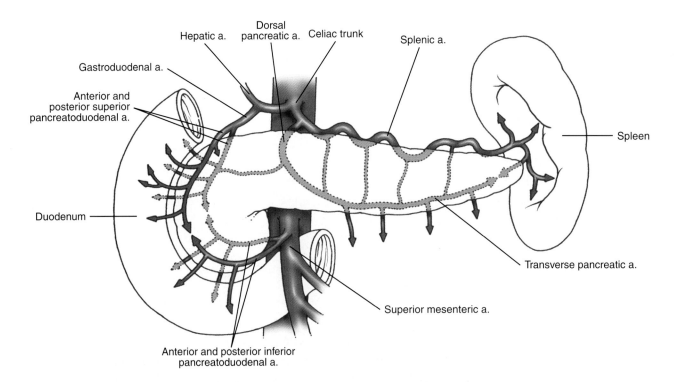

From its origin, the splenic artery crosses the left side of the aorta. It passes along the upper border of pancreas and reaches the tail in front. It then crosses the upper pole of the left kidney. The artery varies in length from 8 to 32 cm, and in diameter from 0.5 to 1.2 cm.

Waizer et al. reported on clinical implications of anatomic variations of the splenic artery. In nine of 26 cadavers the splenic artery made a loop to the right as soon as it emerged from the celiac artery, appearing at the border of the lesser omentum. It would thus be vulnerable to iatrogenic injury during procedures on supracolic organs.

The splenic artery forms the splenic peritoneal fold on its way to the spleen. It ends in the splenorenal ligament, forming a unique and peculiar tree, then reaches and enters the splenic porta.

According to Michels, the artery has four segments: suprapancreatic, pancreatic, prepancreatic, and prehilar segments. When we studied the splenic artery and its branches in toto, we concentrated on the last two distant segments, the prepancreatic and prehilar segments.

When angiography first provided noninvasive access to the vascular system of the spleen, we studied several angiograms, some of them selective splenic artery angiograms. Our conclusion: Not one of these films was a mirror image of another. Each was different, with unlimited variations, unpredictable in the origin of its branches and in length, dilatation (width), tortuosity, and course with regard to the pancreas (above the upper border, in front or behind, or partially or totally within the pancreatic parenchyma).

There is considerable agreement that the splenic artery most commonly bifurcates into two major branches (75% of the time) and less commonly undergoes trifurcation. Any further branching of these primary vessels three or more times yields a widely varying number of branches. These ultimately gain access to the hilus of the spleen. Extremes of branching reported range from 3 to 38.

BRANCHES OF SPLENIC ARTERY

Michels found a superior polar artery originates from the prehilar segment 65% of the time and an inferior polar artery or arteries 82% of the time. Our dissection of the splenic artery in 29 cadavers yielded the following points of origin: 27 from a hepatosplenogastric trunk, one from the common hepatic artery (hepatosplenic trunk), and one from the left gastric artery (gastrosplenic trunk).

The short gastric arteries anastomose with the cardiac branches of the left gastric artery. The short gastric arteries are the collateral circulation of the spleen. Farag et al. stated that because of the short gastric arteries, the upper third of the spleen might survive after a lower two thirds splenectomy in patients with normal size spleens.

Michels found that the left gastroepiploic artery arises from the splenic trunk 72% of the time, from the inferior terminal or its branches 22% of the time, and rarely from the middle splenic trunk or the superior terminal branch.

Other branches of the splenic artery include many small, unnamed branches. The more prominent, named branches are the dorsal pancreatic artery, the great pancreatic artery (pancreatica magna), and the caudal pancreatic artery.

The dorsal pancreatic artery is the "supreme pancreatic artery," posterior to the splenic vein and about 1.5 mm in diameter. Michels considers it the most variable of the celiacomesenteric vessels. The usual origin of the dorsal pancreatic artery is from the proximal 2 cm of the splenic artery (39% of specimens). However, it may arise from other arteries, including an aberrant hepatic artery.

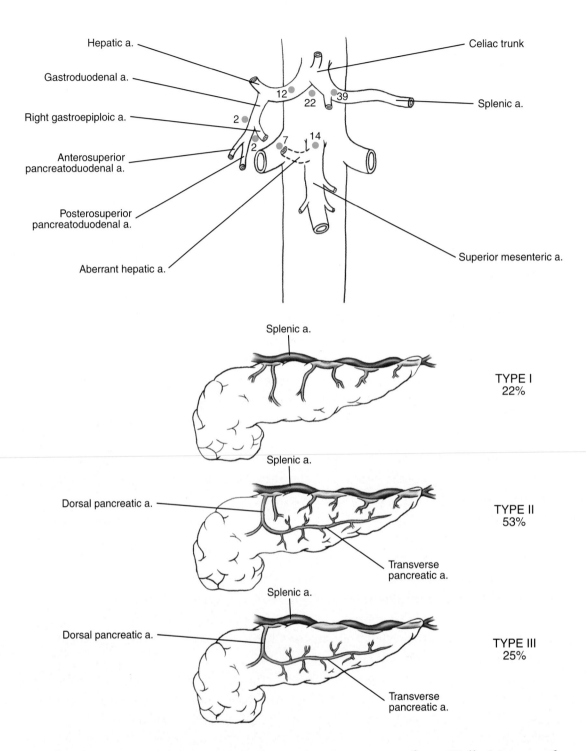

TYPE I
22%

TYPE II
53%

TYPE III
25%

The great pancreatic artery (arteria pancreatica magna of von Haller) is one of the largest branches of the splenic artery. It is the chief blood supply of the distal body and tail of the pancreas.

The caudal pancreatic artery originates from the left gastroepiploic artery or a splenic branch at the hilus of the spleen and anastomoses with branches of the great pancreatic and transverse pancreatic arteries. The caudal pancreatic artery supplies blood to accessory splenic tissue when it is present at the hilus of the spleen.

Collateral Circulation

The splenic artery is not the only artery to supply the spleen with blood. Additional blood supply comes from the inferior or transverse pancreatic artery, short gastric arteries, left gastroepiploic artery, and other pancreatic arteries.

The "main splenic arteries" are for all practical purposes the terminal branches of the splenic artery. They are responsible for the arterial blood supply of the spleen. These arteries originate from the superior and inferior terminal arteries or from the other terminal branches. The superior and inferior polar arteries most often originate from the prehilar segment and should be considered part of the main splenic artery. These arteries penetrate the splenic parenchyma above and below the portas.

The superior polar artery is nearly always present.

Venous Drainage

The splenic vein arises from the trabecular vein. We dissected 27 cadavers to study the splenic vein. The vein was formed by three trunks in 16 cases and by four trunks in eight cases. Three trunks plus the left gastroepiploic formed the splenic vein in the remaining three cases.

It must be remembered that the patterns are highly variable; no one vein resembles the next. Considerable variations are found in the exit points of the veins, their point of confluence in the formation of the main splenic vein, and their entrance into other veins at or outside the hilus.

Douglass et al. reported one point of common ground. The short gastric veins, or most of them, are in direct communication with the spleen. They enter the upper part of the organ rather than the extrasplenic venous vessels. The drainage of the left gastroepiploic vein is into the splenic veins.

The origin of the splenic vein is in the coalescence of five or six tributaries that emerge from the splenic hilus. Although the splenic vein is of large caliber, it does not possess the tortuosity of the splenic artery. The splenic vein passes through the splenorenal ligament with the artery and tail of the pancreas. It passes to the right, usually inferior to the artery and behind the body of the pancreas, receiving pancreatic tributaries. The vein ends deep to the neck of the pancreas by joining the superior mesenteric vein to form the portal vein.

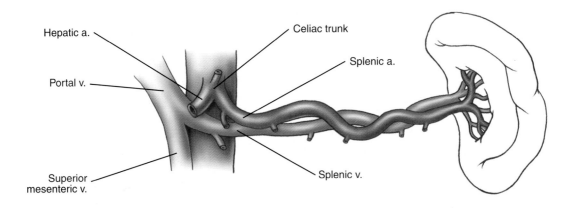

The splenic vein and the splenic artery travel together. Gerber et al. found three anatomic arrangements in 75 consecutive autopsies: vein entirely posterior to the artery, in 54%; vein wrapped around the artery, part posterior and part anterior to it, in 44%; and vein entirely anterior to the artery, in 2%.

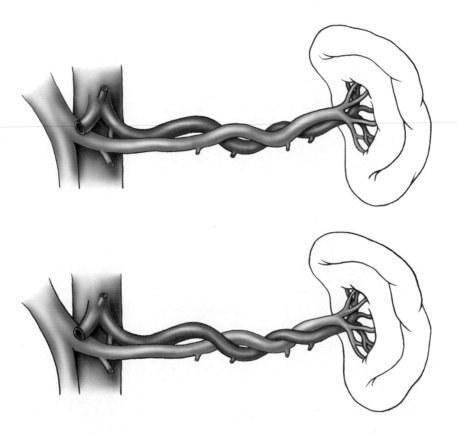

Ligation of the splenic arteries is permissible if the spleen has not been mobilized. The spleen remains viable if the collateral circulation is intact (polar arteries, short gastric arteries, and left gastroepiploic arteries). However, if the color of the spleen is changed and there is evidence of ischemia, splenectomy should be performed. Splenic vein thrombosis is also an indicator for total splenectomy.

As a rule, ligation of the splenic artery should be done only if absolutely necessary (i.e., during splenectomy). It is advisable to perform proximal double ligation of the splenic artery. Ligation of the artery should precede ligation of the vein, which should not be ligated alone. Because the origin and ultimate termination of the terminal arterial and venous branches are unpredictable, these vessels should be isolated and ligated close to the splenic portas to prevent bleeding. The tortuous splenic artery should be ligated with care to prevent pancreatic and splenic vein injury. Elevated segments of the tortuous splenic artery facilitate ligation without anatomic complications.

Nerve Supply

The more medial and anterior portions of the celiac plexus are the source of the splenic plexus. The splenic vessels are accompanied into the hilus by visceral nerve fibers from this plexus. According to Allen, fibers from the right vagus nerve or posterior vagal trunk also pass to the spleen. However, this configuration is questioned on the basis of study results in cats with nerve degeneration after vagotomy.

Myelinated fibers, probably sensory in function, can be identified histologically in a ratio of about 1:20 to unmyelinated autonomic fibers. These few sensory fibers terminate in the spinal cord at the level of the sixth to eighth thoracic vertebrae. The preganglionic sympathetic neurons arise in the intermediolateral cell column from this same level. They pass within the greater thoracic splanchnic nerve to the celiac ganglion and its extensions along the splenic artery. In some mammals, the autonomic fibers terminate in smooth muscle of the capsule, trabeculae, arteries, and veins. However, in humans the distribution of the autonomic fibers appears to be confined mostly to the branches of the splenic arteries.

Lymphatic Drainage

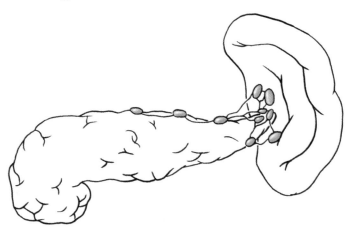

In the classification of the lymphatic vessels as devised by Rouviere, the splenic chain includes suprapancreatic nodes, infrapancreatic nodes, and afferent and efferent lymph vessels. Pancreatic tumors divide the splenic nodes into the hilus of the spleen and the tail of the pancreas.

The splenopancreatic glands are located along the splenic artery. This is the largest group of "splenic lymph nodes." A small number can also be found in the area of the short gastric vessels. The origin of the splenic lymphatic vessels is the splenic capsule and the trabeculae. The splenic nodes accept vessels from the stomach and pancreas.

One of the peculiarities of this enigmatic organ is the lack of provision for lymphatic drainage of the splenic pulp. The lymph nodes described above just happen to be located in the splenic neighborhood. Their destiny is to drain the stomach rather than the spleen. The dilemma of the surgeon is whether the spleen should be removed when the "splenic" lymph nodes are involved with disease. We do not have the answer. Antibiotics and active immunization against pneumococci definitely are of tremendous help against postsplenectomy sepsis. Partial splenectomy may prove to be the answer, even though Dearth et al. discussed the problems of false negative results in staging of Hodgkin's disease.

SURGICAL APPLICATIONS
OPEN SPLENECTOMY
Lee J. Skandalakis, M.D., and Panajiotis N. Skandalakis, M.D., M.S.

Splenectomy performed because of tumor can be divided into two categories. The first type of splenectomy is excision of a massively enlarged spleen. These spleens frequently extend down to the iliac crest. Their sheer weight and size make it difficult to move or lift the organ without rupturing the capsule or one of its attachments. Patience and some special technical maneuvers are required for this type of splenectomy. The second type of splenectomy is performed to stage Hodgkin's disease or to remove the spleen as a margin to adjacent tumors. A special type of splenectomy for staging has many different components.

Incisions

The size of the spleen will dictate the type of incision chosen. Although the subcostal incision gives adequate exposure, the midline incision is preferred in most indications for splenectomy (trauma, hypersplenism with coagulation problems, staging laparotomy for Hodgkin's disease, massive splenomegaly). However, the subcostal incision is appropriate when there is a diagnosis of a splenic mass in a normal or twice normal sized organ or when no additional

Table 15-1   *Indications for Splenectomy*

Control or Stage Primary Disease	Chronic or Severe Hypersplenism
Autoimmune anemia	Agnogenic myeloid metaplasia
Hereditary elliptocytosis	Lymphoproliferative disorder (non-Hodgkin's lymphoma, chronic lymphocytic leukemia, chronic myelocytic leukemia)
Hereditary spherocytosis	Chronic myelocytic leukemia
Immune thrombocytopenic purpura	Hairy cell leukemia
Thrombotic thrombocytopenic purpura	Felty's syndrome
Primary splenic neoplasm	Gaucher's disease
Splenic abscess	Thalassemia major
Splenic cyst	Acquired immunodeficiencies (human immunodeficiency virus)
Hodgkin's lymphoma	Sarcoid
Splenic vein thrombosis	
Splenomegaly caused by hemodialysis	

abdominal procedures are planned. Since these conditions occur infrequently, most surgeons perform splenectomy through a midline incision. Rarely thoracoabdominal incisions are used. The bed of the eighth or ninth rib may be used for massive splenomegaly. There seems to be no difference in postoperative complications with midline and subcostal incisions. Therefore the surgeon should choose the incision that gives the best exposure for the operation planned.

The midline incision offers several important advantages for splenectomy. First, the surgeon can safely remove the spleen, no matter its size, with a large enough incision and adequate exposure of the left upper quadrant. Second, the incision can be made quickly and easily, with minimal blood loss. Third, the midline incision allows the surgeon to explore the entire abdomen.

If there is a well-developed presplenic fold, the anterior approach to the splenic artery at the pedicle may demonstrate six sheets of peritoneum, fat, lymph nodes, and pancreas fused into a single mass. Both the lesser sac and the space between the presplenic fold and the gastrosplenic ligament may be obliterated. Only a single (posterior) leaf of the splenorenal ligament is encountered in a posterior approach to the splenic artery.

Splenectomy for Enlarged Spleen

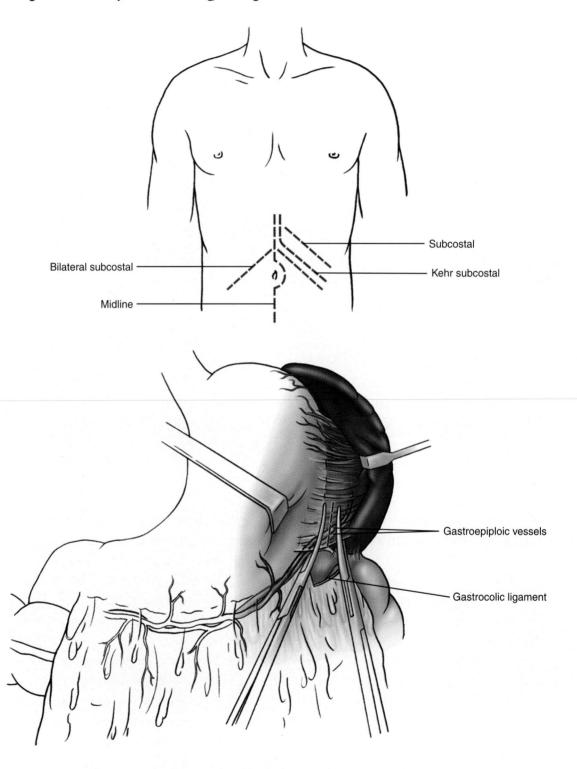

The incision is made. Access to the lesser sac is gained by clamping, incising, and ligating the left part of the gastrocolic ligament and the gastroepiploic artery and vein.

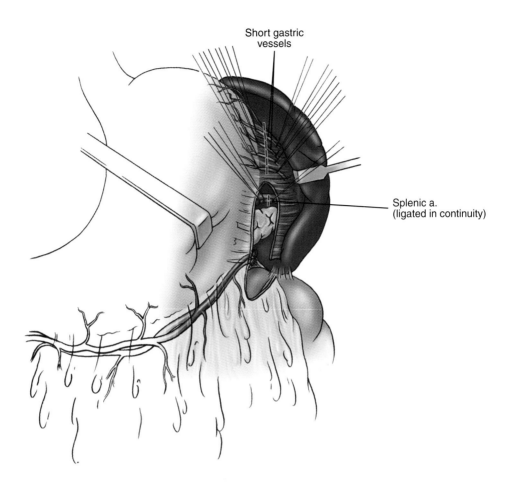

The short gastric arteries and veins are clamped, divided, and ligated one by one. The splenic artery at the superior border of the body of the pancreas is easily located and ligated in continuity, carefully and doubly. Ligatures are placed as distally as possible. Alternatively, the division of the splenic artery may follow mobilization of the spleen.

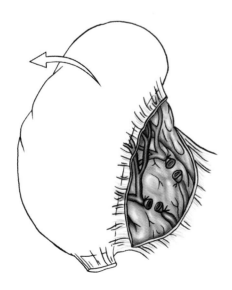

The spleen is mobilized by scissors division of several ligaments. Most of the ligaments are avascular. After a small window is created at the splenorenal ligament, the index finger is inserted deep. Blunt and sharp dissection is used to separate the spleen from the renal covering by proceeding slowly caudad and cephalad. The splenocolic and splenophrenic ligaments are clamped, divided, and ligated.

With a wide window, now large enough to insert four fingers or the hand in toto, the surgeon should elevate the spleen and the tail and part of the body of the pancreas. The spleen is carefully delivered outside the peritoneal cavity, with the only attachment being one of the branches of the splenic arteries and veins. The tail of the pancreas should be handled with care.

All branches of the splenic artery are clamped, divided, and ligated close to the hilum. The splenic vein and its branches are very friable, and clamps should be used with great caution. The main vein is encircled with double suture material, tied carefully with ligature, and the spleen removed.

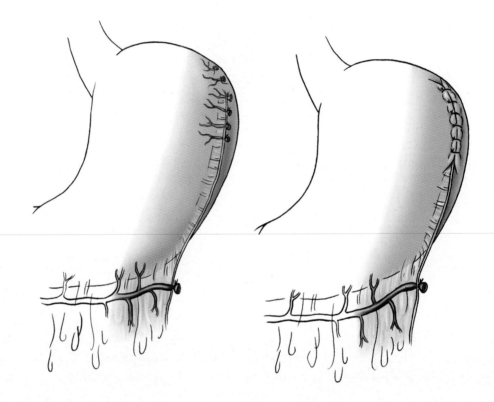

The site is inspected for bleeding and for accessory spleens. Inspection for bleeding proceeds from above downward, starting at the diaphragm and continuing to the greater curvature of stomach, pancreatic tail, gastrosplenic ligament, splenorenal ligament, splenocolic ligament, and splenic bed and other ligaments. Complete hemostasis is essential. The greater curvature may be inverted with continuous 00 suture to prevent postoperative bleeding and possible necrosis in the area of the short gastric arteries. The search for accessory spleens is done after inspection for bleeding.

The use of drains after splenectomy is controversial. The main problem with placing drains in the splenic bed is the possibility of an ascending infection for the skin resulting in an abscess. Thus the drain would cause, rather than prevent, a subphrenic abscess. When drains are used, they should be closed suction drains and should be removed in 2 to 5 days unless a large amount of drainage (more than 50 to 75 ml) indicates the possibility of a fistula.

Splenectomy for Staging Hodgkin's Disease

Improvements in radiologic staging of Hodgkin's disease have virtually eliminated the need for staging procedures for Hodgkin's disease. When performed, they should include the following:

1. Detailed exploratory laparotomy
2. Examination of nodes, and wedge and needle biopsies of both lobes of the liver
3. Total splenectomy with splenic lymph node biopsy
4. Retroperitoneal exploration of the celiac axis, hepatoduodenopancreatic lymph nodes, periaortic lymph nodes, inferior vena caval lymph nodes, iliac lymph nodes, and mesenteric lymph nodes of the small and large intestines for lymph node biopsy
5. Biopsy of iliac crest marrow
6. Search for accessory spleens
7. Placement of metal clips at the splenic pedicle, areas of lymph nodes where biopsies have been done, areas of lymph nodes where biopsies have not been performed, and the site of ovarian translocation

Anatomic Basis of Complications

- Injury to the splenic artery or vein results in severe bleeding. Ligation is necessary.
- Injury to the short gastric vessels causes severe bleeding.
- Injury of the tail or body of the pancreas causes postoperative pancreatitis.
- Imbrication is advised if there is injury to the greater curvature of the stomach.
- Injury to the diaphragm.
- Injury to the left kidney.
- Injury to the left colon or splenic flexure.

KEY REFERENCES

Michels NA. Blood Supply and Anatomy of the Upper Abdominal Organs, With a Descriptive Atlas. Philadelphia: JB Lippincott, 1955.
This book, the product of 20 years' work, was and perhaps still is the "Bible" for the blood supply of the upper abdominal organs.

Michels NA. The variational anatomy of the spleen and the splenic artery. Am J Anat 70:21, 1942.
This is a detailed presentation of the splenic artery, its branches, and their relationships with several other anatomic entities.

Morgenstern L, Rosenberg BA, Geller SA. Tumors of the spleen. World J Surg 9:468, 1985.
Morgenstern is the pioneer of segmental splenic surgery. Together with his associates, he presents a complete essay about splenic tumors and benign and malignant processes of the spleen.

Redmond HP, Redmond JM, Rooney BP, et al. Surgical anatomy of the human spleen. Br J Surg 76(2):198-201, 1989.
This is a beautiful review of the surgical anatomy of the spleen. The emphasis is on blood supply and segmentation.

VanDamme JPJ, Bonte J. Systemization of the arteries in the splenic hilus. Acta Anat 125:217, 1986.
This is an excellent article on the end branches of the splenic artery at the area of the splenic portas. The systematization of the splenic branches at hilum is superb.

VanDamme JP, Bonte J. Vascular Anatomy in Abdominal Surgery. New York: Thieme Medical Publishers, 1990.
This book presents "arterial variations with a surgical eye." It is an excellent description of the vascular anatomy of the intra-abdominal organs from examination of patients and cadavers.

SUGGESTED READINGS

Allen L. The lymphatic system and the spleen. In Anson BJ, ed. Morris's Human Anatomy, 12th ed. New York: McGraw-Hill, 1966, p 907.

Boles ET Jr, Haase GM, Hamoudi AB. Partial splenectomy in staging laparotomy for Hodgkin's disease: An alternative approach. J Pediatr Surg 13:581-586, 1978.

Crosby ED, Humphrey T, Lauer EW. Correlative Anatomy of the Nervous System. New York: Macmillan, 1962, p 545.

Dearth JC, Gilchrist GS, Telander RL, et al. Partial splenectomy for staging Hodgkin's disease: Risk of false-negative results. N Engl J Med 299:345-346, 1978.

Douglas BE, Baggenstoss AH, Hollinhead WH. The anatomy of the portal vein and its tributaries. Surg Gynecol Obstet 91:562, 1950.

Dunphy JE. Splenectomy for trauma. Am J Surg 71:450, 1946.

Farag A, Shoukry A, Nasr SE. A new option for splenic preservation in normal sized spleen based on preserved histology and phagocytic function of the upper pole using upper short gastric vessels. Am J Surg 168(3):257-261, 1994.

Garcia-Porrero JA, Lemes A. Arterial segmentation and subsegmentation in the human spleen. Acta Anat 131:276, 1988.

Gerber AB, Lev M, Goldberg SL. The surgical anatomy of the splenic vein. Am J Surg 82:339, 1951.

Gould FM, Pyle WL. Anomalies and Curiosities of Medicine, 2nd ed. New York: Bell Publishing, 1956, p 657.

Graves FT. Seeing Operative Surgery. London: William Heineman Medical Books, 1979, p 132.

Gupta CD, Gupta SC, Aorara AK, et al. Vascular segments in the human spleen. J Anat 121:613, 1976.

Hamilton WJ, Simon G, Hamilton SGI. Surface and Radiological Anatomy. Baltimore: Williams & Wilkins, 1976.

Katritsis E, Parashos A, Papadopoulos N. Arterial segmentation of the human spleen by post-mortem angiograms and corrosion casts. Angiology 33:720, 1982.

Lord MD, Gourevitch A. The peritoneal anatomy of the spleen, with special references to the operation of partial gastrectomy. Br J Surg 52:202, 1965.

Moody RO. The possibility of the abdominal viscera in healthy young British and American adults. J Anat 61:223, 1927.

Pemberton LB, Manax WG. Complications after vertical and transverse incisions for cholecystectomy. Surg Gynecol Obstet 132:892, 1971.

Rosen A, Nathan H, Luciansky E, et al. The lienorenal ligament and the tail of the pancreas: A surgical anatomical study. Pancreas 3(1):104-107, 1988.

Rouviere H. Anatomy of the Human Lymphatic System. Ann Arbor: Edwards Bros, 1938.

Skandalakis JE, Gray SW, eds. The Spleen. Prob Gen Surg 7:1-150, 1990.

Utterback RA. Innervation of the spleen. J Comp Neurol 81:55, 1944.

Waizer A, Baniel J, Zin Y, et al. Clinical implications of anatomic variations of the splenic artery. Surg Gynecol Obstet 168:57, 1989.

Whitesell FB. A clinical and surgical anatomic study of rupture of the spleen due to blunt trauma. Surg Gynecol Obstet 110:750, 1960.

Williams PL, Warwick R. Gray's Anatomy, 36th ed. Philadelphia: WB Saunders, 1980.

LAPAROSCOPIC SPLENECTOMY
C. Daniel Smith, M.D.

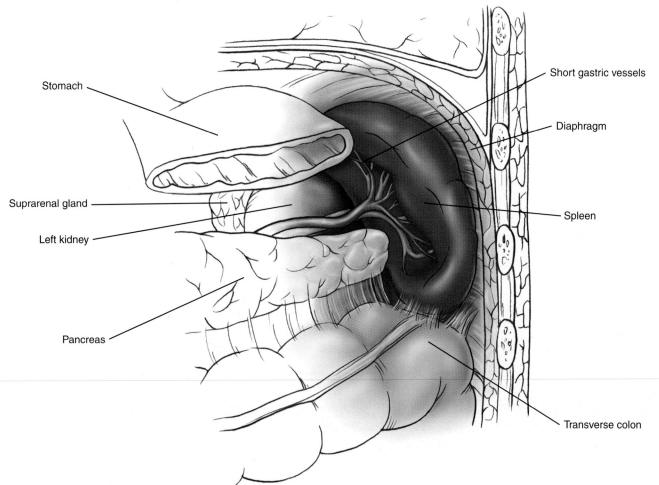

Splenectomy has more recently been performed using minimally invasive techniques. The indications for laparoscopic splenectomy remain the same as those for traditional open splenectomy. Contraindications to the laparoscopic approach include intractable coagulopathy, severe chronic obstructive pulmonary disease (COPD), portal hypertension, inability to tolerate general anesthesia, and massive splenomegaly (>20 cm pole to pole).

By preventing the morbidity associated with upper abdominal incisions, laparoscopic splenectomy decreases the duration of hospitalization and speeds and enhances overall recovery. Over 1000 laparoscopic splenectomies reported in world literature confirm its safety. In many centers laparoscopic splenectomy has become the preferred technique for spleen removal. In our own experience with more than 60 laparoscopic splenectomies, average hospital stay was 2 days, and most patients returned to their usual activities within 3 weeks postoperatively. Minor complications occurred in 3% of patients. Conversion to open splenectomy was necessary in only three patients, one due to bleeding and two due to massive splenomegaly.

Because of its unique anatomic features, with both intraperitoneal and retroperitoneal components, the laparoscopic approach to splenectomy combines a true anterior approach, allowing visualization and exposure of the intraperitoneal anatomy, and a lateral approach, facilitating mobilization and exposure of the retroperitoneal anatomy. This minimally invasive approach has been termed the "leaning spleen" technique of laparoscopic splenectomy.

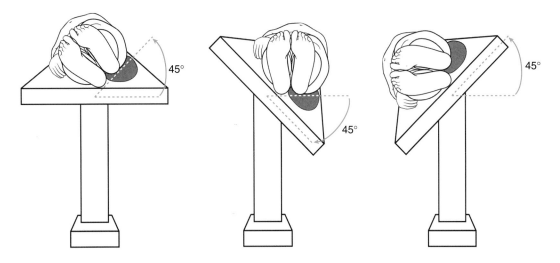

In the leaning spleen laparoscopic approach to splenectomy, the patient is placed in an incomplete right lateral decubitus position at an angle of 45 degrees. This allows the patient's position to be changed from nearly supine to nearly lateral by tilting the operating table. In this way, a combined supine and lateral approach can be realized.

Preoperative Preparation

The patient's preoperative preparation includes administration of polyvalent pneumococcal vaccine at least 2 weeks before surgery. Patients with idiopathic thrombocytopenic purpura and critically low platelet counts (<20,000 μl) receive preoperative immunoglobulin G (IgG) to raise immediate preoperative platelet levels to a safe range. The evening before surgery, patients commence a clear liquid diet and take a mild laxative several hours before bedtime (one bottle of magnesium citrate at 7:00 PM) to decompress the colon and facilitate laparoscopic visualization of the left upper quadrant and spleen. Several units of packed red blood cells are cross matched, and in patients with idiopathic thrombocytopenic purpura, platelets are cross matched for administration after the splenic artery has been ligated intraoperatively.

Immediately preoperatively, pneumatic compression boots are applied and a preoperative antibiotic (1 gm cephazolin) is given. Patients who have been receiving corticosteroids within 6 months of surgery are given stress doses of intravenous corticosteroids. Before transport to the operating room, a beanbag stabilizing bag is placed on the operating table to enable subsequent patient positioning and stabilization.

After endotracheal induction of general anesthesia, a Foley catheter and an orogastric tube are placed.

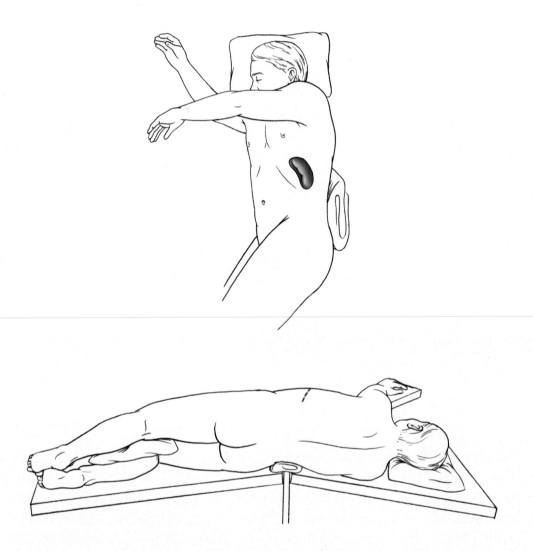

The patient is positioned in the incomplete right lateral decubitus position. It is important to position the patient with the iliac crest immediately over the table's kidney rest and mid–break point. The kidney rest is elevated and the table flexed, allowing more distance between the iliac crest and the left lower costal margin in the midaxillary line. The beanbag stabilizing bag is activated, and the patient's hip is secured to the table with loosely applied tape. Legs are padded with pillows, and an axillary roll is placed. The left arm is hung over the chest on a sling. The arm must be far enough cephalad to clear the operative field and allow obstruction-free use of the laparoscopic instruments. All pressure points are adequately padded.

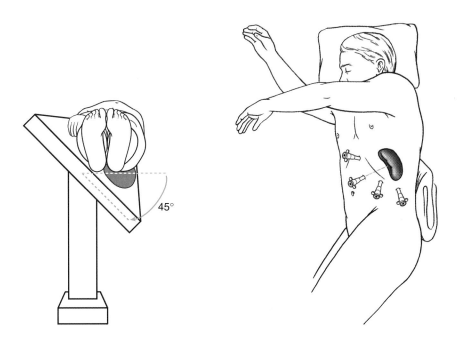

The skin is prepared and draped so that either laparoscopy or open surgery can be performed. The table is tilted 30 degrees to the left to place the patient in the near-supine position. Before incisions are made, the area is anesthetized with long-lasting local anesthetic. Carbon dioxide pneumoperitoneum is initiated using a Veress needle technique through a periumbilical stab incision to a pressure of 15 mm Hg. Cannula sites are marked. The first cannula is 12 mm and is placed through the left rectus sheath in the midclavicular line approximately 15 cm from the cutaneous projection of the splenic hilum. The second port is 12 mm and is placed just below the costal margin in the epigastrium, entering the abdomen just below the left lobe of the liver. The third cannula is 12 mm and is placed in the midaxillary line equidistant between the costal margin and the iliac crest. The fourth cannula is 5 mm and is placed in the posterior axillary line, entering the abdomen just above the superior pole of the left kidney. Before placing this cannula, it is necessary to mobilize the splenic flexure of the colon to prevent injury during cannula placement.

Operative Procedure

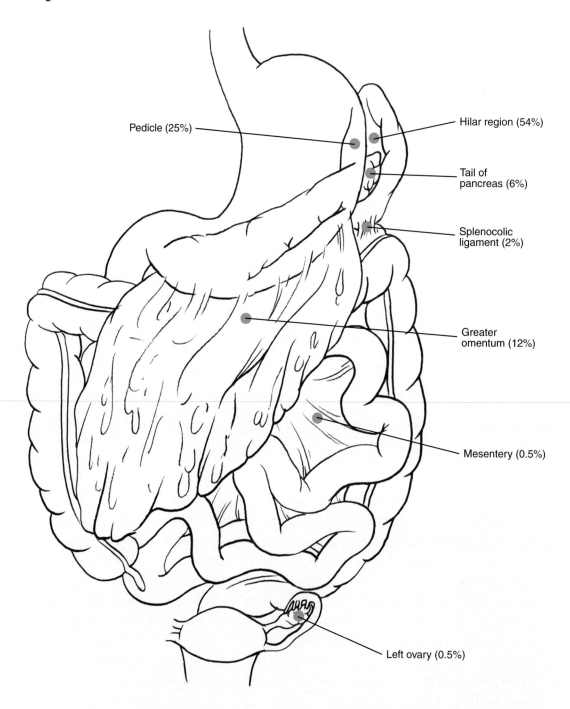

Pedicle (25%)

Hilar region (54%)

Tail of
pancreas (6%)

Splenocolic
ligament (2%)

Greater
omentum (12%)

Mesentery (0.5%)

Left ovary (0.5%)

The operation commences with thorough visual inspection of the omentum
and splenocolic regions, common locations for accessory splenic tissue. The
splenic hilum is then exposed.

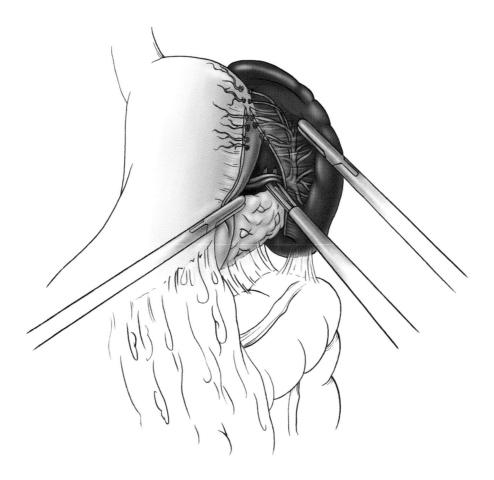

The patient is placed in the reverse Trendelenburg position, and the lesser sac is entered by dividing the greater omentum halfway down the greater curvature of the stomach. Exposure continues by following the greater curve of the stomach cephalad and dividing the short gastric vessels. This is most easily accomplished by having the first assistant retract the omentum ventrally and laterally while the surgeon's left hand retracts the stomach medially and ventrally and the right hand dissects and divides tissue. We have found it helpful to use the Harmonic Scalpel (Ethicon Endosurgery, Cincinnati, Ohio) for this dissection. The splenic artery is identified in the lesser sac and carefully isolated with a blunt-tipped right-angle clamp. This vessel is then ligated with a heavy intracorporeal suture. Similarly, the splenic vein may be ligated at this time if it can be easily isolated. If indicated, platelets are transfused after splenic artery ligation.

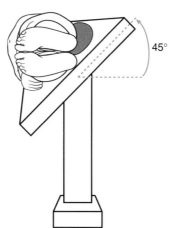

The table is then rotated 30 degrees to the right into the near lateral position. The spleen is rolled medially and ventrally, exposing the lateral and posterior splenic attachments.

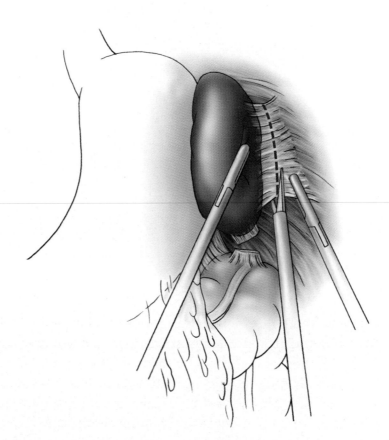

Using monopolar electrocautery or the Harmonic Scalpel, the splenocolic ligament is divided and the posterior and lateral attachments of the spleen released. This mobilization progresses from caudad to cephalad until the spleen is fully mobilized laterally and the left hemidiaphragm is visualized from behind and above the spleen. This gravity-facilitated dissection allows the spleen to fall medially, providing complete visualization of the tail of the pancreas and the splenic hilum. The first assistant elevates the inferior pole of the spleen ventrally, facilitating division of the final attachments to the inferior pole of the spleen. Great care is used when manipulating the spleen to prevent capsular disruption, which could lead to splenosis and recurrent hematologic disease.

The splenic artery and vein can then be easily ligated and divided with a second set of ligatures or a vascular linear cutting stapler. Care is taken to identify and avoid the tail of the pancreas during this final hilar dissection and division.

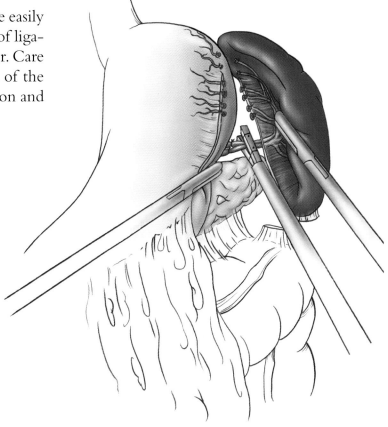

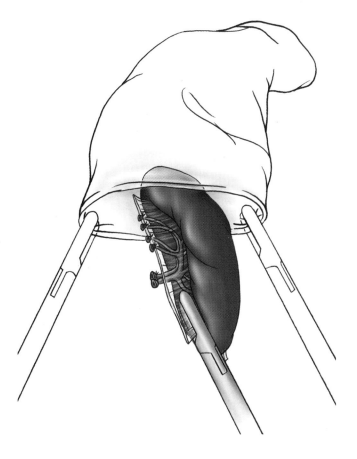

The disconnected spleen is then gently pushed medially and out of the left upper quadrant. The left upper quadrant is inspected for hemostasis. With hemostasis ensured, a nylon reinforced specimen retrieval sac (Cook Surgical, Bloomington, Ind.) is rolled and placed into the abdomen through one of the 12 mm cannulas. The sac is unrolled and positioned in the left upper quadrant with its opening toward the pelvis. The patient is then placed in the steep Trendelenburg position and, with the help of gravity, the spleen is gently pushed or dragged into the sac using perisplenic attachments or the hilar pedicle. The sac is closed by pulling the sac's drawstring, and the mouth of the bag is pulled out through the midclavicular cannula site.

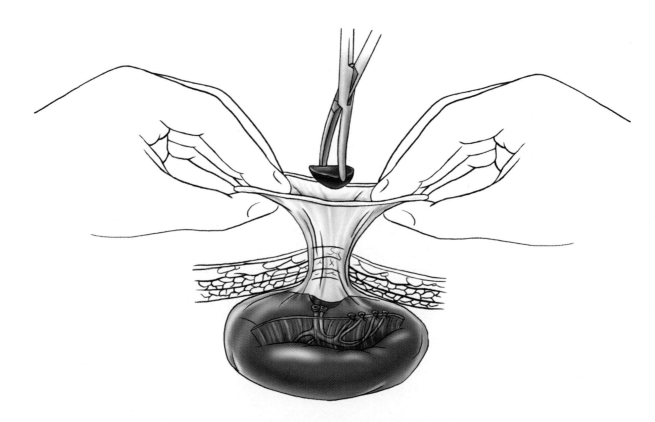

The sac is then entered extracorporeally, and the spleen is morcellated and removed piecemeal from the sac with ring forceps until the sac can be extracted. Intermittent use of a large bore suction device greatly facilitates removal of the morcellatum. In addition, it is helpful to enlarge the incision to 2 cm to facilitate specimen and sac removal. If the splenic architecture needs to be preserved for pathologic assessment, the trocar site incision can be further enlarged to allow removal of the intact spleen. Alternatively, a Pfannenstiel incision can be used to remove the spleen, thereby optimizing the cosmetic results.

The abdomen is then reinsufflated and inspected for hemostasis. When hemostasis is adequate, cannulas are removed under direct vision. The abdomen is desufflated, and the fascia of the primary cannula site (specimen removal site) is closed with absorbable suture. The skin of all cannula sites is closed with a running 4-0 subcuticular stitch. The orogastric tube is removed in the operating room, and the Foley catheter is removed in the recovery room.

Postoperative Care

Postoperatively, the patient is allowed clear liquids orally, and ambulates the night of surgery. Pain is controlled with intermittent parenteral narcotics until the patient is able to take oral pain medication. Diet is advanced on postoperative day 1, and the patient is discharged when oral intake is tolerated and pain is controlled with oral analgesics.

Anatomic Basis of Complications

- Injury to the splenic artery or vein results in significant and rapid blood loss, mandating conversion to an open procedure.
- Injury to the short gastric vessels results in significant and rapid blood loss; if not controlled quickly, mandates conversion to open splenectomy.
- Injury to the tail of the pancreas leads to pancreatic leak, with resulting pancreatitis or pancreatic fistula.

KEY REFERENCE

Smith CD, Meyer TA, Goretsky MJ, et al. Laparoscopic splenectomy by the lateral approach: A safe and effective alternative to open splenectomy for hematologic diseases. Surgery 120:789, 1996.

These authors compare lateral approach to laparoscopic splenectomy with open splenectomy. Time to resumption of oral intake, duration of hospital stay, and duration of nasogastric decompression were all significantly decreased in the laparoscopically treated patients. Laparoscopic splenectomy has become the preferred method of spleen removal.

SUGGESTED READINGS

Brunt LM, Langer JC, Quasebarth MA, et al. Comparative analysis of laparoscopic versus open splenectomy. Am J Surg 172:596, 1996.

Delaitre B, Pitre J. Laparoscopic splenectomy versus open splenectomy: A comparative study. Hepatogastroenterology 44:45, 1997.

Richardson WS, Smith CD, Branum GD, et al. The leaning spleen: A new approach to laparoscopic splenectomy. J Am Coll Surg 185:412, 1997.

Trias M, Targarona EM, Balaque C. Laparoscopic splenectomy: An evolving technique. A comparison between anterior and lateral approaches. Surg Endosc 10:389, 1996.

Yee LF, Carvajal SH, de Lormier AA, et al. Laparoscopic splenectomy. The initial experience at University of California, San Francisco. Arch Surg 130:874, 1995.

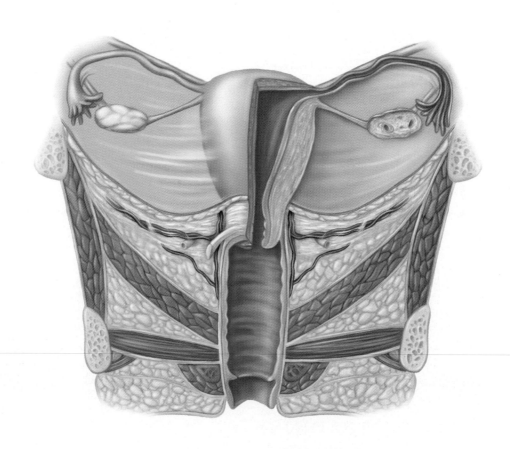

Chapter 16

Female Genital System

Ira R. Horowitz, M.D.

Surgical Applications

- Simple Extrafascial Total Abdominal Hysterectomy With or Without Bilateral Salpingo-oophorectomy
- Laparoscopic Hysterectomy
- Radical Hysterectomy
- Pelvic Lymphadenectomy
- Periaortic Lymph Node Dissection
- Supraclavicular Lymph Node Biopsy
- Omentectomy
- Radical Vulvectomy With Inguinal Femoral Lymphadenectomy

Gynecologic malignancies as a group have an incidence second only to breast cancer. In 1996 approximately 184,300 new breast cancers were diagnosed compared to 82,100 gynecologic malignancies (cervix, 5700; corpus uteri, 34,000; ovary, 26,700; other, 5700). Gynecologic malignancies ranked third in estimated deaths in 1996: lung, 64,300; breast, 44,300; and gynecologic, 26,900 (cervix, 4900; corpus uteri, 6000; ovary, 14,800; other, 1200). The incidence of cervical cancer has markedly decreased over the last 50 years with Papanicolaou (Pap) smear screening and colposcopy. Endometrial carcinoma has also decreased as a result in changes in prescribing hormone supplementation. Unopposed estrogens were responsible for a significant number of well-differentiated carcinomas in the menopausal patient. The addition of progesterone and liberal indications for endometrial biopsy have assisted in decreasing the incidence. In the uterus, tamoxifen is an estrogen agonist compared with being an antagonist in the breast. Uterine stimulation is present with patients receiving tamoxifen to treat breast cancer. All abnormal bleeding in this group of patients is suspect for the presence of endometrial cancer. Endometrial biopsies are required to rule out this malignancy in menopausal patients with abnormal bleeding. Ovarian cancer is difficult to diagnose early. Screening ultrasonography and CA-125 have low sensitivity and specificity when used to diagnose occult ovarian malignances in the asymptomatic patient. As a result, when initially examined these patients have advanced disease, with high mortality.

CLINICAL ANATOMY
Topography
Corpus/Cervix

The uterus is a pear-shaped muscle with a dome-shaped fundus. It consists of two segments: the corpus, or body, and the cervix, or isthmus. In the nulliparous patient the corpus is approximately 8 cm long, 5 cm wide, and 2.5 cm thick. The uterine cavity resembles an inverted triangle, lined with endometrium, which is made up of glandular tissue. The normal thickness of the endometrium is 0.5 cm, with a total thickness of 1 cm. An endometrial cavity larger than 1 cm requires evaluation to rule out the presence of a neoplastic lesion. Office endometrial sampling or hysteroscopy dilation and curettage is adequate for evaluation of the endometria.

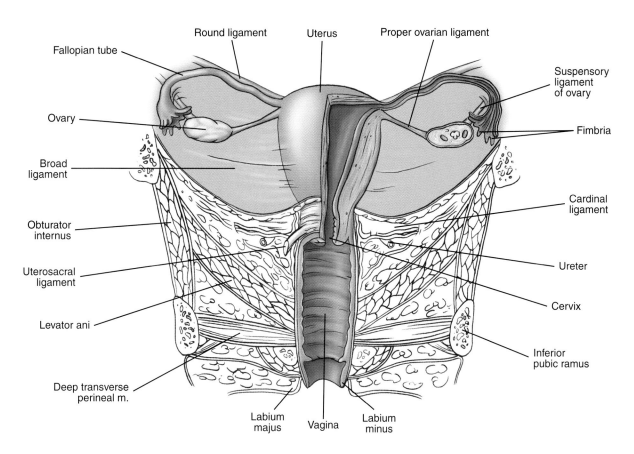

The cervix is divided into the portio vaginalis and the portio supravaginalis cervicis, the latter above the cervix. Surrounding the cervix is a smooth muscle fibrous network with the uterosacral, cardinal, and pubovesical fasciae inserting in it.

Fallopian Tube

Attached to the fundus is the fallopian tube (uterine tube). It is approximately 10 to 12 cm long and divided into four segments. The infundibulum with fimbria distally held by the ampulla is the widest portion of the fallopian tube. The third and fourth segments are the isthmus, which is the narrowest portion, and the interstitial (or intramural) portion, where the fallopian tube passes into the uterus. The fallopian tube is composed of three layers: serosa, muscularis, and mucosa. The muscularis (tunica muscularis) is composed of an inner circular and an outer longitudinal smooth muscle layer. Columnar cells in a sample layer make up the mucosa.

Ovary

Each ovary is 2.5 to 5.0 cm long, 1.5 to 3.0 cm thick, and 0.7 to 1.5 cm wide and is attached by its mesenteric attachment to the broad ligament, the meso-varium. Laterally is the infundibular pelvic ligament, which includes the ovarian artery and vein, and medial the ovarian ligament. The blood vessels enter the hilus of the ovary. Germinal epithelium lines the outside, or capsule, of the ovary. The inner medulla of the ovary is a fibromuscular layer with blood vessels. The cortex, including the stroma, consists of follicles, corpus luteum, and corpus albicans.

Pelvic Suspension

An excavation in the front of the uterus is called the anterior cul-de-sac, and the excavation in the back is called the posterior cul-de-sac, or pouch of Douglas. The cardinal ligaments (Mackenrodt's) provide the lateral attachment from the cervix and superior vagina to the pelvic sidewall and pelvic floor. This is a fibromuscular tissue covered by peritoneum and merges with the uterovaginal and vesicoendopelvic fascial envelope; posteriorly it merges with the uterosacral ligament. The uterosacral (sacral cervical or sacral uterine) ligament is a muscle fiber tissue fanning from the cervix and superior vagina to the lateral sacral borders bilaterally. The broad ligament peritoneal layers envelop the fundus and corpus, the fallopian tube, and the infundibular pelvic ligament, which includes the ovarian artery and veins. Between the layers of the cardinal ligament are the parametria, uterine vessels, ovarian vessels, lymphatic vessels, and nerves. Peritoneum extends anteriorly to cover the bladder and posteriorly to cover the rectum, forming the anterior and posterior cul-de-sacs. The round ligament extends from the fundus through the inguinal canal to form the inguinal ligament. Sampson's vessels course through the round ligament. Suspension of the uterus is also assisted by the levator ani muscles and the pelvic fascial ligaments. An endopelvic fascia envelops the cervix and upper vagina, extending to the pelvic sidewall, and is contiguous with the vesicouterine and rectouterine fascia.

Omentum

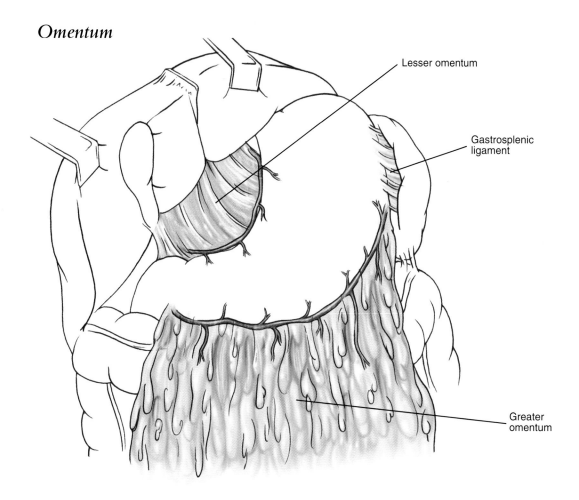

Omentum is a double layer of peritoneum that attaches to the stomach on the greater and lesser curvatures and the transverse colon. The greater omentum is adherent to the greater curvature of the stomach and acts like an apron over the small bowel abdominal contents. It has been called the sentinel of the abdomen. The lesser omentum is adherent to the lesser curvature of the stomach and undersurface of the liver. The gastrosplenic omentum (ligament) connects the spleen and omentum. Omentum contains arteries, nerves, and lymphatic vessels and is composed predominantly of fat. The gastroepiploic vessels traverse the greater omentum inferior to the liver and falciform ligament toward the gallbladder. Additional discussion of the anatomy of the omentum can be found in Chapters 9 and 12.

Vagina

The vagina is a muscular cylinder approximately 8 to 10 cm long. The superior vagina surrounds the portio of the cervix. The most superior recess enveloping the vagina as it envelops the cervix is the anterior and posterior fornices, and laterally the left and right sulci. Lined by epithelium, the vagina has a deeper connective tissue layer called the lamina propria, followed by circular and longitudinal smooth muscle fibers. Adjacent to the anterior vagina is the bladder proximally and the urethra distally. The posterior vagina is divided in three portions: the vaginal portion of the pouch of Douglas superiorly, the rectum in the middle, and the peritoneal body and anus inferiorly. Laterally are the vessels of the ureter and suspensory fibrous tissue to the levator ani. Support of the vagina is predominantly by the levator ani muscles and the endopelvic fascia, which is contiguous with the uterosacral and cardinal ligaments. The middle third of the vagina is suspended laterally by attaching to the arcus tendineus fasciae pelvis on either side, with the inferior portion suspended by the peritoneal body.

Vulva

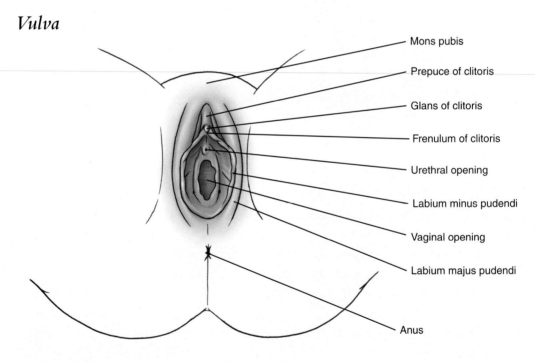

The vulva is that portion of the female genitalia that is external to the perineal region. It includes the mons pubis, anterior commissure, with the clitoris inferiorally, prepuce of the clitoris, and hood of the clitoris, followed by the glans of the clitoris. The urethral orifice is inferior to the frenulum of the clitoris. Adjacent to the urethra are Skene's glands. The hymen is circumferential and is sentinel to the vaginal tube. Lateral to the hymenal ring is the labia minora, followed by the labia majora laterally toward the thighs. Bartholin's glands open at 5- and 7-o'clock positions inferiorly on the vulva. Between the vaginal tube and the anus is the perineal body. The vestibule includes the hymen, vaginal opening, urethral rectus, and Bartholin's and Skene's glands. The labia majora are the major skinfolds of the vulva, with hair extending from the mons pubis to the perineal body. The labia minora are two smaller folds without hair and are the lateral borders of the vestibule. Labia are the anatomic homolog to the scrotum, and the clitoris is homologous to the penis in the male. The glans clitoris, covered by the prepuce, is embryologically similar to the glans of the penis and foreskin. Erectile tissue is present in the clitoris.

Blood Supply

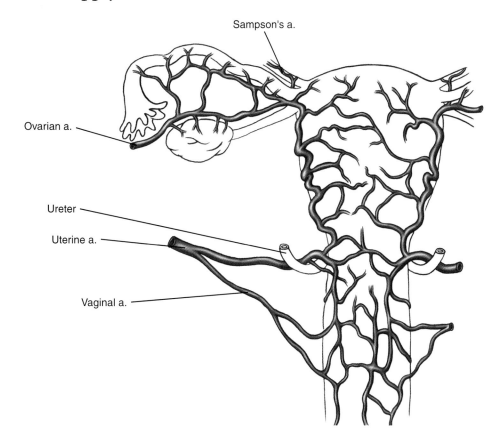

Arterial blood supply to the ovaries is via the ovarian arteries, which have their origin in the anterior surface of the aorta inferior to the renal vessels. The left ovarian vein empties into the left renal vein, which then enters into the vena cava, and the right ovarian vein empties into the vena cava inferior to the right renal vein. These vessels are retroperitoneal. On reaching the most proximal aspect of the ovary closest to the fimbria the vessels break into arcades that supply blood to the fallopian tubes and ovaries. The arcades traverse through the mesentary adherent to these structures. The uterine artery has its origin from the hypogastric (internal iliac) artery, which branches off the common iliac artery. The uterine artery then branches into the vaginal artery and multiple branches from the artery, which measures approximately 10 cm to the cervix and uterus. These branches anastomose with those of the ovarian artery in the area of the utero-ovarian ligament and round ligament, which includes Sampson's artery. The uterine artery crosses over the ureter in the cardinal ligament ("water under the bridge"). Adjacent to the uterine artery are the uterine veins, which drain the corpus and cervix and empty into iliac veins.

The vagina receives its blood supply from the vaginal branch of the uterine artery and the vaginal artery, which originates from the hypogastric artery. The inferior vesical artery off the anterior division of the hypogastric artery provides a cervical and a vaginal branch. These branches anastomose to the superior and middle vesicular arteries of the hypogastric artery. The distal vagina also receives part of its blood supply from the middle and inferior hemorrhoidal arteries, which also have their origin in the anterior branch of the hypogastric artery.

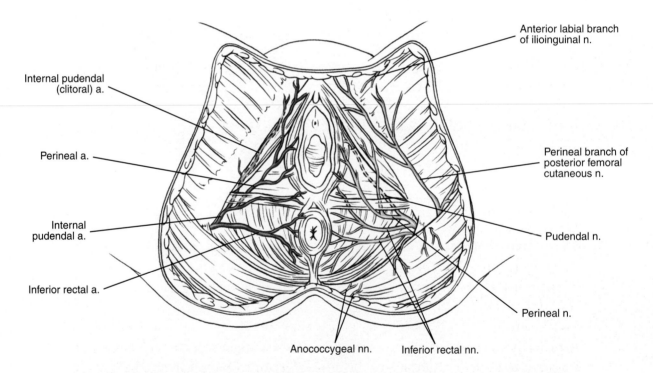

The blood supply to the vulva is predominantly via the internal pudendal artery and exits the pelvis at the ischial spine. The artery branches into the superficial perineal artery, which supplies the labia and artery of the bulb to supply the vestibular bulb and erectile tissue of the vagina, the artery of the corpus cavernosum, and the artery of the clitoris.

Lymphatic Drainage

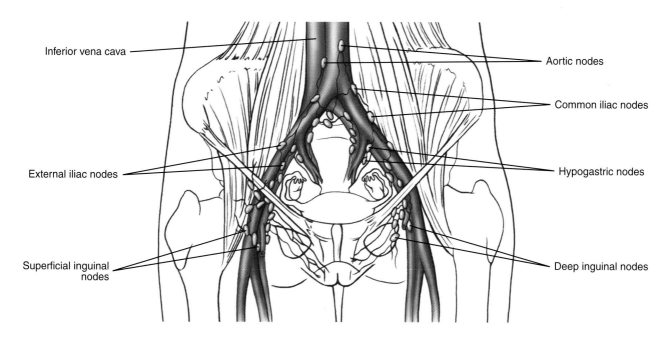

Inferior vena cava

Aortic nodes

Common iliac nodes

External iliac nodes

Hypogastric nodes

Superficial inguinal nodes

Deep inguinal nodes

The lymphatic vessels of the ovary follow the ovarian vessels along the inferior vena cava and aorta to the level of the renal vessels. To perform an adequate lymphadenectomy for ovarian carcinoma, the resection should extend to the level of the renal vessels. Ovarian lymphatic vessels also drain through the iliac vessels, and sometimes through the femoral vessels to the inguinal lymph nodes. Corpus and cervical lymphatic vessels drain along the obturator vessels, the hypogastric, common iliac, and external iliac arteries, and the aorta vena cava. The fundus can also drain along the round ligament to the inguinal region. Posteriorly the cervix and corpus can also drain along the lateral sacral lymph nodes. Vaginal lymphatic vessels divide into two systems that drain the upper two thirds and lower third. The upper two thirds drain as described for the cervix; the inferior third drains to the inguinal femoral lymph nodes in a fashion similar to the vulvar region, which includes drainage of the superficial inguinal lymph nodes, femoral vessels, and deep pelvic lymph nodes.

The lymphatic vessels of the vulva course along the vulva and terminate into the inguinal lymph nodes. Superficial inguinal lymph nodes are located above the cribriform fascia and below Camper's fascia. Femoral vessels are below the cribriform fascia. The lymph node under the inguinal ligament at the entrance of the femoral canal is called the sentinal node, or Cloquet's or Rosenmüller's lymph node. Below that area the lymph nodes follow the femoral vessels to the pelvis.

Nerve Supply

The ovary and fallopian tube receive their innervation from a plexus of nerves that course along the ovarian vessels. Sympathetic innervation is from the tenth thoracic segment and parasympathetic from the branches of the vagus nerve.

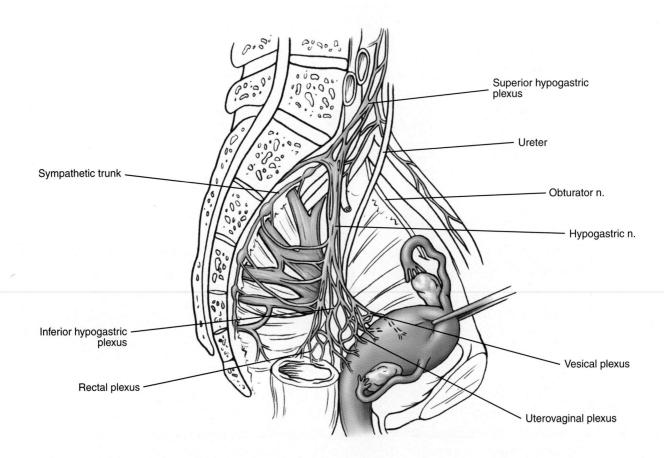

The celiac plexus extends to the level of the superior mesentery artery and courses along the anterior surface of the aorta. These sympathetic fibers are derived from the 12 thoracic and upper lumbar segments. They then form the presacral nerve (hypogastric plexus) at the bifurcation of the aorta. The nerve then divides into the left and right inferior hypogastric plexus (pelvic plexus). The hypogastric nerves then merge with the parasympathetic fibers from S2, S3, and S4. This nerve bundle divides into the vesico plexus in three portions: the vesico plexus, the uterovaginal plexus (Frankenhauser's ganglion), and the middle rectal plexus. The uterovaginal plexus with its nerve supply from T10 to L1, S2, S3, and S4 lies medial to the vessels and extends to the cervix and vagina. The obturator nerve is derived from the anterior division of L2, L3, and L4 and into the pelvis through the psoas muscle along the pelvic sidewall and obturator space. This is the only motor nerve that passes through the pelvis without innervating any of the pelvic organs. If injured during a radical hysterectomy with pelvic lymph node resection or tumor debulking, the patient will have difficulty adducting the thigh muscles. The adductor muscles affected include the adductor magnus, longus, and brevis, the gracilis, and the obturator externus muscles. This can be repaired by suturing the nerve endings with a 4-0 Vicryl suture. Physical therapy is frequently required after repairing the obturator nerve.

The nerve supply to the vulva is via the internal pudendal nerve, which originates from the second, third, and fourth sacral nerves. The perineal nerve divides into three branches: inferior hemorrhoidal nerve, which supplies the anal sphincter and perineal skin; dorsal nerve to the clitoris; and perineal nerve to the labia, perineal muscle, ischiocavernous and bulbocavernosus muscles, and urethral sphincter.

The genitofemoral nerve receives fibers from L1 and L2 and lies on the psoas muscle. Injury to the genitofemoral nerve will result in anesthesia in the medial thigh and lateral labia. Injury to the femoral cutaneous nerve, which receives its nerve supply from L2 and L3, can result in anesthesia over the anterior thigh. Injury to these nerves can occur during tumor resection or pelvic lymphadenectomy. They are frequently injured by retractors in the pelvis or the surgeon's lack of knowledge of the innervation of the pelvis. Femoral cutaneous nerve injury can also occur from overflexion of the hips in the lithotomy position.

TYPES OF MALIGNANCIES
Cervical Carcinoma

In the United States more than 15,000 new cases of cervical carcinoma will be diagnosed, resulting in approximately 4600 deaths. Although the mean age for cervical carcinoma is in the sixth decade, there is a bimodal distribution that peaks in the fourth and seventh decades.

Cervical cancer is clinically staged with the International Federation of Gynecology and Obstetrics (FIGO) Staging System. Staging after diagnosing cervical cancer is with a thorough physical examination, including a bimanual rectovaginal examination to evaluate the parametria, palpate inguinal and scalene lymph nodes, and examine the vagina for contiguous spread. Permissible radiologic evaluations include intravenous pyelography, barium contrast studies, and chest and skeletal x-ray studies. Cervical biopsy, cystoscopy, and sigmoidoscopy are also permitted. Studies such as computed tomography (CT), ultrasonography, magnetic resonance imaging (MRI), radionuclide scanning, and diagnostic laparoscopy are not used in determining the initial stage.

Table 16-1 *Staging of Carcinoma of the Cervix (FIGO 1995)*

TNM Classification: Primary Tumor (T)	FIGO Classification	Definition
TX	—	Primary tumor cannot be assessed.
T0	—	No evidence of primary tumor.
Tis	0	Carcinoma in situ, intraepithelial carcinoma.
T1	I	Cervical carcinoma confined to cervix (extension to the corpus should be disregarded).
T1a	IA	Invasive carcinoma, diagnosed microscopically only. All gross lesions even with superficial invasion are stage IB cancers. Invasion is limited to measured stromal invasion with maximum depth of 5 mm and maximum width of 7 mm.*
T1a1	IA1	Minimal microscopically evident stromal invasion. Measured stromal invasion with maximum depth of 3 mm and maximum width of 7 mm.
T1a2	IA2	Measured stromal invasion with depth from 3 to 5 mm and maximum width of 7 mm.
T1b	IB	Clinical lesions confined to the cervix or preclinical lesions greater than stage IA.
	IB1	Clinical lesions no greater than 4 cm in size.
	IB2	Clinical lesions greater than 4 cm in size.
T2	II	Cervical carcinoma invades beyond the uterus but not to the pelvic wall or to the lower third of the vagina.
T2a	IIA	No obvious parametrial invasion.
T2b	IIB	Obvious parametrial invasion.
T3	III	Extends to the pelvic wall or involves lower third of the vagina or causes hydronephrosis or nonfunctioning kidney.
T3a	IIIA	Tumor involves the lower third of the vagina. No extension to the pelvic wall.
T3b	IIIB	Tumor extends to the pelvic wall or causes hydronephrosis or nonfunctioning kidney.
T4	IV	Carcinoma extends beyond the true pelvis or has clinically involved the mucosa of the bladder or rectum. A bullous edema as such does not permit a case to be allotted to stage IV.
T4a	IVA	Spread of the growth to adjacent organs.
T4b	IVB	Spread to distant organs.

*The depth of invasion should not be more than 5 mm taken from the base of the epithelium, either surface or glandular, from which it originates. Vascular space involvement, either venous or lymphatic, should not alter the staging.

Cervical carcinoma spreads by direct extension into the cervical stroma, vagina cor, and corpus. Lymphatic metastasis, hematogenous metastasis, and rarely coelomic spread may occur. Early invasive cancer of the cervix can be treated with primary surgery. Stage IA with early stroma invasion of less than 1 mm should be treated with cervical conization; if no additional invasion is noted and the patient does not desire fertility, a simple extrafascial hysterectomy is indicated. Stage IA, with 1 to 3 mm of invasion and no lymph vascular invasion, should be treated with conization to rule out further invasion. As with lesions less than 1 mm, an extrafascial hysterectomy is performed when fertility is not an issue. If lymph vascular involvement is present, an extended or radical hysterectomy with pelvic lymph node dissection is required. For stage IA lesions with 3 to 5 mm of invasion, a radical hysterectomy with pelvic lymphadenectomy or primary radiation is recommended. Stage IB carcinoma of the cervix that includes lesions with more than 5 mm of invasion and 7 mm width are surgically resected with a type 3 radical hysterectomy with pelvic lymphadenectomy. Early stage IIA carcinoma of the cervix involving the vaginal fornix is surgically approached in a similar fashion. Large IB barrel lesions may be managed with (1) type 3 radical hysterectomy; (2) preoperative pelvic radiation of lesions more than 4 cm, followed by extrafascial hysterectomy; or (3) primary pelvic radiation. More advanced cervical carcinomas are treated with a combination of brachytherapy and teletherapy. In an attempt to identify those candidates who may benefit from periaortic irradiation, extraperitoneal periaortic lymphadenectomy is performed, with a paramedian incision. If pelvic lymph nodes are palpated, the incision is extended inferiorly to permit resection of enlarged lymph nodes. It is difficult to sterilize markedly enlarged lymph nodes with radiation, and therefore debulking these lymph nodes assists in local control.

Large IB lesions, more than 4 to 5 cm in diameter, also known as IB barrel lesions, can be treated with radical hysterectomy and pelvic lymph node dissection, definitive radiation therapy, or adjuvant radiation therapy followed by a simple extrafascial abdominal hysterectomy. Advanced stage IIA, IIB, IIIA, IIIB, and IV disease should all be treated with definitive radiation therapy. In patients with advanced stage IV disease, adjuvant chemotherapy is frequently used. Chemotherapy in addition to treating metastasis has also been used for large bulky lesions as a radiation sensitizer. Drugs such as hydroxyurea, cisplatin, 5-fluorouracil (5-FU), and paclitaxel (Taxol) have been used with some success.

Central cervical recurrence in patients who have not undergone radiation therapy can be treated successfully with radiation or pelvic exenteration. The latter treatment is usually reserved for patients who have already received definitive radiation therapy. Approximately 25% 5-year survival has been noted in patients treated with radiation for postsurgical recurrence of disease. However, patients who have undergone radiation therapy but have central recurrent cervical carcinoma are candidates for anterior, posterior, or total exenteration. Anterior exenteration includes removal of the upper vagina, anterior of the vagina, bladder, and urethra and construction of a ureteral conduit. Posterior exenteration includes excision of the posterior vaginal wall and the rectum, with colostomy or reanastomosis. It is imperative that attempts be made to perform a diverting loop colostomy to ensure complete healing and closure of the anastomotic site that has been previously irradiated. These patients are at high risk for fistula formation. Five-year survival of 25% to 40% has been quoted with posterior exenteration.

Chemotherapy has not proved efficacious in the treatment of recurrent cervical carcinoma. Active drugs include platinum-containing regimens, with a response rate of 38% to 42%. Paclitaxel, ifosfamide, and topotecan also appear promising as single agents.

Neoadjuvant chemotherapy (i.e., chemotherapy prior to definitive surgery and radiation therapy) has been used in Asia and Europe for the treatment of advanced cervical carcinomas to assist in decreasing tumor bulk and permit a conservative surgical resection.

Uterine Carcinoma

Endometrial carcinoma is a surgically staged cancer, as set forth by FIGO. It is estimated that more than 31,000 cases and 6000 deaths will occur from endometrial carcinoma in the United States. Primary surgical excision remains the most effective treatment. Adjuvant and neoadjuvant radiation therapy also has a role in advanced stages. Endometrial cancer spreads by direct extension, lymphatic dissemination, hematogenous spread, and transtubal migration of tumor cells. Papillary serous lesions spread transcoelomically, like ovarian carcinoma. Lymphatic spread is via the fundus and infundibular pelvic ligament to the periaortic lymph nodes, as well as the hypogastric external iliac and common iliac vessels. Although rare, spread via round ligament to the inguinal region can also occur. Extrafascial hysterectomy (type 1) with pelvic and periaortic lymph node sampling is the recommended surgical procedure for all but grade 1 and 2 carcinomas of the endometrium with no or minimal endometrial-myometrial invasion. Early stages requiring surgical staging include grade 3 lesions, grade 2 lesions greater than 2 cm, and myometrial invasion of more than 50%, cervical extension and aggressive histologic types, such as clear cell carcinoma and papillary serous carcinoma of the endometrium. Patients are at increased risk for nodal and peritoneal metastasis. Known stage II carcinoma of the endometrium can be treated with one of two approaches: (1) type 2 radical hysterectomy, bilateral salpingo-oophorectomy, bilateral pelvic lymphadenectomy, and periaortic lymphadenectomy; and (2) a combination of

FIGO Staging for Carcinoma of the Corpus Uteri

Stage IA G123	Tumor limited to endometrium
Stage IB G123	Invasion to less than one-half the myometrium
Stage IC G123	Invasion to more than one-half the myometrium
Stage IIA G123	Endocervical glandular involvement only
Stage IIB G123	Cervical stromal invasion
Stage IIIA G123	Tumor invades serosa and/or adnexa, and/or positive peritoneal cytology
Stage IIIB G123	Vaginal metastases
Stage IIIC G123	Metastases to pelvic and/or paraaortic lymph nodes
Stage IVA G123	Tumor invasion of bladder and/or bowel mucosa
Stage IVB	Distant metastases including intra-abdominal and/or inguinal lymph nodes

Histopathology—Degree of Differentiation

Cases of carcinoma of the corpus should be classified (or graded) according to the degree of histologic differentiation, as follows:

G1 = 5% or less of a nonsquamous or nonmorular solid growth pattern.

G2 = 6% to 50% of a nonsquamous or nonmorular solid growth pattern.

G3 = more than 50% of a nonsquamous or nonmorular solid growth pattern.

Notes on Pathologic Grading

1. Notable nuclear atypia, inappropriate for the architectural grade, raises the grade of a grade 1 or grade 2 tumor by 1.
2. In serous adenocarcinomas, clear cell adenocarcinomas, and squamous cell carcinomas, nuclear grading takes precedence.
3. Adenocarcinomas with squamous differentiation are graded according to the nuclear grade of the glandular component.

Rules Related to Staging

1. Because corpus cancer is now staged surgically, procedures previously used for determination of stages are no longer applicable, such as the findings from fractional D&C to differentiate between stage I and stage II.
2. It is appreciated that there may be a small number of patients with corpus cancer who will be treated primarily with radiation therapy. If that is the case, the clinical staging adopted by FIGO in 1971 would still apply, but designation of that staging system would be noted.
3. Ideally, width of the myometrium should be measured along with the width of tumor invasion.

From International Federation of Gynecology and Obstetrics. Annual report on the results of treatment in gynecological cancer. Int J Gynecol Obstet 28:189-190, 1989.

preoperative external beam radiation therapy and intracavitary radiation therapy followed by simple extrafascial hysterectomy (type 1), bilateral salpingo-oophorectomy, periaortic lymph node dissection, and postoperative pelvic irradiation, or alternatively, type 1 hysterectomy followed by pelvic teletherapy. Many surgeons forego pelvic lymph node sampling because patients with stage II carcinoma will require pelvic irradiation (collaborative research groups require pelvic node sampling before administering protocol). Patients with stage III and IV carcinoma of the endometrium should undergo surgery to remove all enlarged lymph nodes and maximally debulk the tumor. Depending on the tumor volume, this is followed by adjuvant radiation and chemotherapy or hormone therapy.

Uterine Sarcomas

Uterine sarcomas are not officially staged with the FIGO system for corpus lesions. They are classified as either pure, being of only one mesodermal element;

Classification of Uterine Sarcomas

I. Pure sarcomas
  A. Pure homologous
    1. Angiosarcoma
    2. Fibrosarcoma
    3. Leiomyosarcoma
    4. Stromal sarcoma
  B. Pure heterologous
    1. Chondrosarcoma
    2. Liposarcoma
    3. Osteogenic sarcoma
    4. Rhabdomyosarcoma
II. Mixed sarcomas
  A. Mixed homologous
  B. Mixed heterologous
  C. Mixed homologous and heterologous
III. Malignant mixed müllerian tumors
  A. Malignant mixed müllerian tumor, homologous type; carcinoma plus one or more of the homologous sarcomas listed in IA
  B. Malignant mixed müllerian tumor, heterologous type; carcinoma plus one or more of the heterologous sarcomas listed in IB; homologous sarcoma(s) may also be present
IV. Sarcoma, unclassified
V. Malignant lymphoma

or mixed, with malignant mesodermal and malignant epithelial components (i.e., carcinosarcoma). Mixed mesodermal tumors have both an epithelial and stromal component and can be homologous or heterologous. Homologous types have a native stromal component such as muscle; heterologous types are consistent with rhabdomyosarcoma, chondrosarcoma, liposarcoma, or neuroendocrine differentiation. Heterologous tumors are much more aggressive. Müllerian adenosarcomas consist of a benign epithelial element, usually a fibrosarcoma or endometrial sarcoma, and rarely heterologous elements.

Endometrial stromal sarcomas are tumor cells resembling that of the stroma surrounding proliferative endometrium. Low-grade lesions have fewer than 10 mitoses per 10 high-power field; high-grade lesions have more than 10 mitoses per 10 high-power field. High-grade lesions frequently are found in postmenopausal patients and are usually estrogen and progesterone receptor negative.

Leiomyosarcomas are uterine smooth muscle tumors. Tumors are evaluated histologically from mitoses per 10 high-power field. Fewer than 5 mitoses per 10 high-power field indicates a benign lesion; 5 to 9 mitoses per 10 high-power field, an intermediate lesion; and more than 10 mitoses per 10 high-power field, aggressive lesions that frequently recur.

Although there is no official staging, the FIGO system for corpus carcinoma is frequently used. Metastasis occurs by direct extension and lymphatic and hematogenous spread. Surgical treatment of uterine sarcomas is type 1 extrafascial hysterectomy and bilateral salpingo–oophorectomy. In young patients with leiomyosarcomas, ovarian preservation is at times maintained. Additional surgical staging such as lymphadenectomy and omentectomy has not proved efficacious in increasing survival. Studies of adjuvant radiation chemotherapy have demonstrated mixed results in patients with sarcomas.

Epithelial Ovarian Carcinomas

In the United States, approximately 24,000 new epithelial carcinomas, with 14,000 deaths, are expected to occur in 1999. Ovarian carcinoma, as endometrial carcinoma, is surgically staged in accordance with the criteria of the FIGO system. Surgical staging includes removal of all peritoneal fluid from the cul-de-sac, which is then submitted for cytologic evaluation. If no fluid is present, peritoneal washings obtained with normal saline solution are collected for cytologic evaluation. The anterior and posterior cul-de-sac, pericolic gutters, epigastrium, and hemidiaphragms should be sampled. The latter specimens are sent separately. After the abdominal washings are obtained, the abdomen should be thoroughly evaluated for transcoelomic spread of ovarian carcinoma. The diaphragms as well as the liver, spleen, and viscera are palpated. The small intestines should be exteriorized, and the entire length as well as the large intestine should be examined. Areas suspicious for carcinoma should be excised and sent to the pathology laboratory for histologic evaluation. If no gross tumor is

FIGO Staging for Carcinoma of the Ovary

Staging of ovarian carcinoma is based on findings at clinical examination and by surgical exploration. The histologic findings are to be considered in the staging, as are the cytologic findings as far as effusions are concerned. It is desirable that a biopsy be taken from suspicious areas outside of the pelvis.

Stage I — Growth limited to the ovaries.

Stage IA — Growth limited to one ovary; no ascites present containing malignant cells. No tumor on the external surface; capsule intact.

Stage IB — Growth limited to both ovaries; no ascites present containing malignant cells. No tumor on the external surfaces; capsules intact.

Stage IC* — Tumor classified as either stage IA or IB but with tumor on the surface of one or both ovaries; or with ruptured capsule(s); or with ascites containing malignant cells present or with positive peritoneal washings.

Stage II — Growth involving one or both ovaries, with pelvic extension.

Stage IIA — Extension and/or metastases to the uterus and/or tubes.

Stage IIB — Extension to other pelvic tissues.

Stage IIC† — Tumor either stage IIA or IIB but with tumor on the surface of one or both ovaries; or with capsule(s) ruptured; or with ascites containing malignant cells present or with positive peritoneal washings.

Stage III — Tumor involving one or both ovaries with peritoneal implants outside the pelvis and/or positive retroperitoneal or inguinal nodes. Superficial liver metastasis equals stage III. Tumor is limited to the true pelvis but with histologically proven malignant extension to small bowel or omentum.

Stage IIIA — Tumor grossly limited to the true pelvis with negative nodes but with histologically confirmed microscopic seeding of abdominal peritoneal surfaces.

Stage IIIB — Tumor of one or both ovaries with histologically confirmed implants of abdominal peritoneal surfaces, none exceeding 2 cm in diameter; nodes are negative.

Stage IIIC — Abdominal implants greater than 2 cm in diameter and/or positive retroperitoneal or inguinal nodes.

Stage IV — Growth involving one or both ovaries, with distant metastases. If pleural effusion is present, there must be positive cytologic findings to allot a case to stage IV. Parenchymal liver metastasis equals stage IV.

From International Federation of Gynecology and Obstetrics. Annual report on the results of treatment in gynecological cancer. Int J Gynecol Obstet 28:189-190, 1989.
*To evaluate the impact on prognosis of the different criteria for allotting cases to stage IC or IIC, it would be of value to know whether the rupture of the capsule was spontaneous or caused by the surgeon and if the source of malignant cells detected was peritoneal washings or ascites.

present in the omentum, an infracolic omentectomy is performed. The greater omentum adherent to the transverse colon is excised. Retroperitoneal spaces are evaluated for nodal enlargement, pelvic lymph nodes are sampled, and peri-aortic lymphadenectomy to the level of the renal veins is performed. Random peritoneal biopsy specimens are taken for staging ovarian lesions that are macroscopically confined to the ovaries. Ovarian tumors with metastasis are surgically debulked. Optimal cytoreduction (debulking) has been attained when each piece of tissue is less than 2 cm in diameter. Survival, however, continues to improve if cytoreduction is to tumor volume less than 5 mm.

Early stage IA, grade 1 tumors in women who desire to preserve fertility can be treated with unilateral oophorectomy. The uterus and contralateral ovary are preserved to permit future childbearing. It is controversial whether stage IA, grade 1 lesions require complete staging, which would increase the risk for adhesions. Stage IA and IB, grade 2 and 3, and stage IC carcinomas are treated with total abdominal hysterectomy, bilateral salpingo-oophorectomy, and surgical staging. Stage IA, grade 1 tumors do not require chemotherapy. The remaining stage I carcinomas are treated with four to six courses of chemotherapy.

Stages II, III, and IV tumors are managed similarly, with the ultimate goal to remove all macroscopic disease. Cytoreduction markedly increases response to adjuvant chemotherapy and improves survival. Intestinal resection and splenectomy are indicated if a bowel obstruction or pending obstruction is present or resection will permit optimal debulking of tumor to less than 2 cm. With the recent advent of the ultrasonic surgical aspirator, the need for a diaphragm resection has become infrequent. The ultrasonic surgical aspirator has also permitted surgeons to electively remove tumor from the abdominal viscera and hence decrease the need for resection. All stage II, III, and IV carcinomas are treated with six courses of chemotherapy. The combination of agents most active is cisplatin plus paclitaxel.

Second-Look Laparotomy

All disease greater than stage IA, grade 1 requires adjuvant chemotherapy. Second-look laparotomy is advocated for advanced ovarian carcinoma in patients who undergo adjuvant chemotherapy and have no evidence of disease on completion of the initial therapy. CT or MRI of the abdomen and pelvis is performed to rule out the presence of persistent disease. CA-125 if elevated at diagnosis can provide a measure of response. Markedly elevated levels at the completion of therapy or increased levels during initial chemotherapy are indicative of persistent disease or poor response. Second-look laparotomy entails performing a laparotomy and evaluating all coelomic peritoneal surfaces for gross disease. If any gross tumor is present, attempts are made to resect the remaining tumor, and adjuvant chemotherapy is continued. If no tumor is identified macroscopically, peritoneal biopsy specimens are obtained from all surfaces, including the anterior and posterior cul-de-sacs, lateral pelvic sidewalls, pericolic gutters, anterior abdominal wall, and abdominal pelvis and hemidiaphragms, and the infragastric omentum is excised. Representative samplings of the peritoneal and bowel adhesions are sent to the pathology laboratory for histologic evaluation. If no disease is present, pelvic and periaortic lymph node sampling is performed. Any enlarged nodes are excised and sent for histologic evaluation. Ovarian carcinoma will recur by 5 years in 40% to 50% of patients in whom second-look laparotomy yielded normal findings. A national collaborative group study (Gynecologic Oncology Group) is randomizing patients to observation vs. *p32* therapy. It is hoped that *p32* will destroy microscopic disease not identified at second-look laparotomy. In patients with positive findings or recurrent disease, topotecan, etoposide, or hexamethamelamine, in descending order, are administered as single agents.

Second-look laparoscopy has become increasingly common. It is strongly recommended that open laparoscopy be performed because of the nature of ovarian carcinoma. If laparoscopic findings are positive, all attempts are made to remove the remaining disease via laparoscopy or laparotomy. If there is no evidence of disease at laparoscopy, laparotomy is recommended for thorough evaluation of the peritoneal cavity, including palpation of the peritoneal surfaces, to assist in identifying persistent disease.

Vulvar Carcinoma

Vulvar carcinoma is uncommon, accounting for less than 5% of all gynecologic malignancies.

The use of radical procedures to treat vulvar carcinoma has decreased markedly during the past decade. Attempts are made to perform radical hemivulvectomies and unilateral inguinal femoral lymph node dissections through separate incisions, rather than en bloc resection of the vulva and lymph nodes. Of importance is the depth of invasion as well as width of the lesion. Lesions of less than 1 mm of invasion and 2 cm in width can be treated conservatively with wide local radical excision and no inguinal lymph node dissection. With less than 1 mm of invasion, risk of inguinal lymph node metastasis is essentially zero. T1 lesions of less than 2 cm with invasion of more than 1 mm should be treated with radical vulvectomy. If the tumor is a lateralizing lesion, hemivulvectomy is appropriate, preferably with 2 cm tumor margins. Attempts should be made to spare the clitoris, urethra, and anal sphincter. Ipsilateral inguinal femoral lymph dissection should be performed, and if suspect nodes are positive for metastasis at frozen-section analysis, contralateral lymph node dissection is required. The Gynecologic Oncology Group has shown that pelvic lymphadenectomy in patients with positive inguinal femoral lymph nodes was not superior to pelvic irradiation. T2 and early T3 lesions are surgically treated with a radical vulvectomy and bilateral inguinal femoral lymph node dissection. Two methods are available for performing this technique. The first, traditional method, initially described by Way, involves en bloc resection. The second, preferred method, involves three separate incisions: the radical vulvec-

FIGO Staging of Vulvar Carcinoma

Stage 0 TIS	Carcinoma in situ, intraepithelial carcinoma
Stage I T1 N0 M0	Tumor confined to the vulva and/or perineum—2 cm or less in greatest dimension, no nodal metastasis
Stage II T2 N0 M0	Tumor confined to the vulva and/or perineum—more than 2 cm in greatest dimension, no nodal metastasis
Stage III T3 N0 M0 T3 N1 M0 T1 N1 M0 T2 N1 M0	Tumor of any size with . . . (1) Adjacent spread to the lower urethra and/or the vagina or the anus, and/or . . . (2) Unilateral regional lymph node metastasis
Stage IVA T1 N2 M0 T2 N2 M0 T3 N2 M0 T4 any N M0	Tumor invades any of the following: upper urethra, bladder mucosa, rectal mucosa, pelvic bone, and/or bilateral regional node metastasis
Stage IVB Any T Any N M1	Any distant metastasis including pelvic lymph nodes

TNM Classification of Carcinoma of the Vulva (FIGO)

T		*Primary tumor*
	TIS	Preinvasive carcinoma (carcinoma in situ)
	T1	Tumor confined to the vulva and/or perineum—2 cm or less in greatest dimension
	T2	Tumor confined to the vulva and/or perineum—more than 2 cm in greatest dimension
	T3	Tumor of any size with adjacent spread to the urethra and/or vagina and/or to the anus
	T4	Tumor of any size infiltrating the bladder mucosa and/or the rectal mucosa, including the upper part of the urethral mucosa and/or fixed to the bone
N		*Regional lymph nodes*
	N0	No lymph node metastasis
	N1	Unilateral regional lymph node metastasis
	N2	Bilateral regional lymph node metastasis
M		*Distant metastasis*
	M0	No clinical metastasis
	M1	Distant metastasis (including pelvic lymph node metastasis)

Adapted from International Federation of Gynecology and Obstetrics. Annual report on the results of treatment in gynecological cancer. Int J Gynecol Obstet 28:189-190, 1989.

tomy with attempts to spare the urethra and anus and two additional groin incisions below the inguinal ligament for inguinal lymph node dissection. Separate groin incisions should not be used in patients with large midline or clitoral lesions. In patients with T4 lesions and lesions that appear to be invading the rectum or proximal urethra, a combination of chemotherapy and teletherapy is used to shrink the tumor and permit more conservative surgical resection of the tumor.

SURGICAL APPLICATIONS
Simple Extrafascial Total Abdominal Hysterectomy With or Without Bilateral Salpingo-oophorectomy

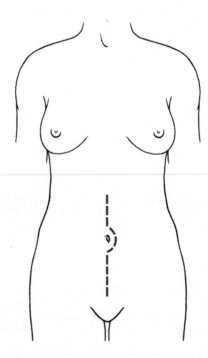

Exploratory laparotomy is performed through a midline or transverse incision. Kelly clamps are utilized to clamp the cornial areas of the uterus, which decreases the theoretical risk for transtubal migration of tumor cells in the presence of an endometrial lesion.

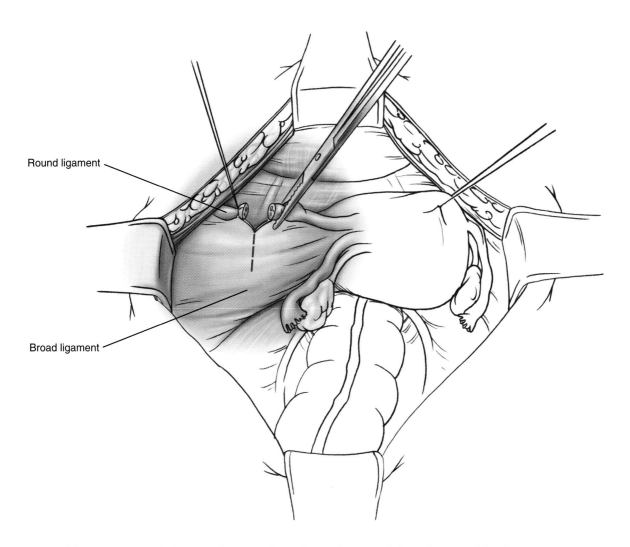

Two atraumatic Kelly clamps placed on the cornial region enable the surgeon to elevate the uterus and place traction on it. The round ligament is identified, grasped with a Kelly clamp, and ligated distally. The round ligament contains Sampson's artery, which can produce postoperative bleeding if the pedicle is not ligated with a Metzenbaum scissors or cautery. The posterior leaf of the broad ligament is then incised. Pelvic vessels, including the infundibular pelvic ligament, the common iliac, hypergastric, and external iliac vessels, and the ureter, are identified. The infundibular pelvic ligament is isolated in the medial leaf of the peritoneum and sharply incised throughout its entire length from the pelvic brim to the uterus. It is then double clamped and ligated with 0 Vicryl suture. If the ovaries are to be conserved, the utero-ovarian (suspensory) ligaments adjacent to the uterus are clamped and ligated. The ovaries are then suspended out of the pelvis to prevent adherence to the cuff and placed outside the potential radiation field.

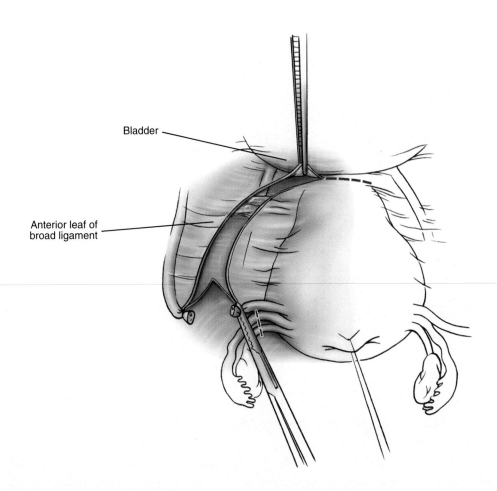

The anterior cul-de-sac bladder peritoneum is grasped with atraumatic forceps and sharply incised. The vesicovaginal space is then sharply incised, with tension placed medially to avoid the lateral vascular bladder pillars. If no extrauterine disease is present, sharp dissection of the peritoneal reflection of the posterior cul-de-sac is not required. If additional mobilization is required, the peritoneum is sharply incised and the rectovaginal plane sharply and bluntly dissected. The vesicovaginal and rectovaginal planes are avascular planes of the pelvis.

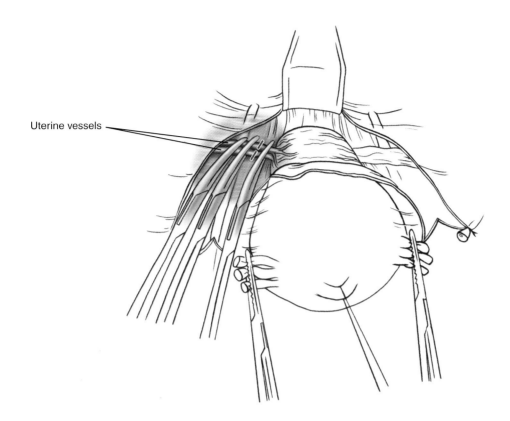

Uterine vessels

The uterus is now freely mobile. The uterine vessels can be seen adjacent to the cervix and uterus, with the ureter coursing under the uterine artery to its insertion in the bladder. Each artery is approximately 10 cm long, and the ureters are 30 cm long. The uterine vessels are then doubly clamped and ligated at the level of the internal os. A third clamp is used distally to prevent backbleeding from the uterine specimen. Uterosacral ligaments are easily identifiable and palpated at this time. The pubovesical cervical fascia is part of the endopelvic fascia, which surrounds and supports the cervix. This pubovesical fascia becomes contiguous with the cardinal and broad ligaments, extending to the lateral pelvic sidewall. In patients with malignancy this fascia is left intact during hysterectomy. Atraumatic hysterectomy clamps are used to clamp the cardinal ligaments to the level of the external os. Each pedicle is suture ligated at the level of the external os, and a curved clamp is placed that includes the vaginal apex and the uterosacral ligament. Transfixion stitches are used to assist in vault suspension by attachment of the vaginal cuff to the uterosacral ligament. Alternatively, the vagina can be entered and the specimen sharply excised. Ochsner clamps are used to secure the vaginal margins. Angle sutures are placed in a figure-of-eight fashion including the vaginal apex and uterosacral ligaments. The remainder of the vaginal cuff is closed with interrupted sutures. In the past, it was customary to suture the vaginal edges for hemostasis and leave the cuff open, but with the present availability of closed drainage systems and antibiotics this is no longer required.

Laparoscopic Hysterectomy

Laparoscopy initially was used to assist in performing a difficult vaginal hysterectomy, and also enabled vaginal removal of the adnexa. Surgeons have returned to using the supracervical hysterectomy via a laparoscopic approach. After ligation of the vessels and cardinal ligaments the uterus is morcellized. The morcellized fragments are then extracted through the trocar site. A supracervical hysterectomy is rarely indicated for gynecologic malignancies. A laparoscopy-assisted hysterectomy and bilateral salpingo-oophorectomy is an accepted substitute for abdominal or vaginal hysterectomy in the treatment of stage I and II carcinoma of the endometrium or stage IA carcinoma of the cervix.

Radical Hysterectomy

Piver et al. identified five classes of extended hysterectomy for cervical carcinoma. Type I hysterectomy is an extrafascial, simple hysterectomy. In type II, or modified radical hysterectomy, described by Wertheim, the medial 50% of the cardinal ligament and uterosacral ligaments are excised. Type III hysterectomy includes removal of most of the uterosacral and cardinal ligaments and the upper third of the vagina. Type IV, or extended radical hysterectomy, includes excision of the periurethral tissue, superior vesical artery, and up to 75% of the vagina. Type V, or partial exenteration, includes removal of the distal ureter and bladder. This technique is rarely used because stage IV carcinomas are most properly treated with definitive radiation therapy. Stage IA2 carcinoma of the cervix with invasion more than 3 mm below the basement membrane and/or lymph vascular involvement, stage IB carcinoma of the cervix, and early stage IA carcinoma of the cervix with extension to the upper third of the vagina are treated with type II or III radical hysterectomy.

The patient is placed in a modified dorsal supine lithotomy position, with the legs in Allen stirrups. The abdomen, perineum, and vagina are prepared to make sterile and draped, and a urethral Foley catheter is placed in the bladder. An abdominal wall incision is made, either a vertical midline, Maylard, or Cherney incision. Upon entering the peritoneal cavity the peritoneum is inspected for tumor infiltration. The upper abdomen, including the diaphragm, liver, spleen, periaortic and pelvic lymph nodes, is palpated to ensure that no areas suspicious for metastasis are present. The abdominal visceral contents are then packed out of the pelvis with a Balfour retractor or Buckwalter retractor. The fundus is grasped with a Lahey thyroid clamp to permit traction of the uterus and cardinal ligaments. Two philosophies exist regarding order of performing an extended abdominal hysterectomy (radical) and bilateral pelvic lymph node dissection. Some gynecologic oncologists prefer to perform a pelvic lymph node dissection with frozen-section evaluation prior to the extended hysterectomy. In the absence of suspect lymph nodes, I prefer to perform the hysterectomy, then pelvic lymph node dissection. If multiple lymph nodes are microscopically positive, adjuvant radiation therapy is required. With tension on the uterus, the round ligament is grasped distally and ligated with 0 Vicryl suture. The proximal limb is either clipped or suture ligated.

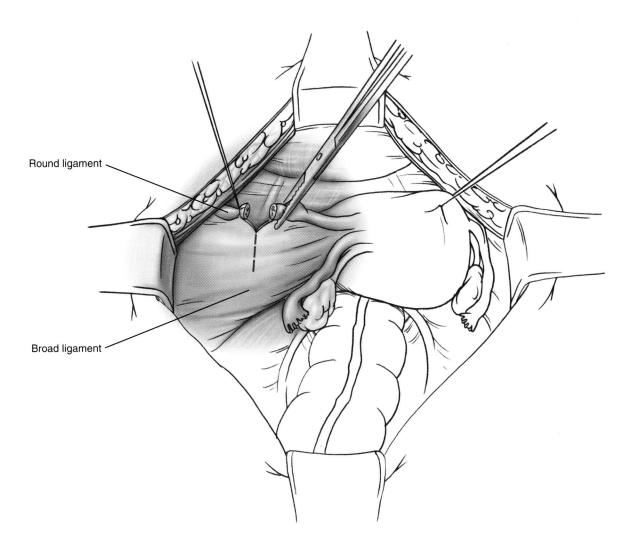

Round ligaments are then incised and the incision extended cephalad. This permits identification of the common iliac, external iliac, and hypogastric vessels and the ureter. If the patient is older than 40 years the ovaries are frequently not preserved and an oophorectomy is performed. After the infundibulopelvic ligament is identified medially, the peritoneum is sharply incised distally to the uterine vessels. This thoroughly isolates the adnexa and the infundibulopelvic ligament, which includes the uterine artery and veins. The infundibulopelvic ligament is then doubly clamped and ligated with 0 Vicryl suture. The proximal ligation may be a double 0 Vicryl tie or a single 0 Vicryl tie, followed by a 0 Vicryl suture tie distal to the free tie. The peritoneum overlying the bladder sharply is incised.

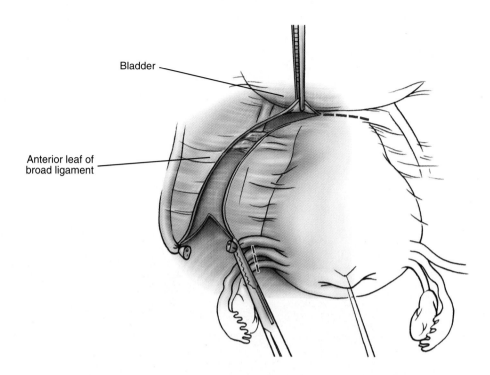

The anterior leaf of the broad ligament is lifted along the vesicouterine peritoneal fold, and the vesicovaginal space is dissected sharply, with the bladder mobilized anteriorly. This space is avascular. Attempts should be made to dissect in the midline and avoid perforating vessels present in the bladder pillars laterally.

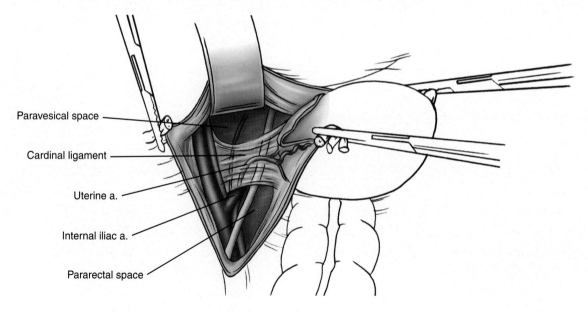

Two additional avascular spaces are then dissected free. The paravesical space is bordered medially by the obliterated artery, laterally by the obturator internus muscle, posteriorly by the cardinal ligament, and anteriorly by the pubic symphysis. The pararectal space is bordered medially by the rectum, laterally by the hypogastric artery, anteriorly by the cardinal ligament, and posteriorly by the sacrum.

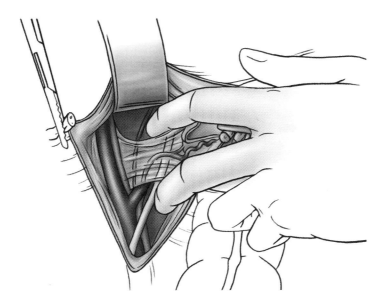

Placing the index finger and the middle finger in the perirectal space, the surgeon can palpate the lateral extent of the cardinal ligament or web. Nodularity or tumor is a contraindication to type II or III hysterectomy. Cardinal ligaments contain branches of the internal iliac vein and the sympathetic nerve fibers to the bladder superiorly and parasympathetic nerve fibers inferiorly. The pelvic lymph nodes are inspected again. If the dissection is performed prior to hysterectomy, the lymph node dissection is performed at this point.

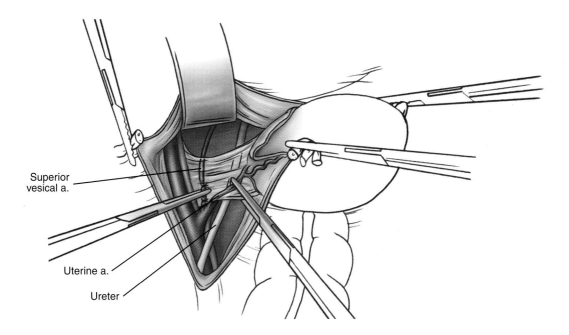

Superior
vesical a.

Uterine a.

Ureter

During an extended hysterectomy the uterine artery is identified at its origin on the anterior division of the hypogastric artery. Frequently the superior vesical artery requires dissection from the cardinal ligament to assist in isolating the uterine artery. The artery is then clamped and ligated bilaterally at its origin.

Clamping the distal pedicle of the uterine artery affords us the ability to have additional traction. The ureter is then sharply dissected from the medial peritoneum. Additional traction may be obtained with atraumatic forceps. The filmy adhesions about the ureter are sharply incised.

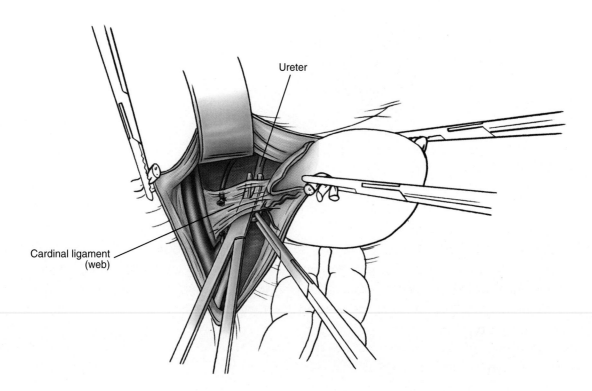

The cardinal ligament engulfs the uterine artery and ureter. A procedure called "untunneling" the ureter is then performed. With traction on the uterine artery, the ureter is sharply dissected free of the web to its insertion in the uterus. The ureter is freed with a combination of sharp and blunt dissection of the tunnel with a right-angle clamp. Reinhoff-type clamps are used to clamp the roof of the tunnel. This should be done in several steps, ligating each pedicle. The remainder of the roof at the tunnel is the anterior vesicouterine ligament, which is also incised.

The uterus is retracted caudad and medially. A fourth avascular plane of the pelvis, the rectovaginal space, is dissected.

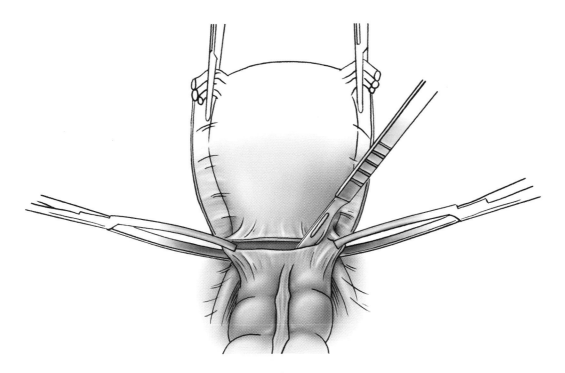

The peritoneal reflection of the rectum and uterus is grasped with two Allis clamps and retracted cephalad. The peritoneum is then sharply incised and the rectovaginal space dissected. Parametria, cardinal ligaments, uterosacral ligament, and vagina can now be freely palpated and the extent of tumor evaluated. In a type II hysterectomy the ureter is retracted laterally and 50% of the cardinal ligament is excised. Parametrial clamps such as Wertheim clamps are used in this procedure. It is recommended that a transfixion stitch be placed on the pedicles. This procedure is then repeated on the uterosacral ligament.

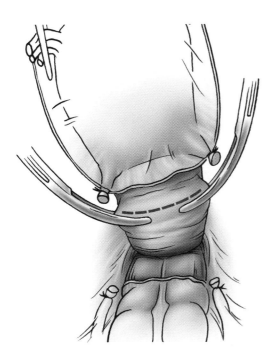

The procedure is completed bilaterally. The vaginal tube is isolated, and up to one third is excised in a type III hysterectomy. The majority of the cardinal ligament and uterosacral ligament is excised. Interrupted sutures are used to close the vaginal cuff. One complication of this surgery is febrile morbidity in 25% to 50% of patients. Blood loss is frequently less than 1 L. Retrovaginal or vesicovaginal fistula occurs in approximately 1% to 2% of patients. As with any laparotomy for invasive malignancy, pulmonary embolism and small bowel obstruction occur in 1% to 2% of patients. A late complication is bladder dysfunction secondary to incising the sympathetic and parasympathetic nerves coursing through the uterosacral and cardinal ligaments. Bladder sensitivity is markedly diminished, and as a result the patient is unable to initiate voiding. Management includes bladder drainage by one of three methods. In the first methods an indwelling suprapubic or transurethral catheter is placed intraoperatively and removed after the patient has demonstrated resolution of bladder dysfunction. The method I prefer is intermittent catheterization. If postvoiding residual urine is more than 150 ml, the patient is taught to perform intermittent catheterization and discharged with instructions to catheterize herself every 4 to 6 hours prior to resumption of micturition. On resumption of micturition, the patient collects postvoiding residual urine until the volume is less than 100 ml. In patients who have difficulty identifying the urethra, gentian violet or methylene blue is used to paint the urethral orifice to guide the patient in catheterization. Lymphocysts may develop and can be followed up expectantly or drained under ultrasound guidance.

Extended, or type II or III, radical hysterectomies have been attempted laparoscopically, but the procedure is controversial among gynecologic oncologists. Many believe dissection via laparoscopy is not extensive enough. The combination of laparoscopy and radical vaginal hysterectomy (Schauta type) did not gain popularity in the United States until laparoscopic pelvic lymphadenectomy was accepted. The initial dissection is performed laparoscopically, and the procedure is completed via a vaginal approach.

Pelvic Lymphadenectomy

Pelvic lymphadenectomy is performed prior to or after radical hysterectomy. Stage IA, IB, and IIA carcinomas of the cervix, and stage IIA and IIB carcinomas of the endometrium can be treated with radical (extended) hysterectomy and bilateral pelvic lymph node dissection with periaortic lymph node evaluation.

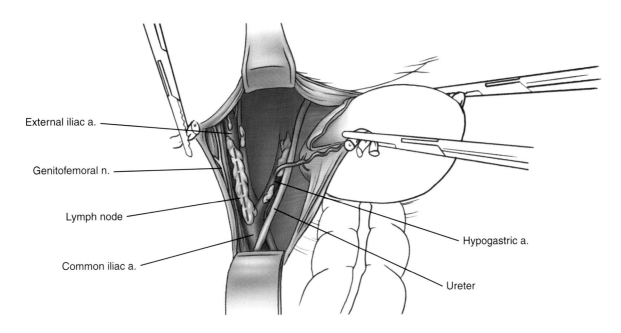

External iliac a.

Genitofemoral n.

Lymph node

Common iliac a.

Hypogastric a.

Ureter

The round ligament is ligated and incised. This permits the surgeon to incise the lateral leaf of the peritoneum toward and above the bifurcation of the common iliac artery. A Deaver retractor is used to expose the majority of the common iliac artery cephalad. A small Richardson retractor is used distally to assist in exposing the inferior epigastric vessels. On entering the retroperitoneal space, the ureter and the hypogastric, external iliac, and common iliac vessels are identified. At the bifurcation of the common iliac chain the external iliac node is divided into lateral and medial portions.

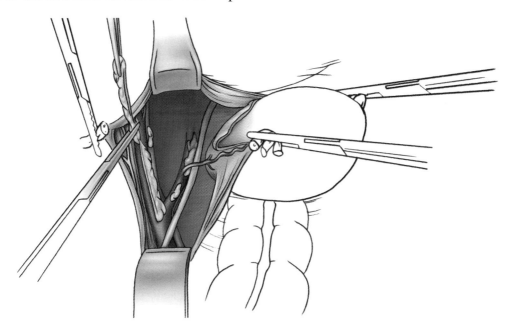

The lateral chain is stripped free from the artery, stripped along the artery to the circumflex iliac vein. Hemoclips may be placed along the length of the proximal and distal pedicles.

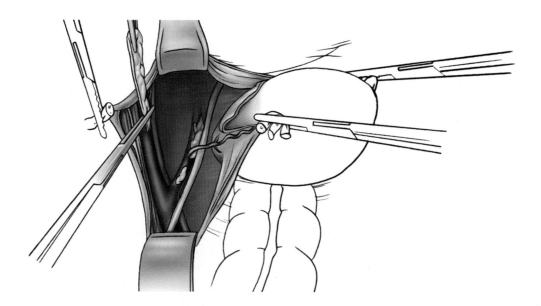

The medial chain is then dissected. It is important to note that the genitofemoral nerve courses along the psoas muscle and can be injured if care is not taken to spare this nerve. The hypogastric lymph nodes are also dissected, and clips are placed caudad and cephalad. Tension is then placed on the obturator space and obturator lymph nodes. Special attention must be taken to not injure the external iliac vein. The iliac vein is retracted laterally with a vein retractor.

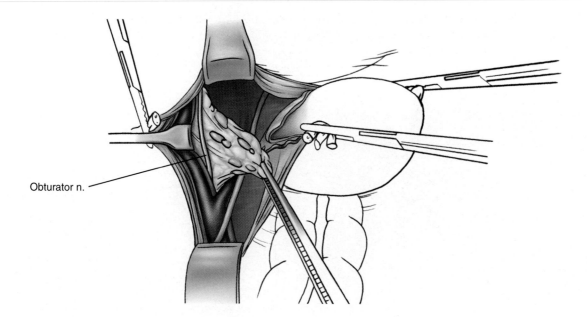

Obturator n.

The lymphatic tissue and fat in the obturator space are gently teased, and the obturator nerve is identified before excising or clipping any tissue. If the obturator nerve is incised, a plexus of vessels can be seen posterior to the obturator nerve. Careful dissection will assist in avoiding these vessels. Damage to the obturator nerve results in inability to adduct the thighs. The nerve should be repaired with 4-0 Vicryl interrupted sutures. Physical therapy is frequently required for complete rehabilitation. The obturator artery and vein are usually dorsal to the obturator nerve. In approximately 10% of patients, an aberrant vein arises from the external iliac vein.

Pelvic lymph node dissections can be performed laparoscopically without difficulty. The common iliac, external, and hypogastric lymph nodes are exposed after making an incision in the lateral leaf of the peritoneum. An obturator lymph node resection is performed similarly to a laparotomy. Prior to excising the nodes, it is imperative to identify the obturator nerve. Laparoscopic vein retractors are used to assist in reflecting the hypogastric vein laterally.

Periaortic Lymph Node Dissection

There are two approaches for periaortic lymph node dissection. In early stage cervical carcinoma large periaortic lymph nodes should be biopsied and sent for frozen-section analysis. If results are negative, the radical hysterectomy (extended hysterectomy) should proceed. It is controversial whether periaortic lymph node dissection should be performed in early cervical carcinoma if the pelvic lymph nodes test negative. Traditionally, early cervical carcinoma and endometrial carcinoma was treated with a limited periaortic lymph node dissection approximately 2.5 cm above the inferior mesenteric artery. Two approaches are taken. In one, an incision is made lateral to the ascending colon, the retroperitoneal space is entered, and the bowel is reflected medially.

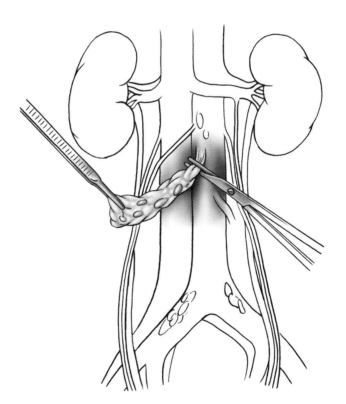

An alternative method, which I prefer in most patients, is to exteriorize the small bowel medially and enter the retroperitoneum by incising the medial peritoneal reflection over the mesenteric vessels, vena cava, and aorta. A Deaver retractor is used cephalad, the ureter is identified bilaterally, and a lymph node dissection is performed starting at the bifurcation of the aorta and extending approximately 2.5 cm above the inferior mesenteric artery for endometrial and cervical carcinoma and to the renal veins for ovarian carcinoma. Ligation clips are used during this procedure to decrease the possibility of losing a perforating vessel. Note that the left and right ovarian arteries have their origin on the aorta below the superior mesenteric artery and renal vessels. The right ovarian vein empties directly into the inferior vena cava, and the left ovarian vein enters into the left renal vein prior to emptying into the inferior vena cava. When performing a lymph node dissection, the pericaval and periaortic lymph nodes are removed. It is imperative that the lymph nodes on the right and left sides of the vena cava be excised and sent to the pathology laboratory for histologic evaluation. If the ureters are not identified bilaterally, the surgeon is at risk of ligating and incising the ureter. Occasionally during an extensive lymph node dissection, as a result of marked fibrosis or enlarged lymph nodes, the inferior mesenteric artery might not be identified and ligated. The inferior hemorrhoidal vessels and the superior mesenteric artery via the marginal artery of Drummond provide collateral circulation to the bowel that was dependent on the inferior mesenteric artery.

Laparoscopic periaortic lymphadenectomy can be performed with minimal difficulty to the level of the inferior mesenteric artery. Extensive dissection to the level of the renal vessels is difficult and should be attempted only by surgeons with significant laparoscopic experience. It is imperative that the laparoscopic surgeon be prepared to deal with the potential complications inherent in excising periaortic lymph nodes.

Supraclavicular Lymph Node Biopsy

In patients with cervical cancer with positive periaortic lymph nodes, 5% to 30% will have positive supraclavicular (scalene) lymph nodes. If a lymph node is palpable, needle aspiration can be performed, thereby averting the necessity for excisional biopsy. If no enlarged lymph nodes are palpated, a supraclavicular lymph node biopsy is performed. An incision is made transversely 1 to 2 cm above and parallel to the clavicle. After the subcutaneous tissue is incised, a scalene fat pad containing lymph nodes is identified and resected.

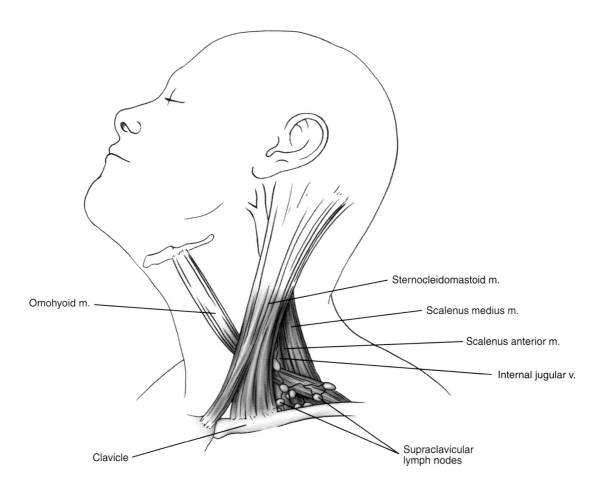

The anatomic landmarks include the clavicle inferiorly, the omohyoid muscle laterally and posteriorly, and the sternocleidomastoid muscle medially. The triangle consists of the scalenus anterior and medius muscles. Injury can occur if attention is not paid to the adjacent structures such as the internal jugular vein posterior to the scalenus medius muscle, which lies beyond the internal carotid artery, beyond the scalenus muscle. The phrenic nerve courses through the subclavicular triangle, frequently on the surface of the scalenus muscles. Damage to the phrenic nerve decreases diaphragm movement. In addition to these adjacent structures, injury to the thoracic duct or lung can occur. Complications include chylothorax or pneumothorax, respectively.

Omentectomy

In staging of ovarian cancer, omentectomy is required even if no gross tumor is present. In the presence of gross disease debulking may require infracolic and supracolic omentectomy. Omentectomy is also indicated in endometrial papillary serous carcinoma.

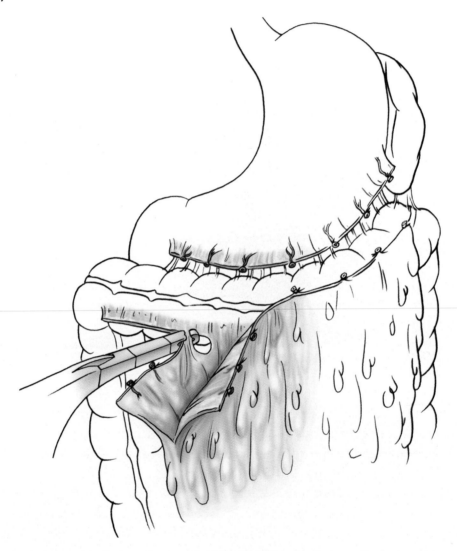

The omentectomy begins at the hepatic flexure of the colon. Initially the omentum is dissected free from the transverse colon with a cautery or Metzenbaum scissors. Vascular pedicles are ligated with free ties, ligation clips, or the CO_2 Power L.D.S. stapler (U.S. Surgical Corp., Norwalk, Conn.). The lesser sac is exposed during this procedure. If a supracolic omentectomy is required, the omental branches of the gastric artery are ligated as previously described. The dissection is carried out to the level of the splenic hilum, with the gastroepiploic artery left intact to supply blood to the greater curvature of the stomach. A nasogastric tube should be in place postoperatively.

Laparoscopic resection of the omentum can be performed with a combination of laparoscopic ligation clips through a 10 to 12 mm port and cautery.

Radical Vulvectomy With Inguinal Femoral Lymphadenectomy

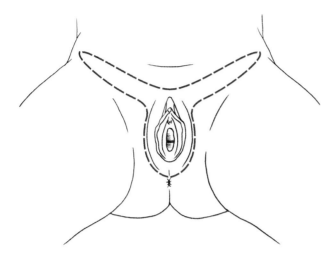

The patient is placed supine with the legs in candy cane or moveable stirrups. The abdomen and perineum are prepared and draped. A groin incision is made approximately 2 cm above the inguinal ligament and carried down to the aponeurosis of the external oblique muscles.

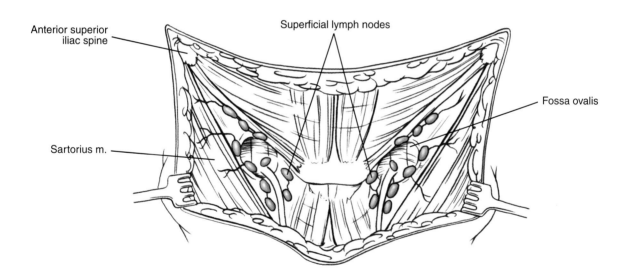

Anterior superior iliac spine

Superficial lymph nodes

Fossa ovalis

Sartorius m.

The skin flap is then mobilized, preserving Camper's fascia. It should be noted that the incision is carried from the anterosuperior iliac spine across the mons to the contralateral anterosuperior iliac spine. A combination of cautery and sharp dissection with the Metzenbaum scissors is utilized. The superficial lymph nodes are removed. Each inguinal ligament is then identified. Lymph nodes at the inguinal ring, that is, Cloquet's, Rosenmüller's, and sentinel lymph nodes, frequently are sent separately for histologic evaluation; if positive, deep lymph nodes are sampled in all cases. The saphenous vein can be identified at this time. The vein has been traditionally doubly clamped and incised, then ligated with 2-0 suture. Attempts are now made not to sacrifice this vessel. It is believed that by preserving the saphenous vein venostasis will be decreased, and hence leg edema postoperatively.

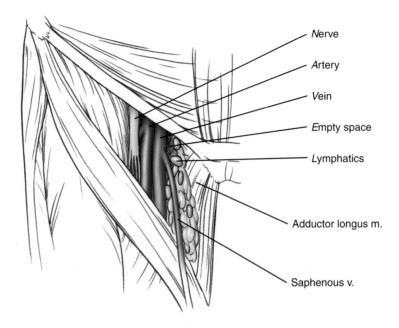

Nerve
Artery
Vein
Empty space
Lymphatics
Adductor longus m.
Saphenous v.

At this point the surgeon can identify all of the inguinal structures. The mnemonic navel (*n*erve, *a*rtery, *v*ein, *e*mpty space, *l*ymphatics) is used to assist in identification of the femoral and lymphatic vessels. Approximately 1 to 2 cm above the origin of the saphenous vein is the circumflex artery. The adductor longus muscle is identified below the saphenous vein. This muscle and the area around the saphenous vein are stripped of all lymphatic tissue. The fascia lata is split with approximal femoral vein. Femoral lymph nodes are situated medial to the femoral vein within the opening of the fascia ovalis.

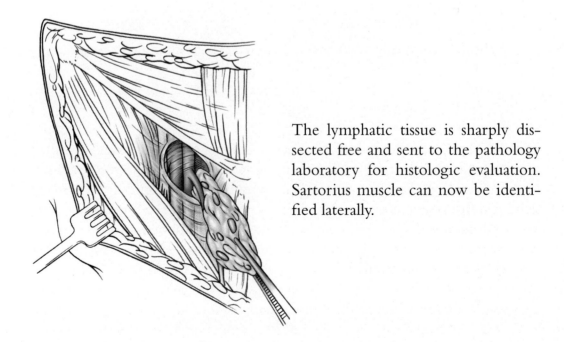

The lymphatic tissue is sharply dissected free and sent to the pathology laboratory for histologic evaluation. Sartorius muscle can now be identified laterally.

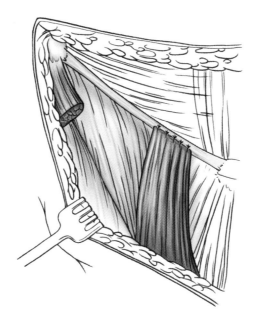

To protect the femoral vessel it is transected at its insertion with a cautery and transposed over the femoral artery and vein. If the fascia can be sutured closed there is no need to perform this maneuver. In 50% to 90% of en bloc resections primary closure results in wound breakdown. Sartorius muscle transposition will protect the vessels and nerve during granulation. It is controversial whether this is required when a transverse rectus abdominis musculocutaneous (TRAM) flap or gracilis flap is used to cover the vulvectomy and lymph node defects, because these myocutaneus flaps bring additional muscle into the field to protect the vessels. On completion of the lymph node dissection the vulvar and vaginal incisions are marked with a marking pen. Metzenbaum scissors and a cautery are used to dissect the specimen down to the urogenital diaphragm. The pudendal artery and vein are identified, clamped, and ligated. Superiorly at the clitoris careful attention must be placed so as not to clamp the proximal urethra. A catheter is placed into the bladder. The dorsal bundle and clitoral vessels are isolated and clamped with a Kocher clamp. The specimen is then incised and 0 absorbable suture placed. The specimen is dissected off the pubic periosteum and adducted fascia. Laterally the incision is made in the labiocrural fold or 2 cm from the lesion. This incision is dissected down to the fascia of the urogenital diaphragm. The ischiocavernosus muscles can then be transsected. Posteriorly it is imperative that the vulva and distal vagina be sharply dissected from the rectum. A medial margin of the vulvar specimen is then incised with a No. 10 blade and sent to the pathology laboratory for histologic evaluation. Although 2 cm margins are attempted, the specimen is sent for frozen-section evaluation of the lateral and medial margins of the tumor resection.

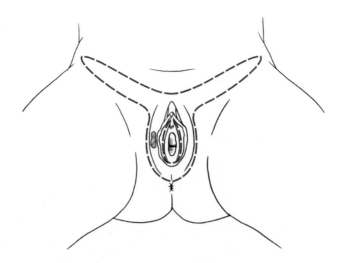

The pathologist should also be made aware that the en bloc vulvar specimen includes the superficial lymph nodes in the mons tissue. This en bloc resection is frequently called the rabbit or longhorn incision. Although one can mobilize the adjacent tissue and primarily close it, I have found the use of TRAM or gracilis flaps to be advantageous in decreasing wound separation and breakdown. The three incisions, however, can be closed primarily if vulvar resection is not extensive.

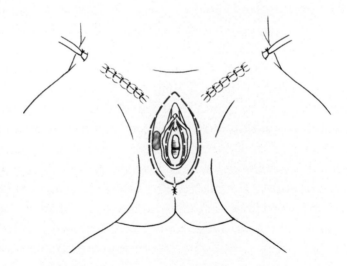

Two closed suction drains are placed in the groin and vulvar region. Both sides of the groins are incised and the mons left intact. The vulva or hemivulvectomy incisions are made separately.

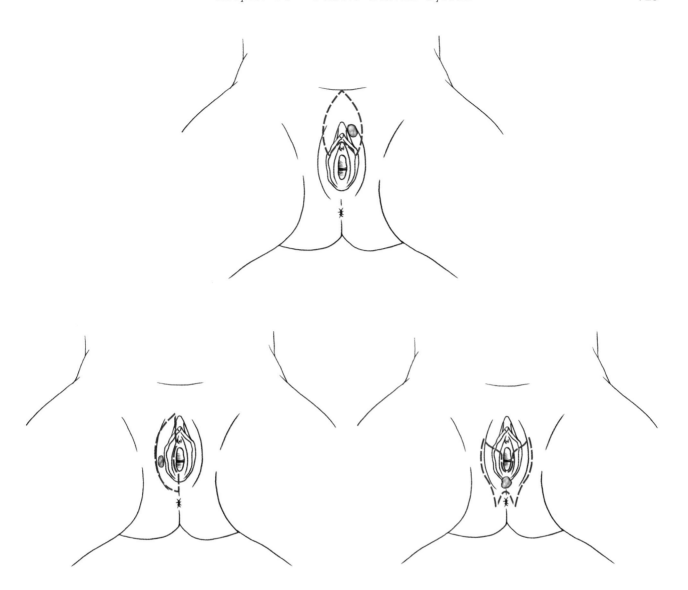

Hemivulvectomies are used in small isolated lesions. Radiation therapy has been used as neoadjuvant therapy in patients with advanced disease who would otherwise require pelvic exenteration. Radiation therapy is usually administered with chemotherapy, such as cisplatin, 5-FU, and myomycin-C. With the combination of chemotherapy and radiation the lesion can be shrunk to a size that permits conservative therapy rather than total pelvic exenteration. Adjuvant pelvic radiation therapy is used when two or more ipsilateral inguinal lymph nodes are positive for cancer. Additional indications may be tumors with margins less than 5 mm and women who are not medically able to undergo inguinal lymph node dissection. Lymph node metastasis is the most important prognostic feature in vulvar cancer, followed by tumor ploidy and size.

Anatomic Basis of Complications

MAJOR

- Major suture placement through bladder and vagina results in vesicovaginal fistula.
- Extensive devascularization and dissection of ureter results in ureterovaginal fistula.
- Ureteral ligation can occur if vessels and ureter are not identified during hysterectomy or lymph node dissection.
- Extensive inguinal femoral lymph node dissection can result in lymphadenectomy of the leg.

MINOR

- Bladder atony results from denervation during radical hysterectomy.
- Obturator injury during pelvic lymphadenectomy can result in difficulty adducting thighs, even after repair.
- Injury to the genitofemoral nerve results in anesthesia to the medial thigh and lateral labia.
- Injury to the femoral cutaneous nerve results in anesthesia over the anterior thigh.

KEY REFERENCES

DeLancey JOL. Surgical anatomy of the female pelvis. In Rock JA, Thompson JD, eds. TeLinde's Operative Gynecology, 8th ed. Philadelphia: Lippincott-Raven, 1997, pp 63-94.

This chapter provides an extensive review of pelvic anatomy. In addition to comprehensive coverage of the pelvic viscera, vessels, nerves, and lymphatic vessels, Dr. DeLancey introduces the surgeon to musculature of the pelvis.

Griffiths CT, Silverstone A, Tobias J, et al, eds. Gynecologic Oncology. London: Mosby-Wolfe, 1977.

This book reviews the treatment of gynecologic malignances. In addition, the etiology, epidemiology, pathologic presentation, and staging are discussed.

Hoffman MS, Cavanagh D. Malignancies of the vulva. In Rock JA, Thompson JD, eds. TeLinde's Operative Gynecology, 8th ed. Philadelphia: Lippincott-Raven, 1997, pp 1331–1384.
This chapter is a thorough analysis of the surgical treatment of vulvar malignancies and the data supporting it. This is a classic text in gynecologic surgery.

Thompson JD, Warshaw JS. Hysterectomy. In Rock JA, Thompson JD, eds. TeLinde's Operative Gynecology, 8th ed. Philadelphia: Lippincott-Raven, 1997, pp 771–854.
Most gynecologic surgeons read about the simple hysterectomy for the first time in this text. This chapter keeps the tradition alive with its discussion and illustrations of abdominal and vaginal hysterectomies.

Wheeless CR Jr. Atlas of Pelvic Surgery, 2nd ed. Philadelphia: Lea & Febiger, 1988.
This surgical atlas is a must for the surgeon interested in pelvic surgery. Each procedure is illustrated in stepwise fashion.

SUGGESTED READINGS

Netter FH. The CIBA Collection of Medical Illustrations, vol 2. Reproductive System. New York: RR Donnelley, 1984.

Thompson JD. Operative injuries to the ureter: Prevention, recognition and management. In Rock JA, Thompson JD, eds. TeLinde's Operative Gynecology, 8th ed. Philadelphia: Lippincott-Raven, 1997, pp 1135–1174.

Thompson JD. Vesicovaginal and urethrovaginal fistulas. In Rock JA, Thompson JD, eds. TeLinde's Operative Gynecology, 8th ed. Philadelphia: Lippincott-Raven, 1997, pp 1175–1206.

Uterine Cancer

Bloss JD, Berman ML, Bloss LP, et al. Use of vaginal hysterectomy for the management of stage I endometrial cancer in the medically compromised patient. Gynecol Oncol 40:74, 1991.

Currie JL. Malignant tumors of the uterine corpus. In Rock JA, Thompson JD, eds. TeLinde's Operative Gynecology, 8th ed. Philadelphia: Lippincott-Raven, 1997, pp 1501–1556.

Hacker NF. Uterine cancer. In Berek JS, Hacker NF, eds. Practical Gynecologic Oncology, 2nd ed. Baltimore: Williams & Wilkins, 1994, pp 285–326.

Horowitz IR, De La Cuesta RS. Benign and malignant tumors of the ovary. In Carpenter SEK, Rock JA, eds. Pediatric and Adolescent Gynecology. New York: Raven, 1992.

Horowitz IR, Shingleton HM. The role of chemotherapy and radiotherapy in the treatment of endometrial carcinoma. Curr Obstet Gynaecol 7:22–29, 1997.

Hricak H, Burinstein LV, Gerhman GM, et al. MR imaging evaluation of endometrial carcinoma: Results of an NCI Cooperative Study. Radiology 179:829, 1991.

Lurain JR. The significance of positive peritoneal cytology in endometrial cancer. Gynecol Oncol 46:143, 1992.

Morrow CP, Bundy BN, Kurman RJ, et al. Relationship between surgical-pathologic risk factors and outcome in clinical stage I and II carcinoma of the endometrium: A Gynecologic Oncology Group study. Gynecol Oncol 40:55, 1991.

Shingleton HM, Thompson JD. Cancer of the cervix. In Rock JA, Thompson JD, eds. TeLinde's Operative Gynecology, 8th ed. Philadelphia: Lippincott-Raven, 1997, pp 1413-1500.

Cervical Cancer

Bachsbaum JH, Lifshitz S. The role of scalene lymph node biopsy in advanced carcinoma of the cervix uteri. Surg Gynecol Obstet 143:246, 1976.

Hatch KD. Cervical cancer. In Berek JS, Hacker NF, eds. Practical Gynecologic Oncology, 2nd ed. Baltimore: Williams & Wilkins, 1994, pp 243-284.

Hatch KD, Parham G, Shingleton HM, et al. Ureteral strictures and fistulae following radical hysterectomy. Gynecol Oncol 19:17, 1984.

Piver M, Rutledge F, Smith J. Five classes of extended hystrectomy for women with cervical cancer. Obstet Gynecol 44:265, 1974.

Weiser GB, Bundy BN, Hoskins WJ, et al. Extraperitoneal versus transperitoneal selective paraaortric lymphadenectomy in the pretreatment surgical staging of advanced cervical carcinoma (GOG Study). Gynecol Oncol 33:283, 1989.

Ovarian Cancer

Berek JS. Epithelial ovarian cancer. In Berek JS, Hacker NF, eds. Practical Gynecologic Oncology, 2nd ed. Baltimore: Williams & Wilkins, 1994, pp 327-376.

Berek JS, Griffith CT, Leventhal JM. Laparoscopy for second-look evaluation in ovarian cancer. Obstet Gynecol 58:192, 1981.

Deppe G, Malviya VK, Boike G, et al. Use of Cavitron Surgical Aspirator for debulking of diaphragmatic metastases in patients with advanced carcinoma of the ovaries. Surg Gynecol Obstet 168:458, 1989.

Hacker NF, Berek JS, Lagasse LD. Gastrointestinal operations in gynecologic oncology. In Knapp RE, Berkowitz RS, eds. Gynecologic Oncology, 2nd ed. New York: McGraw-Hill, 1993, pp 361-375.

Hoskins WJ, Bundy BN, Thigpen TJ, et al. The influence of cytoreductive surgery on recurrence-free interval and survival in small volume stage III epithelial ovarian cancer: A Gynecologic Oncology Group study. Gynecol Oncol 47:159, 1992.

Hunter RW, Alexander NDE, Soutter WP. Meta-analysis of surgery in advanced ovarian carcinoma: Is maximum cytoreductive surgery an independent determinant of prognosis? Am J Obstet Gynecol 166:504, 1992.

McGuire WP, Hoskins WJ, Brady MF, et al. A phase III trial comparing cisplatin/cytoxan (PC) and cisplatin/taxol (PT) in advanced ovarian cancer. Proc Am Soc Clin Oncol 29:808, 1993.

Omura GA, Brady MF, Homesley HD, et al. Long-term follow-up and prognostic factor analysis in advanced ovarian carcinoma: The Gynecologic Oncology Group experience. J Clin Oncol 9:1138, 1991.

Piver MS, Hempling RE. Ovarian cancer: Etiology, screening, prophylactic oophorectomy, and surgery. In Rock JA, Thompson JD, eds. TeLinde's Operative Gynecology, 8th ed. Philadelphia: Lippincott-Raven, 1997, pp 1557-1568.

Rubin SC, Hoskins WJ, Hakes TB, et al. Recurrence after negative second-look laparotomy for ovarian cancer: Analysis of risk factors. Am J Obstet Gynecol 159:1094, 1988.

Vulvar Cancer

Berek JS, Heaps JM, Fu YS, et al. Concurrent cisplatin and 5-fluorouracil chemotherapy and radiotherapy for advanced stage squamous carcinoma of the vulva. Gynecol Oncol 42:197, 1991.

Burke TW, Stringer CA, Gershenson DM, et al. Radical wide excision and selective inguinal node dissection of squamous cell carcinoma of the vulva. Gynecol Oncol 38:328, 1990.

Hacker NF. Vulvar cancer. In Berek JS, Hacker NF, eds. Practical Gynecologic Oncology, 2nd ed. Baltimore: Williams & Wilkins, 1994, pp 403-440.

Hacker NF, Berek JS, Lagasse LD, et al. Individualization of treatment for stage I squamous cell vulvar carcinoma. Obstet Gynecol 63:155, 1984.

Hacker NF, Leuchter RS, Berek JS, et al. Radical vulvectomy and bilateral inguinal lymphadenectomy through separate groin incisions. Obstet Gynecol 58:574, 1981.

Homesley HD, Bundy BN, Sedlis A, et al. Radiation therapy versus pelvic node resection for carcinoma of the vulva with positive groin nodes. Obstet Gynecol 68:733, 1986.

Rotmensch J, Rubin SJ, Sutton HG, et al. Preoperative radiotherapy followed by radical vulvectomy with inguinal lymphadenectomy for advanced vulvar carcinomas. Gynecol Oncol 36:181, 1990.

Stehman F, Bundy N, Bell J, et al. Groin dissection versus groin radiation in carcinoma of the vulva: A Gynecologic Oncology Group study. Int J Radiat Oncol Biol Phys 24:389, 1992.

Stehman FB, Bundy B, Droretsky PM, et al. Early stage I carcinoma of the vulva treated with ipsilateral superficial inguinal lymphadenectomy and modified radical hemivulvectomy: A prospective study of the Gynecologic Oncology Group. Obstet Gynecol 79:490, 1992.

Taussig FJ. Cancer of the vulva: An analysis of 155 cases. Am J Obstet Gynecol 40:764, 1940.

Way S. Carcinoma of the vulva. Am J Obstet Gynecol 79:692, 1960.

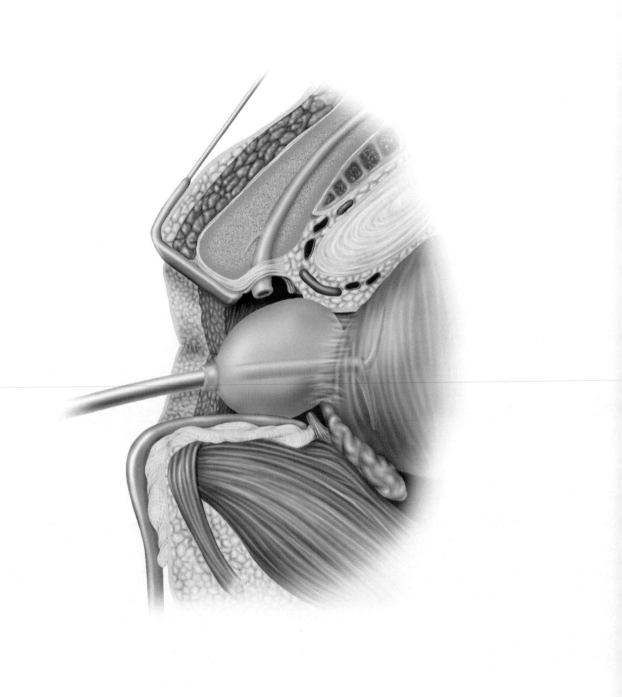

Male Genital System

Sam D. Graham, Jr., M.D., and Allen A. Futral III, M.D.

Surgical Applications

C ancer surgery has always been one of the major surgical procedures performed by the practicing urologist. As prostate cancer has become the most common cancer found in men, radical prostatectomy has become an accepted and effective therapy for this diagnosis. Other less common forms of urologic cancers in the male genitalia can also be cured with timely surgical treatment. Surgery of the genitourinary tract is well tolerated by the patient as long as a thorough knowledge of the anatomic nuances is understood. This chapter covers the more important anatomic aspects of the male genital system.

Prostate Gland

The incidence of adenocarcinoma of the prostate gland has risen dramatically over the past 10 years to become the most commonly reported solid carcinoma, with an estimated 330,000 new cases in 1996. This has been primarily a result of the identification of prostate-specific antigen (PSA) as a useful adjunct in the early detection of prostate cancer, which in turn has led to diagnosis at an earlier average age and earlier stage of disease than has been seen in the past. Because patients are younger and healthier, and the cancer likely is localized, the trend for the past 10 years has been more toward radical prostatectomy as the primary form of therapy.

SURGICAL ANATOMY
Topography

The prostate gland is located inferior to the bladder, where it rests on a sling of pelvic musculature known collectively as the "pelvic floor." It is comprised histologically of two forms of glandular epithelium: the peripheral or true prostatic tissue, which arises from Wolffian elements, and the periurethral glands, which arise from the urogenital sinus as a continuation of the bladder with age.

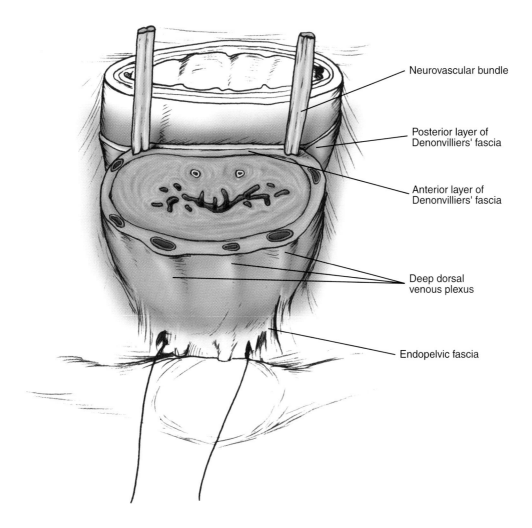

Neurovascular bundle

Posterior layer of
Denonvilliers' fascia

Anterior layer of
Denonvilliers' fascia

Deep dorsal
venous plexus

Endopelvic fascia

The prostate is separated from the rectum by the capsule of the gland, which is a coalescence of fibromuscular tissue that develops in the embryo, and by Denonvilliers' fascia, an extension of the peritoneal sac with anterior and posterior leaves. Anteriorly the prostate is attached to the symphysis pubis by a coalescence of the endopelvic fascia known as the puboprostatic ligaments. Between the prostate and the symphysis pubis is a freely anastomosing plexus of veins known as the plexus of Santorini or the dorsal venous complex, which is a continuation of the dorsal venous drainage of the penis. The prostatic urethra is that portion from the bladder to the pelvic floor and traverses the prostate with an anterior deflection approximately midprostate to end at the anterior apex of the prostate. The rectourethralis muscle, a coalescence of muscular and fibrous tissue, joins the rectum to the urethra.

Blood Supply

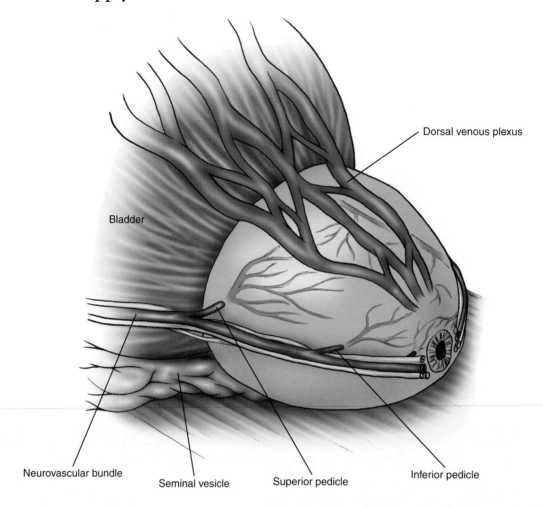

The vascular supply of the prostate is via branches of the anterior division of the hypogastric artery that continue into the pelvic floor to vascularize the corpora cavernosa and therefore contribute to erectile function. The primary vascular pedicle enters the prostate in a hilum near the base of the gland (superior prostatic pedicle), with variable expression of pedicles at the apex of the prostate. The pathway of the vascular pedicles parallels the autonomic nerves on the posterolateral border of the prostate between the anterior and posterior layers of Denonvilliers' fascia. Near the apex, the neurovascular bundle crosses the apex and enters the pelvic floor just posterior to the membranous urethra.

Lymphatic Drainage

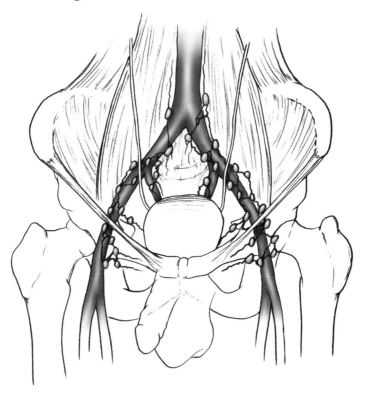

The lymphatic drainage from the prostate is initially via the intraprostatic lymphatic vessels, which coalesce into microtubules that exit the prostate in a vascular hilum located at the base and apex of the gland. These microtubules freely anastomose in the areolar tissue around the prostate at its base and the seminal vesicles, coalescing into lymphatic vessels that empty into the obturator nodes along the hypogastric vessels and at the bifurcation of the common iliac artery. Lymphatic drainage continues along the common iliac vessels to enter the general retroperitoneal lymphatic drainage. Lymphatic connections in the presacral space may be independent of the obturator chain.

Pelvic Floor Anatomy and Continence

The pelvic floor is a sling of muscle that provides support for the perineum and is important in urinary continence. The perineum can be divided into two parts: the anterior (urogenital) triangle and the posterior (anal) triangle. The line dividing the two parts extends from the two ischial tuberosities. Under the skin and superficial fascia is Colle's fascia, which overlies the pelvic musculature and is a continuation of the dartos fascia of the scrotum and membranous fascia of the abdominal wall. The superficial structures in the male perineum include the bulbospongiosus musculature, which covers the corpora spongiosum (bulb of the penis). On either side of the bulbospongiosus muscle are the ischiocavernosus muscles, which cover the crura of the penis as they attach to the ischial tuberosities. The perineal body, which is the anterior attachment of the anal sphincter to the urogenital triangle, is also joined by the superficial transversus perinei muscles, which also attach to the inferior pubic rami and form the posterior border of the urogenital triangle. Deep to these superficial structures is the perineal membrane, and deep to the membrane is the deep perineal musculature, which in the male is divided into two parts: the anterior (periurethral) portion, forming the sphincter urethrae, and the posterior portion, comprising the deep transversus perinei muscles. Buried in this latter musculature are the paired Cowper's glands. Removal of this deep perineal layer reveals a deep pelvic fascia overlying the obturator internus muscles, which also overlie the levator ani muscle.

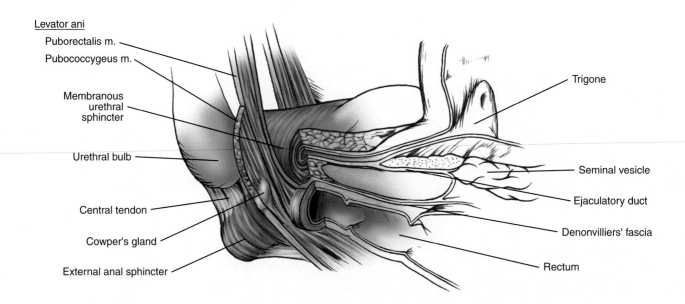

The anal triangle is covered by a superficial subcutaneous fascia that is continuous with the superficial abdominal fascia and the fascia of the urogenital triangle. In the center of the triangle is the opening of the anal canal, through which traverses the anus. To either side are the fibrofatty spaces known as the ischiorectal fossae, bounded by the ischial tuberosities laterally and the levator ani muscle. The pudendal nerve, inferior rectal artery and vein, and internal pudendal artery all cross the ischiorectal fossa as they exit the pelvis via Alcock's canal. The anal canal is composed of three layers of muscle (subcutaneous, superficial, and deep) that constitute the anal sphincter. The subcutaneous portion is beneath the skin and completely encircles the anus. The superficial portion attaches to the coccygeal ligament and the coccyx posteriorly and the perineal body anteriorly. The deep portion fuses to the levator ani muscle and completely encircles the anal canal. This striated outer sphincter mechanism of the anal canal encircles the smooth muscle component of the internal anal sphincter.

The vascular supply of the perineum is derived from the internal pudendal artery, which exits from Alcock's canal (pudendal canal) along with the pudendal nerve. The artery branches to form the inferior hemorrhoidal artery posteriorly and the superficial (posterior scrotal) and deep (between the perineal membrane and deep fascia) anterior branches.

Continence in the male is controlled by smooth muscle that lines the prostatic and membranous urethra, known as the internal mechanism. These fibers are a continuation of the detrusor fibers from the bladder.

SURGICAL APPLICATIONS
Transrectal Needle Biopsy

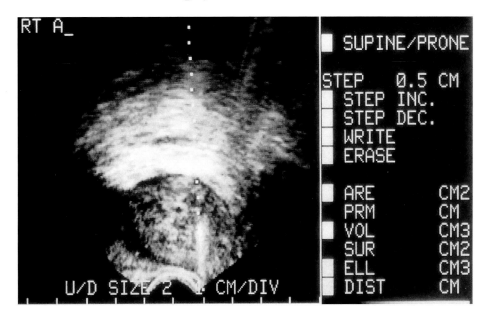

Transrectal biopsy of the prostate is indicated in patients who have either an elevated PSA level or suspect findings at digital rectal examination, which would include a nodule or more subtle finding such as asymmetry of shape or consistency of the gland. In most centers transrectal biopsy is performed with ultrasound as a guide (transrectal ultrasonography). Generally the operator scans the prostate longitudinally and transversely to look for variations within the prostatic stroma such as areas of decreased echogenicity (hypoechogenic foci) and to calculate the volume of the prostate, which when divided into the PSA allows the operator to calculate PSA density. This technique is used to take into account the contribution to the serum PSA by benign prostatic tissue and estimate the probability that the PSA level, along with the ratio of PSA to free PSA, is elevated as a result of cancer.

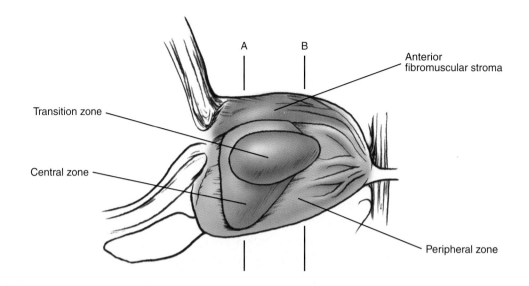

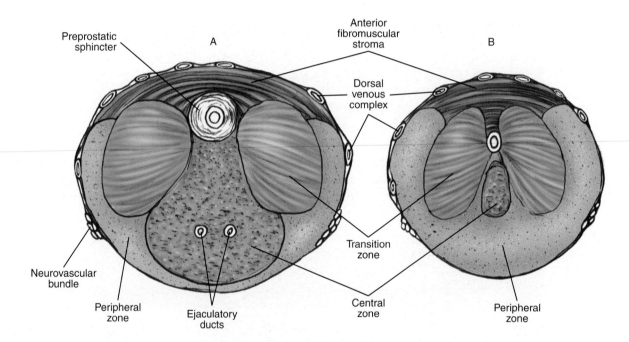

The prostate can be divided into well-defined zonal anatomy during ultrasonography. These zones include the peripheral zone, transition zone, and central zone, corresponding to the histologic anatomy of the periphery of the prostate (true prostatic glands), the periurethral prostate (periurethral glands), and the tissue around the ejaculatory ducts, respectively.

The biopsy is performed with an automated biopsy device (e.g., Biopty, CR Bard, Covington, Ga.) using an 18-gauge needle. The sites for the biopsy are visualized with ultrasound and, with the biopsy alignment software in most units, the needle can be guided accurately. Sites selected include any abnormal ultrasonographic finding that may represent a malignancy, any site that is palpably suspect despite the ultrasonographic findings, and, if no specific site is seen, systematic biopsy of the prostate in each of six, eight, or 10 sectors. The cores are examined and sent in separate containers to allow pathologic localization of the cancer and to enable estimation of the volume of the cancer, which will be useful in planning further therapy. In addition, if the operator detects any abnormality in the seminal vesicles, such as deformity of the angle of the seminal vesicles compared with the prostate, biopsy of the seminal vesicles may be warranted to enable staging of the cancer. Since most of the cancers arise in the periphery of the prostate, the biopsy sites are usually toward the peripheral zone, yet if prior biopsies yielded negative results and the PSA level is significantly elevated, biopsy of the periurethral (transition zone) prostate may be indicated.

Pelvic Lymph Node Dissection

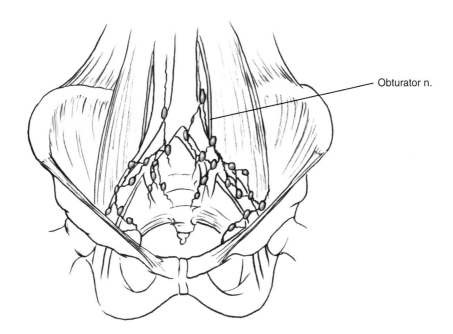

Obturator n.

Pelvic lymph node dissection is limited to the nodes within the obturator fossa, which is considered the first tier of significant lymphatic tissue. While most patients with positive nodes will have metastases to the obturator nodes, the presacral nodes may occasionally be the only site of positive nodes. Furthermore, it should be noted that pelvic node dissection is done only for staging and is not intended to be therapeutic, because (1) removal of the intervening lymphatic tissue from the prostate to the nodes is not feasible, (2) it is not possible to remove all pelvic lymphatic tissue without severe and debilitating lower extremity complications, and (3) lymphatic metastases should be considered systemic disease.

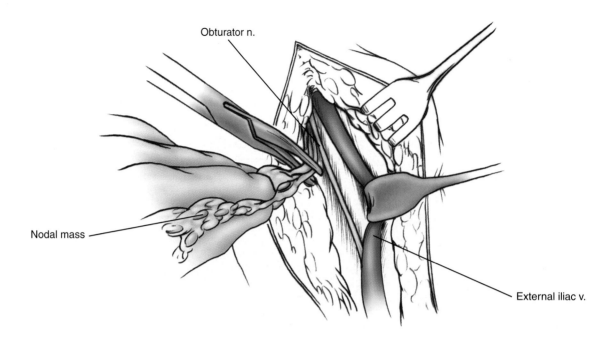

The surgical approach to the pelvic lymph nodes is transabdominal and can be performed as an open procedure either intraperitoneally or extraperitoneally, or via laparoscopy. The technique is the same with any approach, however, once the abdomen is entered. The limits of the node dissection should be the external iliac vein laterally, Cooper's ligament inferiorly, the hypogastric artery posteriorly, and the bifurcation of the common iliac artery cranially. The dissection is begun by identifying the external iliac vein and incising the lymphatic tissue-fat along the path of the vein. Once the adventitia of the vein is exposed, the dissection can be carried caudally using blunt dissection to the junction of the vein with Cooper's ligament. At this point, there is generally a circumflex vein, which can be avoided. At Cooper's ligament the dissection is carried posteriorly, and by staying close to the vein the surgeon can identify an avascular plane that will allow isolation of the inferior limit of the nodal mass. Care must be taken to prevent injury to the obturator nerve and vessels, and a hemoclip is applied across the lymphatic mass, which is divided. With a vein retractor under the external iliac vein, the dissection is carried superiorly to the bifurcation of the common iliac artery and laterally to the pelvic sidewall. The prostatic and vesicular branches of the hypogastric artery are exposed during this dissection. At the superior margin of dissection, care must be taken to prevent injury to the ureter.

Radical Retropubic Prostatectomy

The patient is positioned in a supine position with the table flexed 10 to 20 degrees. A 20 Fr Foley catheter is passed through the urethra, the balloon is inflated, and gravity drainage is initiated. A midline incision is made from the umbilicus to the symphysis pubis, and the pelvis is exposed extraperitoneally. Bilateral pelvic lymph node dissection is performed. The endopelvic fascia is incised bilaterally, and the puboprostatic ligaments are divided close to the pubis, exposing the dorsal venous complex.

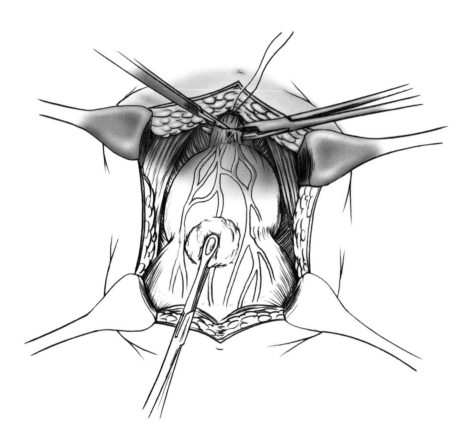

With an angled dissector, the dorsal venous complex is isolated and ligated over the urethra with a large absorbable ligature. The dorsal venous complex is then divided and membranous urethra exposed, which is also isolated and divided with the catheter in place.

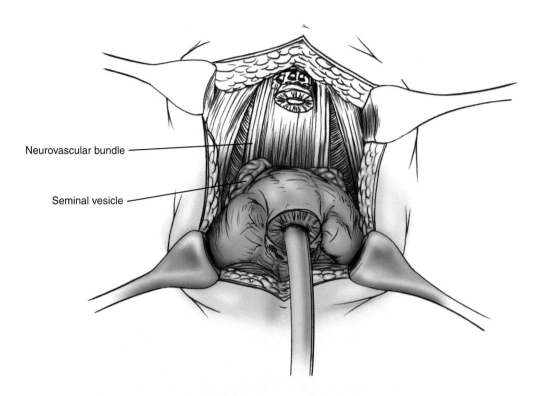

With the distal catheter and inflated balloon as a retraction device, the apex of the prostate is elevated, taking care to prevent injury to the neurovascular bundles at the apex. The prostate is then dissected from the apex to the base, dividing the lateral pedicles close to the prostate and taking care to prevent injury to the neurovascular bundles. The ampullae of the vas deferens and the seminal vesicles are identified and dissected free.

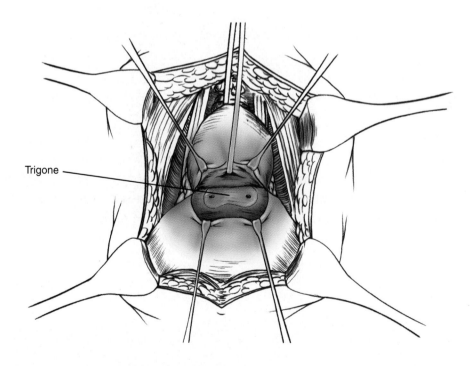

The prostate is dissected from the bladder neck and removed.

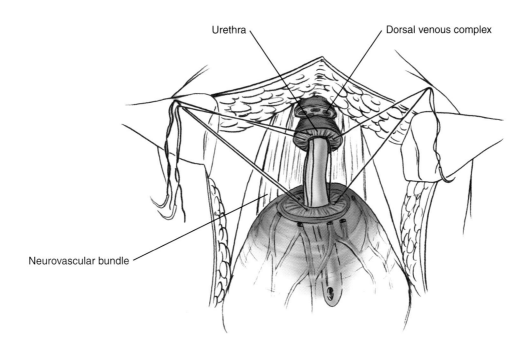

If the bladder neck is patulous, the opening is tapered from posterior to anterior with an absorbable suture. The vesicourethral anastomosis is accomplished over a 20 Fr Foley catheter by placing quadrant absorbable sutures in the urethra and corresponding areas of the bladder neck. Depending on the surgeon's preference or the tension on the anastomosis, vest sutures may be placed in the lateral bladder and into the pelvic floor. Pelvic drains are placed, and the abdominal fascia is closed with interrupted sutures.

Radical Perineal Prostatectomy

The perineal approach to radical prostatectomy requires that the patient be placed in an exaggerated lithotomy position with the perineum parallel to the floor. The patient's weight is entirely supported by a roll under the sacrum, with no tension on the hamstrings and taking care to prevent injury to the brachial plexus by not using shoulder braces. An inverted U-shaped incision is made from ischial tuberosity to ischial tuberosity anteriorly, crossing the perineum at the mucocutaneous border of the rectum. The ischial rectal fossae are identified and the central tendon divided. The dissection is then carried along the anterior rectal wall under the anal sphincter mechanism and beneath the levator ani.

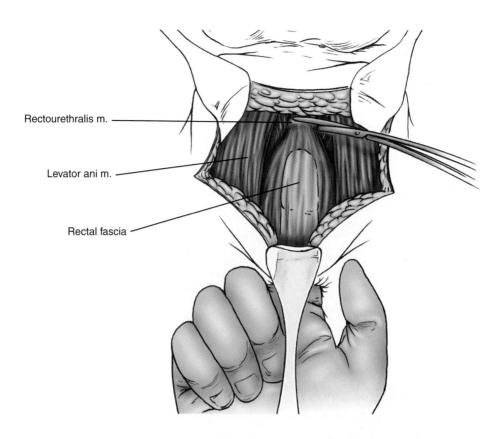

Rectourethralis m.

Levator ani m.

Rectal fascia

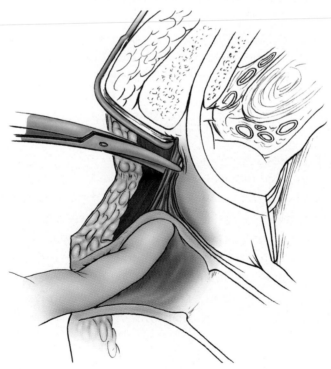

The rectourethralis muscle is identified and divided, allowing access to the apex of the prostate. The posterior layer of Denonvilliers' fascia is incised, and the dissection is carried cranially along the posterior prostate between the layers of Denonvilliers' fascia.

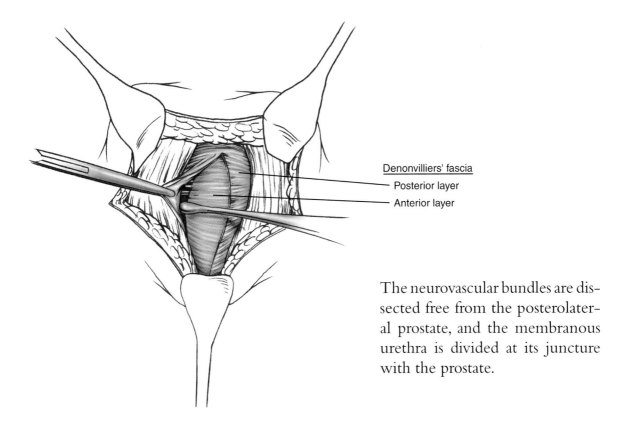

The neurovascular bundles are dissected free from the posterolateral prostate, and the membranous urethra is divided at its juncture with the prostate.

With a Young prostatic retractor, the dissection is directed along the anterior prostate, dividing the endopelvic fascia and avoiding the dorsal venous complex. The prostate is dissected free from the bladder neck, the urethra is divided at the bladder neck, and the superior prostatic pedicles are divided.

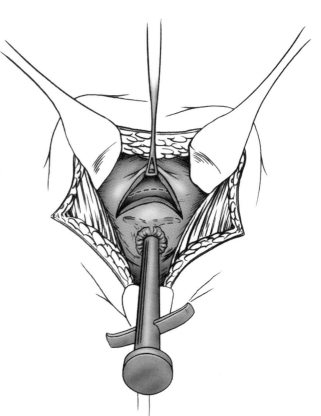

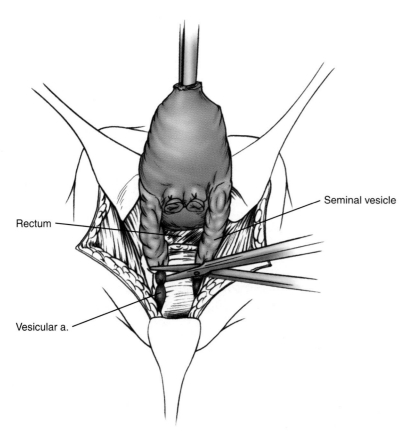

The seminal vesicles are dissected free and the ampullae of the vas deferens are divided, allowing removal of the specimen. Care should be directed at the tips of the seminal vesicles to control the seminal vesicular artery, which may retract on division.

The bladder neck is reconstructed to approximately 22 Fr posteriorly to anteriorly and anastomosed to the urethra with interrupted absorbable sutures. A 22 Fr Foley catheter is placed through the urethra and connected to gravity drainage, a Penrose drain is placed, and the skin is closed with 3-0 chromic interrupted horizontal mattress sutures.

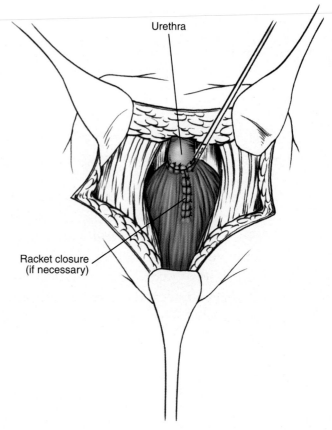

Testes

Carcinoma of the testes is uncommon in the general practice of urology, yet is the most common tumor in men between the ages of 20 and 40 years. These tumors are almost exclusively germ cell tumors arising from the totipotential germ cells in the seminiferous tubules and may represent one or more histologic types: seminoma, embryonal cell, teratoma, or choriocarcinoma. Detection is usually by physical examination of a solid mass in the testicle, although it can be confused with epididymitis or orchitis. Any testicular mass that is not clearly due to epididymitis or other pathologic condition should be considered a possible testicular carcinoma and treated accordingly. Potentially useful adjuncts in the diagnosis include transscrotal ultrasonography and serum markers, but if clinical suspicion is sufficiently raised despite equivocal results of ultrasound or even negative serum markers, inguinal exploration is indicated. Violation of the scrotum such as by needle aspiration or scrotal exploration is mentioned only in condemnation, since this may result in alteration of the lymphatic drainage, contaminate the scrotal compartment, and complicate further therapy.

SURGICAL ANATOMY
Topography

The testis is a paired organ that is important for both hormonal and germ cell functions. The adult testis is approximately 4 to 5 cm long and 2 to 3 cm thick. Anatomically a testis resides in a compartment in the scrotum separated from the other testis by a central septum. The testicular compartment is lined with a visceral and parietal layer of tunica vaginalis, which embryologically is a continuation of the peritoneum. The testis itself is divided into multiple lobules by septations that are invaginations of the tunica albuginea, coalescing in the upper pole at the rete testis. Each lobule contains two or more seminiferous tubules, which converge at the rete testis to join a tubular network, joining the globus major (caput) of the epididymis. The seminiferous tubules are lined by germinal epithelium, with supporting stromal (Sertoli and Leydig cells), components that are responsible for the hormonal function of the testes.

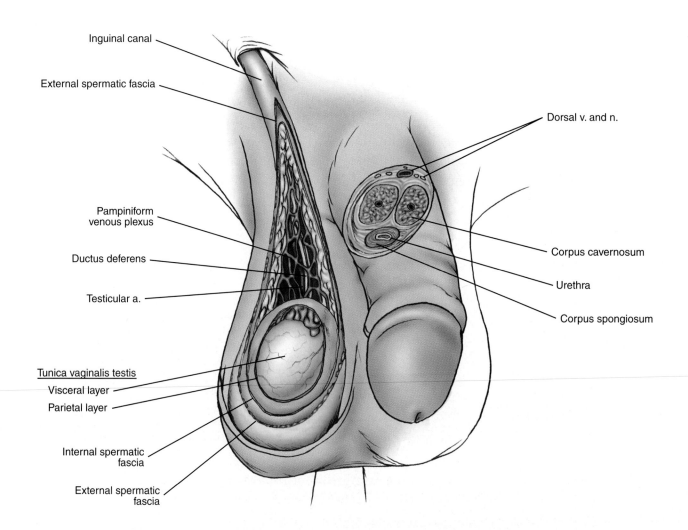

The spermatic cord carries all of the vascular and lymphatic structures of the testis from the retroperitoneum through the inguinal canal into the scrotum. As it passes through the inguinal canal, it acquires coverings that correspond to the various layers of the abdominal wall. These coverings, known as the internal spermatic fascia, cremasteric muscle, and external spermatic fascia, correspond to the transversus abdominis, internal oblique, and external oblique muscles, respectively. Within the spermatic cord the testicular veins form a plexus of veins (pampiniform plexus) that freely anastomose until they coalesce into the spermatic vein.

Blood Supply, Lymphatic Drainage, and Nerve Supply

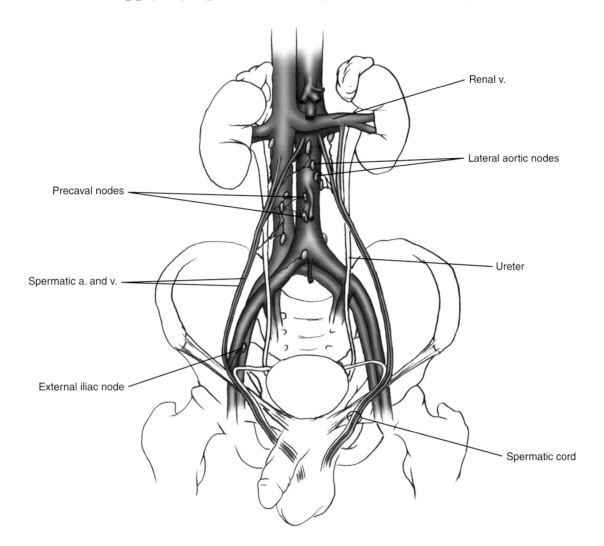

The blood supply to the testes is derived embryologically from the site of origin on the urogenital ridge near the kidneys. The internal spermatic arteries emanate from the aorta just below the renal arteries and proceed retroperitoneally into the pelvis, where they freely anastomose with the cremasteric and vasal arteries, exiting through the internal inguinal ring into the inguinal canal and onto the testes. The venous return parallels the arterial supply except that the right spermatic vein enters the vena cava below the renal vein, and the left spermatic vein enters the central venous system by its anastomosis with the left renal vein.

The lymphatic drainage of the testes parallels the vascular supply, with its primary lymph nodes in the retroperitoneum adjacent to the renal vein.

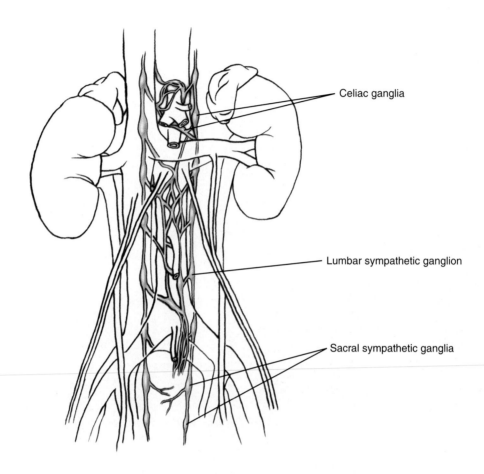

Celiac ganglia

Lumbar sympathetic ganglion

Sacral sympathetic ganglia

The autonomic innervation of the pelvic floor is derived from the sympathetic chain (L1-5) and the sacral roots (S1-4). The sympathetic chain is located lateral and adjacent to the aorta and vena cava at the lumbar region, closely applied to and intertwined among the lumbar arteries and veins. In addition, the preganglionic nerves exit via the lumbar splanchnic nerves, course over the aorta, and join the sympathetic ganglia within the sympathetic chain.

SURGICAL APPLICATIONS
Radical Inguinal Orchiectomy

An incision is made over the inguinal canal extending from approximately the lateral border of the symphysis pubis superolaterally to the internal inguinal ring. The external inguinal ring is identified, and the inguinal canal is opened from the external to the internal ring, exposing the spermatic cord. The cord is isolated and a ½-inch Penrose drain is applied as a tourniquet near the internal inguinal ring. With manual compression on the scrotum combined with sharp dissection of the spermatic cord, the testis is delivered into the field along with the visceral and parietal tunica vaginalis. The attachments from the tunica to the scrotum are divided and the cord dissected into its components, the vas and the vessels, and each is ligated and divided just inside the internal ring. The external oblique is closed in interrupted 3-0 silk, and the skin is reapproximated.

Retroperitoneal Lymph Node Dissection

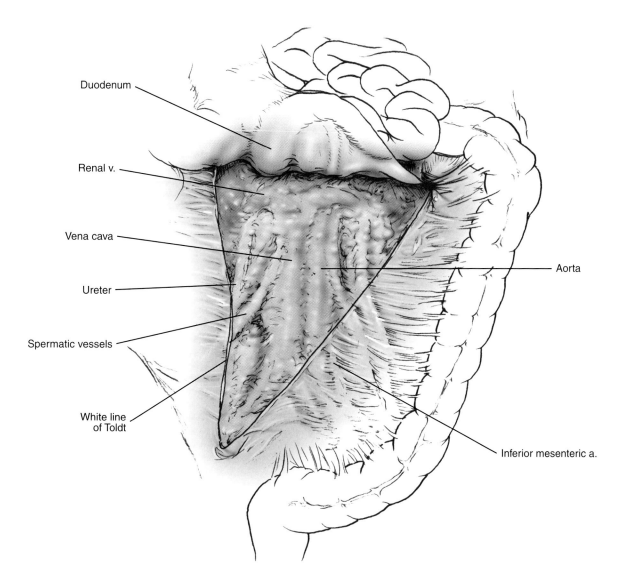

A midline incision is made from the xiphoid process to the symphysis pubis, and the peritoneal cavity is entered. An incision is made along the white line of Toldt and carried superiorly to the hepatic flexure of the colon and medially and superiorly along the root of the mesentery of the small intestine to the ligament of Treitz. The entire small bowel and right colon are retracted superiorly to expose the retroperitoneum.

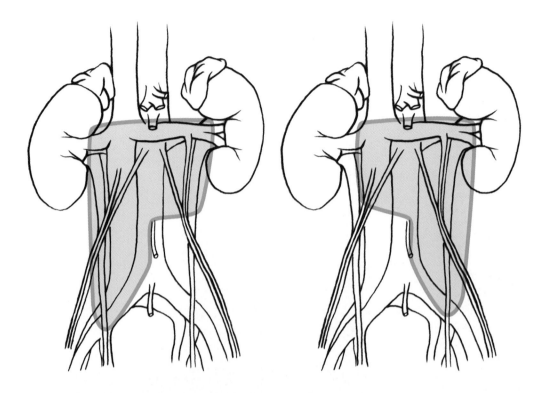

The observation that the primary site for metastases is the renal hilum and the minimal chances of crossover from side to side, combined with the marked effectiveness of chemotherapy, have allowed modification of the formal complete retroperitoneal node dissection to spare the sympathetic chain, which is important to prevent retrograde ejaculation. The ability to perform a nerve-sparing operation is predicated on the fact that the patient has no known retroperitoneal adenopathy and has not had prior chemotherapy for testicular cancer. If a nerve-sparing procedure is contemplated, either the dissection along the great vessels will follow a template designed to prevent disruption of the sympathetic chain on the side contralateral to the tumor or a selective nerve-sparing procedure will be performed. In a template dissection, the lateral border of dissection is the ipsilateral ureter, and the medial border is the lateral vena cava (left-sided tumor) or lateral aorta (right-sided tumor). The superior border is the superior edge of the renal vein, and the inferior margin is the end of the spermatic cord on the ipsilateral side and the bifurcation of the common iliac artery on the contralateral side. Care should be taken in dissection at the bifurcations of the great vessels to prevent injury to the presacral artery and the parasympathetic nerves, which would result in the patient becoming anejaculatory.

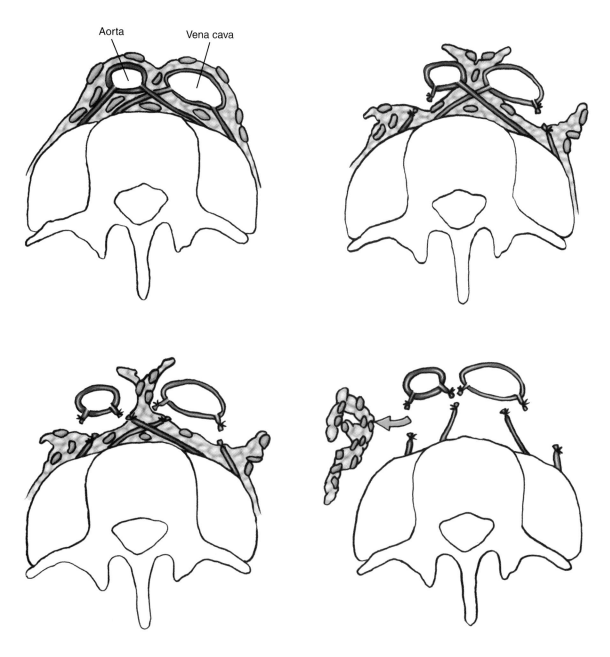

The dissection is begun on the anterolateral surface of the contralateral great vessel and carried along the vessel to the inferior margin of dissection, where the fatty-lymphatic tissue is divided. Similarly, the superior margin is divided and the packet rolled medially. The packet is dissected from the interaortocaval space, taking care to prevent injury to the lumbar arteries and veins. Generally these can be taken with no consequences, and division of the lumbar arteries facilitates dissection and reduces blood loss. The packet is split longitudinally and the lymphatic tissue dissected from behind the ipsilateral great vessel and anterior to the vessel. The dissection is carried inferiorly to the end of the spermatic cord (previously marked with a silk ligature during the inguinal orchiectomy), laterally to the ureter, and superiorly to the superior border of the renal vein. The spermatic vein is ligated at the juncture with the vena cava in right-sided tumors and at the juncture with the renal vein in left-sided tumors. The surgeon must be aware that the left renal vein frequently has a posterior lumbar branch that will complicate dissection behind the left renal vein.

Potential hazards from this operation include ejaculatory disturbance due to disruption of the autonomic nerves, spinal cord ischemia with aggressive sacrificing of the lumbar arteries, and lymphoceles, which can be avoided with liberal use of ligatures and hemoclips. The only vessel of significance on the anterior surface of the artery is the inferior mesenteric artery, which may be left intact, although it is occasionally necessary to resect a segment. In the latter scenario, the surgeon should be aware that, although most patients have sufficient collateral vessels to continue perfusion of the distal colon, a small proportion (>20%) will experience ischemia of the distal colon.

The posterior peritoneum is closed with a running absorbable suture, and the abdominal cavity is closed with interrupted figure-of-eight sutures. Generally neither drains nor gastrointestinal tubes are required.

Penis

Carcinoma of the penis is a rare cancer that is directly preventable by neonatal circumcision. This cancer is more common in developing countries where good hygiene is not practiced and may be linked to human papillomavirus (HPV) infection. Although the cancer is uncommon, the most effective therapy in localized cancer is surgical excision, which, except in the rare case of the small lesion on the foreskin that requires only circumcision, generally requires partial penectomy, a psychologically devastating procedure.

SURGICAL ANATOMY
Topography

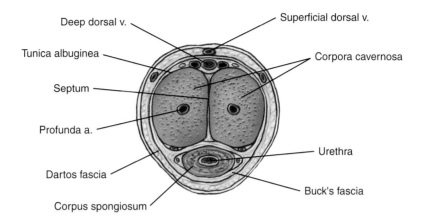

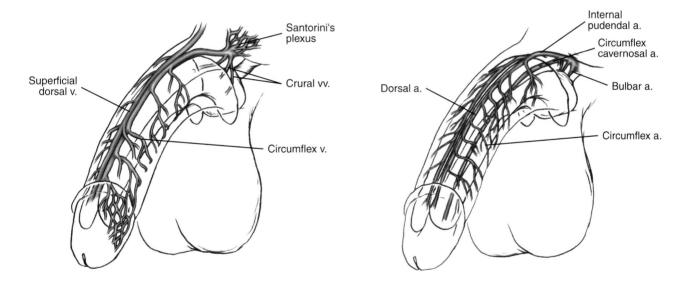

The penis is a midline structure composed of the paired corpora cavernosa and the ventral corpus spongiosa. Anatomically the penis can be divided into three regions: the root (provides fixation and stability in the superficial perineum), the body (the majority of the penis), and the glans (a distal expansion of the corpus spongiosa). The corpora cavernosa are sponge-like masses of vascular tissue covered by a double layer of Buck's fascia (tunica albuginea) and separated by a central septum. At the perineum, however, they diverge into the crus of the penis to attach to the ischium. The corpus spongiosum is likewise composed of a rich vascular space and completely surrounds the urethra during its course through the penis. Anatomically the corpus spongiosum is divided into three portions: proximal (bulbar), body, and distal (glans). The bulbar portion is larger than the body and is surrounded by the bulbospongiosus muscle, which aids in propelling fluid through the distal urethra. The penis is fixed to the pelvis via the attachment of the crura to the ischia and via the suspensory ligament of the penis attaching the corpora to the symphysis pubis.

Blood Supply and Lymphatic Drainage

The vascular supply of the penis includes the three distal branches of the pudendal artery: the deep penile artery, bulbar artery, and urethral artery. The deep penile artery supplies the corpora cavernosa via the dorsal artery and cavernous artery. The corpus spongiosum is supplied by the bulbar artery and the urethral artery. Venous drainage of the penis is via the superficial, intermediate, and deep venous systems. The superficial system consists of the superficial dorsal vein, draining the skin and subcutaneous tissues. The intermediate system comprises the lateral and circumflex veins that drain the corpora cavernosa into the deep dorsal vein and into the prostatic plexus after it enters the pelvis beneath the symphysis pubis. The deep venous system includes the bulbar veins draining the corpus spongiosus, the crural and cavernosal veins draining the corpora cavernosa, and the internal pudendal vein, all of which empty into the prostatic plexus. The glans is further drained via a retrocoronal plexus into the deep dorsal vein.

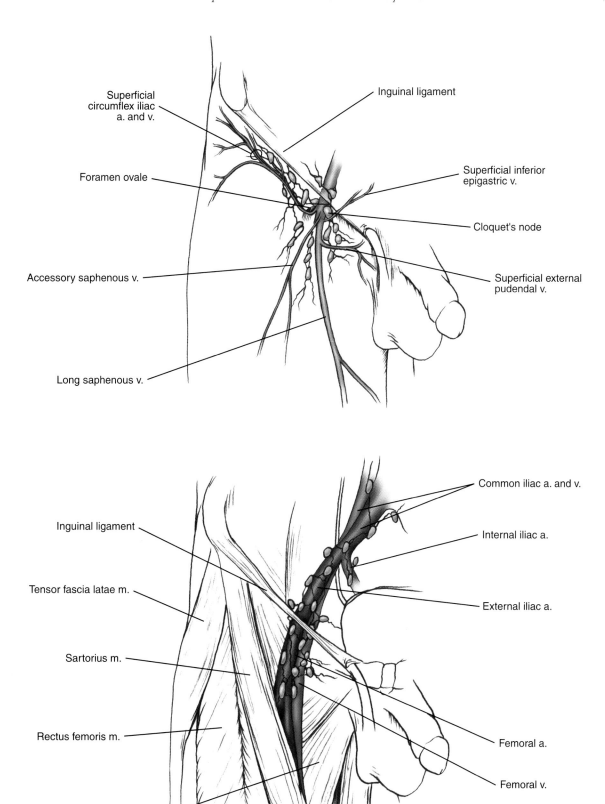

The lymphatic drainage of the penis parallels the venous drainage both into the pelvis and into the superficial inguinal nodes.

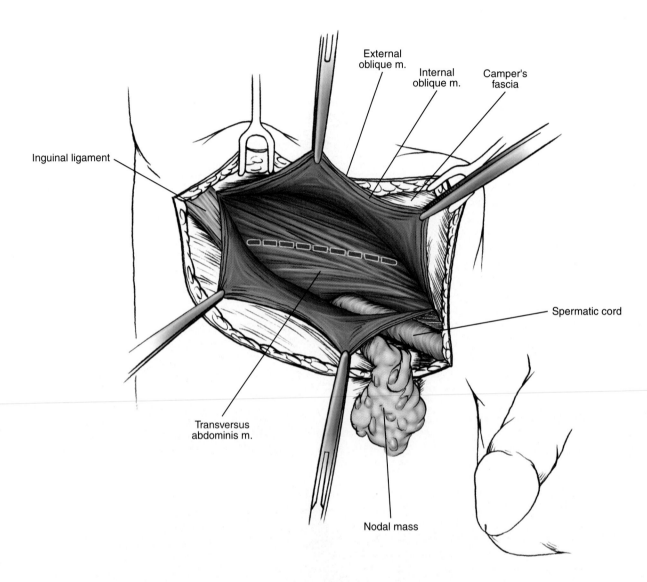

Site of incision for procedures involving the penis are shown.

SURGICAL APPLICATIONS
Total Radical Penectomy

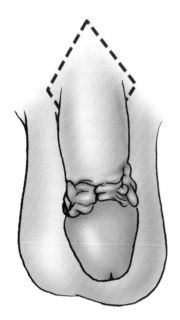

An elliptical incision is made around the base of the penis.

The corpora cavernosa are resected from the ischia taking care to ligate the corporal arteries. The urethra and corpus spongiosum are resected to the distal bulbar urethra and divided.

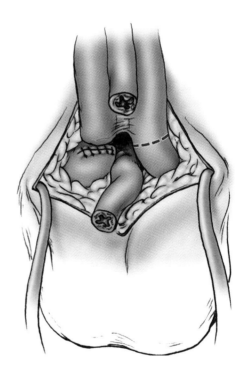

Partial Penectomy

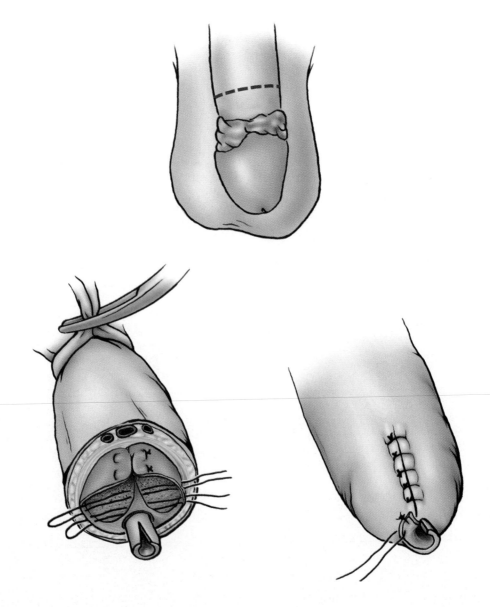

The patient is placed in a supine position, and the distal penis is examined and palpated to determine a 3 cm margin from the tumor. The skin is incised circumferentially approximately 0.5 cm distal to the planned margin and retracted proximally. The corpora cavernosa is incised at the planned margin and divided on either side. The corpus spongiosum (and urethra) is divided and the specimen removed. Hemostasis is obtained by suturing the distal corpora together.

The inferior skin is button-holed in the midline approximately 1 to 1.5 cm from the edge with an inverted V incision and the urethra spatulated ventrally. With absorbable suture, direct anastomosis of the urethra is performed, with the spatulation inlaid with the tongue of the V skin flap. The skin edges are closed with absorbable sutures.

Reconstruction

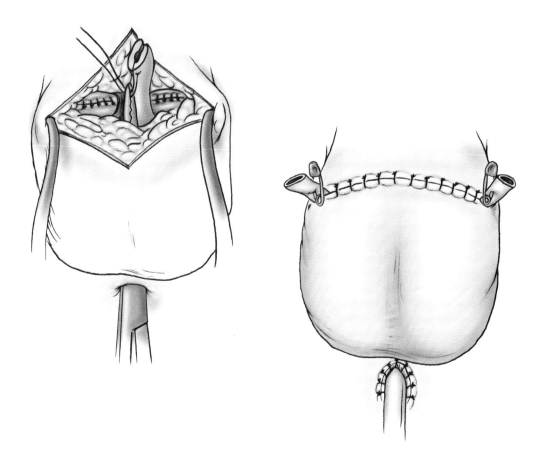

The scrotal and abdominal skin are closed and the urethra is brought out through the perineum in a separate incision.

Anatomic Basis of Complications

Pelvic Lymph Node Dissection
- Injury to external iliac vein or bifurcation can result in significant blood loss.
- Injury to obturator nerve will cause loss of adduction of thigh.
- Lack of adequate control of major pelvic lymphatic vessels will result in symptomatic lymphocele.

Radical Retropubic Prostatectomy
- Injury to neurovascular bundle of the prostate while dissecting the postero-lateral capsule of the prostate will cause impotence.
- Failure to preserve the external sphincter during dissection of the prostatic apex will cause significant incontinence.
- Loss of internal sphincter and injury to the bladder neck during removal of the prostate will often cause retrograde ejaculation.
- Injury to anal sphincter during perineal prostatectomy will occasionally cause temporary fecal incontinence.

Inguinal Orchiectomy
- Injury to herniated bowel.
- Failure to adequately ligate the cord or obtain hemostasis will result in scrotal hematoma.

Retroperitoneal Lymph Node Dissection
- Damage to lumbar sympathetic vessels may result in infertility secondary to failure of seminal emission.
- Major blood loss due to dissection of the great vessels or their tributaries.

KEY REFERENCES

Donahue JP, Maynard B, Zachary JM. The distribution of nodal metastasis in the retroperitoneum from nonseminomatous testis cancer. J Urol 128:315, 1982.
   The authors map the differences and percentage of nodal areas that more commonly receive metastatic lymphatic spread in regard to left and right testis involvement. They suggest templates of nodal dissection that can preserve the lumbar sympathetic chain in an effort to preserve seminal emission.

Donahue JP, Rowland RG. Complications of retroperitoneal lymph node dissection. J Urol 125:338, 1981.

Due to the location of the lumbar sympathetic chain, the authors describe the common occurrence of failure of seminal emission after bilateral dissection of the retroperitoneal nodes. This work led to the development of the described nerve-sparing techniques, which can preserve potency in approximately 90% of patients.

Myers RP, Goellner JB, Cahill DR. Prostate shape, external striated urethral sphincter and radical prostatectomy. The apical dissection. J Urol 138:543, 1987.

This reference delineates the anatomic relationship of the external striated urethral sphincter to the prostate apex and commissure. The authors noted that sphincteric tissue extended from the bladder base to the tunica albuginea of the corpus cavernosum. The proximal extent of the sphincter was found by the presence of an anterior apical notch. If there, the sphincter was shown to function due to presence of sphincteric fibers. The authors recommend urethral transection as far proximal as possible without including the apex but preserving the verumontanum.

Skinner DG, Leadbetter WF, Kelley SB. The surgical management of squamous cell carcinoma of the penis. J Urol 107:2783, 1972.

This remains the classic description of the surgical and anatomic considerations in treatment and staging of the relatively uncommon squamous cell carcinoma of the penis.

Walsh PC, Lepor H, Eggleston JC. Radical prostatectomy with preservation of sexual function: Anatomical and pathological considerations. Prostate 4:473, 1983.

Having identified the location of the branches of the pelvic plexus that innervate the corpora cavernosa and their relationship with the prostate vascular supply and the lateral pelvic fascia, the authors describe a modified technique of radical retropubic prostatectomy used to preserve the critical branches of the pelvic plexus and preserve potency in more than 80% of their patients.

SUGGESTED READINGS

Graham SD Jr. Radical perineal prostatectomy. In Graham SD Jr, ed. Glenn's Urologic Surgery. New York: Lippincott (in press).

Hinman F Jr. Atlas of Urosurgical Anatomy. Philadelphia: WB Saunders, 1993.

McNeal JE. The prostate and prostatic urethra: A morphologic study. J Urol 104:443, 1970.

McNeal JE. The zonal anatomy of the prostate. Prostate 2:35, 1981.

Myers RP. Improving exposure of the prostate in radical retropubic prostatectomy: Longitudinal branching of the deep venous plexus. J Urol 142:1282-1284, 1987.

Tanagho EA. The anatomy and physiology of micturition. Surg Gynecol Obstet 5:3, 1978.

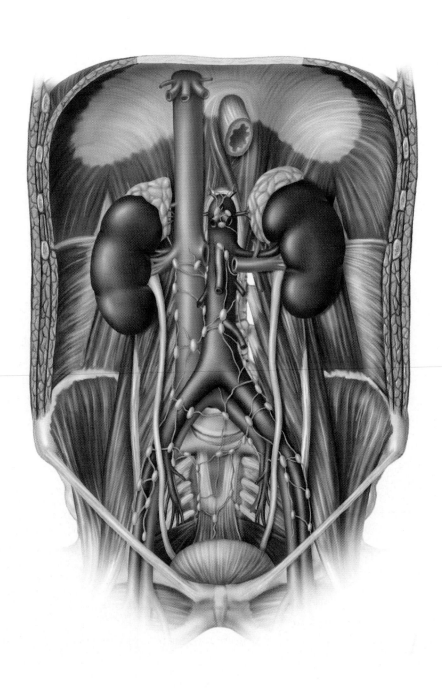

Retroperitoneum

Roger S. Foster, Jr., M.D., and John E. Skandalakis, M.D., Ph.D.

Surgical Applications

R etroperitoneal soft tissue sarcomas are uncommon tumors, comprising 10% to 20% of all soft tissue sarcomas in adults. Of the malignancies arising in the retroperitoneal space but not from the kidneys or adrenal glands, soft tissue sarcomas account for 40% to 70%. Lymphomas account for 15% to 30% of the total, and the less common tumors such as paragangliomas and malignant teratomas account for the remainder. The most frequent histologic types of retroperitoneal sarcoma are liposarcoma and leiomyosarcoma, followed by fibrosarcoma and malignant fibrous histiocytoma. Less common histologic types include malignant peripheral nerve tumor, lymphangiosarcoma, rhabdomyosarcoma, and hemangioendothelioma.

Soft tissue sarcomas arising in the retroperitoneal space present a challenge to the surgeon because they tend to grow silently to a large size before detection, tend to invade adjacent organs, and the anatomic location tends to limit the surgeon's ability to resect them with adequate margin. Chemotherapy for soft tissue sarcomas is of limited effectiveness, and therapeutic doses of radiation therapy are difficult to deliver because of the limited tolerance of the visceral organs. Thus, despite the difficulties of surgical resection, aggressive complete or near complete resection is the mainstay of current treatment. Survival is related to the extent of resection. Unresected or unresectable disease is uniformly fatal. Complete resection of retroperitoneal sarcomas leads to a 5-year survival rate of more than 50%, and even partial resection (defined as resection of more than 80% to 90% of the tumor) has led to a 5-year survival rate of more than 40%. Additional patients will die of recurrent disease after 5 years. Patients with recurrent local disease without evidence of distant metastases are candidates for aggressive repeat resection, which may lead to 5-year survival rate after repeat resection of approximately 20%.

It is important that the surgeon who performs the first definitive resection be prepared to carry out the widest possible resection, with removal of adjacent organs as necessary to obtain a clear margin. Breaking into and spilling the tumor leads to multifocal local recurrence that is unlikely to be resectable. An en bloc resection of the sarcoma may require resection of any invaded adjacent organs such as the kidney and adrenal gland, colon, small intestine, pancreas, stomach, or pelvic organs. Complete resection of a retroperitoneal sarcoma requires removal of one or more involved organs in more than three fourths of procedures. In a few patients resection of portions of the abdominal wall, diaphragm, or pelvic wall is necessary. Portions of the vena cava or iliac vessels may require resection. Involvement of the aorta or superior mesenteric vessels tends to limit the margin of resection. Reports from experienced surgeons indicate that complete excision (no clinical evidence of residual tumor) can be accomplished in one half to two thirds of patients with tumor deemed resectable on preoperative evaluation. If it appears that a generous margin of resected tissue cannot be obtained, preoperative radiation therapy, especially for higher grade soft tissue sarcomas, offers the best opportunity to sterilize the periphery of the tumor prior to resection.

Anatomic Basis of Tumor Surgery

SURGICAL ANATOMY
Retroperitoneal Space

The retroperitoneal space is the area of the posterior abdominal wall located between the posterior parietal peritoneum and the posterior part of the transversalis fascia. Within this space are embryologically related organs such as the adrenal glands, kidneys, and ureters, referred to as the retroperitoneal viscera. Also within the retroperitoneal space is the neurovascular apparatus, formed by the aorta and its branches, the inferior vena cava and its tributaries, the lymphatic vessels and lymph nodes, and the lumbar plexus with its branches and the sympathetic trunk.

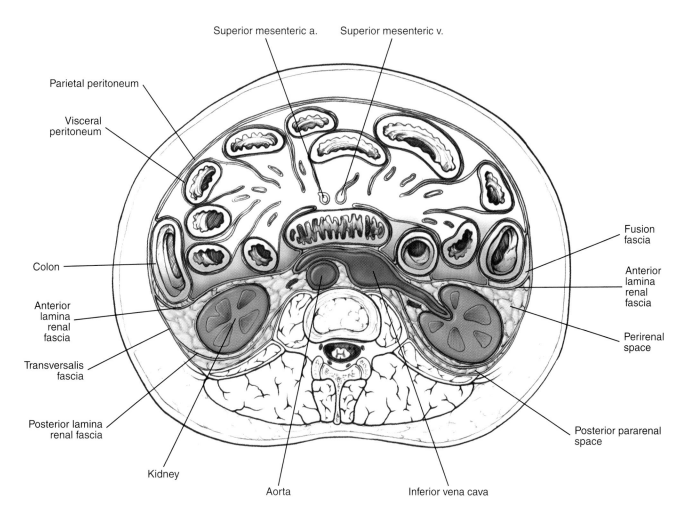

The parietal peritoneum is in continuity with the visceral peritoneum and vice versa. Because the parietal peritoneum is not fixed or fused, it can be readily dissected. Only the transversalis fascia is fixed. It is fused with the subdiaphragmatic fascia above, the psoas fascia laterally, and the fascia of the quadratus lumborum to form the anterior lamina of the lumbodorsal fascia. The transversalis fascia attaches medially to the vertebrae's spinous processes and later continues with the iliac and the fascia of the pelvic diaphragm.

Several separate spaces (or compartments) can be defined within the greater retroperitoneal space. The fascial layers and the spaces in the renal area are, from anterior to posterior, the peritoneum, anterior pararenal space (fat), anterior lamina of Gerota's fascia, perirenal space (fat, adrenal, kidney, ureter), posterior lamina of Gerota's fascia, posterior pararenal space (fat), and lumbodorsal fasciae and fasciae of the psoas muscle.

Boundaries

The retroperitoneal space is covered anteriorly by the parietal peritoneum and posteriorly by the transversalis fascia. The retroperitoneal space extends from the twelfth thoracic vertebra and the twelfth rib cephalad to the base of the sacrum, the iliac crest, and the pelvic diaphragm caudally. The lateral borders may be considered to be extended from an imaginary line from the tip of the twelfth rib down to the junction of the anterior half of the iliac crest with the posterior half of the iliac crest.

Compartments

Within the upper retroperitoneal space are the three compartments created by the renal fascia of Gerota: anterior pararenal, posterior pararenal, and perirenal. The lower retroperitoneal space is contiguous with the two areas that must be considered from a surgical standpoint: the iliac fossa and the pelvic wall of the true pelvis.

The renal fascia has a peculiar pathway. It covers the fat of the anterior and posterior surfaces of the kidney, having some fixation medially with the adventitial coverings of the renal vessels, with extension to the aorta on the left and the inferior vena cava on the right. Above and toward the adrenal glands and diaphragm the anterior and posterior laminae unite, or perhaps fuse, and finally join the subdiaphragmatic fascia. However, at the upper pole of the kidney a fascia separates the adrenal gland from the kidney.

Psoas Muscle

For all practical purposes the psoas muscle extends from the posterior mediastinum to the thigh. On its way downward, it is closely associated with the perirenal space and the posterior pararenal space.

Lymphatic Drainage

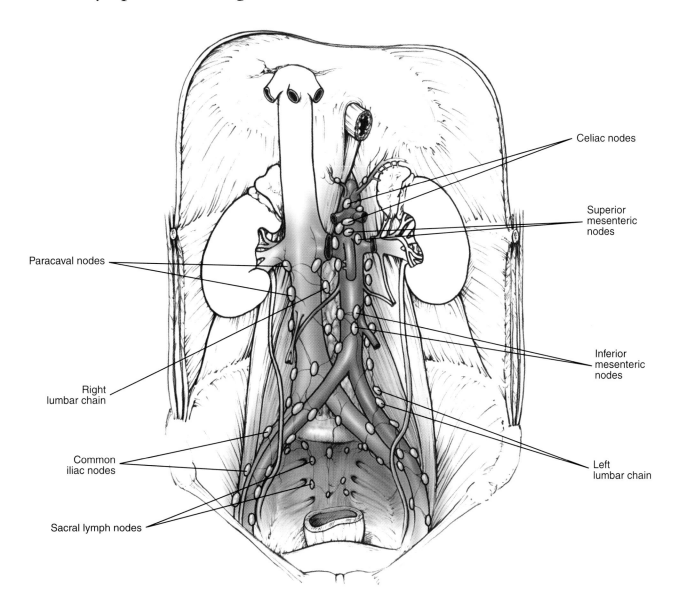

The retroperitoneal lymph nodes form a rich and extensive chain from the inguinal ligament to the diaphragm and the posterior mediastinal nodes. The nodes are classified simply, logically, and anatomically as follows:

Aortic group
    Preaortic: celiac axis, superior mesenteric artery, inferior mesenteric artery
    Para-aortic: right lateral, left lateral
Caval group
    Precaval
    Retrocaval
    Paracaval: right lateral, left lateral
Pelvic group
    Common iliac
    External and internal iliac
    Obturator
    Sacral

Aortic Group

One to three celiac nodes are located around the base of the celiac artery. They are closely related to the celiac ganglion and the lymph nodes of the superior mesenteric artery. These nodes receive lymph from the stomach, liver, pancreas, and superior mesenteric nodes. Two or three superior mesenteric nodes receive lymph from the small bowel, right colon, part of the transverse colon, and pancreas. They communicate with the celiac and inferior mesenteric nodes. The two nodes of the inferior mesenteric artery receive lymph from the left colon. The right lateral paraaortic nodes along with the left paracaval nodes form the right lumbar chain of nodes, which may be found around the inferior vena cava. The left para-aortic (left lumbar) lymph nodes are a group of five to 10 lymph nodes that communicate with the common iliac nodes and drain into the thoracic duct.

Caval Group

Precaval lymph nodes are located at the anterior wall of the inferior vena cava. Two of these nodes, one at the aortic bifurcation and one at the termination of the left renal vein, are fairly constant.

Retrocaval lymph nodes are located on the psoas muscle and the right crus of the diaphragm. The right paracaval nodes are found at the right lateral side of the inferior vena cava. The one at the entrance of the right renal vein to the inferior vena cava is the metastatic node for right testicular malignancy. The left paracaval nodes are in close association with the right aortic nodes.

Pelvic Group

There are four to six common iliac lymph nodes, located around the iliac artery. There are eight to 10 external iliac lymph nodes, located laterally and medially, and occasionally anteriorly. The internal iliac lymph nodes are located around the internal iliac vessels. There are one or two obturator lymph nodes, located at the obturator foramen close to the obturator neurovascular apparatus. The sacral lymph nodes are located close to the median and lateral sacral vessels.

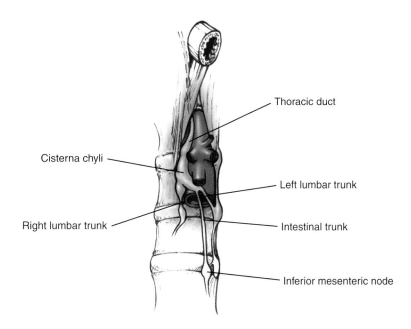

The cisterna chyli is formed at approximately the L2 vertebra by the confluence of the right and left lumbar lymphatic trunks with the intestinal trunk.

Nerve Supply

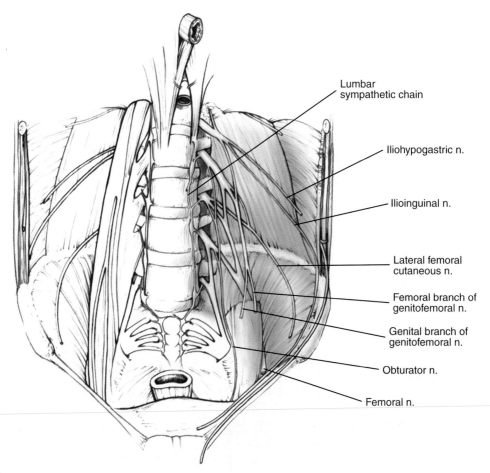

Lumbar
sympathetic chain

Iliohypogastric n.

Ilioinguinal n.

Lateral femoral
cutaneous n.

Femoral branch of
genitofemoral n.

Genital branch of
genitofemoral n.

Obturator n.

Femoral n.

Six nerves are present in the retroperitoneal space: iliohypogastric, ilioinguinal, genitofemoral, lateral femoral cutaneous, obturator, and femoral. All are branches of the lumbar plexus, which is formed by a branch of T12 and by the anterior primary divisions of L1 to L4.

The iliohypogastric nerve, from T12–L1, or L1 only, is the first nerve of the lumbar plexus. It emerges from the lateral border of the psoas muscle. After relating to the quadratus lumborum muscle, it travels downward between the internal oblique and the transversus abdominis muscles. The iliohypogastric nerve produces two branches. The lateral cutaneous nerve supplies the posterolateral skin of the gluteal area and the anterior cutaneous nerve supplies the skin over the symphysis pubis.

The ilioinguinal nerve from L1 has the same general pathway as the iliohypogastric nerve, but on its way downward it transverses the inguinal canal together with the spermatic cord. In the thigh it innervates the triangle of Scarpa, part of the scrotal or labia majora skin.

The genitofemoral nerve from the L1 and L2 nerves pierces the psoas muscle anteriorly. It gives origin to two branches: the genital branch and the femoral branch. The genital branch, within the inguinal canal, is related to the ilio-pubic tract and supplies the cremaster muscle and part of the scrotal skin. The femoral branch passes below the inguinal ligament and participates in innervation of the skin of the triangle of Scarpa.

The lateral femoral cutaneous nerve from L2 and L3 emerges from the lateral border of the psoas muscle approximately at the area of the fourth lumbar vertebra. After perforating the inguinal ligament close to the superoanterior iliac spine, it passes into the lateral aspect of the thigh.

The obturator nerve from L2 to L4 emerges from the medial border of the psoas muscle. It enters together with the obturator vessels into the obturator foramen, continuing downward to innervate the medial part of the thigh.

The femoral nerve from L2 to L4 emerges from the lateral border of the psoas muscle. It passes under the inguinal ligament and is closely associated with the iliopsoas muscle.

The lumbar sympathetic chain lies right and left along the medial border of the psoas muscle. It is located anterior to the lumbar vertebrae and is covered by the inferior vena cava on the right and the right para-aortic nodes on the left. It is formed by four ganglia, which vary in size and position. They communicate with each other and with the thoracic trunk above and the pelvic trunk below.

Iliac Fossa

The iliac fossa is lined by peritoneum, which covers subperitoneal fat. It continues medially to the retroperitoneal space (lumbar area), then downward to the pelvic wall and to the anterior abdominal wall. Just behind the subperitoneal fat is the transversalis fascia. This narrow space is the home of the right and left iliac vessels, right and left ureters, right and left genitofemoral nerves, right and left gonadal vessels, and lymphatic vessels and lymph nodes.

The floor of the iliac fossa is the iliacus muscle, covered by the iliac fascia. On the way up after covering the psoas major muscle, the fascia is attached to the brim of the pelvis or to the linea terminalis. On the way down, it is attached to the inguinal ligament together with the transversalis fascia.

SURGICAL APPLICATIONS

Retroperitoneal sarcomas are almost always best approached by the transperitoneal route. The surgical anatomy of these routes is described, with presentation of the surgical anatomy related to excision of sarcomas in the right and left lumbar areas.

Biopsy

Biopsy is frequently important to distinguish whether a lesion is (1) a soft tissue sarcoma for which surgical resection is the primary therapy, (2) a lymphoma for which surgical resection is inappropriate, or (3) an embryonal rhabdomyosarcoma or testicular carcinoma for which preoperative chemotherapy is appropriate. Attention to the technique of biopsy is critical to provide adequate material for pathologic diagnosis and to minimize the chance of tumor seeding of uninvolved tissue or the peritoneum.

A representative piece of tumor needs to be provided to the pathologist. Areas of necrosis or hemorrhage should be excluded.

Needle Biopsy

Core needle biopsy may be the simplest way to obtain a tissue sample, but the small size of the sample may limit the pathologist's ability to provide a diagnosis. Formerly there was a tendency to avoid needle biopsy, but when a representative sample of tissue is obtained experienced pathologists are becoming increasingly capable of providing an accurate diagnosis. Needle biopsy may be particularly useful for the diagnosis of obviously unresectable tumors, for establishing that a retroperitoneal tumor is something other than a soft tissue sarcoma, or for confirming the histologic features of a recurrent tumor.

Concern has been raised that needle biopsy will contaminate normal tissue planes or the peritoneal cavity. The concern is real, but the risk is probably small. Open biopsy of retroperitoneal sarcomas probably carries the same or greater risk of contamination. If the diagnosis can be established with percutaneous needle biopsy, the possibility of preliminary general anesthesia and laparotomy simply to establish a tissue diagnosis is averted.

Open Biopsy

If it is not possible to obtain a definitive diagnosis of soft tissue sarcoma with percutaneous needle biopsy, incisional biopsy with frozen-section analysis is carried out at laparotomy. The pathologist may be unable to give a definitive reading from frozen-section analysis. Sometimes other malignancies such as lymphomas, malignant germ cell tumors, and anaplastic carcinomas may be distinguishable only on permanent sections.

The open biopsy of a retroperitoneal tumor is planned so that there is the least chance of spillage into the peritoneal cavity and so that any tissue plane contamination is excised in the definitive operation. A 1 × 1 × 1 cm portion of nonnecrotic tumor should provide the pathologist with adequate material. Prior to obtaining the biopsy the area is packed off with sterile sponges to catch any tumor spillage. After the biopsy, meticulous hemostasis is obtained and the area cauterized.

Resection of Left-Sided Retroperitoneal Sarcoma

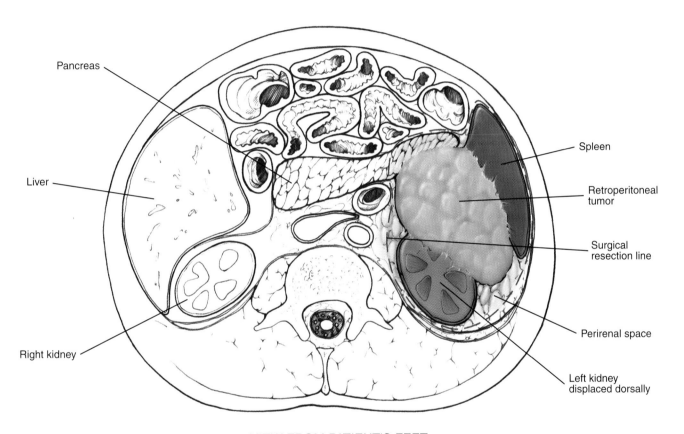

VIEW FROM PATIENT'S FEET

Computed tomography (CT) scans or magnetic resonance imaging (MRI) studies will suggest the extent of involvement of adjacent organs. The retroperitoneal sarcoma shown involves the spleen, pancreas, and kidney. There is no obvious involvement of the colon or colonic mesentery; however, preoperative bowel preparation is carried out in case colonic resection is necessary.

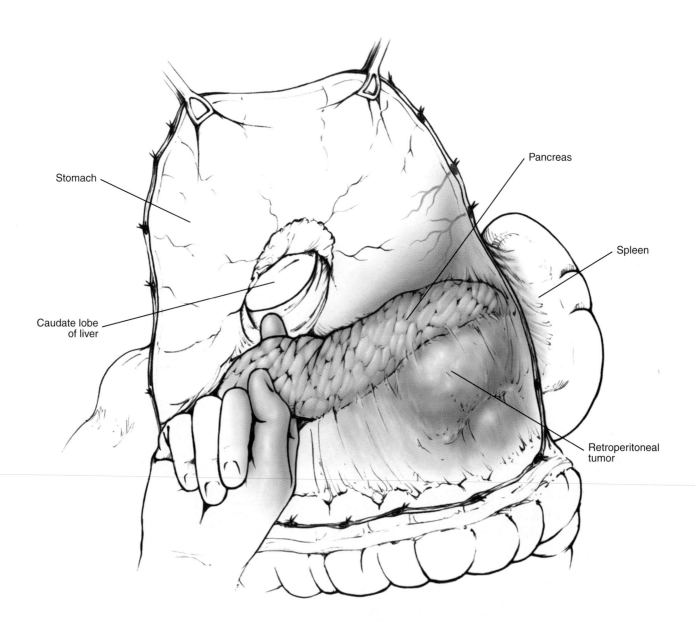

Stomach

Pancreas

Spleen

Caudate lobe
of liver

Retroperitoneal
tumor

After a long midline incision is made, general exploration of the abdomen is carried out. The greater omentum is dissected from the transverse colon, the vasa brevia from the spleen to the stomach are divided, and the uninvolved stomach is retracted superiorly to expose the lesser sac. The retroperitoneal sarcoma has displaced the pancreas superiorly. The spleen and pancreas are adherent to the tumor. The tumor is lateral to the aorta, and the colon and colonic mesentery are free from tumor involvement.

The left colon is freed laterally by incision along the white line of the peritoneal reflection. After division of the splenocolic ligament and the ligament of Treitz, the left colon and the duodenum are swept medially. Palpation of the retroperitoneum reconfirms that the aorta is free, but there is firm adherence of the sarcoma to the kidney.

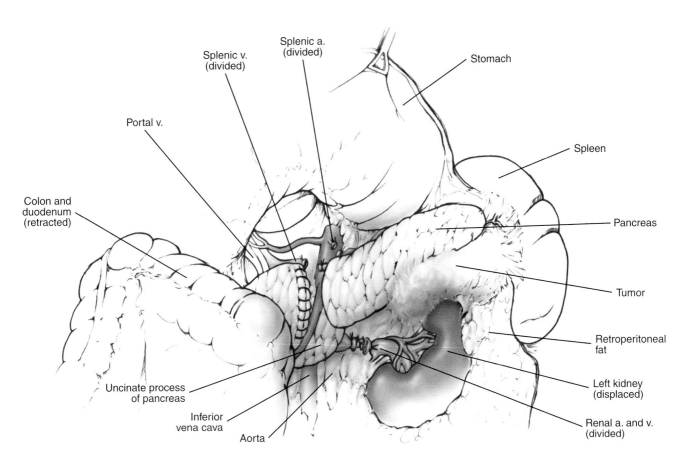

At the left lateral border of the aorta the splenic artery and vein are isolated and divided. The pancreas is transected, and if possible the pancreatic duct is identified and individually ligated. The renal artery and vein are ligated and divided, as are the ureter and gonadal vein. The lateral peritoneal attachments of the spleen are divided, and the spleen and tail of the pancreas are mobilized inferiorly.

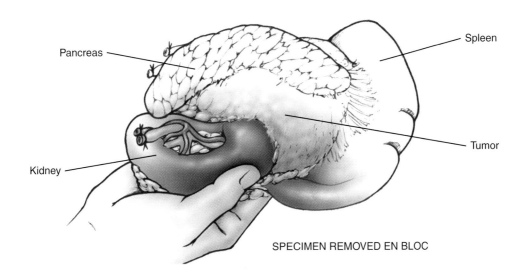

SPECIMEN REMOVED EN BLOC

With blunt dissection in the retroperitoneal plane behind the kidney and the sarcoma, the specimen containing the sarcoma, the kidney, adrenal gland, spleen, and tail of the pancreas are mobilized from the diaphragm and posterior abdominal wall and delivered. Additional hemostasis is obtained as needed.

If the mesocolon were involved, it would have been left attached to the tumor mass and the colon mobilized with preservation of the marginal artery. Involvement of the marginal artery or of the colon itself would have led to en bloc resection of the colon with the sarcoma.

Resection of Right-Sided Retroperitoneal Sarcoma

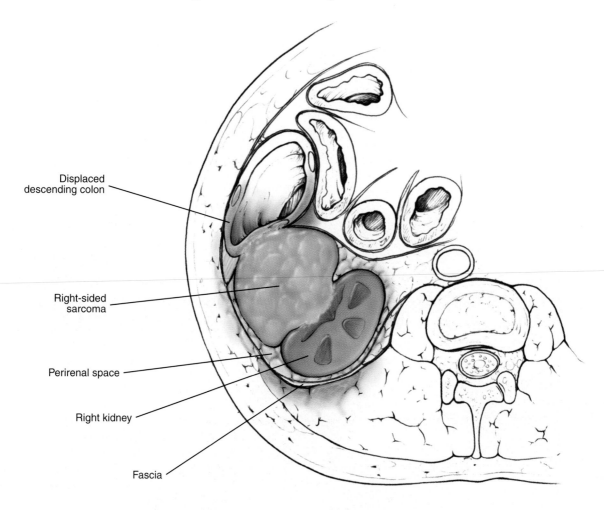

CT scans and MRI studies suggest the retroperitoneal sarcoma involves the lower pole of the right kidney and the right colon. The duodenum and vena cava appear not to be involved with the tumor.

A long midline incision is made. After general exploration of the abdomen confirms the location of the tumor and the absence of metastases, the relationship of the tumor to the superior mesenteric vessels and the vena cava is explored through an incision in the mesocolon.

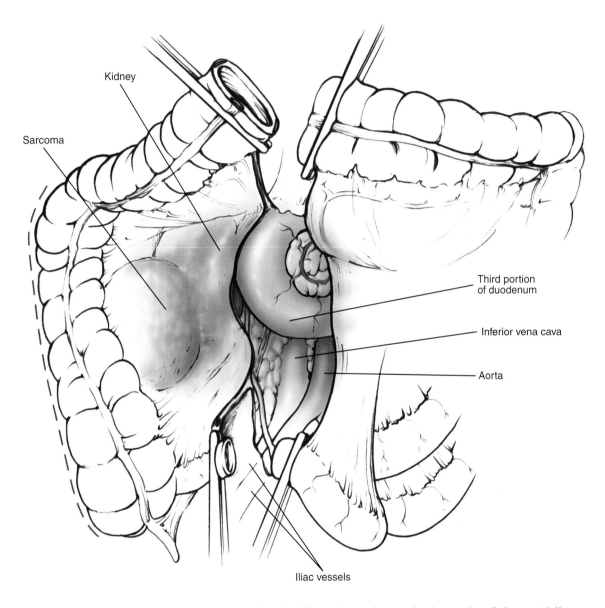

The transverse mesocolon is divided lateral to the right branch of the middle colic artery. The transverse colon and the distal ilium are clamped and divided. The medial border of the dissection is defined by exposing the third portion of the duodenum, the vena cava, and the iliac vessels.

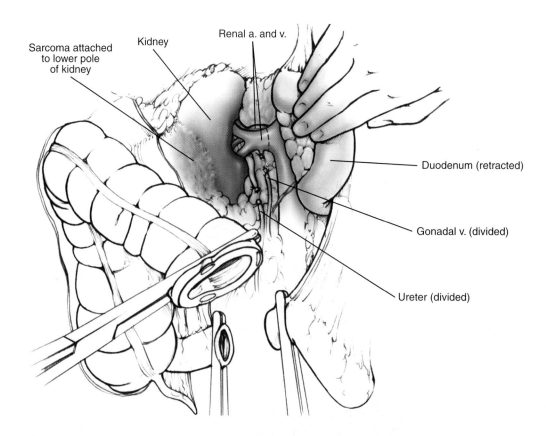

The peritoneal reflection of the right colon is incised, and the hepatic flexure of the colon is mobilized caudad. With an extended Kocher maneuver the duodenum and head of the pancreas are mobilized medially. Attachment of the tumor to the inferior pole of the kidney is confirmed, and the renal artery and vein are exposed, isolated, and divided. The ureter and gonadal vein are ligated and divided.

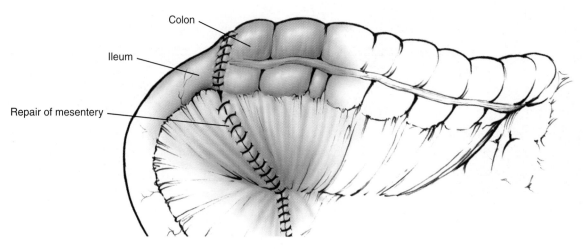

With blunt dissection in the retroperitoneal plane, the sarcoma, kidney, and colon are mobilized free from the posterior abdominal wall. If tumor is adherent to an area of the posterior abdominal wall muscle, that portion of muscle is excised. The procedure is completed with an ileocolostomy and repair of the mesenteric window. After secure hemostasis is confirmed, the abdomen is closed without drains.

Anatomic Basis of Complications

- The most commonly reported major complications of resection of retroperitoneal sarcomas are intra-abdominal abscess, enterocutaneous fistula, and intra-abdominal bleeding. Specific structures that can be injured include the pancreas, small and large bowels, ureter, retroperitoneal lymphatic vessels, including the cisterna chyli, and retroperitoneal nerves.
- Manipulation of the pancreas may induce pancreatitis. Injury to or partial resection of the pancreas that opens the ductal system may lead to a pancreatic leak and fistula.
- Entry into the intestine or compromise of the blood supply to the bowel that is not recognized and satisfactorily repaired can lead to abdominal sepsis or fistula. Sepsis in the area of a major vessel, particularly if the vessel has been injured, may be accompanied by bleeding.
- If an extensive pelvic dissection interrupts the iliac and pelvic lymphatic vessels, permanent leg edema may develop. Dissection behind the aorta on or cephalad to L2 may injure the cisterna chyli or lymphatic trunk and, if unrecognized, lead to a lymphatic fistula. If necessary, these structures may be ligated with impunity.
- Injury to the ureter may lead to hydronephrosis or urinary fistula.
- Injury to any of the six peripheral nerves coursing through the lumbar space (iliohypogastric, ilioinguinal, genitofemoral, lateral femoral cutaneous, obturator, femoral) can lead to dysesthesia or anesthesia over the cutaneous sensory distribution of the nerve. Injury to the femoral or obturator nerves may, in addition, result in motor loss in the anterior and medial thigh muscles, respectively.
- During extensive retroperitoneal dissection it is important to maintain the patient's body temperature to prevent the coagulopathy that can occur with hypothermia.

KEY REFERENCES

Glenn J, Sindelar WF, Kinsella T, et al. Results of multimodality therapy of resectable soft-tissue sarcomas of the retroperitoneum. Surgery 97:316-325, 1985.

Chemotherapy did not appear to improve survival and was associated with major morbidity. Radiation therapy was also associated with major morbidity, and the authors believe it remains to be established that this modality is beneficial in improving survival.

Jaques DP, Coit DG, Hajdu SI, et al. Management of primary and recurrent soft-tissue sarcoma of the retroperitoneum. Ann Surg 212:51-59, 1990.

This review of the 1982 to 1987 experience at Memorial Sloan-Kettering could show no significant effect of adjuvant radiation therapy and chemotherapy on survival. The authors emphasize a concerted attempt at complete resection of both primary and recurrent retroperitoneal soft tissue sarcomas.

Nathanson SD, Sonnino R. An anatomic approach to tumors of the psoas major muscle. Surgery 101:763-766, 1987.

The authors clearly describe and illustrate a technique for the excision of the entire psoas muscle through a retroperitoneal route when primary tumors are confined to the psoas muscle.

Pack GT, Tabah EJ. Collective review; Primary retroperitoneal tumors: Study of 120 cases. Int Abstr Surg 99:209-231, 313-341, 1954.

This classic paper defines the natural history of retroperitoneal sarcomas and outlines the approach to complete or near complete resection.

Sindelar WF, Kinsella TJ, Chen PW, et al. Intraoperative radiotherapy in retroperitoneal sarcomas. Arch Surg 128:402-410, 1993.

High-dose intraoperative radiation therapy plus postoperative low-dose external beam radiation therapy led to a decrease in local recurrence, compared with randomized high-dose external beam radiation therapy, but median survival times were no higher for the intraoperative radiation therapy group. Ten of 20 patients who received high-dose external beam radiation therapy had disabling radiation enteritis vs. two of 15 who received intraoperative radiation therapy plus low-dose external beam radiation therapy, but radiation-related peripheral neuropathy was more frequent among those patients who received intraoperative plus low-dose external beam radiation therapy (nine of 15) vs. one of 20 healed with external beam radiation therapy only.

Willett CG, Suit HD, Tepper JE, et al. Intraoperative electron beam radiation therapy for retroperitoneal soft tissue sarcoma. Cancer 68:278-283, 1991.

Of 10 patients treated initially with external beam radiation therapy followed by surgical resection who also received intraoperative radiation therapy because of microscopic residual disease, seven remained free of disease. The authors conclude that aggressive radiation therapy and surgical resection provide satisfactory resectability rates and local control with acceptable tolerance.

SUGGESTED READINGS

Alvarenga JC, Ball AB, Fisher C, et al. Limitations of surgery in the treatment of retroperitoneal sarcoma. Br J Surg 78:912-916, 1991.

Angermeier KW, Ross JH, Novick AC, et al. Resection of nonrenal retroperitoneal tumors with large vena caval thrombi using cardiopulmonary bypass and hypothermic circulatory arrest. J Urol 144:735-739, 1990.

Bevilacqua RG, Rogatko A, Hajdu SI, et al. Prognostic factors in primary retroperitoneal soft-tissue sarcomas. Arch Surg 126:328-334, 1991.

Cohan RH, Baker ME, Cooper C, et al. Computed tomography of primary retroperitoneal malignancies. J Comput Assist Tomogr 12:804-810, 1988.

Dalton RR, Donohue JH, Mucha P Jr, et al. Management of retroperitoneal sarcomas. Surgery 106:725-732, discussion 732-733, 1989.

Desai AL, Gilbert JM, Charig M. Excision of the inferior vena cava in the surgical management of retro-peritoneal sarcomas. J R Soc Med 87:170-171, 1994.

Eitan S, Szold A, White DE, et al. High-grade retroperitoneal sarcomas: Role of an aggressive palliative approach. J Surg Oncol 53:197-203, 1993.

Karakousis CP, Gerstenbluth R, Kontzoglou K, et al. Retroperitoneal sarcomas and their management. Arch Surg 130:1104-1109, 1995.

McGrath PC, Neifeld JP, Lawrence W Jr. Improved survival following complete excision of retroperitoneal sarcomas. Ann Surg 200:200, 1984.

Neifeld JP, Walsh JW, Lawrence W Jr. Computed tomography in the management of soft tissue tumors. Surg Gynecol Obstet 155:535, 1982.

Schmidt B, Schmiedl U, Kegel T, et al. CT of primary retroperitoneal soft tissue masses. Digitale Bilddiagn 9:114-118, 1989.

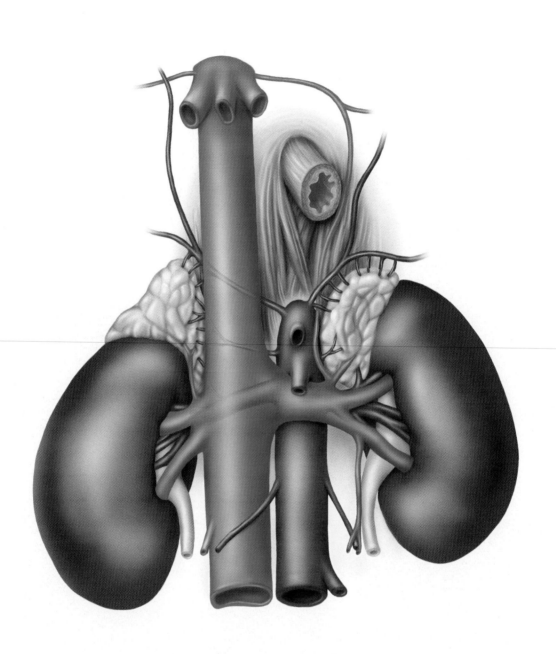

Chapter 19

Adrenal Glands

Open Adrenalectomy

Roger S. Foster, Jr., M.D., John G. Hunter, M.D.,
Hadar Spivak, M.D., and C. Daniel Smith, M.D.

Laparoscopic Adrenalectomy

C. Daniel Smith, M.D., Hadar Spivak, M.D., and
John G. Hunter, M.D.

Surgical Applications

Open Adrenalectomy

Roger S. Foster, Jr., M.D., John G. Hunter, M.D., Hadar Spivak, M.D., and C. Daniel Smith, M.D.

The availability of highly sensitive preoperative localizing procedures along with biochemical testing permits the surgeon to select from a variety of operative approaches to the adrenal glands, depending on the size of the lesion and the pathologic process. There was a time when the anterior transabdominal approach was the standard operative procedure for almost all adrenal lesions. This chapter describes alternative approaches that may provide better exposure for specific types of tumors or permit excision of the adrenal tumor with decreased morbidity. In addition to the anterior abdominal approach, alternative surgical approaches discussed are the posterior approach, posterolateral extraperitoneal approach, thoracoabdominal approach, thoracolumbar approach, and laparoscopic approach. One of us (R.S.F.) has found each of the open procedures useful for specific adrenal tumors, and three of us (J.G.H., H.S., C.D.S.) have performed endoscopic adrenalectomies.

SURGICAL EMBRYOLOGY

Knowledge of adrenal development aids in understanding of the potential locations of heterotopic adrenal glands and nodules of cortical tissue, as well as the locations of extra-adrenal chromaffin tissue.

The adrenal cortex begins to develop during the fourth or fifth week of gestation, when coelomic mesothelial cells located at the root of the dorsal mesentery and the developing gonad begin to divide and proliferate. Concordant with the development of the adrenal cortex is the development of the autonomic nervous system and the adrenal medulla.

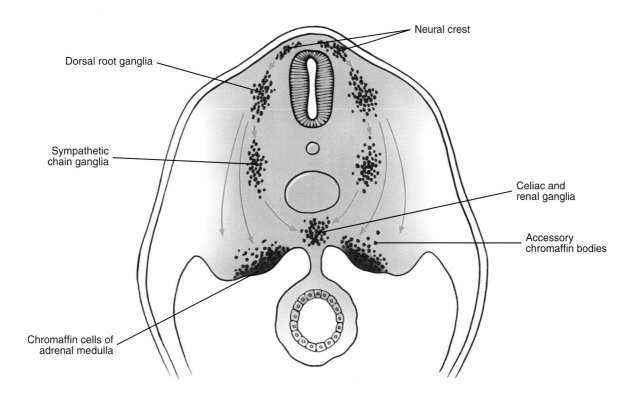

Ectodermal neural crest cells in the thoracic region migrate ventrally to reside on both sides of the spinal cord just behind the aorta. By caudal and rostral migration these cells form primitive sympathetic ganglia from T1 to L2. During migration of the sympathetic neuroblasts to form the sympathetic ganglia, small islands of cells become detached and form independent glandular elements along the vertebral column. Most of these islands of chromaffin cells spontaneously regress. However, a large group of chromaffin cells migrate along the adrenal vein and invade the adrenal cortex, and eventually are surrounded by the primitive adrenal cortex. Preganglionic sympathetic fibers synapse directly on these developing chromaffin cells, which form the adrenal medulla. A second group of neuroblasts form the aortic glands, or the glands of Zuckerkandl. The glands of Zuckerkandl, which have no known function, are located laterally to the aorta at the level of the inferior mesenteric artery. On occasion the glands of Zuckerkandl are the site of development of an extra-adrenal pheochromocytoma or a neuroblastoma.

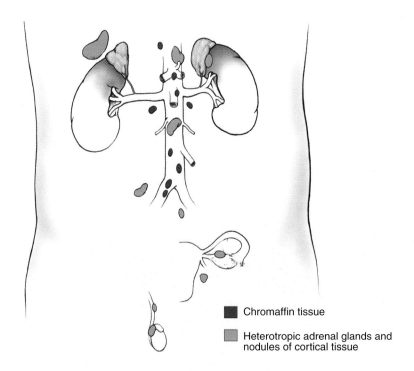

■ Chromaffin tissue

▨ Heterotropic adrenal glands and
nodules of cortical tissue

Heterotopic adrenal glands and nodules of cortical tissue may be found at a variety of sites. Occasionally an otherwise normal adrenal gland is totally separate from the kidney (suprarenal gland). Heterotopic cortical tissue may be found along the course of the aorta, iliac vessels, or gonadal vessels. This heterotopic tissue usually does not have a significant function.

Extra-adrenal chromaffin tissue at the sites of rest of neuroblasts along the vertebral column anterior to the aorta may be the sites of pheochromocytomas, "nonfunctioning" paragangliomas without clinical evidence of hormonal activity, and neuroblastomas.

SURGICAL ANATOMY
Topography

The adult adrenal glands weigh from 4 to 8 gm and measure about 4 × 3 × 1 cm. The adrenal glands, on average, are larger in women than in men. They are composed of two distinct and highly specialized endocrine tissues, the cortex and the medulla, which are embryologically, anatomically, biochemically, and pathologically distinct. The cortex is the larger portion, eight to 10 times the volume of the medulla.

The cortex is composed of the outer zona glomerulosa, the middle zona fasciculata, and the inner zona reticularis layers. The approximate proportion of cortex occupied by each zone is 15%, 78%, and 7%, respectively.

A wide variety of steroid molecules are made in the adrenal cortex; however, only a few hormones are secreted and biologically active. Aldosterone, the major mineralcorticoid, is made in the zona glomerulosis. The zona fasciculata produces the major glucocorticoid, cortisol, and also produces smaller amounts of corticosterone and the weak androgen dehydroepiandrosterone (DHEA). The major hormone produced by the zona reticularis is DHEA, but small amounts of glucocorticoids and estrogens are also made here.

The adrenal medulla, which is surrounded by the adrenal cortex, is composed of chromaffin cells, which synthesize dopamine, epinephrine, and norepinephrine.

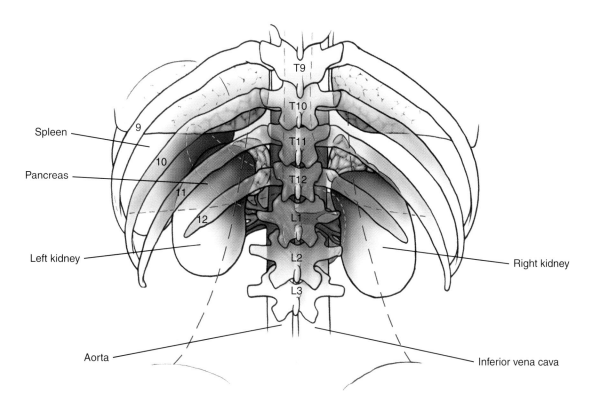

The adrenal glands lie on the anteromedial surfaces of the kidneys near the superior poles. Both the adrenal glands and the kidneys are retroperitoneal. The adrenal glands differ in shape. The left is more flattened and in more extensive contact with the kidney. The left adrenal gland may extend onto the medial surface of the kidney, almost to the hilum. The right gland is more pyramidal and lies higher on the kidney. Because of its shape and location, the right adrenal gland is higher than the left adrenal gland, the reverse of the relative position of the kidneys. Each adrenal gland is covered by a thin connective tissue stroma, capsule-like.

The adrenal gland, together with the associated kidney, is enclosed in the renal fascia (of Gerota) and surrounded by fat. This perirenal fat is more yellow and more firm than fat elsewhere in the abdomen.

The adrenal glands are firmly attached to the renal fascia, which in turn is attached firmly to the abdominal wall and to the diaphragm. Coresponsible for holding the adrenal glands in situ are several violin string–like cords, as well as its arteries and veins. A layer of loose connective tissue separates the capsule of the adrenal gland from that of the kidney. Because the kidney and adrenal gland are thus separated, the kidney may be ectopic or ptotic without corresponding displacement of the gland. Fusion of the kidneys (horseshoe kidney), however, is often accompanied by fusion of the adrenal glands. Occasionally the adrenal gland is fused with the kidney such that separation is almost impossible. Adrenalectomy in such cases requires at least partial nephrectomy.

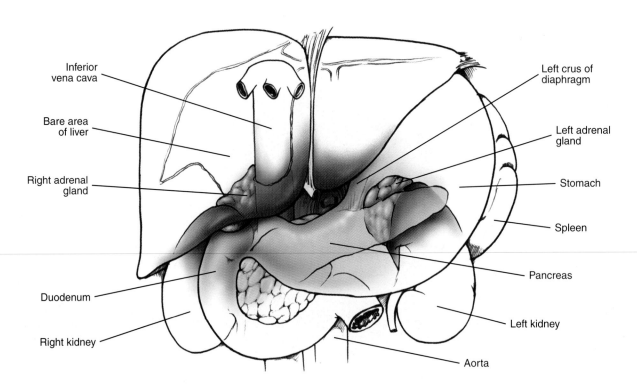

For all practical purposes, each adrenal gland has only an anterior and a posterior surface. Their relationships to other structures are as follows. For the right adrenal gland, the anterior surface is in contact superiorly with the "bare area" of the liver, medially with the inferior vena cava, laterally with the bare area of right lobe of the liver, and inferiorly there is occasional contact with the first part of the duodenum and rarely the peritoneum. The posterior surface of the right adrenal gland is in contact superiorly with the diaphragm and inferiorly with the anteromedial aspect of the right kidney. For the left adrenal gland, the anterior surface is in contact superiorly with the peritoneum (posterior wall of the omental bursa) and the stomach and inferiorly with the body of the pancreas. The posterior surface is in contact medially with the left crus of the diaphragm and laterally with the medial aspect of the left kidney.

The medial borders of the right and left adrenal glands are about 4.5 cm apart. In this space, from right to left, are the inferior vena cava, the right crus of the diaphragm, part of the celiac ganglion, the celiac trunk, the superior mesenteric artery, part of the celiac ganglion, and the left crus of the diaphragm.

Important aspects of adrenal anatomy include the following:

1. For all practical purposes, the right adrenal gland is located posterior to the duodenum and the right lobe of the liver.
2. The medial part of the right adrenal gland often is related to the inferior vena cava.
3. The right adrenal vein is short and enters the posterolateral surface of the vena cava, and thus may be difficult to ligate.
4. The right adrenal is anterior to the diaphragmatic and pleural reflections.
5. The left adrenal gland is located posterior to the stomach and pancreas and medial to the splenic portas.
6. The left adrenal gland is located inferior to the reflections of the diaphragm and pleura.
7. The left adrenal gland is related to the medial aspect of the upper pole of the left kidney, occasionally extending to the left renal vascular pedicle.

Blood Supply

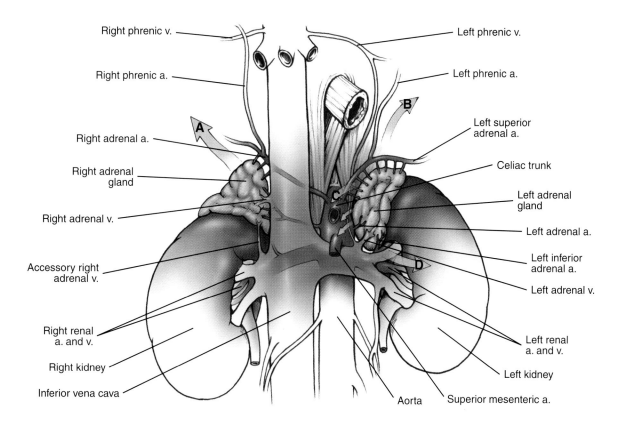

The adrenal glands vie with the thyroid gland for having the greatest blood supply per gram of tissue. The arterial supply to the adrenal glands is from three general sources:

1. A group of six to eight arteries arises separately from the inferior phrenic arteries. One artery may be larger than the others or all may be of similar size.
2. A middle adrenal artery arises from the aorta at or near the level of the origin of the superior mesenteric artery. It may be single, multiple, or absent. It may supply the perirenal fat only.
3. One or more inferior adrenal arteries arise from the renal artery, an accessory renal artery, or a superior polar renal artery. Small twigs may arise from the upper ureteric artery.

All of these arteries branch freely before entering the adrenal gland; thus 50 to 60 small arteries penetrate the capsule over the entire surface.

The adrenal venous drainage does not accompany the arterial supply and is much simpler. Usually a single vein drains the adrenal gland, emerging at the hilum. The left adrenal vein passes downward over the anterior surface of the gland and is joined by the left inferior phrenic vein before entering the left renal vein. The short right adrenal vein passes obliquely to open into the inferior vena cava posteriorly. It does not have any tributaries. Occasionally there are two veins, one having a normal course and the accessory vein entering the inferior phrenic vein. Accessory veins have been encountered several times in our 40 years in the dissecting room.

When using the posterior approach to the adrenal gland, the left adrenal vein is found on the anterior surface of the gland. The right adrenal vein is found between the inferior vena cava and the gland. Careful mobilization of the gland is necessary for good ligation of the vein.

Lymphatic Drainage

The lymphatic vessels of the adrenal gland consist of a subcapsular plexus that drains with the arteries and a medullary plexus that drains with the veins. Lymphatic drainage from both adrenal glands is to renal hilar nodes, periaortic nodes, and by way of the diaphragmatic orifices for the splanchnic nerves to nodes of the posterior mediastinum above the diaphragm. Rouviere stated that lymphatic vessels from the upper pole of the right adrenal gland may enter the liver.

Nerve Supply

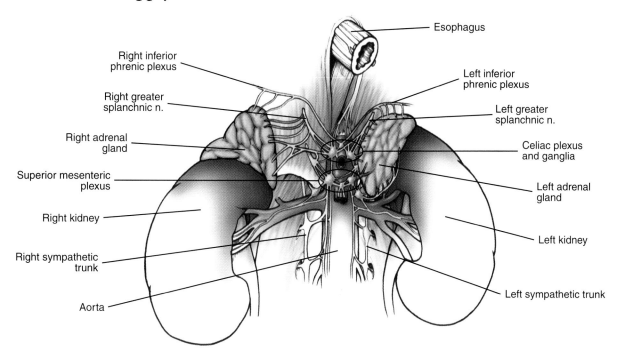

The adrenal cortex appears to have only vasomotor innervation. Most of the fibers reaching the gland from the splanchnic nerves, lumbar sympathetic chain, celiac ganglion, and celiac plexus go to the medulla. These nerve fibers are preganglionic and end on the medullary chromaffin cells. This arrangement is not so anomalous as it might appear; chromaffin cells arise from the same embryonic source as do the postganglionic neurons elsewhere. Most of these preganglionic fibers in humans are nonmyelinated.

SURGICAL APPLICATIONS

The anterior approach for adrenalectomy may be preferred when the adrenal disease is bilateral (10% of patients), the tumor is larger than 10 cm, or the adrenal tumor has invaded surrounding structures. Both glands can be inspected, palpated, or biopsied with the anterior approach. In spite of these advantages, improvements in preoperative diagnosis, such as computed tomography (CT), adrenal scintigraphy, and selective adrenal venous sampling, have increased the use of other approaches. The evolving procedure of minimal access endoscopic adrenalectomy may prove to have the lowest morbidity. The posterior approach has the least postoperative morbidity of the open adrenalectomy approaches.

The posterolateral extraperitoneal approach also has a relatively lower morbidity than transabdominal or thoracoabdominal approaches. The thoracolumbar approach through the chest and then through the diaphragm is relatively well tolerated for large high-lying tumors. Under rare circumstances, thoracoabdominal and abdominosternal approaches may be necessary for large tumors, tumors with nodal metastases, or tumors that have invaded adjacent organs or the vena cava. A few surgeons have developed the skills to remove benign adrenal tumors endoscopically.

Anterior Approach

The incision chosen for the anterior approach may be midline, transverse, chevron, or extended Kocher. The use of a table-attached retractor, such as the upper hand retractor, greatly improves exposure and decreases the necessity of using a thoracoabdominal incision.

Exposure and Mobilization of the Left Adrenal Gland

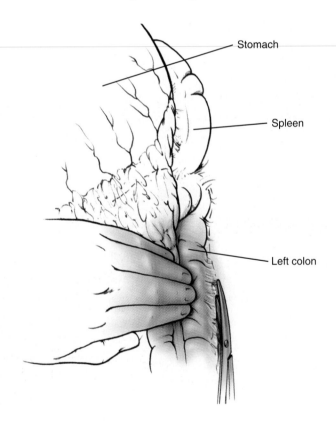

Exposure of the left adrenal gland usually begins with incision of the posterior parietal peritoneum lateral to the left colon. The incision is carried upward, dividing the splenorenal ligament. Care must be taken to prevent injury to the spleen or the splenic capsule, or to the splenic vessels and the tail of the pancreas. The latter are enveloped by the splenorenal ligament.

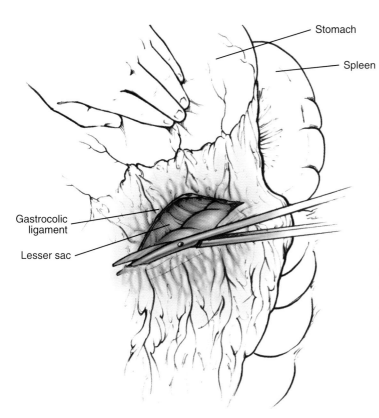

Another approach to the left adrenal gland is by opening the lesser sac through the gastrocolic omentum, which may be incised longitudinally outside the gastroepiploic arcade. Care must be taken to prevent traction on the spleen or on the splenocolic ligament. The ligament may contain tortuous or aberrant inferior polar renal vessels or a right gastroepiploic artery.

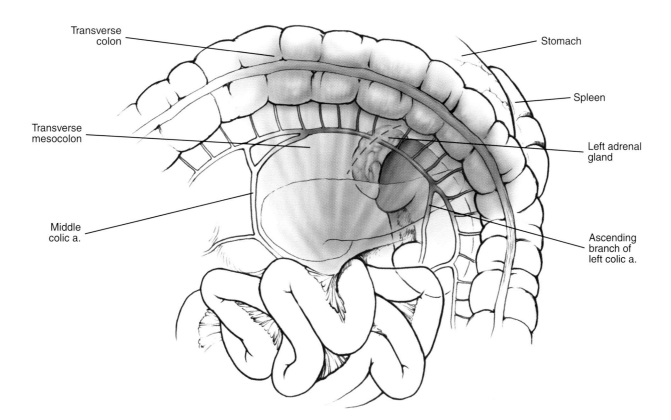

A third approach to the left adrenal gland, which may occasionally be useful when an adrenal lesion is anterior, is to gain exposure by an oblique incision of the left mesocolon. The arcuate vessels may be divided, but the major branches of the middle and left colic arteries must be preserved. Taking care to avert excessive retraction will prevent injury to the wall of the left colon.

Following any of the approaches to get exposure posterior to the colon, the peritoneum under the lower border of the tail of the pancreas is incised medially about 10 cm. The pancreas can then be gently retracted upward, preventing injury. This maneuver will expose the left adrenal gland on the superior pole of the left kidney; both are covered with the renal fascia (of Gerota). The gland will be lateral to the aorta, about 2 cm cranial to the left renal vein. Incision of the renal fascia completely exposes the adrenal gland and permits access to the adrenal vein. If the operation is to remove a pheochromocytoma, the adrenal vein should be ligated first to decrease the release of catecholamines into the circulation during subsequent manipulation of the gland. Retraction on the mesocolon must be gentle to prevent tearing the inferior mesenteric vein from the splenic vein. Although the inferior mesenteric vein may be ligated without sequelae, it is prudent to avoid this complication if possible.

In some lesions with high metabolic rates, such as primary aldosteronism, the adrenal gland is hypervascular and friable; meticulous attention to hemostasis is essential. The adenoma may be disguised or mimicked by hematomas caused by "operative trauma." The surgeon may use part of the adjacent periadrenal fascia to manipulate the gland. Manipulation should be with fine forceps only. Hemostasis from the numerous arteries can be maintained by clips, ligatures, or electrocoagulation.

Dissection should start at the inferolateral aspect of the left adrenal gland and proceed superiorly. The surgeon should keep in mind the possible presence of a superior renal polar artery. The adrenal gland may be retracted superiorly. Remember that the left adrenal gland extends downward, close to the left renal artery and vein.

After removal of the adrenal gland, its bed should be inspected for bleeding points. Surrounding organs, especially the spleen, should be inspected for injury. Splenic injury may be repaired with sutures over a piece of retroperitoneal fat, gelatin sponge (Gelfoam), or Avitene. More severe injury may require partial or even total splenectomy.

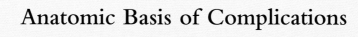

Anatomic Basis of Complications

VASCULAR INJURY

- The inferior mesenteric vein may be avulsed by excessive traction at its junction with the splenic vein. Bleeding is difficult to control, and the vessel may have to be ligated.
- The middle and left colic arteries, or their larger branches, may be severed by sharp dissection through the left mesocolon. A segmental colectomy may be necessary if the blood supply is compromised.
- Superior renal polar arteries are present in about 15% of patients. Their position, superior to the renal arteries, renders them vulnerable. They may be ligated if necessary.
- The left adrenal gland extends down the medial surface almost to the hilum; hence injury to the renal vessels while mobilizing the gland is possible. Careful repair is required. If repair is not possible, nephrectomy may be necessary. Remember, however, that the left kidney may be saved if the left renal vein is ligated proximal to its junction with the adrenal and gonadal veins. If ligation must be distal to these tributaries, venous infarction will occur, and repair of the vein or nephrectomy is mandatory. If nephrectomy is performed, the renal and gonadal veins should be ligated separately. Extensive experience has demonstrated that major divisions of the renal vein at the hilus may be ligated with impunity. The intrarenal collateral circulation will compensate for the segmental venous ligation.

ORGAN INJURY

- Excessive traction on the spleen with tearing of the capsule is the greatest single operative risk in anterior left adrenalectomy. Splenic injury requiring splenectomy has been reported in up to 20% of adrenalectomies. We believe that the splenic injury rate should be much lower. When there is injury to the spleen, repair or partial splenectomy should be performed whenever possible.
- The pancreatic parenchyma may be injured during upward reflection of the organ. This may lead to postoperative pancreatic pseudocysts or clinical pancreatitis. Injury to the tail of the pancreas requires ligation and drainage or ligation, resection, and drainage. If injury to the inferior border is minor, drain; if major, repair and drain or resect the entire distal pancreas and drain.
- Sharp dissection of the inferior medial margin of the left adrenal gland can injure the capsule of the left kidney. Capsular tears need not be repaired, but parenchymal injuries should be repaired.
- Incision of the left mesocolon or excessive retraction of the colon could injure the colon wall or even perforate it.

Exposure and Mobilization of the Right Adrenal Gland

On the right, the anterior approach to the adrenal gland begins with mobilization of the hepatic flexure of the colon. Sharp dissection is necessary to divide posterior adhesions of the liver to the peritoneum. Remember that medial attachments may contain hepatic veins.

Mobilization of the colon will expose the duodenum. The second portion of the duodenum is freed by incision of its lateral, avascular peritoneal reflection. It may now be separated from retroperitoneal structures and reflected forward and to the left (Kocher maneuver).

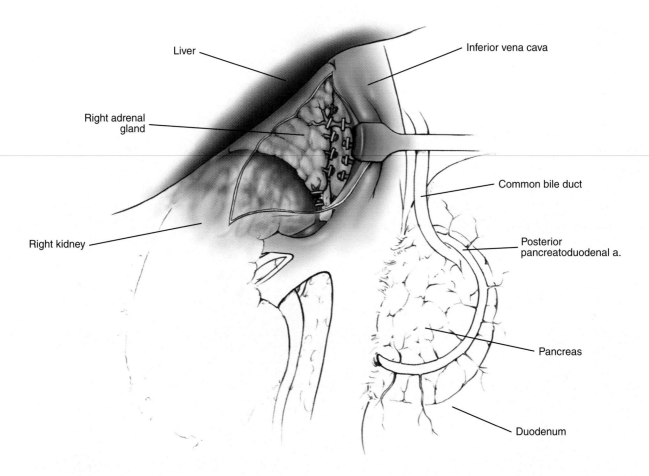

Mobilization of the hepatic flexure of the colon and the Kocher maneuver on the duodenum will expose the vena cava, the right adrenal gland, and the upper pole of the right kidney. The surgeon must remember that the common bile duct and the gastroduodenal artery are also in this area.

Unlike the left adrenal gland, the right gland rarely extends downward to the renal pedicle. The right adrenal vein usually leaves the gland on its anterior surface close to the cranial margin and enters the vena cava on its posterior surface. Rather than attempting to expose the right adrenal vein by retracting the adrenal gland laterally and inferiorly, the vena cava should be dissected away from the gland. To prevent the release of catecholamines, when operating on a pheochromocytoma, hemostatic clips should be placed as soon as both borders of the vein are visible. Excessive stretching of the vein invites hemorrhage from the vena cava.

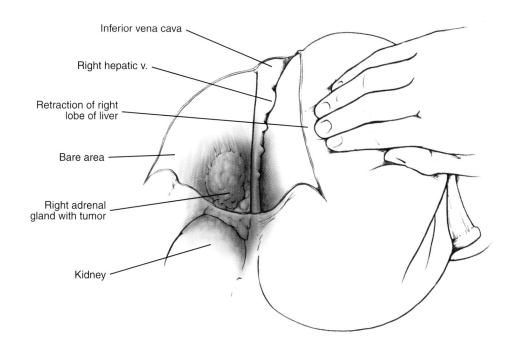

If the adrenal tumor is large or is obscured by the right lobe of the liver, additional exposure can be gained by reflecting the right lobe of the liver medially. The falciform and triangular ligaments are incised anteriorly, laterally, and superiorly. Dissection of the bare area of the right lobe of the liver permits reflection of the right lobe medially. Care must be taken not to injure the right hepatic vein.

Anatomic Basis of Complications

VASCULAR INJURY

- Remember that the medial posterior attachments of the liver contain the hepatic veins. Retract with care. A right hepatic vein may be ligated. Hepatic resection after major hepatic vein ligations is necessary in some animals but not in humans.
- Avoid aggressive lateral retraction of the adrenal gland. Traction on the right adrenal vein may rupture the vena cava; hemorrhage here is difficult to control, and immediate repair is necessary.
- As on the left, the occasional superior renal polar artery lies close to the operative field and may be injured. If injured, it may be ligated.
- The gastroduodenal artery should be identified and avoided during the Kocher maneuver. If injured, ligation is necessary.

ORGAN INJURY

- Injury to the liver may result from excessive retraction. Pressure, cautery, Gelfoam, or Avitene may be used for repair.
- Mobilization and reflection may injure the duodenum and result in catastrophic postoperative duodenal fistula. Avoid sharp dissection, and be prepared to repair any defect.

Posterior Approach
Exposure and Mobilization of the Adrenal Gland

The posterior approach may be used for any adrenalectomy unless a large or ectopic tumor is a strong possibility.

With the patient prone, a curvilinear incision is made through the latissimus dorsi muscle to the posterior lamella of the lumbodorsal fascia. This exposes the sacrospinalis muscle. Lumbar cutaneous vessels must be ligated or cauterized. The usual posterior approach is through the bed of the twelfth rib. Some surgeons have advocated removing the eleventh rib in approaching the right adrenal gland. However, dissecting the pleural fold and preventing pneumothorax is more difficult through the eleventh rib bed.

The sacrospinalis muscle attachments to the dorsal aspect of the twelfth rib should be detached, exposing the rib. The rib must be removed subperiosteally to avoid damaging the underlying pleura. The periosteum should be stripped on the superior surface from medial to lateral and on the inferior surface from lateral to medial. Avoid injury to the twelfth intercostal nerve bundle at the inferior angle of the rib. The nerve is separate from but parallel to the blood vessels. The vessels may be ligated if necessary.

The pleura must be separated from the upper surface of the diaphragm, and the diaphragm should be incised from lateral to medial. Gerota's fascia may be opened, and the upper pole of the kidney identified. Inferior retraction of the kidney will usually bring the adrenal gland into the field. Care must be taken to avoid tearing the renal capsule or stretching a possible superior polar artery.

Dissection of the left adrenal gland should begin on the medial aspect, with clips applied to the arteries as they are encountered. Remember that the pancreas lies just beneath the gland and is easily injured. The last step in the posterior approach is to identify the left adrenal vein, which usually emerges from the medial aspect of the gland and courses obliquely downward to enter the left renal vein. Undue traction on the gland can tear the renal vein.

The right adrenal gland is approached by retracting the superior pole of the right kidney inferiorly; the posterior surface of the adrenal gland can then be dissected free from fatty tissue. The liver must be retracted upward as the apex of the gland is reached. The lateral borders are freed, leaving only the medial margins attached.

The right adrenal gland should be retracted laterally, and arterial branches from the aorta and right renal artery to the gland should be ligated. The right adrenal vein should also be ligated. We recommend freeing up the vena cava far enough to ensure room for an angle clamp should hemorrhage from the vena cava or adrenal vein require it. After removal of the gland, careful inspection for air leaks and bleeding should be made before closing the incision.

Anatomic Basis of Complications

VASCULAR INJURY

- Vascular injury with bleeding can be difficult to manage through the limited exposure of the posterior approach. If necessary, extra exposure can be obtained by extending the incision cephalad, at the lateral edge of the sacrospinalis muscle, and transecting the eleventh rib, the pleura, and the diaphragm. Transection of the tenth rib should give additional exposure if necessary.

- As in other approaches, the superior renal polar arteries, which are inconstant, are vulnerable to inadvertent injury. They may be ligated if necessary.

- A hepatic vein lies just cephalad to the right adrenal vein. It may be torn by excessive traction, and may be ligated if necessary.

- In a right adrenalectomy, the vena cava may be injured by retraction or sharp dissection. Such injury must be repaired.

ORGAN INJURY

- The pleura at the twelfth rib must be identified and pushed out of the way. If perforation occurs, evacuation of air from the pleural cavity by catheter with pulmonary inflation will be necessary. Repair the pleural defect if possible.

- The twelfth intercostal nerve should be protected. Its injury will result in annoying postoperative hypesthesia.

- Excessive retraction may tear the renal capsule. Repair if necessary.

- Remember that in the posterior approach the pancreas lies just beneath the adrenal gland. For details of pancreatic injury, see p. 795.

Posterolateral Extraperitoneal Approach

The extrapleural, extraperitoneal, eleventh rib resection approach is an excellent approach for either left or right adrenal tumors, when the tumors are judged to be too large (>4 cm) to resect through the posterior approach.

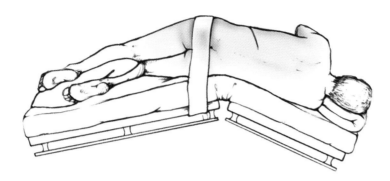

The patient is positioned in the lateral decubitus position with the flank area over the break in the table, with appropriate support in the axilla and a pillow between the knees.

The incision is made over the eleventh rib through the latissimus dorsi muscle and external oblique muscle, and the rib is excised after the periosteum has been stripped. The incision is then carried through the periosteal bed and the internal oblique muscle with care to push the peritoneum and the structures within it medially. With dissection from lateral to medial along the posterior abdominal and diaphragmatic musculature, Gerota's fascia containing the kidney and adrenal gland is swept medially and traction is maintained on the kidney in an inferomedial direction. To maintain the usefulness of traction on the kidney for exposure, dissection of the inferior surface of the adrenal gland off the kidney is the last part of the adrenalectomy.

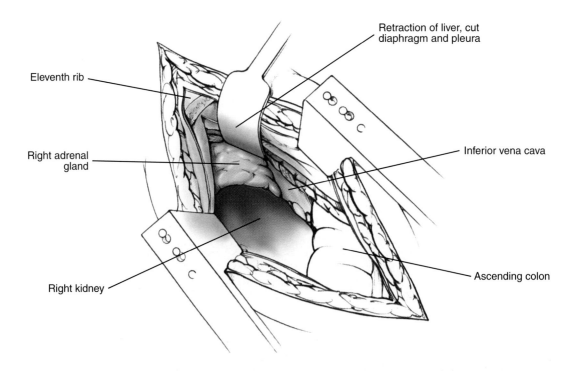

Retraction of liver, cut
diaphragm and pleura

Eleventh rib

Right adrenal
gland

Inferior vena cava

Right kidney

Ascending colon

For resection of the right adrenal gland the liver within the peritoneum is retracted anteriorly and superiorly off the anterior surface of the gland. The dissection is carried from lateral to medial behind the superior portion of the
gland along the posterior abdominal and diaphragmatic musculature. The multiple adrenal arteries superiorly are clipped as traction on the kidney is maintained inferiorly. Release of superior vasculature and attachments improves exposure of the adrenal gland, making it possible to clip the medial arteries and
expose and mobilize the vena cava. The adrenal vein, which is relatively high
and posterior, is doubly clipped or ligated. At this point dissection of the adrenal gland from the superior pole of the kidney is usually quite simple unless a
malignancy has directly invaded the kidney, in which case en bloc nephrectomy may be necessary.

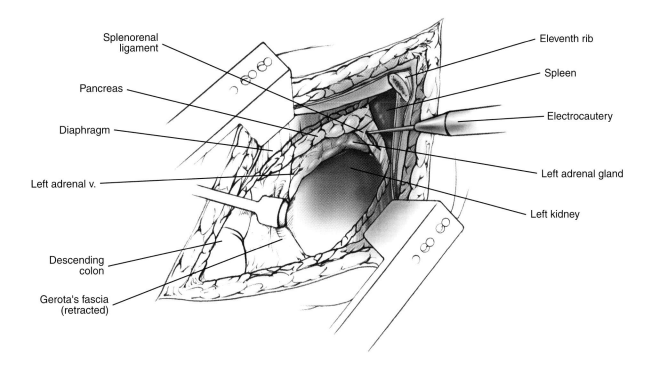

For the left adrenal gland, sweeping Gerota's fascia medially exposes the splenorenal ligament, which is divided so the spleen and pancreas within the peritoneum can be lifted cephalad to expose the anterior surface of the gland.

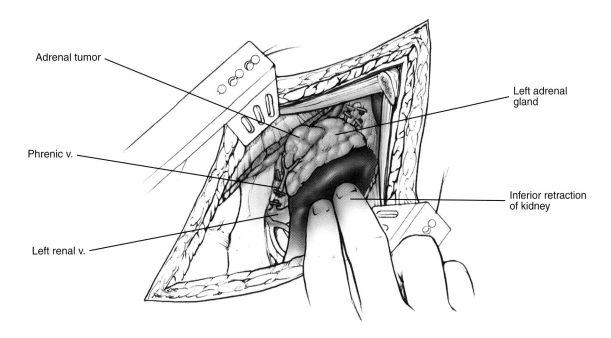

With inferior traction on the kidney, the superior arteries are clipped first. Superiorly and medially the adrenal-phrenic vein should be divided. With further dissection along the aorta and crus of the diaphragm and clipping of small arteries entering the gland medially, the renal vein is encountered, and the adrenal vein emptying into the renal vein is doubly ligated. Then the adrenal is removed from the kidney. The incision is closed without drainage.

Anatomic complications of the posterolateral extraperitoneal extrapleural approach to adrenalectomy include bleeding and organ injury, as with the anterior and posterior approaches. The area of the diaphragm should be inspected for any pleural tears.

Thoracoabdominal Approach

The thoracoabdominal approach may occasionally provide better exposure for a very large tumor of a single adrenal gland. It enables removal of the spleen, distal pancreas, or a portion of the liver if they are involved with the adrenal tumor.

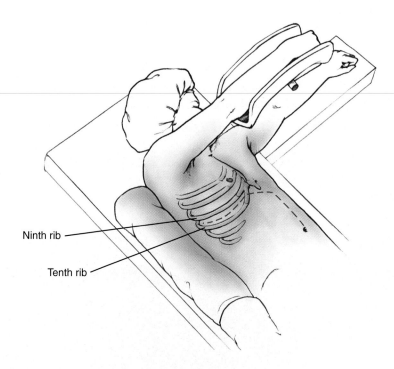

Ninth rib

Tenth rib

The incision extends from the angle of the ninth or tenth rib, across the midline to the midpoint of the contralateral rectus muscle just above the umbilicus. The underlying rib is removed. The pleura may be opened or may be carefully dissected off the chest wall and diaphragm. The diaphragm is incised radially. The remainder of the procedure is similar to the anterior approach.

Most potential vascular and organ injuries are similar to those described for the anterior approach to adrenalectomy. In addition, the lung and the phrenic nerve are at risk for injury in the thoracolumbar approach. An injury to the lung should be repaired to provide an airtight closure. Incision of the diaphragm must be planned to prevent section of the major branches of the phrenic nerve (see pp. 814 and 815).

Large adrenal carcinomas, particularly on the right side, may grow into the adrenal vein with extension into the vena cava and occasionally as far as the right atrium. The tumor is usually not adherent to the vascular endothelium and, with the proper operative approach, can be removed in continuity with the primary tumor in the adrenal gland. The abdominosternal approach can be ideal when there is need to gain control of the vena cava or the right heart atrium and ventricle, or when the tumor is extremely large and extending medially.

The midline abdominal incision is extended into a standard median sternotomy. Excellent exposure to both the subdiaphragmatic and supradiaphragmatic vena cava is provided. If necessary the right side of the heart can be cannulated and hypothermic circulatory arrest induced.

Thoracolumbar Approach

The transthoracic transdiaphragmatic approach provides excellent exposure to the left adrenal gland and on occasion very good exposure to the right adrenal gland when a high-lying tumor has pushed the liver medially.

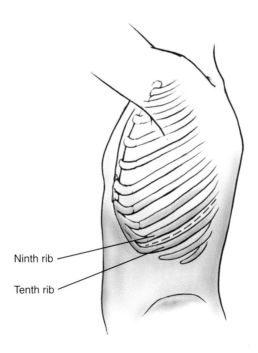

Either an intercostal incision is made or, after excision of the rib, incision is made through the bed of the ninth or tenth rib.

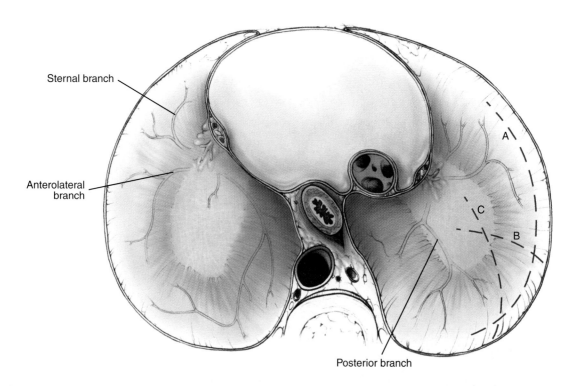

Sternal branch

Anterolateral branch

Posterior branch

The main branches of the phrenic nerves on the cranial surface of the diaphragm are illustrated. The dashed lines indicate the possible incisions that can be used to avoid the phrenic nerves. For the thoracolumbar approach to the adrenal gland, incision B provides excellent exposure. The incision is made approximately 2 to 3 cm from the chest wall to minimize transection of phrenic nerve fibers. Adrenalectomy is carried out much as described for the posterolateral eleventh rib approach.

KEY REFERENCES

Carpenter PC. Diagnostic evaluation of Cushing's syndrome. Endocrinol Metab Clin North Am 17:445-472, 1988.
This is an excellent summary of the workup of patients with Cushing's syndrome, based on Mayo Clinic experience.

Doppman JL. Adrenal imaging. In DeGrott LJ, Besser M, Burger HG, et al., eds. Endocrinology. Philadelphia: WB Saunders, 1995, pp 1711-1730.
This excellent summary of adrenal imaging is based on the extensive experience of a clinician at the National Cancer Institute.

Keiser HR. Pheochromocytoma and related tumors. In DeGrott LJ, Besser M, Burger HG, et al., eds. Endocrinology. Philadelphia: WB Saunders, 1995, pp 1853-1877.
This chapter provides an excellent summary of the physiology and pathology of pheochromocytoma.

Ross NS, Aron DC. Hormonal evaluation of the patient with an incidentally discovered adrenal mass. N Engl J Med 323:1401-1405, 1990.

The recommended evaluation for patients with incidentally discovered adrenal masses is measurement of urinary catecholamines or their metabolites in all patients and serum potassium in patients with hypertension, with evaluation for hyperaldosteronism in those patients found to be hypokalemic. Laboratory evaluations for hypercortisolism and excess androgen secretion are recommended only in those patients with specific clinical evidence of hypersecretion. However, other authorities recommend in all patients that after adrenal metastases, pheochromocytomas, myelolipomas, and cysts have been ruled out, morning serum and evening cortisol levels be measured to detect any loss of diurnal variation.

SUGGESTED READINGS

Bravo EL, Gifford JW Jr. Pheochromocytoma: Diagnosis, localization and management. N Engl J Med 311:1298-1303, 1984.

Chino ES, Thomas CG. An extended Kocher incision for bilateral adrenalectomy. Am J Surg 149:292-294, 1985.

Davie TB. Renal-adrenal adherence. Br J Surg 22:428-432, 1935.

Gagner M, Lacroix A, Prinz R, et al. Early experience with laparoscopic approach of adrenalectomy. Surgery 114:1120-1125, 1993.

Guz BV, Straffon RA, Novick AC. Operative approaches to the adrenal gland. Urol Clin North Am 16(3):527-534, 1989.

Horky K, Widimsky A, Hradec E, et al. Long-term results of surgical and conservative treatment of patients with primary aldosteronism. Exp Clin Endocrinol 90:337-346, 1987.

Irony I, Kater CE, Biglieri EG, et al. Correctable subsets of primary aldosteronism: Primary adrenal hyperplasia and renin responsive adenoma. Am J Hypertens 3:576-582, 1990.

Irvin GL III, Fishman LM, Sher JA, et al. Pheochromocytoma: Lateral versus anterior operative approach. Ann Surg 209:774-778, 1989.

Laimore TC, Ball DW, Baylin SB, et al. Management of pheochromocytomas in patients with multiple endocrine neoplasia type 2 syndromes. Ann Surg 217:595-603, 1993.

Mampalam TJ, Tyrrell JB, Wilson CB. Transsphenoidal microsurgery for Cushing disease. Ann Intern Med 109:487-493, 1988.

Merendino KA. The intradiaphragmatic distribution of the phrenic nerve. Surg Clin North Am 44:1217-1226, 1964.

Merklin RJ, Michels NA. The variant renal and suprarenal blood supply with data on inferior phrenic, ureteral and gonadal arteries: A statistical analysis based on 185 dissections and review of the literature. J Int Coll Surg 29:41-76, 1958.

Pommier RF, Brennan MF. An eleven-year experience with carcinoma. Surgery 112:963-971, 1992.

Prinz RA. Mobilization of the right lobe of the liver for right adrenalectomy. Am J Surg 159:336-338, 1990.

Sarkar R, Thompson NW, McLeod MK. The role of adrenalectomy in Cushing's syndrome. Surgery 108:1079-1084, 1990.

Schwartz RJ, Schmidt N. Efficient management of adrenal tumors. Am J Surg 161:576-579, 1991.

Shahian DM, Nieh PT, Libertino JA. Resection of atriocaval adrenal carcinoma using hypothermic circulatory arrest. Ann Thorac Surg 48:421-422, 1989.

Sheps SG, Jiang NS, Klee GG, et al. Recent developments in the diagnosis and treatment of pheochromocytoma. Mayo Clin Proc 65:88-95, 1990.

Welbourn RB. Survival and causes of death after adrenalectomy for Cushing's disease. Surgery 97:16-20, 1985.

Laparoscopic Adrenalectomy

C. Daniel Smith, M.D., Hadar Spivak, M.D., and John G. Hunter, M.D.

The technique of laparoscopic adrenalectomy was first introduced in 1992 and has rapidly gained popularity, largely because of the many advantages of minimally invasive surgery. Diminished pain, rapid rehabilitation and short hospitalization are all realized with endoscopic adrenalectomy.

There are three vital considerations in selecting patients for endoscopic adrenalectomy. First, malignant tumors or large pheochromocytomas are best treated by transabdominal or thoracoabdominal exposure. The potential reduction in operative trauma is insufficient justification for endoscopic access when radical resection is necessary. Second, the indications for surgery, perioperative biochemical testing, and pharmacologic coverage should be the same regardless of the method chosen for adrenal access. Third, only surgeons who have adequate experience in open adrenalectomy and have mastered the techniques of advanced laparoscopic surgery should perform the procedure endoscopically.

Although there are few absolute contraindications to laparoscopic adrenalectomy, tumors larger than 10 cm should not be approached laparoscopically, primarily because of the difficulty tumors of this size create in exposure and mobilization, rather than cancer risk. Other contraindications are those of any laparoscopic operation: uncorrectable coagulopathy, prior abdominal surgery preventing safe laparoscopic access or exposure, and cardiopulmonary disease preventing general anesthesia or pneumoperitoneum.

Two minimal access approaches to the adrenal gland are described: the lateral transperitoneal approach and the posterior retroperitoneal approach. The transabdominal lateral laparoscopic adrenalectomy, as described by Gagner, provides the best overall access to the adrenal gland and the areas of adrenal exposure and dissection. This approach enables gravity retraction of the surrounding organs and simplifies exposure of the adrenal gland, and enables the surgeon to inspect the entire abdomen and use familiar anatomic landmarks. Although it is less popular, endoscopic retroperitoneal adrenalectomy may be ideal for nonobese patients who have had previous abdominal surgery and for patients undergoing bilateral adrenalectomy. This discussion focuses on the lateral transperitoneal technique.

Endoscopic surgery is an access method; therefore anatomic considerations and recognition of tissue planes, as well as the principles of careful dissection, are similar to those for open adrenalectomy.

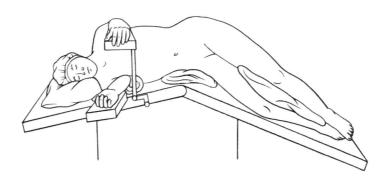

In the transabdominal lateral approach to adrenalectomy the patient is placed in the lateral decubitus position (right or left, depending on the side to be operated on) with knees bent to enable gravity-facilitated exposure of the adrenal glands. In this position, tissue and organs overlying the adrenal glands do not need to be manipulated with laparoscopic instruments, but fall away from the retroperitoneum with the help of gravity. With this gravity-facilitated exposure, the complications and bleeding associated with such manipulation are avoided.

SURGICAL APPLICATIONS
Left Adrenalectomy

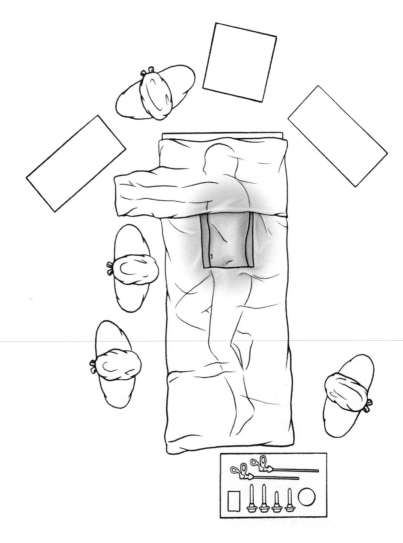

The operating room is set up. After induction of general, endotracheal anesthesia, a Foley catheter and an orogastric tube are placed and the patient is placed in the lateral decubitus position with the left side exposed. The patient is positioned with the iliac crest immediately over the table's kidney rest, and the kidney rest is elevated and the table extended. This maximizes the distance between the iliac crest and the costal margin in the midaxillary line for subsequent cannula insertion. Use of a beanbag on the operating table facilitates stabilization of the patient in this position. The left arm is positioned over the chest on a sling. All pressure points are adequately padded. The patient's skin is prepared and draped so that either laparoscopy or open surgery can be performed.

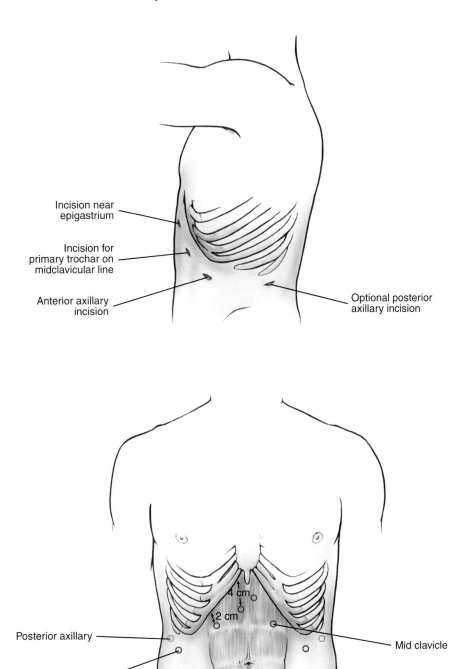

Incision near
epigastrium

Incision for
primary trochar on
midclavicular line

Anterior axillary
incision

Optional posterior
axillary incision

4 cm

2 cm

Posterior axillary

Anterior axillary

Mid clavicle

LEFT
ADRENALECTOMY

RIGHT
ADRENALECTOMY

Cannula sites and uses are illustrated. Preincisional local anesthesia is used. Moderate reverse Trendelenburg positioning is used. Carbon dioxide pneumoperitoneum to 15 mm Hg is initiated with a Veress needle inserted at the midclavicular line 2 cm below the left costal margin (cannula site for the camera).

This primary trocar may be placed with the Hasson technique if desired. A 30-degree angle scope is introduced, and a complete inspection of the abdomen is performed. Under direct vision, two additional 11 mm trocars are positioned about 2 cm below the costal margin near the epigastrium and at the anterior axillary line. Placement of the most lateral trocar requires sufficient mobilization of the hepatic flexure of the colon. A fourth trocar is placed in 50% of left-sided adrenalectomies and should be located in the posterior axillary line.

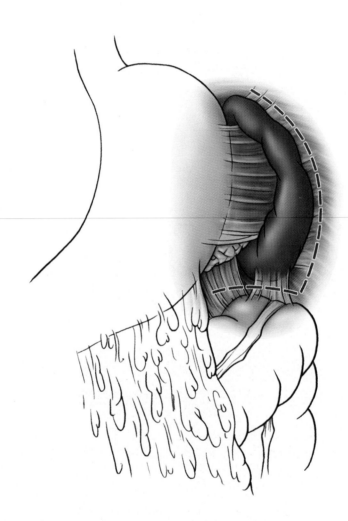

The first step of the operation is to establish the plane along the anterior surface of the left kidney just lateral and dorsal to the spleen and tail of the pancreas. This is accomplished by incising the splenorenal ligament and mobilizing the spleen laterally. Decubitus positioning facilitates this dissection and mobilization.

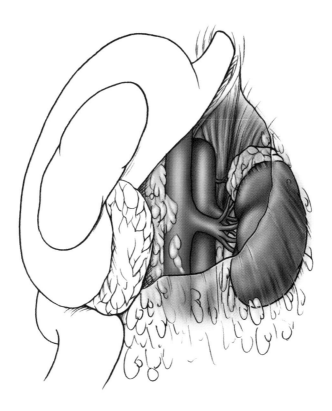

With gravity pulling the spleen medially and away from the anterior surface of the kidney, the spleen and tail of the pancreas are dissected away from the retroperitoneum and the superior pole of the kidney is exposed. The left adrenal gland, an orange-yellow gland nested in the perinephric fat, often is visible at this point.

This dissection plane is relatively avascular. If excessive bleeding is encountered, the wrong plane of dissection is being developed. It is important to continue the mobilization up to the diaphragm and close to the greater curve of the stomach and short gastric vessels. The dissection along the anterior surface of the kidney and adrenal gland continues until the inferior pole and medial border of the adrenal gland are exposed.

The exposure is analogous to opening a book, with the pages of the book being the spleen–pancreatic tail and the anterior surface of the kidney–adrenal gland, and the spine of the book being a line just beyond the medial edge of the adrenal gland. Depending on the adrenal pathology and amount of retroperitoneal body fat, the lateral and anterior surfaces of the adrenal gland will become visible during this dissection. It is important not to mobilize the adrenal gland along its lateral edge too early in the exposure. If this mistake is made, gravity will allow the mobilized adrenal gland to fall medially, preventing visualization and access to the medial and inferior edges of the gland where the left adrenal vein is most likely encountered.

When the retroperitoneal fat prevents clear visualization of the gland, its medial and inferior edges can be localized by ballottement of the retroperitoneal tissue along the anterior surface of the kidney. In even the most obese patients or those with Cushing's syndrome, both situations where localization can be difficult, this technique has enabled identification of the dissection plane between the anterior surface of the kidney and the inferior border of the adrenal gland. Once this cleavage plane is estimated, careful dissection with a hook cautery eventually exposes the inferior and medial edge of the gland. In these difficult situations, some have advocated the routine use of intraoperative laparoscopic ultrasonography to localize the gland. While we have been prepared to apply this, with the techniques described above, we have never needed to rely on ultrasound for gland localization.

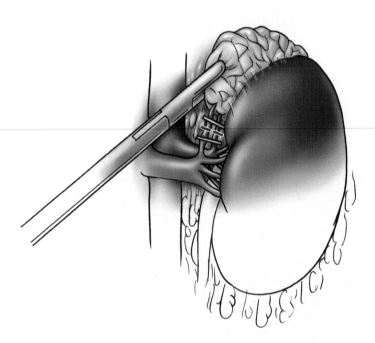

The next step is isolation of the left adrenal vein, typically located at the inferior pole of the adrenal gland and draining into the left renal vein. With small tumors (<5 cm), this is most easily accomplished by first dissecting the inferior and medial aspects of the adrenal gland, staying close to the gland until the vein is isolated and clipped. A right-angle dissector greatly facilitates this exposure and isolation. By staying close to the gland, risk to the left renal vein is minimized. The vein is then clipped with a medium to large ligature clip. We have found a 5 mm clip applier adequate for this ligation. Once the vein is transected, dissection continues from inferior and medial to superior and lateral following the anterior surface of the kidney. For large tumors, early identification of the adrenal vein may be difficult. In these cases, we mobilize the gland laterally and inferiorly to find the inferior border of the gland and the adrenal vein.

Final dissection and gland excision progresses from medial to lateral and inferior to superior. While some have advocated use of an ultrasonic dissector to dissect the soft tissues surrounding the adrenal gland, we have found monopolar electrocautery with a hook dissector the most effective method in the confined space and relatively avascular planes of dissection. The inferior phrenic artery is frequently encountered along the superior edge of the adrenal gland and should be sought and ligated with clips. Alternatively, the numerous left adrenal arteries can be individually secured with bipolar electrosurgery, an ultrasonic dissector, or vascular clips. Dissection continues until the adrenal gland is completely free.

Before specimen extraction, the operative field is carefully inspected for hemostasis. The area is irrigated and suctioned dry. Points of bleeding from retroperitoneal fat are coagulated with electrocautery. Areas of bleeding from visible vessels are clipped.

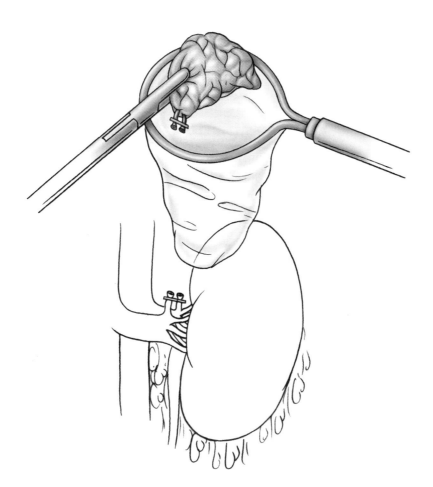

When hemostasis is ensured, the adrenal gland is placed in a specimen retrieval sac inserted through the medial 10 mm cannula. Sac size will depend on the specimen to be removed. The sac must be stout enough so as not to rupture during extraction.

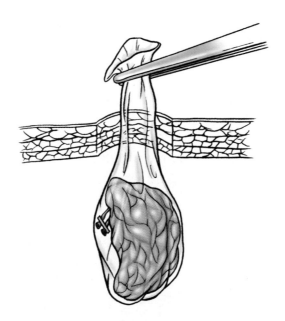

The sac is removed through one of the 10 mm cannula sites. The fascia of the cannula site of extraction may need to be stretched with a Kelly clamp to facilitate removal. For large tumors, the entire incision may need to be extended. The adrenal gland should not be morcellated, because histologic architecture must be preserved for pathologic analysis.

The operation is completed by closing the fascia of the 10 mm incisions with absorbable suture. If a significant amount of irrigation was used during the procedure, it will tend to disperse to the lower and right abdomen, out of the reach of suction. It may be difficult to aspirate all of this irrigant and, when the patient is again supine, it will tend to drain from the lateral cannula site. In these cases, a soft Silastic drainage catheter positioned in the left upper quadrant and exiting the lateral-most cannula site may help control and evacuate this fluid during the first 12 hours postoperatively. This drain is removed on the first postoperative morning. If irrigation is minimal (<500 ml) no drain is necessary.

Right Adrenalectomy

The patient is placed in the lateral decubitus position, with the right side up. Pneumoperitoneum to 15 mm Hg is initiated with a Veress needle inserted at the midclavicular line below the right costal margin (cannula site for the camera). After establishing pneumoperitoneum, the remaining cannula sites are marked. A fourth cannula in the epigastrium is necessary for a retractor to elevate the right lobe of the liver. This cannula site needs to be several centime-ters below the costal margin, allowing the angle of retractor insertion to be par-allel to the underside of the right lobe of the liver. Insertion too far cephalad will create an acute angle to the undersurface of the liver, making positioning of the liver retractor difficult. We use a 5 mm liver retractor, allowing trocar sites to remain as small as possible. The liver retractor can be held by the first assistant or camera operator. We use a table-mounted liver retractor, allowing the first assistant to stand at the surgeon's left side.

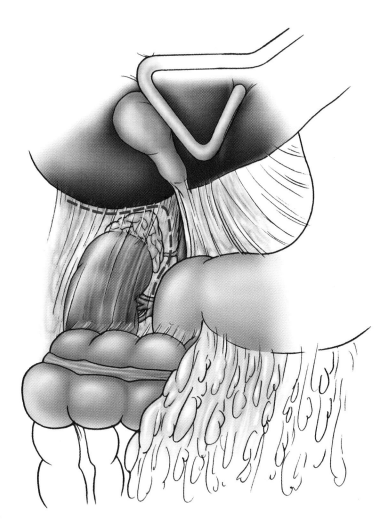

With the liver retractor positioned, the anterior surface of the right kidney and the lateral edge of the inferior vena cava can be clearly seen. The duodenum falls medially with gravity. The dissection commences by creating a hockey stick–shaped incision along the retroperitoneal attachment of the right lobe of the liver and the medial border of the inferior vena cava. This mobilizes the right lobe of the liver posteriorly and allows exposure of the anterior surface of the adrenal gland as the liver is pushed cephalad. If necessary, the hepatic flexure of the colon is mobilized and reflected inferomedially, and the duodenum is mobilized medially, exposing Gerota's fascia and perinephric fat surrounding the upper pole of the right kidney and adrenal gland.

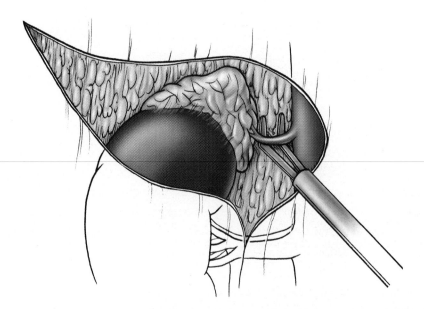

The medial border of the inferior vena cava is carefully exposed while looking for the right adrenal vein. This vein is typically broad, short, and enters the cava at a right angle and slightly posteriorly. We have found using a blunt-tipped right-angle dissector most useful for this dissection. Once the adrenal vein has been isolated, it is ligated with three medium to large ligature clips proximally and two distally. Because of the short length of this vein, the most proximal clip should be immediately at the edge of the vena cava.

After the right adrenal vein has been controlled and divided, the dissection continues laterally, dividing small vessels and attachments until the gland is completely mobilized. As with the left adrenalectomy, the lateral edge of the gland should not be dissected too early, because gravity will cause the laterally mobilized gland to hang over the medial edge, making visualization difficult.

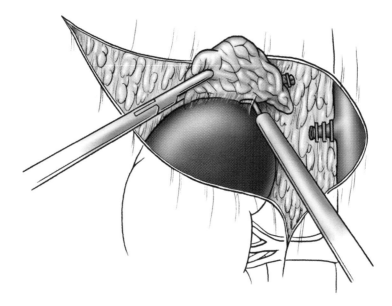

By dissecting from medial to lateral and inferior to superior, the superior pole of the kidney can be used as a dissection plane, and the dissection progresses away from any anatomic concerns (inferior vena cava and renal vein). As with left adrenalectomy, monopolar electrocautery is adequate for the majority of the dissection. Visible vessels are clipped, and the inferior phrenic vessels are commonly encountered at the superior and lateral borders of the gland.

After completion of the dissection, the adrenal bed is inspected for hemostasis. The incision is dilated or extended as necessary to remove the specimen. Trocars should be removed under visual inspection, and the fascia is approximated with absorbable sutures.

Bilateral Adrenalectomy

Bilateral adrenalectomy is performed as described for each individual side. Since right adrenalectomy is at a higher risk for conversion to open adrenalectomy because of the immediate consequences of adrenal vein or caval injury, we perform left adrenalectomy first. Thus the patient has the greatest likelihood of benefiting from a laparoscopic approach. Before repositioning for right adrenalectomy the entire left adrenalectomy is completed, including wound closure and abdominal desufflation (minimizing duration of carbon dioxide pneumoperitoneum). Average operative time for bilateral adrenalectomy is about 5 hours, including turnover time between sides.

Postoperative Care

The orogastric tube and Foley catheter are removed before the patient awakens. Postoperatively the patient is given clear liquids, and ambulates the night of surgery. Pain is controlled with intermittent parenteral narcotics until the patient is able to take oral pain medication. Diet is advanced on postoperative day 1, and the patient is discharged when oral intake is tolerated and pain is controlled with oral analgesics.

SPECIAL CONSIDERATIONS

Debate continues regarding the management of adrenal incidentalomas. Traditionally, nonfunctioning adrenal tumors discovered during abdominal CT or ultrasound for other indications have been managed based on tumor size: tumors ≥6 cm are removed; tumors ≤3 cm are considered inconsequential and require no further management; incidentalomas in the 3 to 6 cm range are typically observed with serial CT and removed if they increase in size. With the success of laparoscopic adrenalectomy and the dramatically improved patient recovery, we are beginning to see more referring physicians requesting adrenalectomy for 3 to 6 cm incidentalomas. It has been suggested that this may be a more cost-effective management strategy, avoiding multiple CT evaluations or the potential for patients being lost to follow-up and returning with advanced lesions later in their course. While this may be appropriate in selected patients, more data are necessary before recommending adrenalectomy for all nonfunctioning tumors 3 to 6 cm in size.

COMPLICATIONS AND OUTCOMES

Bleeding from small vessels that have not been properly ligated or cauterized is the most frequent complication of endoscopic adrenalectomy. Injury to the pancreas, spleen, or colon is also possible. The most devastating injuries are avulsions or tears of the renal vein, inferior mesenteric vein, or even the vena cava. These major venous injuries are extremely rare. When encountering such an injury, the surgeon must quickly convert to an open procedure if the repair is not straightforward and easy. Grasping of the friable adrenal gland should be avoided as much as possible. However, gentle grasping with an oval ring grasper may occasionally be required. Alternatively, placement of EndoLoops around the gland and pulling on the loops may prevent avulsion of the gland.

Endoscopic clips are sufficient for ligating the adrenal vessels. However, laparoscopic suturing should be one of the surgeon's skills. The right adrenal vein usually enters the vena cava on the posterolateral aspect and may be difficult to ligate. Mobilization of the lateral and superior margins of the gland, followed by dissection along the renal vein and vena cava, provides good exposure of the right adrenal vein. It should also be kept in mind that the vein may have anomalous drainage to the right hepatic or renal vein.

We have performed 28 laparoscopic adrenalectomies for a variety of adrenal pathologic conditions, using the approach as described. Outcomes from this small group have been favorable. The one conversion to an open adrenalectomy was in a patient with lung cancer and metastasis to the right adrenal gland that was found to be invading the right lobe of the liver. This patient experienced the greatest intraoperative blood loss in the series.

Laparoscopic Adrenalectomy at University of Cincinnati/Emory University

Number	28
Left:right	14:14

Indications

Hyperaldosteronism	9
Hypercortisolism	4
Pheochromocytoma	3
Incidentaloma	6
Metastasis	3
Lymphoma	1
Angiomyolipoma	1
Other	1

Outcomes

Tumor size (cm)	3.3 (1.4 to 12.2)
Operative time (min)	152 (110 to 210)
Left	156
Right	145
Converted	1*
Blood loss (ml)	62 (20 to 250*)
Intraoperative complications	0
Duration of hospital stay (day)	2.3 (1 to 6)
Postoperative complications	1

*Metastatic lung cancer invading liver (greatest blood loss).

Table 19-1 *Summary of Outcomes of Selected Experience With Laparoscopic Adrenalectomy*

Author	Year	No. of Patients	OR Time (min)	Converted to Open Procedure	Complications	Duration of Stay (day)
Vargus	1997	20	155	2	2 (10%)	3.2
Brunt	1996	24	183	0	—	3.2
Duh	1996	23	226	0	1* (4%)	2.2
Gagner	1996	85	130	2	13 (15%)	3.0
Marescaux	1996	26	200	5	3 (12%)	4.6
Miccoli	1995	25	109	0	0	3.0
Nakagawa	1995	25	254	0	0	—
Smith	1997	28	151	1	1 (4%)	2.2
Total		256	176	10 (6)	20 (8%)	2.7

*Patient died.

Several authors have similarly detailed their experience with laparoscopic adrenalectomy. Those series with 20 or more laparoscopic adrenalectomies are summarized. With nearly 600 laparoscopic adrenalectomies reported in the world literature showing similar results, the feasibility and safety of this technique are proved.

KEY REFERENCE

Smith CD. Laparoscopic adrenalectomy: The new gold standard. World J Surg (in press).

The laparoscopic technique of adrenalectomy is reviewed, including its development and the variety of techniques available. Outcomes of the various techniques are compared with their open counterparts. The lateral approach to laparoscopic adrenalectomy is favored by most surgeons performing this operation; a description of the technique, including indications and outcomes, is detailed.

SUGGESTED READINGS

Brunt LM, Doherty GM, Norton JA, et al. Laparoscopic adrenalectomy compared to open adrenalectomy for benign adrenal neoplasms. J Am Coll Surg 183:1, 1996.

Duh QY, Siperstein AE, Clark OH, et al. Laparoscopic adrenalectomy. Comparison of the lateral and posterior approaches. Arch Surg 131:870, 1996.

Gagner M. Laparoscopic adrenalectomy. Surg Clin North Am 76:523, 1996.

Gagner M, Lacroix A, Bolte E, et al. Early experience with laparoscopic approach for adrenalectomy. Surgery 114:1120, 1993.

Jacobs JK, Goldstein RE, Geer RJ. Laparoscopic adrenalectomy. A new standard of care. Ann Surg 225:495, 1997.

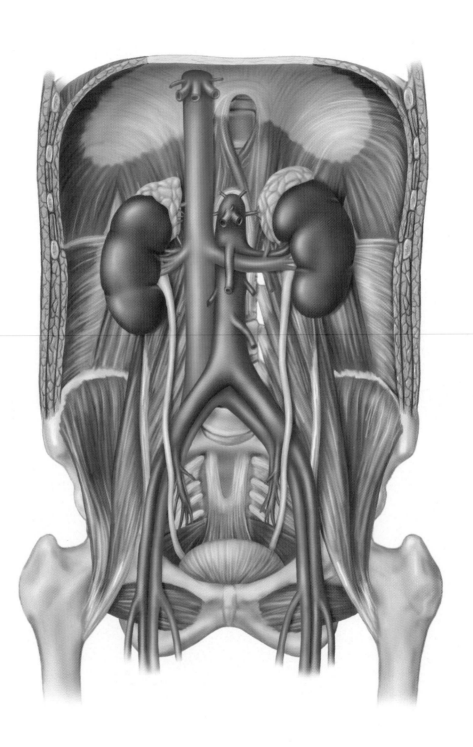

Chapter 20

Kidneys, Ureters, and Bladder

Rizk E.S. El-Galley, M.B., B.Ch., F.R.C.S.(Edin), and
Thomas E. Keane, M.B., B.Ch., F.R.C.S.(Ire)

Surgical Applications

The genitourinary tract is composed of the kidneys, ureters, bladder, prostate gland, and urethra. The first three organs together compose the upper urinary tract (kidneys and ureters) and the upper part of the lower urinary tract (bladder). The main focus of this chapter is on the clinical and surgical anatomy and variants that can be encountered when dealing with neoplasms of these organs. Current techniques for the diagnosis and optimal imaging of various pathologic conditions also are discussed.

Upper Urinary Tract
SURGICAL ANATOMY
KIDNEYS
Topography

The kidneys are paired, reddish brown, solid organs situated on each side of the midline in the retroperitoneal space. Their weight depends on body size, averaging 150 and 135 gm each in the adult male and female, respectively. Kidneys in mature adults vary in length from 11 to 14 cm, in width from 5 to 7 cm, and in thickness from 2.5 to 3.0 cm. Due to the effect of the hepatic mass, the right kidney is shorter and broader and lies 1 to 2 cm lower than the left kidney.

Gerota's Fascia

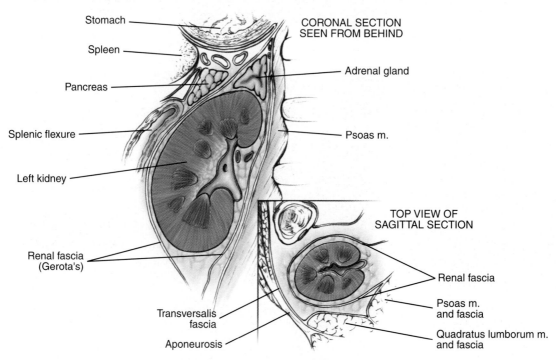

Each kidney is surrounded by a layer of fat, covered by the Gerota's fascia. Gerota's fascia is completely fused above and lateral to the kidney; medially and inferiorly fusion is incomplete. This incomplete fusion is of clinical importance in determining the possible routes of spread of bleeding or infection around the kidneys. Both layers of Gerota's fascia probably continue across the midline, with the posterior layer crossing behind the great vessels and the anterior layer extending in front of the great vessels. The parietal peritoneum fuses with the anterior layer of Gerota's fascia to form the white line of Toldt laterally. During surgical approaches to the kidneys, incision along this line enables the surgeon to reflect the peritoneum with the mesocolon through a relatively bloodless plane and gives access to the renal hilum.

Anatomic Relationships

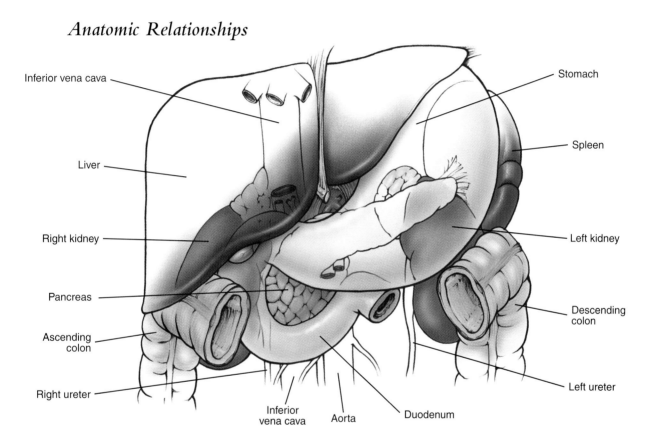

The upper pole of the left kidney lies at the level of the twelfth thoracic vertebral body and the lower pole at the level of the third lumbar vertebra. The right kidney usually extends from the top of the first lumbar vertebra to the bottom of the third lumbar vertebra. Due to the free mobility of the kidneys, these relationships change with both body position and respiration.

The right adrenal gland covers the uppermost part of the anteromedial surface of the right kidney. The anterior relationships of the right kidney include the liver, which overlies the upper two thirds of the anterior surface, and the hepatic flexure of the colon, which overlies the lower third. The right renal hilum is overlaid by the second part of the duodenum. The anterior surface of the kidney beneath the liver is the only area covered by peritoneum. The anteromedial surface of the left kidney is also covered by the left adrenal gland in its uppermost part. The spleen, body of the pancreas, stomach, and splenic flexure of the colon are all anterior to the left kidney. The area of the kidney beneath the small intestine, the spleen, and the stomach is covered by peritoneum.

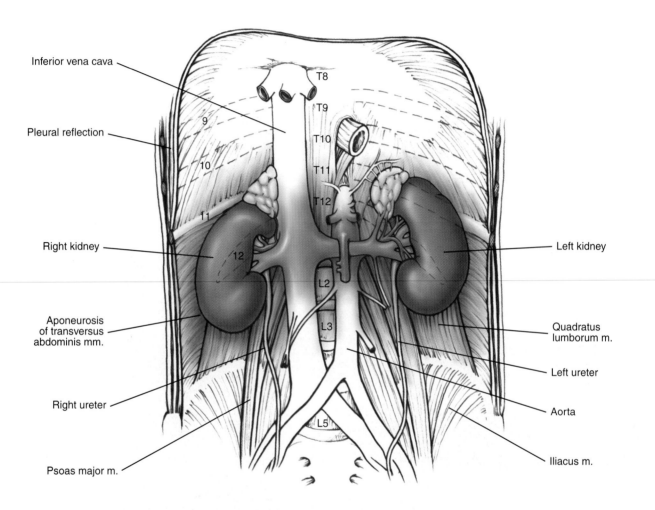

Both kidneys share relatively symmetric relations to the posterior abdominal wall. The upper third or upper pole of each kidney lies on the diaphragm, behind which is the pleural reflection. An operative approach to this area with a high incision above the eleventh or tenth rib risks entering the pleural space. The upper border of the left kidney usually extends to the upper border of the eleventh rib, and the upper pole of the right kidney, which is lower, is usually at the level of the eleventh intercostal space. The lower two thirds of the posterior surface of both kidneys lies on three muscles, which from medial to lateral are the psoas major, quadratus lumborum, and the aponeurosis of the transversus abdominis muscles. The renal vessels and pelvis lie against the contour of the psoas muscle, which tilts the lower pole of each kidney away from the midline. Alterations in this alignment may be seen with space-occupying lesions and should prompt careful assessment.

Renal Parenchyma

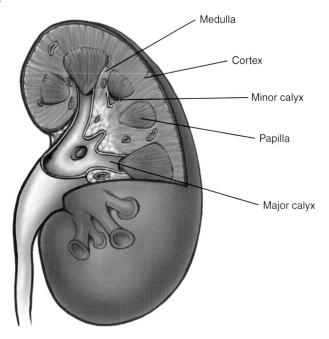

The renal parenchyma is divided into an internal darker medulla and an external lighter-hued cortex. The medulla is composed of eight to 18 conical structures called the renal pyramids, which are made of ascending and descending loops of Henle and collecting ducts. The round tip of each pyramid is known as the renal papilla. These papillae cannot be seen during surgical dissections because each papillary projection is encompassed by a smooth muscular sleeve called a minor calyx. These minor calyces coalesce to form two or three major calyces, which in turn join to form the renal pelvis. The renal pelvis extends through the renal hilum behind the renal vessels and continues as the ureter. Anatomic variations in the renal pelvis are not uncommon. The renal pelvis, which is usually partially extrarenal, may lie completely outside or within the kidney. Occasionally the renal pelvis may be duplicated, with duplication of the renal units. Anatomic variations of the renal pelvis tend to occur bilaterally, which should be considered when evaluating urographic studies to differentiate pathologic conditions from normal variations.

The renal cortex lies between the bases of the pyramids and the renal capsule. The tongues of cortical tissue that extend between the renal pyramids are called the columns of Bertin and, when enlarged, can closely resemble a renal mass. The outer border of the renal cortex should be smooth. Indentations on the cortical surface might represent persistent fetal lobulations, previous scarring, and infection or space-occupying lesion.

Blood Supply

Each kidney is classically supplied by a renal artery and a larger renal vein, arising from the aorta and the inferior vena cava, respectively, at the level of the second lumbar vertebra below the takeoff of the superior mesenteric artery. These vessels enter the renal hilum medially, with the vein anterior to the artery and both anterior to the renal pelvis. Although the right kidney is lower than the left kidney, the right renal artery arises from the aorta at a higher level and takes a longer course than the left renal artery. It travels downward behind the inferior vena cava to reach the right kidney, whereas the left renal artery passes slightly upward to reach the left kidney. Due to the posterior position of the kidneys, both renal arteries course slightly posterior.

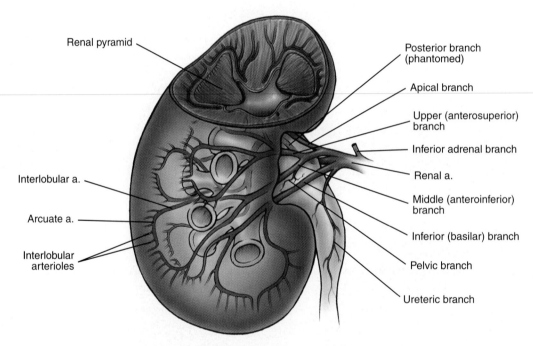

Renal pyramid

Posterior branch (phantomed)

Apical branch

Upper (anterosuperior) branch

Inferior adrenal branch

Renal a.

Interlobular a.

Middle (anteroinferior) branch

Arcuate a.

Inferior (basilar) branch

Interlobular arterioles

Pelvic branch

Ureteric branch

RIGHT KIDNEY, ANTERIOR SURFACE

Two small but important branches arise from the main renal artery before its termination in the hilum: the inferior adrenal artery and the artery that supplies the renal pelvis and upper ureter. Ligation of this branch may result in ischemia to the area of the upper ureter with stricture formation. The main renal artery divides into five segmental arteries at the renal hilum. Each segmental artery is an end artery; therefore occlusion will lead to ischemia and infarction of the corresponding renal segment. The first branch is the posterior artery, which arises just before the renal hilum and passes posterior to the renal pelvis to supply a large posterior segment of the kidney. The main renal artery then terminates into four anterior segmental arteries at the renal hilum: the apical, and upper, middle, and lower anterior segmental arteries. Both the apical and inferior arteries supply the anterior and posterior surfaces of the upper and lower poles of the kidneys, respectively. The upper and middle arteries supply two corresponding segments on the anterior surface of the kidney. Renal vascular segments are also identified.

The segmental arteries course though the renal sinus and branch into the lobar arteries, which are usually distributed one for each pyramid. Each lobar artery divides into two or three interlobar arteries that pass between the renal pyramids to the corticomedullary junction, where they become the arcuate artery. The arcuate arteries, as their name implies, arch over the bases of the pyramids and give rise to a series of interlobular arteries, which in turn take a straight course to the renal cortex, with some terminal small branches anastomosing with the capsular arteries. This anastomosis can enlarge to supply a significant amount of blood to the superficial cortical glomeruli, particularly in cases of gradual narrowing of the renal arteries.

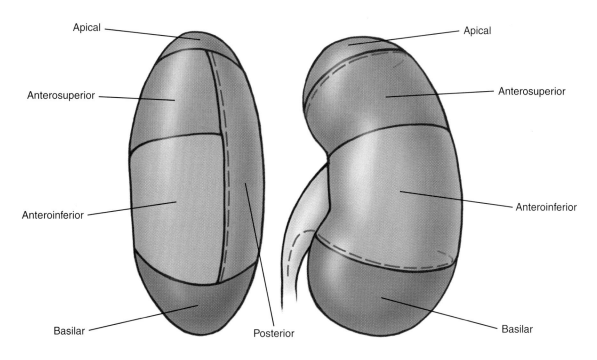

Apical — Apical

Anterosuperior — Anterosuperior

Anteroinferior — Anteroinferior

Basilar — Posterior — Basilar

LEFT KIDNEY, VASCULAR SEGMENTS

Of importance to the urologist is the relatively avascular plane on the posterior surface of the kidney located approximately one third the distance between the posterior and anterior surfaces. Incision through this line toward the renal pelvis is unlikely to traverse any major vessels. Similarly, transverse incisions are usually possible between the posterior segmental circulation and polar segments supplied by the apical or lower segmental arteries of the anterior circulation to gain access to upper or lower pole calyces.

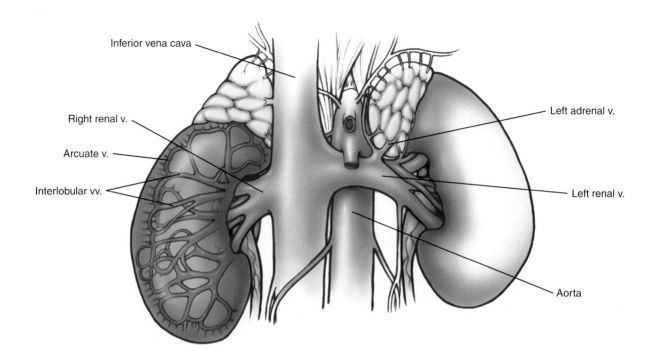

The renal cortex is drained by the interlobular veins, which, unlike the renal arteries, anastomose freely with the arcuate veins at the base of the medullary pyramids and with the capsular and perirenal veins on the surface of the kidney. The arcuate veins drain through the interlobar veins to the lobar veins, which join to form the renal vein. The right renal vein, 2 to 4 cm long, joins the lateral aspect of the inferior vena cava, usually without receiving any tributaries. The left renal vein, 6 to 10 cm long, crosses anterior to the aorta and ends in the left aspect of the inferior vena cava. It receives three tributaries lateral to the aorta: the left adrenal vein superiorly, left gonadal vein inferiorly, and a lumbar vein posteriorly. At the renal hilum the renal vein usually lies in front of the renal artery. However, passing more medially the renal artery may be a centimeter or more higher or lower than the vein.

Lymphatic Drainage

Lymphatic vessels within the renal parenchyma consist of cortical and medullary plexuses that follow the renal vessels to the renal sinus and form several large lymphatic trunks. The renal sinus is the site of numerous communications between lymphatic vessels from the perirenal tissues, renal pelvis, and upper ureter. Initial lymphatic drainage runs to the nodes present at the renal hilum lying close to the renal vein. These nodes form the first station for lymphatic spread of renal cancer. On the left side, lymphatic trunks from the renal hilum drain to the para-aortic lymph nodes from the level of the inferior mesenteric artery to the diaphragm. Lymphatic vessels from the right kidney drain into the lateral paracaval and interaortocaval nodes from the level of the common iliac vessels to the diaphragm. Lymphatic vessels from both sides may extend above the diaphragm to the retrocrural nodes or directly into the thoracic duct.

Nerve Supply

The kidneys have both sympathetic and parasympathetic innervation, yet the function of these nerves is poorly understood. Sympathetic fibers are derived from the greater and lesser splanchnic nerves, which link the celiac and superior mesenteric ganglia. Both sympathetic and parasympathetic fibers travel around the renal artery to the renal pelvis.

URETERS
Topography

The ureter is a muscular tube that follows a gentle S-shaped course in the retroperitoneum. The muscle fibers are arranged in three separate layers: inner and outer longitudinal and middle circular. The length of the ureter in the adult is 28 to 34 cm, varying in direct relation with the height of the person. The average diameter of the ureter is 10 mm in the abdomen and 5 mm in the pelvis.

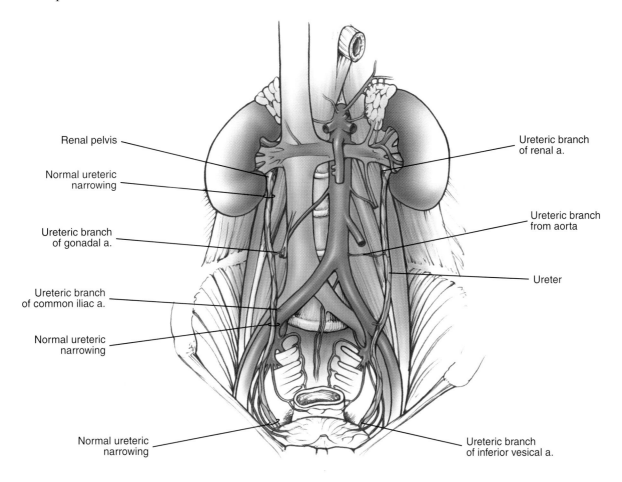

However, three areas of physiologic narrowing in the ureter should not be considered abnormal unless the proximal ureter is significantly dilated: the ureteropelvic junction, the point where the ureter crosses the iliac vessels, and the ureterovesical junction.

Both ureters have the same posterior relations, lying on the medial aspect of the psoas major muscle and traveling downward adjacent to the transverse processes of the lumbar vertebrae. They enter the pelvis medial to the sacroiliac joints, cross over the bifurcation of the common iliac vessels, and follow the hypogastric artery in a gentle lateral curve on the pelvic wall. At the level of the greater sciatic foramen, they turn medially again to enter the bladder obliquely and course submucosally for 2 to 3 cm, ending in the ureteral orifices.

Just proximal to their midpoints, both ureters cross behind the gonadal vessels. The right ureter passes behind the second part of the duodenum, lateral to the inferior vena cava, and is crossed by the right colic and ileocolic vessels. The left ureter passes behind the left colic vessels, descends parallel to the aorta, and passes under the pelvic mesocolon. In the male, the ureter crosses under the vas deferens in close proximity to the upper end of the seminal vesicle before entering the urinary bladder. In the female, the ureter travels in the posterior border of the ovarian fossa, passes forward under the lower part of the broad ligament lateral to the cervix and underneath the uterine artery. This area is a common site for ureteric injury during hysterectomy.

Blood Supply

The upper ureter derives its blood supply from a ureteric branch of the renal artery. During their course in the abdomen, the ureters receive blood from the gonadal vessels, aorta, and retroperitoneal vessels. In the pelvis they receive additional branches from the hypogastric artery, vasal artery, and vesical arteries. The abdominal portion of the ureter has a medial vascular supply; the pelvic portion receives its blood vessels from the lateral side. This should be taken into consideration during partial mobilization of the ureter to preserve as much as possible of the blood supply.

Venous drainage follows the arterial blood supply.

Lymphatic Drainage

Lymphatic drainage of the ureters follows the arterial blood supply.

Nerve Supply

The ureteric muscle fibers contain both α-adrenergic (exitatory) and β-adrenergic (inhibitory) receptors. However, peristaltic contractions occur in denervated ureters and can be altered by sympathomimetic or sympatholytic medications. This indicates that the role of nerve supply to the ureter is to modulate peristalytic activity, not initiate it.

SURGICAL APPLICATIONS

The kidneys can be approached though various incisions: lumbar, anterior transperitoneal, thoracoabdominal, and posterior lumbar. Factors that should be taken into consideration before selecting an incision include type of operation and pathologic condition, body habitus, and pulmonary or spinal deformities. The most important factor is the operation to be performed.

Operations for benign kidney disease (e.g., simple nephrectomy, partial nephrectomy, deroofing of a renal cyst, stone extraction) can be performed through an extraperitoneal flank incision. This approach has the advantages of being extraperitoneal, with a shorter period of ileus, and in obese patients most of the panniculus falls away from the kidney. However, exposure of the renal pedicle with lateral lumbar approaches is not so good as an anterior approach, and runs the risk of entering the pleural cavity, particularly if a supracostal incision is performed. This incision can be performed above the twelfth or eleventh rib, either extrapleural or intrapleural, to expose the suprarenal gland or the upper pole of the kidney, and can also be extended downward to expose the ureter.

For good exposure of the renal vessels, particularly for vascular procedures or operation for advanced tumors, an anterior transperitoneal approach is preferred. It can be performed through an anterior subcostal, midline, or paramedian incision. The midline incision is faster to perform and to close, but the incidence of incisional hernia is higher than with paramedian incisions. Posterior lumbar incisions are easy to perform and are easier on the patient, but the exposure is limited, particularly with respect to renal vessels. However, good access is provided to the renal pelvis and upper third of the ureter for stone surgery, but this approach is not recommended for malignancies.

Lumbar Approaches
Subcostal Approach

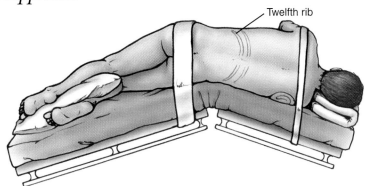

After induction of general anesthesia and endotracheal intubation, the patient is placed in the lateral decubitus position on the operating table so that the center of the kidney rest or the table brake is just below the tip of the twelfth rib. The kidney rest is elevated and the table flexed to place tension on the incision site. Both arms should be supported in a horizontal position on well-padded armrests to prevent pressure injuries to the vessels and nerves. A soft pad or wrapped towel should be placed under the lower axilla to support the weight of the body away from the axillary vessels and nerves. The lower knee and hip are flexed, and the upper limb is fully extended. A soft pillow is placed between the knees. Prophylaxis against deep venous thrombosis with pressure stockings or pneumatic compression devices should be considered if the operation is expected to be lengthy. Adhesive tape (3 inch) can be applied to the upper shoulder and thigh to secure position.

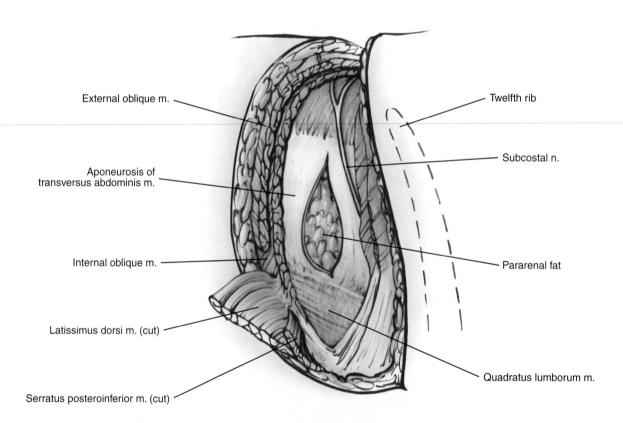

The skin is incised one fingerbreadth below the distal half of the twelfth rib and carried over the flank toward the umbilicus, where it can be extended as far as the opposite rectus abdominis muscle. The incision is deepened through the subcutaneous fat to the first fascial layer, which is incised to expose the external oblique muscle anteriorly and the latissimus dorsi muscle posteriorly. These muscles are sharply divided to expose the fibers of the internal oblique muscle anteriorly and the serratus posterior muscle, which is sometimes seen below the latissimus dorsi muscle. These muscles are incised sharply in the line of the wound to expose the transversus abdominis muscle.

The subcostal nerve runs between the internal oblique and the transversus abdominis muscles, and care should be taken during incision of the internal oblique muscle to identify the nerve, dissect it free, and retract it away. Injury to the subcostal nerve can lead to numbness in a small area of the skin in the suprapubic region and weakness of the lower segment of the ipsilateral rectus abdominis muscle.

The transversalis (thoracolumbar) fascia in the depth of the wound is sharply incised to allow entrance into the retroperitoneal space. A finger is passed in this space, and the peritoneum is dissected medially away from the undersurface of the transversus abdominis muscle. The fibers of the transversus abdominis muscle can then be separated or incised to expose Gerota's fascia covering the perirenal fat.

Transcostal Approach

The transcostal approach can be performed through the tenth, eleventh, or twelfth ribs. However, the higher the level the more risk for pleural injury.

The patient is positioned as for the subcostal approach. The rib chosen for the incision is palpated and may be marked before the skin is incised. The skin and subcutaneous fat are incised as for the subcostal incision approach. However, the incision should pass over the outer surface of the rib. The latissimus dorsi and external oblique muscles are incised to expose the outer surface of the rib. The periosteum is incised the whole length of the rib. A periosteal elevator is used to strip the periosteum of the rib on the outer surface, followed by the upper and lower borders. This removes the attachments of the abdominal and intercostal muscles from the rib. Care should be taken not to injure the intercostal vessels when dissecting the lower edge of the rib.

A Doyen rib elevator is passed between the posterior surface of the rib and the periosteum and is moved backward and forward to free the rib from its attachments. A rib cutter is used to cut the rib posteriorly as far as the dissection allows.

The muscular slips of the corresponding crus of the diaphragm, still attached to the periosteum, are sharply incised, and the transversalis fascia is dissected to expose Gerota's fascia.

Supracostal Approach

In contrast to the transcostal approach, the supracostal incision provides good exposure to the suprarenal gland and the upper pole of the kidney without the need for rib excision.

The patient is positioned as for the subcostal or transcostal approaches.

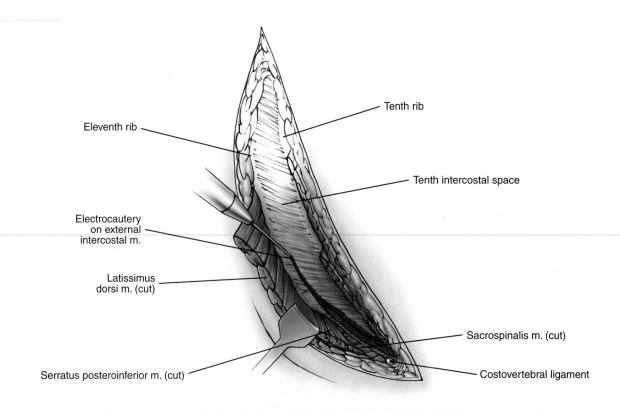

The skin is incised from the posterior axillary line, passing over the eleventh or tenth intercostal space to the rectus sheath. Subcutaneous fat and fascia are divided.

The latissimus dorsi muscle and the serratus posterior inferior muscle are incised to uncover the intercostal muscles, which can be freed from the upper border of the rib with an electrocautery. Great care should be taken while dissecting the intercostal muscles to prevent pleural injury or damage to the more cephalad intercostal vessels and nerve. The sacrospinalis muscle, covering the intercostal muscle in the posterior part of the wound, should be mobilized or divided to enable complete dissection of the intercostal muscles.

The costovertebral ligament is divided to allow hinge-like movement of the rib so that it can be retracted without breaking.

The diaphragmatic fibers attached to the posterior part of the periosteum are divided and the pleura mobilized superiorly. Then the transversalis fascia is incised sharply to display Gerota's fascia.

Downward Extension of Lumbar Incision

Lateral lumbar incisions, both subcostal and transcostal, can be extended downward to the suprapubic region. This is particularly useful for exposure of the ureter and kidney, as for nephroureterectomy utilizing the same incision. However, this approach is difficult in obese patients, and two separate incisions may be needed.

Positioning is similar to that for the lumbar approach, but the patient is tilted backward and a long towel is rolled under the back to give access to the suprapubic area, where the incision will be carried. The incision is similar to the typical lumbar approach, cutting toward the umbilicus, then gently curving toward the lateral border of the rectus abdominis muscle to the pubis. Care should be taken not to extend the incision parallel to the lateral border of the rectus sheath to avert denervation of the rectus muscle. The abdominal wall muscles are cut in the direction of the wound, and the extraperitoneal space is entered as in the subcostal approach. The transversalis fascia is incised, and blunt dissection is used to mobilize the retroperitoneal fat and display the ureter.

Thoracoabdominal Approach

Thoracoabdominal incision offers good exposure of the kidney and adrenal gland in cases of upper pole kidney tumors, suprarenal tumors, or large renal tumors in a highly positioned kidney. The morbidity with this incision is higher than that with other approaches because of opening the pleural cavity and the need for a chest tube in the postoperative period.

The patient is placed in a semioblique position with the involved flank elevated 30 to 45 degrees with rolled towels or sandbags. The operating table is extended to put the abdominal wall muscles under stretch. A soft pillow or a fluid-filled bag is placed under the contralateral axilla, and the arms are supported on armrests.

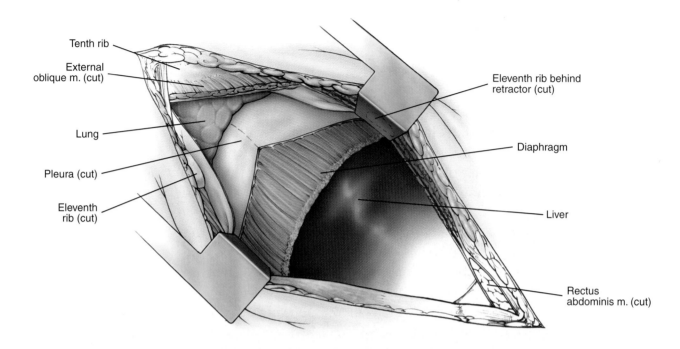

The incision is started at the angle of the ninth, tenth, or eleventh rib and continued downward and anteriorly toward the midpoint of the ipsilateral rectus muscle. It can be extended to the contralateral rectus muscle if necessary.

The subcutaneous fat and fascia are incised. The latissimus dorsi muscle overlying the serratus posterior muscle will be seen in the posterior part of the wound, as well as the external and internal oblique muscles covering the anterior part of the wound. The muscles are sharply incised in the direction of the wound to uncover the rib and the intercostal muscles. The intercostal muscles are divided sharply, and the costal cartilage of the corresponding rib is divided. The posterior end of the rib should be freed posteriorly by dividing the costovertebral ligaments to facilitate retraction, or the rib can be excised.

The pleura is usually opened during dissection of the intercostal muscles, which is completed to expose the thoracic surface of the diaphragm. Care should be taken to avoid injuring the lung. With two fingers inserted under the diaphragm anteriorly, blunt dissection is carried out to separate the abdominal surface of the diaphragm from the upper surface of the liver on the right and the spleen on the left. The diaphragm is divided from its thoracic surface, taking care not to injure the phrenic nerve. The internal oblique and transversus abdominis muscles, which pass medial to the ribs, are also divided.

If the procedure is to be performed extraperitoneally, the peritoneum is mobilized medially and freed from the undersurface of the diaphragm, transversalis fascia, and anterior rectus fascia. The allows the liver on the right side and the spleen and pancreas on the left side to be moved medially away from the dissection.

Anterior Midline Approach

The anterior midline incision is usually transperitoneal. While this approach is associated with a longer period of postoperative ileus, it is required when careful inspection of intra-abdominal viscera is needed or when access to the renal vessels is desired before manipulating the kidney. This incision is usually chosen for exploration for urologic trauma because it is quick to perform and enables simultaneous exposure of the upper and lower urinary tracts, in addition to good exposure of the abdominal vasculature.

The patient is placed supine. Exposure of the kidney is improved by placing a cushion or a sandbag under the ipsilateral flank, extending the table, and tilting it in slight Trendelenburg position.

A complete midline incision is started at the xiphoid and carried down to curve around the umbilicus, usually on the left side to avoid the falciform ligament, and is continued to the symphysis pubis. If the surgery is limited to the kidney or upper ureter, the incision can be extended only to the umbilical level. Similarly, incision from the umbilicus to the symphysis pubis is adequate for exposure of the lower part of the ureter and the pelvic organs.

The incision is deepened through the subcutaneous fat and fascia to expose the decussating fibers of the linea alba. In patients without previous history of abdominal surgery, the safest area at which to enter the peritoneal cavity is 5 cm above the umbilicus. The linea alba is incised at this level, the transversalis fascia is incised, and the fat is cleared. Then the peritoneum is grasped with two hemostats and incised carefully with a scalpel.

A finger is passed through into the peritoneal cavity to palpate for bowel or omentum adherent to the abdominal wall. Once this is cleared, two fingers are passed in the incision, and the abdominal wall is opened to the full length of the skin incision. If adhesions to the anterior abdominal wall are encountered, the wound is opened in stepwise fashion and adhesions are divided by sharp dissection.

Anterior Paramedian Approach

The anterior paramedian incision, an alternative to midline incision, has the theoretical advantage of producing a stronger scar and less chance of incisional hernia, but it is time consuming to perform and close. It is preferred in operations where a stoma is created so that the subsequent scar will not interfere with the adhesive part of the urinary appliance.

The patient is placed supine. The skin is incised on the ipsilateral side 2 to 5 cm lateral to the midline. The incision can be carried from the costal margin to the pubis. The anterior rectus fascia is incised along the length of the wound. The rectus muscle is dissected from its attachment to the fascia and displaced laterally. The posterior rectus sheath and the peritoneum are then incised about 2 to 3 cm from the midline.

Anterior Subcostal Approach

The anterior subcostal incision provides good exposure of the adrenal gland and the upper pole of the kidney, in addition to adequate access to other upper abdominal organs such as the liver on the right and the spleen and pancreas on the left. Bilateral subcostal incision (Chevron incision) is an excellent approach when simultaneous exposure of both kidneys or adrenal glands is required.

The patient is placed supine with a rolled sheet or sandbags under the ipsilateral flank, shoulder, and pelvis. The table is flexed to about 20 degrees to put the abdominal wall muscles in stretch. If bilateral incision is planned, the patient is placed supine with a rolled sheet beneath the upper lumbar spine, and the table is flexed.

The skin incision starts at the midaxillary line at the tip of the twelfth rib and is carried medially in a gentle curve about 2 to 3 cm below the costal margin. It is usually ended at the lateral border of the rectus muscle, but can be extended to the midline or the contralateral side as required. The incision is deepened through the subcutaneous fat and fascia, and the external oblique muscle and anterior rectus sheath are incised.

An electrocautery is used to cut the rectus abdominis, internal oblique, and transversus abdominis muscles. Care should be taken to identify and ligate the branches of the superficial epigastric artery, which lies on the posterior rectus sheath. The posterior rectus sheath, transversalis fascia, and the peritoneum are picked up in layers between two hemostats and are incised with the knife carefully to avoid injuring the abdominal organs. The opening is widened, and the surgeon's finger is used to palpate for adhesive structures to the abdominal wall. Then the peritoneal cavity is opened to the full length of the incision.

KIDNEY TUMORS
Radical Nephrectomy

Renal cell carcinoma is a relatively rare tumor, accounting for approximately 3% of malignancies in adults, but is the most common tumor of the kidney and the third most common tumor seen by urologists. The classic symptom triad of pain, hematuria, and flank pain is certainly a reliable clinical symptom complex. However, more recently the majority of renal cell carcinomas are diagnosed at earlier stages and are frequently found incidentally at radiologic investigation done for other reasons.

Indications

Renal cell carcinoma is refractory to most traditional oncologic treatment, including chemotherapy, radiation therapy, and hormonal therapy. Therefore radical nephrectomy, removing all the contents of Gerota's fascia, is considered the standard treatment for localized tumors. However, more recent data indicate that in carefully selected patients partial nephrectomy may be an option. The role of radical nephrectomy in patients with metastatic disease is controversial and is not indicated unless the patient has intractable bleeding or pain, or it is necessary to debulk the tumor for immunotherapy or other systemic therapies. Local extension into the renal vein or inferior vena cava is not considered a contraindication to radical nephrectomy. However, tumor extension beyond Gerota's fascia involving other organs is associated with poor prognosis, and nephrectomy should be considered only for palliation or as part of an adjuvant therapy protocol.

Preoperative Evaluation

Due to the recent advances in sophisticated radiologic studies, the surgeon can now make an accurate preoperative assessment of the nature and extent of kidney tumors. The diagnosis of renal cell carcinoma is generally made with computed tomography (CT), showing a solid mass in the parenchyma of the kidney. Fewer than 5% of all renal cell carcinomas have a cystic appearance with septations, irregular borders, dystrophic calcification, or other features that distinguish it from a simple renal cyst.

The differential diagnosis of solid kidney masses includes oncocytoma (granular oncocytes on histologic analysis, with a central scar in the tumor), angiomyolipoma (contains fat, seen on CT scans), xanthogranulomatous pyelonephritis (usually in patients with diabetes, with a concurrent stone in a poorly functioning kidney), fibromas, or metastasis. In spite of the diagnostic clues seen at radiologic investigation, the histologic nature of these masses cannot be confirmed without tissue biopsy, which is generally avoided because of the risk for seeding malignant cells through the needle track or the possibility of obtaining benign tissue approximating a malignant area. Accordingly, in most of these patients radical nephrectomy is required before the kidney pathologic entity is finally diagnosed.

CT and magnetic resonance imaging (MRI) are the imaging studies most commonly used to stage renal tumors. Abdominal CT is particularly useful to show local extension of tumor and the presence of enlarged para-aortic lymph nodes. MRI is superior to CT for determining the superior extent of a vena caval thrombus; however, the new generation of CT scanners with rapid image acquisition are as accurate as MRI in vena caval imaging. These new imaging studies have replaced, to large extent, venocavography and arteriography, which are more invasive. Chest radiography or chest CT is routinely done to rule out pulmonary metastasis; bone scanning is required only in the presence of a large tumor or if clinical evaluation suggests metastasis to bone.

Incision

The eleventh or twelveth rib supracostal incision, with attempt to remain extrapleural, is recommended for most cases. It provides good exposure of the kidney, renal pedicle, and adjacent organs. Thoracoabdominal incision is preferable in patients with large upper pole tumors or tumors that extend into the inferior vena cava, although median sternotomy is an option for high caval thrombi. Unilateral anterior extraperitoneal incision provides adequate exposure in noncomplicated cases. Bilateral tumors can be approached with a midline or Chevron incision; however, such lesions are best approached one side at a time.

Right Radical Nephrectomy

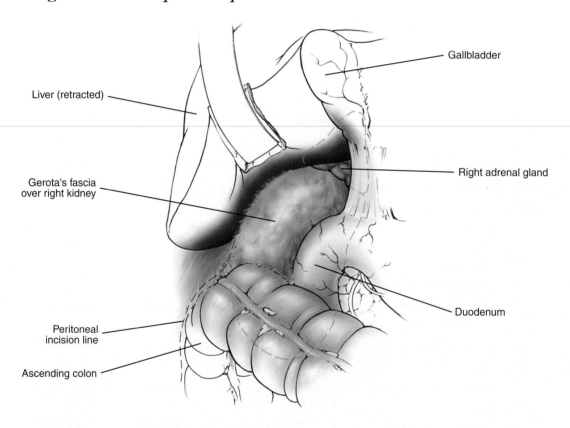

Once the peritoneum is entered, the intra-abdominal contents, mainly the liver, are inspected for unrecognized metastasis, and the tumor is carefully examined for resectability. The diaphragm is retracted superiorly with a self-retaining retractor, and countertraction is applied to the superior border of the rib below after releasing the costochondral ligament. The liver is kept out of the way by gentle retraction to prevent hepatic injury. During extensive inferior vena cava mobilization care must be taken not to injure the short caudate veins.

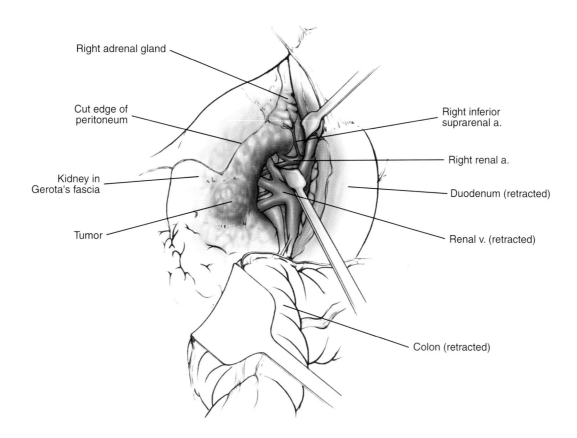

Attention should be given to the renal pedicle, which can be approached ventrally by retracting the ascending colon and dividing the lateral paracolic peritoneum. The hepatic flexure and duodenum are mobilized medially to expose the renal pedicle and the renal veins lying in front of the artery. As an alternative, with the dorsal approach to the renal pedicle the renal artery is readily accessible for ligation and division. This maneuver significantly reduces potential blood loss. It can be performed by dissecting the kidney and surrounding tissues free from the posterior abdominal wall and rotating it medially, after which the renal artery can be identified, ligated, and divided.

The ureter, gonadal vessels, and periureteral fat are dissected free of the posterior peritoneum and divided in two or three separate bundles. The dissection is then carried superiorly along the inferior vena cava on its anterior surface, where there are few, if any, significant branches.

Superior to the renal vessels the peritoneum fans out laterally, and the dissection is carried out to the lateral border of the peritoneum. In most larger tumors and some smaller tumors, the peritoneum cannot be dissected free of Gerota's fascia, and the surgeon is forced to remove a window of peritoneum with the specimen. Care should be taken to avert injury to the bowel, especially the C portion of the duodenum.

The superior portion of the specimen, including the adrenal gland, should be dissected free of the retroperitoneum and liver. As there may be branches of the phrenic and other vessels at this point, we generally use a series of large hemoclips, dividing the tissue below the clips to enhance hemostasis.

The specimen should be free at this point except for the venous structures. The adrenal vein is short and easily avulsed, and drains directly into the inferior vena cava. It should be identified and ligated carefully. The renal vein should be collapsed because the renal artery is divided. If the renal vein is still full, beware of branch arteries that may still be perfusing the specimen. The vein should be palpated for possible unsuspected thrombi, divided, and ligated. The specimen is then removed and the wound closed, without a drain in most cases. Recent evidence suggests that when dealing with lower pole tumors adrenalectomy is frequently unnecessary.

Left Radical Nephrectomy

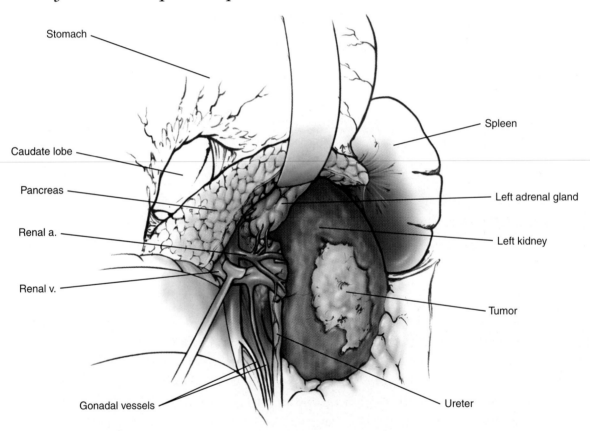

The intra-abdominal contents are inspected for unrecognized metastasis, and the tumor is carefully examined for resectability. The diaphragm is then retracted superiorly with a self-retaining retractor.

The descending colon is retracted medially, and the lateral reflection of the peritoneum is incised. The mesentery is dissected bluntly from the anterior surface of Gerota's fascia. Care should be taken to prevent injury to the tail of the pancreas, which is mobilized medially. If the tumor extends into the colonic mesentery, this part of the mesentery can be resected with the specimen without great risk for colonic ischemia as long as the marginal artery is not disrupted. The kidney and surrounding tissues are dissected free from the posterior abdominal wall and rotated medially, and the renal artery is identified, ligated, and divided. In bulky tumors the superior mesenteric artery might be displaced laterally; therefore great care should be taken to distinguish the superior mesenteric artery from the renal artery on either side.

The ureter, gonadal vessels, and periureteral fat are dissected free of the posterior peritoneum and divided in two or three separate bundles. The dissection is then carried superiorly along the aorta on its anterior surface, where there are few significant branches. The splenorenal ligament is identified, ligated, and divided to avert splenic injury during mobilization of the kidney. The superior portion of the specimen should be dissected free of the retroperitoneum.

The specimen should be free at this point except for the venous structures. The left adrenal vein drains into the renal vein and is ligated and divided. The back surface of the renal vein should be carefully inspected for any lumbar veins, which if present should be ligated and divided. Then the renal vein should be palpated for possible unsuspected thrombi, divided, and ligated. Large tumors on either side frequently develop parasitizing vessels, which are abnormal in structure and can frequently lead to troublesome bleeding if not ligated or clipped with great care. In some cases where it is difficult to identify the renal artery the vein may be ligated and divided first, accepting the fact that the kidney will quickly become engorged, but identification of the artery will be much facilitated. The specimen is then removed, and the wound is closed without a drain in most cases.

Management of Tumor Extension in the Vena Cava

The presence of a solid mass in the vena cava might represent tumor extension into the lumen, blood thrombus, or less commonly tumor invasion of the vena cava wall. Tumor extension into the vena cava occurs in 4% to 10% of cases, and tumor-free survival equivalent to survival for stage II disease is achieved by complete removal of tumor extension in patients without lymph node involvement. Exploration of the vena cava is a major procedure, and a complete set of vascular instruments should be available. The extent of the tumor extension into the vena cava should be delineated preoperatively to help in planning the surgical approach. Right-sided renal tumors with limited vena caval extension can be approached with a right flank incision. A thoracoabdominal incision is utilized for high right-sided tumor extension, whereas a midline incision with a median sternotomy extension is frequently required for patients with left renal tumors and vena caval extension to the level of the hepatic veins or above.

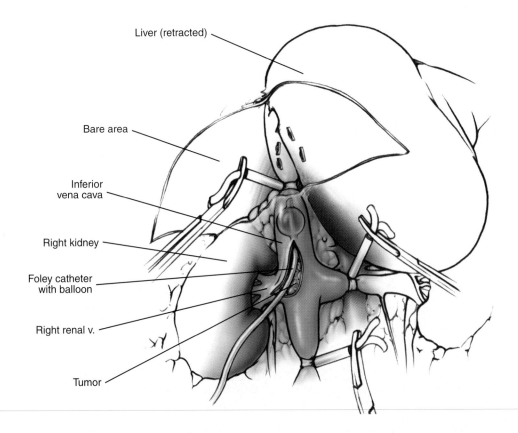

Liver (retracted)

Bare area

Inferior
vena cava

Right kidney

Foley catheter
with balloon

Right renal v.

Tumor

Exposure of the retrohepatic vena cava is started with division of the right tri-angular and coronary ligaments of the liver and ligation of the small hepatic (caudate) veins. The liver is then mobilized medially to expose the vena cava, and a cardiac tourniquet is applied around the vessel for temporary occlusion. The contralateral renal vein and the infrarenal vena cava are also occluded with a Rumel tourniquet. Since about one fourth of the venous return in the vena cava comes from the liver, clamping the porta hepatis through the foramen of Winslow with a noncrushing vascular clamp reduces the blood loss remark-ably. A cavotomy is made adjacent to the hepatic veins and extended inferiorly to the origin of the affected renal vein. A 20 Fr Foley catheter with a 30 ml balloon is introduced into the vena cava, and the balloon is inflated above the level of the thrombus and is withdrawn gently to extract the thrombus out of the vena cava. In the rare occasion when the tumor invades the wall of the vein, partial or complete resection of the vein is considered.

Air should be evacuated from the vena cava before closure. A Satinsky clamp is applied to the cavotomy, and the edges of the vena cava are approximated gently with Allis clamps. The tourniquet on the contralateral renal vein and infrarenal vena cava and the clamp on the porta hepatis are released, leaving the tourniquet on the suprahepatic vena cava in place. The Satinsky clamp is briefly vented to allow the air in the venal cava to be evacuated; then the clamp is closed again, and the last tourniquet on the vein is released. The affected renal vein is transected flush with the vena cava. The entire cavotomy is then closed with a continuous 5-0 polypropylene suture.

Lymphadenectomy

The prognosis of renal cell carcinoma is mostly affected by presence or absence of nodal metastasis. Due to the position of the kidney just inferior to the cisterna chylae, tumor spread from the renal lymphatic vessels to the cisterna chylae and widespread dissemination of the disease is common. Therefore curative lymphadenectomy is not possible in most cases, and the value of lymphadenectomy is limited to the diagnosis of lymph node involvement. Limited dissection of the tissue around the junction of the renal vessel to the nearest great vessel and resection of the visible or palpable nodes is usually sufficient.

Nephroureterectomy

Transitional cell carcinoma of the calyces, pelvis, or ureter usually is treated with nephroureterectomy, provided the contralateral collecting system is normal and no evidence of distant metastasis exists. Preoperative evaluation should include cystoscopy and bilateral retrograde pyelography for better evaluation of the collecting system. The operation can be performed through a flank incision with downward extension, or alternatively two separate incisions or a midline incision can be made. The technique of nephrectomy is the same. The ureter is mobilized with blunt and sharp dissection down to its insertion in the bladder. A cuff of the bladder must be removed with the lower ureter because this is the most common site for tumor recurrence after nephroureterectomy. The bladder is then closed in two layers with 2-0 chromic catgut sutures. A Foley catheter is left in the bladder for drainage, as well as a drain in the pelvis next to the suture line.

Partial Nephrectomy

Renal cell carcinoma in a solitary functioning kidney or bilateral tumors are best treated with partial nephrectomy. Full preoperative evaluation should be carried out to confirm that the disease is localized. The arterial anatomy of the affected kidney should be carefully studied with preoperative angiography.

Flank incisions through the bed of the eleventh or twelfth rib, with attempt to stay extrapleural and extraperitoneal, provide an excellent exposure of the peripheral renal vessels. Then the kidney is mobilized within Gerota's fascia. Temporary occlusion of the renal artery and surface cooling of the kidney with iced slush during the procedure will allow 30 minutes of operating time without significant ischemic injury to the kidney. For longer procedures the kidney should be perfused with cold Collin's solution through an arterial catheter, which allows 3 hours for surgery. However, small polar or peripheral renal tumors may not require renal artery occlusion, and the segmental artery can be identified and divided instead. Simple enucleation for malignant lesions should be avoided even if the tumor looks well defined, because of the probable presence of microscopic extensions of these tumors beyond the pseudocapsule. Tumors of the upper or lower pole of the kidney are best resected by polar nephrectomy (guillotine resection), whereas mid-renal tumors are resected with wedge resection.

Polar Nephrectomy

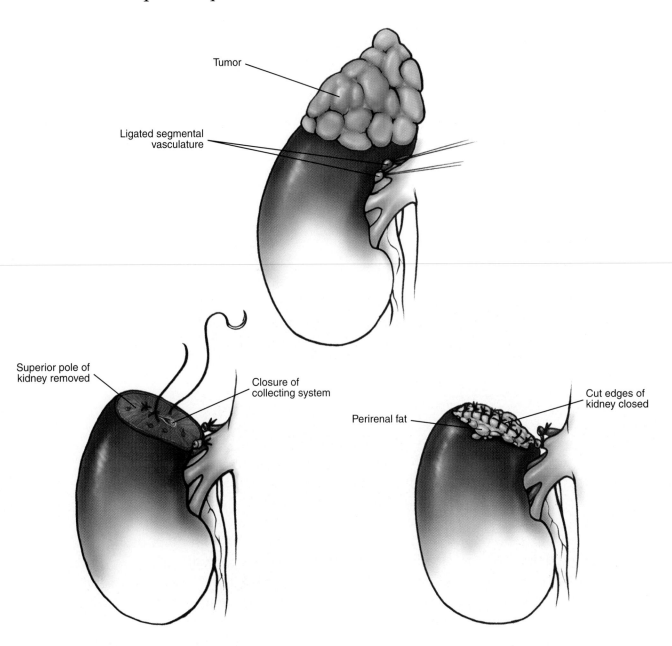

After mobilization of the kidney, the renal artery and vein are dissected free from surrounding structures. Dissection of the branches of the renal artery will delineate the segmental artery of the affected pole of the kidney, which is ligated and divided. Often a corresponding venous branch is present, which is similarly ligated and divided. The kidney is inspected for the ischemic line of demarcation, which outlines the segment of the kidney to be excised. If this area is not obvious, injection of a few milliliters of methylene blue in the distal part of the apical artery gives a better outline of the area to be resected. This segment of the kidney and the covering Gerota's fascia is then excised by sharp and blunt dissection, making sure that the incision is at least 1 to 2 cm from the visible edge of the tumor.

The collecting system is then closed with interrupted or continuous 4-0 chromic catgut sutures to ensure a watertight closure. Small vessels are identified and controlled with figure-of-eight 4-0 chromic sutures. The edges of the kidney are then approximated with 2-0 chromic sutures, passing through the capsule and superficial parenchyma, with some perirenal fat applied to the edge of the kidney, and the sutures are tied on top of it. A drain should be left in the perirenal space, particularly if the collecting system is opened. A double J stent also is frequently placed.

Wedge Resection

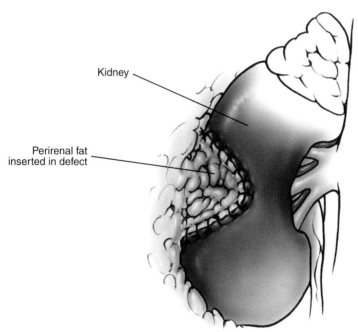

Temporary renal artery occlusion and surface cooling are usually required for wedge resection. A wedge of Gerota's fascia and renal parenchyma is resected with 1 to 2 cm of surrounding grossly normal renal parenchyma. The collecting system and the vessels are closed with 4-0 chromic sutures. Portions of the perirenal fat are mobilized and inserted in the defect, and the edges are closed with interrupted 2-0 or 3-0 chromic sutures. Alternatively, if the defect is small, the edges can be approximated with insertion of fat with a small piece of oxidized cellulose (Oxycel) placed at the base of the defect for hemostasis. There should be no tension on the sutures, and the renal vessels should not be significantly kinked after closure.

URETERIC TUMORS

Transitional cell carcinoma accounts for more than 95% of ureteric tumors. The surgeon should be aware that this tumor is commonly multicentric, and careful search for other tumors in the urinary tract should be considered in every case before the diagnosis of solitary ureteric tumor is made. Squamous cell carcinoma, adenocarcinoma, and sarcoma account for less than 5% of ureteric tumors.

Total ureterectomy is most frequently done in combination with nephrectomy for treatment of renal pelvic or ureteric neoplasms. Localized solitary tumors of the ureter can be treated with partial ureterectomy.

Preoperative Evaluation

Gross hematuria is the most common symptom of ureteric tumors. Most patients have hematuria throughout urination, and passage of vermiform clots. Gradual ureteric obstruction by tumor may lead to dull flank pain in about a third of patients. However, the passage of blood clots might cause severe ureteric colic, and care should be taken not to summarily diagnose stone disease, particularly if the patient has a history of bladder urothelial tumors.

The majority of ureteric tumors are demonstrated as a filling defect on excretory urograms. Other causes of filling defects are blood clot, air bubble, radiolucent stone, sloughed renal papilla, and less commonly fibroepithelial polyp, fungus ball, granuloma, leukoplakia, and hemangioma.

Cystoscopy should be performed in all patients with ureteric tumors to rule out bladder tumors, found in approximately 40% of patients. Retrograde urography provides better visualization of the upper urinary tract and can be performed in patients with deteriorated renal function. After x-ray films have been obtained, urine should be collected for cytologic analysis. It is important to use a nonionic contrast material to prevent the cytologic artifact that results from cell dehydration when hyperosmolar contrast materials are used. In some cases ureteroscopy and brush biopsies are necessary to establish the diagnosis.

CT is useful for diagnosis and staging, but small tumors can be missed due to volume averaging. Ureteric stones are opaque on CT scans and can be easily differentiated from tumors. Abdominal CT, chest radiography, bone scan, and liver function tests should be considered to rule out metastasis.

Endoscopic Treatment

Over the past decade, due to the advances in the ureteroscopic instruments, ureteroscopy and laser ablation of ureteric tumors have been described as an alternative to open surgery. Tumors should be solitary, superficial, and accessible with the ureteroscope. There are few reports on the long-term results of this treatment, with recurrence rates of about 25%. Complications include ureteric perforation, extravasation, and stricture formation.

Partial Ureterectomy
Indications

Conservative treatment of localized ureteric tumors is especially indicated in patients with solitary kidney, functionally dominant kidney, or bilateral tumors. Upper and middle third ureteric tumors should be treated with segmental resection if they are solitary and low grade, and with nephroureterectomy if they are multifocal or high grade. Distal ureteric tumors should be treated by distal ureterectomy, removing a cuff of tissue from the bladder around the ureteric orifice.

Incision

Surgical approaches to the ureter depend on the part of the ureter to be operated on. Upper third tumors can be accessed with a subcostal flank incision; middle third tumors can be removed through a muscle-splitting incision in the appropriate position; and lower third tumors can be approached through a lower midline, paramedian, or hockey stick incision. The decision whether the incision should be transperitoneal or extraperitoneal depends on whether exploration of the abdominal viscera is necessary and the type of urinary reconstruction planned.

Technique

Extraperitoneal exposure of the ureter is achieved by incising the abdominal muscles and the transversalis fascia. It is important to enter the plane between the transversalis fascia and the parietal peritoneum. The peritoneum is mobilized medially with blunt dissection, and the ureter should be looked for in the retroperitoneal space. Sometimes the ureter is mobilized with the parietal peritoneum and can be palpated as a cord-like structure on the peritoneum surface. It is important to know that the femoral nerve and the tendon of the psoas minor muscle, if present, can be palpated as a cord-like structure in the pelvis and can be confused with the lower third of the ureter. Careful observation for peristaltic activity is helpful in these situations. The ureter enters the pelvis medial to the sacroiliac joint, and in front of the bifurcation of the common iliac artery this anatomic landmark may prove helpful in identifying the ureter more readily. A chronically obstructed ureter can be dilated and hypertrophied enough to be confused with the colon, but it lacks the tinea coli and appendices epiploica that characterize the colon.

Once the ureter is identified and the tumor is palpated, a decision is made on the length of segment to be removed. The ureter is then closed with non-crushing vascular clamps both proximal and distal to this segment to prevent spillage of tumor cells. This segment is then excised.

Primary anastomosis of the ureter should be considered only if the segment removed is short enough to allow ureteric anastomosis without tension on the suture line. Both ends of the ureter should be spatulated to prevent anastomotic strictures. Absorbable interrupted sutures (e.g., 4-0 Vicryl) should be used.

If the resection is limited to the lower third of the ureter, ureteric reimplantation into the bladder with or without a psoas hitch and anterior bladder wall flap (Boari flap) should be attempted. In some situations the segment removed precludes reimplantation. In these circumstances the ureter can be mobilized proximally and anastomosed to a suitable length of mobilized ileum, which is then reimplanted into the bladder.

Whenever the ureter is incised, a stent should be left in situ to allow the anastomosis to heal. It is recommended that a drain be left near the anastomotic site. Whenever the ureter is mobilized, consideration must be given to its blood supply and the alternating directions from which it is derived, depending on which area of the ureter is involved.

Urinary Bladder
SURGICAL ANATOMY
Topography

The bladder is a hollow muscular organ that functions as a reservoir. When empty, the bladder is situated in the pelvis, behind the pubic symphysis. As the urine content increases, the bladder rises above the pubic ramus and, in cases of urinary retention, can be palpated above the umbilicus. The bladder has a number of areas or surfaces that enable the position of lesions or abnormalities to be accurately documented. There are two anterolateral, a superior, and a posterior (base) surface. Other named areas include the apex (dome) of the bladder and the neck. At the apex a short fibrous cord is present, which is the remnant of the urachus; this structure originally connected the allantois to the bladder. This cord runs from the apex to the umbilicus between the transversalis fascia and the peritoneum, raising a ridge of peritoneum called the median umbilical ligament. The urachus should be removed in continuity with the bladder during radical cystectomy for bladder cancer. It can also be the original site of malignancy, in which case the lesion is usually an adenocarcinoma as opposed to a transitional cell lesion. The superior surface of the bladder is the only surface covered by peritoneum, except for a small part of the base in the male.

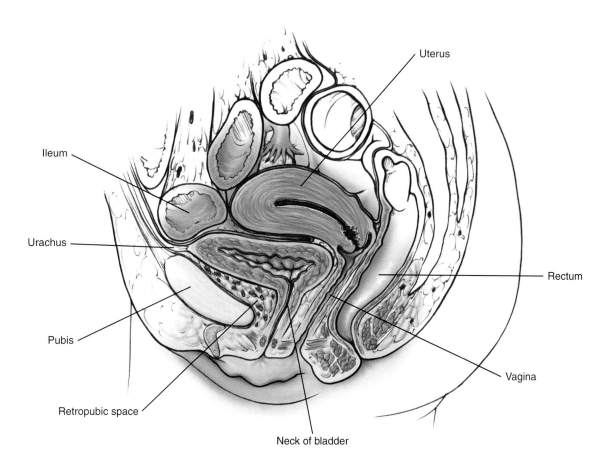

In the female the ileum and uterus lie against the superior surface of the bladder, whereas in the male the ileum and pelvic colon occupy this area. The antero-lateral surfaces are related to the pubic bone and the levator ani and obturator internus muscles. The bladder is separated from the pubis by the retropubic space, which contains vessels and abundant fat. The base of the bladder is posteriorly separated from the rectum by the uterus and vagina in the female, and the vasa deferentia, seminal vesicles, and ureters in the male. The most inferior part of the bladder is the neck, which leads directly into the urethra. The neck remains fairly constant in position as the bladder fills, except when the supporting structures have been damaged, such as in complicated childbirth, when the entire organ can prolapse as a result of variations in position and intra-abdominal pressure.

The mucosal surface of the bladder is composed of layers of transitional epithelium. The underlying connective tissue allows considerable stretching of the mucosa except in the trigonal area; thus when empty the bladder has numerous mucosal folds, whereas when full the mucosa is stretched flat. The trigonal area, which stretches from the bladder neck to both ureteric orifices and the area in between, is always flat.

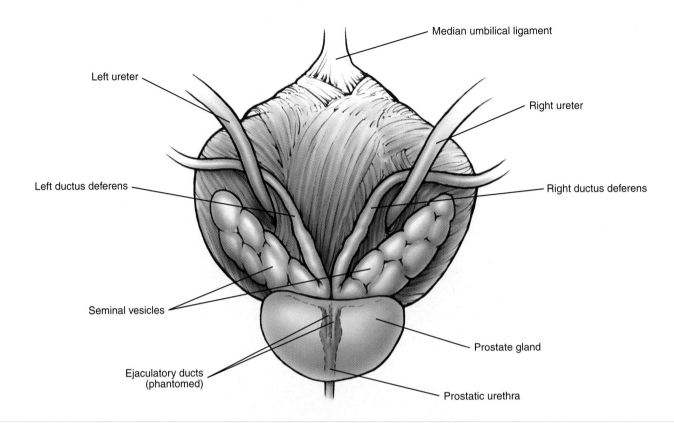

The muscles of the bladder are arranged in crude muscle bundles with no particular layering arrangement except in the area of the bladder neck and outlet. In other areas the bundles interdigitate freely without orientation, varying from circular to longitudinal. At the neck of the bladder a circular layer of muscle is sandwiched between two longitudinal layers; these layers rapidly intermingle as they move cranially, with muscle bundles from an inner to middle to outer level and back again to form a definite mesh pattern. The overall impression of the bladder musculature, with the exception of the bladder neck, is of one large muscle with component bundles weaving in and out of varying planes and directions.

Condensations of loose subserous fascia, which is continuous superiorly over all pelvic organs, form attachments between the bladder and the anterior abdominal wall and lateral pelvic wall. Dorsolaterally this condensation is called the dorsolateral ligament, and through it the main vascular and neurologic supply enters the bladder base. The median umbilical ligament connects the bladder to the umbilicus via the urachal remnant. The inferior condensations in the male are the puboprostatic ligaments, and in the female the pubovesical ligaments. These attachments run from the levator ani muscle and the pubic bone to the bladder.

Blood Supply

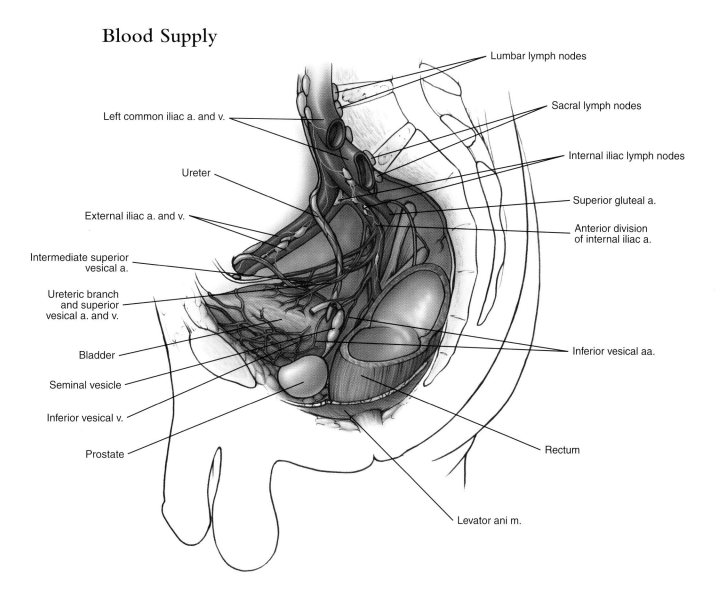

Arterial branches come from the superior, middle, and inferior vesical arteries, which are branches of the anterior division of the internal iliac artery. During cystectomy care should be taken to prevent high ligation of the anterior division, which may result in buttock claudication secondary to ligation of one of the main gluteal arteries, which also originate in this area. Excessive bleeding can be temporarily controlled by placing a vascular clamp on the main internal iliac trunk. Smaller branches from the obturator and inferior gluteal arteries also supply the bladder. In the female the uterine and vaginal vessels also contribute to the rich blood supply.

The bladder is drained by a rich plexus of veins situated between the bladder wall and its adventitial covering. These vessels drain to the internal iliac veins after coalescing into main trunks, some of which run with accompanying arteries. In the male the vesical plexus communicates with the plexus of Santorini (retropubic) and can cause significant bleeding if not adequately secured.

Lymphatic Drainage

The external iliac, internal iliac, and common iliac lymph nodes constitute the primary lymphatic drainage of the bladder. There is an extensive lymphatic anastomosis between the pelvic, genital, and lower intestinal organs.

Nerve Supply

The neural supply to the bladder is composed of the two components of the autonomic system. The sympathetic supply originates primarily from T11–12 and L1–2. These fibers run via the sympathetic trunk to the lumbar splanchnic plexus and the superior hypogastric plexus, which divides into the right and left hypogastric nerves. These nerves then run inferiorly to join the pelvic plexus of parasympathetic fibers and innervate the bladder and urethra. The parasympathetic nerve supply arises from S2–4 and forms the pelvic parasympathetic plexus. After mixing with the sympathetic fibers to form the pelvic plexus, vesical branches run toward the bladder base. These fibers reach the lateral sides of the bladder to innervate the bladder and urethra. The prostate gland receives a segment to form the prostatic plexus, from which runs the cavernous nerves responsible for penile erection and clitoral erection. These nerves are combined motor and sensory. The vesical plexus gives many branches to the bladder that intermingle in the adventitia and penetrate the muscular wall to supply the entire bladder. Ganglia are formed along the nerve trunks of the vesical plexus and in its deeper branches. These nerves continue to branch and ultimately are distributed throughout the muscular coat. The ratio of nerve fiber to muscle fiber varies, roughly 1:1 for parasympathetic cholinergic fibers and considerably lower for the sympathetic fibers, which in contrast to the parasympathetic fibers are unevenly distributed throughout the bladder, with maximal concentration in the bladder base and proximal urethra. Since the nerves branch frequently and run a tortuous course, they are not damaged by bladder filling (stretching) except at extreme volumes. The majority of the bladder muscle (detrusor) is innervated primarily by parasympathetic fibers (stretch and fullness), and the trigone, bladder neck, and lower end of the ureters mainly by sympathetic fibers (pain, touch, and temperature). Nerve damage may occur during any radical pelvic procedure, with varying clinical manifestations ranging from hyperreflexia (frequency, nocturia, urgency) to hyporeflexia (decreased stream, retention), depending on the fibers damaged.

SURGICAL APPLICATIONS
Radical Cystectomy
Indications

Bladder cancer is the second most common tumor, after prostate adenocarcinoma, treated by urologists. The most common histologic pattern of bladder cancer in the United States is transitional cell carcinoma. Less common are carcinoma in situ, adenocarcinoma, squamous cell carcinoma, anaplastic carcinoma, and sarcomatous tumors. Superficial bladder tumors can be treated with transurethral resection, BCG (bacille Calmette-Guérin) vaccine or other chemotherapeutic installations, or radiation therapy. However, invasive bladder cancer, in the absence of metastasis, is best treated with radical cystectomy. More than half of muscle-invasive transitional cell carcinomas and 20% to 30% of tumors penetrating the perivesical fat are cured with radical cystectomy.

Preoperative Evaluation

Cystoscopy should be performed and bladder biopsy specimens taken with cup forceps or a resectoscope. Care should be taken to obtain representative samples from the tumor and from bladder muscle to determine the depth of tumor invasion. Samples should be taken from any abnormal area in the bladder, which might represent secondary tumors or carcinoma in situ, as well as random samples from the bladder and prostatic urethra. The presence of urethral invasion with tumor is an indication for cystourethrectomy. Tumor extension into prostatic stroma is a bad prognostic sign, and the need for radical cystectomy is debatable.

Upper urinary tract evaluation with intravenous pyelography or retrograde pyelography should be performed to define the anatomy of the upper urinary tract and to rule out the presence of any filling defects that might represent coexisting tumors. A radiograph of the chest, CT scan of the pelvis and abdomen, and bone scan should be obtained to rule out distant metastases. A sterile urine culture should be documented before hospital admission.

The method of urinary diversion should be discussed with the patient before surgery. Multiple techniques of continent urinary diversions have evolved over the past decade, with good results. However, in patients with subnormal kidney function (serum creatinine >2 mg/dl) an ileal loop conduit is better because continent diversion leads to kidney deterioration in the majority of these patients. The proper site for the abdominal stoma should be marked the day before surgery and a urinary collection device, half filled with water, fitted to the site for trial the night before surgery.

Most patients are admitted the day before surgery for mechanical and antibiotic bowel preparation. Prophylaxis against deep venous thrombosis should be considered, particularly in patients at increased risk. The patient should be kept well hydrated, particularly with the bowel preparation and increased fluid loss. Intravenous prophylactic antibiotics should be administered just before surgery. If the patient is admitted with a urethral catheter, the catheter should be changed and the bladder irrigated the day before surgery, and the intravenous antibiotics started at the same time. Two to three units of blood should be available because this is major surgery and some blood loss should be expected, especially if previous pelvic surgery has been performed or radiation has been delivered to the pelvis.

Technique in Male Patients

The patient is placed supine with the legs in a modified lithotomy position with foot stirrups. The abdomen, perineum, and genitalia are prepared and draped, and a catheter is inserted into the patient's bladder.

A midline incision is made from the symphysis pubis to a point several centimeters above the umbilicus or to the xiphoid, if necessary, and is carried through the midline fascia.

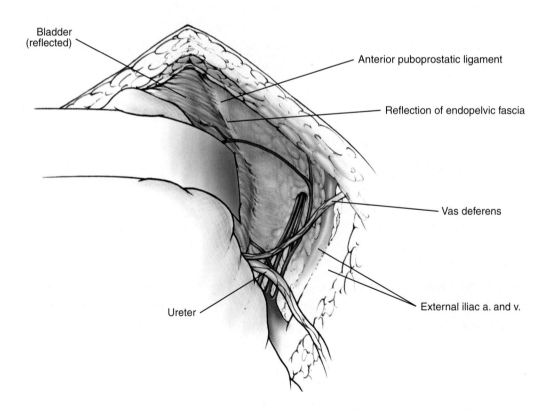

The bladder is reflected medially with blunt dissection to develop a plane between the bladder and the lateral pelvic wall; then the retropubic fat is mobilized with sharp and blunt dissection to display the puboprostatic ligaments.

This dissection is performed on both sides of the pelvis because it is easier done before the peritoneal cavity is opened. The external iliac vessels are seen on the lateral pelvic wall, and the fat and lymph nodes in the obturator fossa can be palpated for any enlarged lymph nodes. The obturator nerve should be palpated or viewed in the depth of the obturator fossa, and care should be taken during lymph node dissection to prevent injury to this nerve that supplies motor fibers to the adductor muscles of the thigh. The bladder is examined carefully to evaluate the extent and resectability of the tumor. The peritoneal cavity is then opened through the whole length of the incision, and the intra-abdominal contents are examined for any metastasis. The vas deferens and gonadal vessels are encountered during lateral dissection. The vas is divided and the pelvic segment excised with diathermy; the gonadal vessels are mobilized laterally.

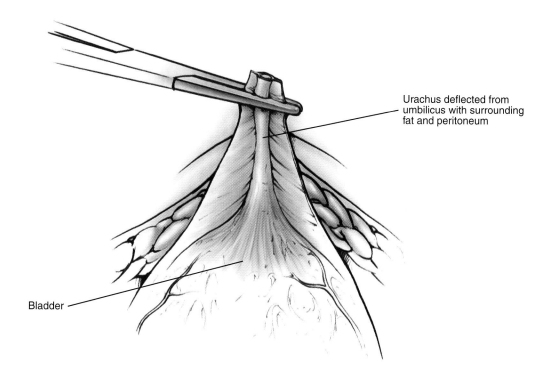

Urachus deflected from umbilicus with surrounding fat and peritoneum

Bladder

Once the resectability of the tumor and the absence of metastasis are confirmed, the bladder dissection is started by dividing the urachus between two clamps and freeing the apex of the bladder of the abdominal wall. The peritoneal reflection on the lateral walls of the bladder is then incised in the depth of the wound on each side of the umbilical ligament to free the lateral sides of the bladder from the pelvic wall.

Pelvic lymphadenectomy is performed to remove the lymphatic tissues related to the iliac vessels and obturator fossa. The dissection is started by incising the areolar tissue on the external iliac artery and extending the dissection to the bifurcation of the common iliac artery proximally, the internal iliac artery medially, and the femoral canal distally.

The wound is retracted with a self-retaining retractor. The peritoneal reflection on the posterior wall of the bladder is incised, and the small bowel and the ascending colon are retracted superiorly and kept in position with moist abdominal packs and the malleable arm of the self-retaining retractor. On the left side the sigmoid colon is mobilized medially to display the ureter where it crosses the bifurcation of the common iliac artery, which is tied several centimeters proximal to the bladder and incised above the tie. A specimen from the proximal end of the ureter is excised and sent for frozen-section analysis to confirm the absence of tumor extension. The same procedure is repeated for the right ureter. Devascularization of the ureter can be prevented by mobilizing it within the periureteric fat and by remembering that the ureteric blood vessels in the pelvis enter the ureter from the lateral side. Good ureteric length is important to facilitate subsequent reconstruction.

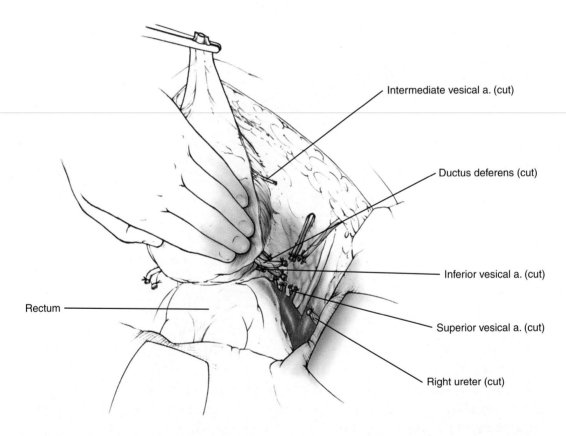

Intermediate vesical a. (cut)

Ductus deferens (cut)

Inferior vesical a. (cut)

Superior vesical a. (cut)

Right ureter (cut)

Rectum

The anterior branches of the internal iliac artery are then divided in sequence, beginning with the obliterated umbilical artery. Each pedicle is isolated and divided, with the artery being divided prior to division of the vein. This includes the superolateral vesical pedicle, middle lateral vesical pedicle, and inferolateral vesical pedicle. A plane is then developed bluntly between the rectum, the seminal vesicles, and the prostate gland to enable identification of the posterior pedicles, which are serially clipped and divided. The isolation of individual vessels is time consuming and unnecessary. Branches of the pelvic plexus that ennervate the corpora cavernosae and are required for erection are usually in-

jured during division of the anterolateral vascular pedicle or the internal pudendal artery, which arises from the distal internal iliac artery. If a nerve-sparing
technique is attempted, care should be taken to prevent injury to the inferior
branches of the hypogastric artery, which form the pudendal artery. As the dissection is carried down to the prostate gland it enters the plane between the
two layers (parietal and visceral) of Denonvilliers' fascia to the apex of the
prostate. The prostatic pedicles are divided and ligated.

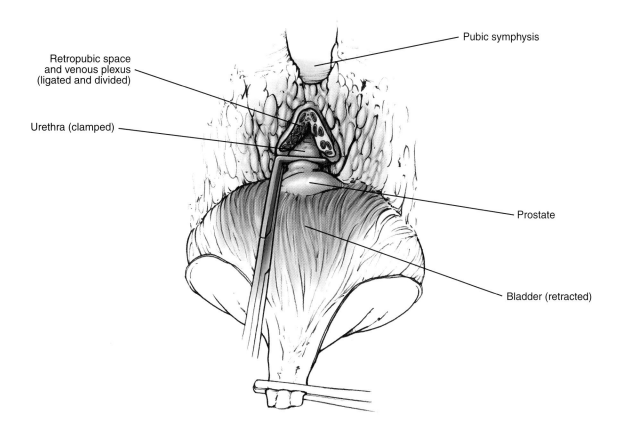

Pubic symphysis

Retropubic space
and venous plexus
(ligated and divided)

Urethra (clamped)

Prostate

Bladder (retracted)

The endopelvic fascia is identified superolateral to the prostate gland and incised to expose the puboprostatic ligaments. The ligaments are divided at the
posterior surface of the symphysis pubis to enable identification of the venous
plexus, which drains the deep dorsal veins of the penis (plexus of Santorini). A
large right-angle clamp (McDougal clamp) is passed under the venous plexus
to develop a plane between the venous complex and the urethra. The venous
plexus is then tied with heavy nonabsorbable sutures and divided. The ure-
theral catheter is removed, and the urethra is retracted from the urogenital diaphragm, clamped with a large clamp beyond the apex of the prostate to prevent tumor spillage, and divided if no concomitant urethrectomy is planned.
Some surgeons prefer to introduce 50 to 100 ml of 10 % formaline solution in
the bladder for 10 minutes before catheter removal to reduce the viability of
potentially contaminating tumor cells.

   Hemostasis is secured, and the pelvis is packed with moist packs. Attention
is then given to the urinary diversion.

Technique in Female Patients

The patient is placed supine with the legs in the modified lithotomy position with Allen stirrups.

The perineum and abdomen are prepared and draped, and a catheter placed in the bladder. A midline incision is made from the xiphoid process to the symphysis pubis, and carried through the midline fascia to the lower limit of the posterior rectus fascia. A pelvic lymph node dissection is performed with the same boundaries as above.

The peritoneum is incised with an inverted V incision extending inferolaterally on both sides to the juncture of the external iliac artery and along the external iliac artery to the bifurcation of the iliac arteries, as in male patients. The ureter is identified and dissected free of the retroperitoneum, traced to its point of entry under the superior vesical pedicle, and divided. Frozen sections of the distal ureter are sent for analysis while the rest of the operation proceeds.

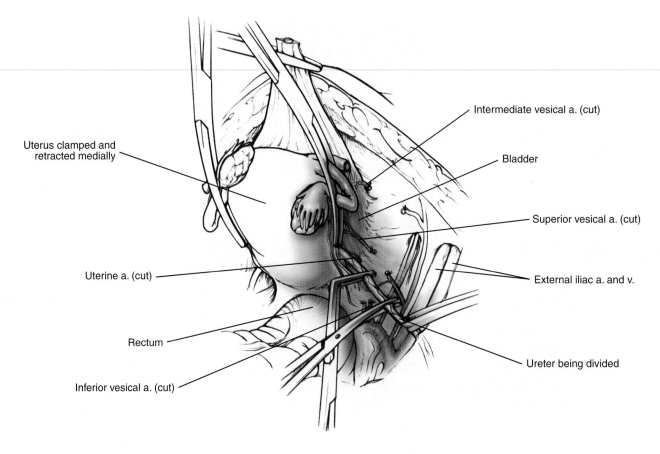

If the patient has not had a prior hysterectomy, the ovarian arteries and veins are divided and the fallopian tubes and ovaries retracted medially on both sides. The round ligament is also divided and retracted medially. The superior, middle, and inferior vesical pedicles are divided, as in cystectomy in male patients, and the peritoneal incision is carried across the midline at the fornix of the vagina.

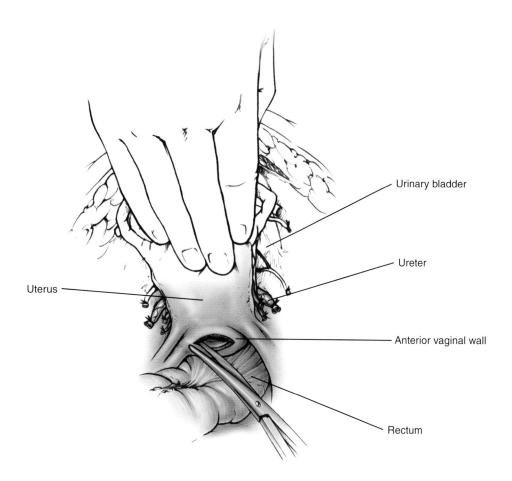

The uterine pedicles are divided and ligated. A swab on a stick is inserted into the vagina, and the vagina is entered at the fornix. With sharp dissection, the anterior vaginal wall is excised with the specimen to the urethra. At the urethra the anterior vaginal incisions are carried medially to encircle the urethral meatus, and the specimen is removed. Allis clamps are placed along the incision in the vagina to provide temporary hemostasis, which is usually obtained as part of the vaginal reconstruction with 2-0 Vicryl running sutures.

Partial Cystectomy

Partial cystectomy has been used in the management of bladder cancer for many years, although its exact role today is not well defined. Improvements in the management of localized bladder tumors have dramatically reducd the frequency of this procedure.

Certain advantages such as the sparing of potency in male patients, retention of a functioning urinary reservoir, and the ability to achieve full-thickness resection of bladder tumors and sample perivesical nodal tissue make partial cystectomy an attractive procedure in selected patients. The major drawback to partial cystectomy in the treatment of bladder cancer is the high tumor recurrence rates, which range from 40% to 80% in reported series.

Indications

Certain criteria which must be met before a patient can be considered for partial cystectomy. First, the tumor must be a solitary, primary lesion located in a part of the bladder that allows for complete excision with adequate margins of at least 3 cm. Second, in patients who are not candidates for endoscopic resection due to a combination of body habitus, hypomobility of the hips secondary to osteoarthritis, or a fixed prostatic urethra, partial cystectomy may be required for complete diagnosis. Third, it has been recommended that tumors located in bladder diverticuli be managed with partial cystectomy because bladder diverticuli have attenuated walls that may be easily perforated with transurethral resection, allowing tumor spillage into the perivesical space. Finally, other indications for partial cystectomy include management of genitourinary sarcomas, urachal carcinomas involving the dome of the bladder, involvement of the bladder by tumors in adjacent organs, and palliation of severe local symptoms.

Contraindications to partial cystectomy include patients with multiple lesions, recurrences or tumors located on the trigone where adequate excision is not possible due to the proximity of the ureteral orifices and bladder neck. In addition, patients must have biopsy-proven absence of cellular atypia or carcinoma in situ in the remainder of the bladder and prostatic urethra. If there is evidence of fixation of the tumor to adjacent pelvic structures or if segmental resection of the tumor would require removal of so much of the bladder as to necessitate augmentation cystoplasty, then a partial cystectomy should not be performed.

Technique

The patient is placed on the operating room table in the supine position with the break of the table at the anterosuperior iliac spine, which allows adequate flexion and elevation of the bladder into the wound. The sterile field includes the penis in men and the vulva and vagina in women to allow sterile insertion of a Foley catheter into the bladder after resection of the tumor and before closure of the incision.

A lower midline incision or a transverse suprapubic incision can be utilized. The rectus abdominis muscle is divided in the midline and the space of Retzius is entered. The patient is then placed in the Trendelenburg position to elevate the abdominal contents out of the pelvis. Depending on the location of the tumor in the bladder, an extraperitoneal or intraperitoneal approach can be performed. For tumors on the dome or anterior part of the bladder an extraperitoneal approach is optimal; for tumors on the posterior aspect of the bladder an intraperitoneal approach is preferred.

Extraperitoneal Partial Cystectomy

The anterior surface of the bladder is exposed through the space of Retzius, and the peritoneum is mobilized where it is easily separated from the bladder. A bilateral pelvic lymph node dissection is performed. The bladder is freed laterally and posteriorly well beyond the site of the tumor. The superior vesicle pedicle can be divided if necessary. The fat over the site of the tumor is left attached to the bladder.

Several stay sutures are then placed in the bladder at a site known from cystoscopy to be distant from the tumor. The wound edges are packed away from the bladder with laparotomy pads or plastic drapes, and the bladder is entered between the stay sutures with an electrocautery, taking care to minimize the amount of urine spillage in order to reduce the risk for tumor implantation. The incision is extended several centimeters anteriorly and posteriorly to allow adequate visualization of the tumor and its relationship to the ureteric orifices and bladder neck.

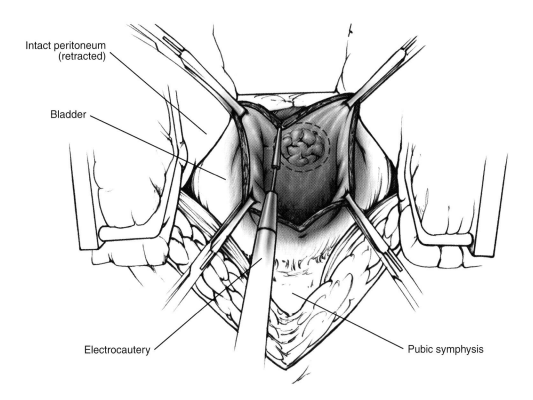

The tumor is then excised, taking care to leave a 3 cm margin of normal-appearing bladder around the tumor. The tumor should be removed en bloc with the overlying perivesical fat and peritoneum, with an electrocautery or with sharp dissection. If the tumor lies less than 3 cm from the ureteric orifice, the orifice should be resected and the ureter reimplanted elsewhere. If excision of the tumor involves the bladder neck, it is possible to excise the bladder neck and the surrounding prostatic capsule after enucleation of the prostate gland. However, it is probably safer to perform radical cystectomy in such a situation. The bladder neck should not be resected in female patients because of the high risk for incontinence.

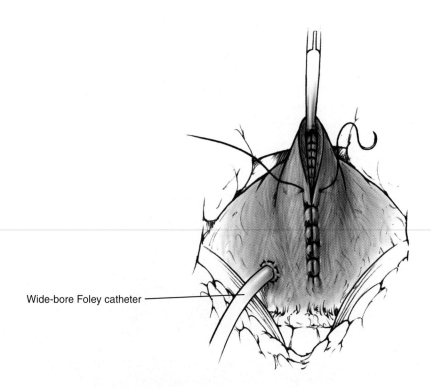

Wide-bore Foley catheter

After removal of the tumor, the bladder should be closed in two layers with 3-0 Vicryl sutures to close the urothelium and 2-0 Vicryl sutures to close the muscular layer. A suprapubic cystostomy catheter is contraindicated because of the risk for tumor spillage, so it is essential that a wide-bore Foley catheter be used. The perivesical space is drained for 3 to 4 days or until drainage is minimal. The abdominal wall is then closed in the standard fashion.

Postoperatively the urethral catheter should be left in place for 7 to 10 days. If there is any doubt as to the integrity of the repair, gentle gravity cystography may be performed.

Intraperitoneal Partial Cystectomy

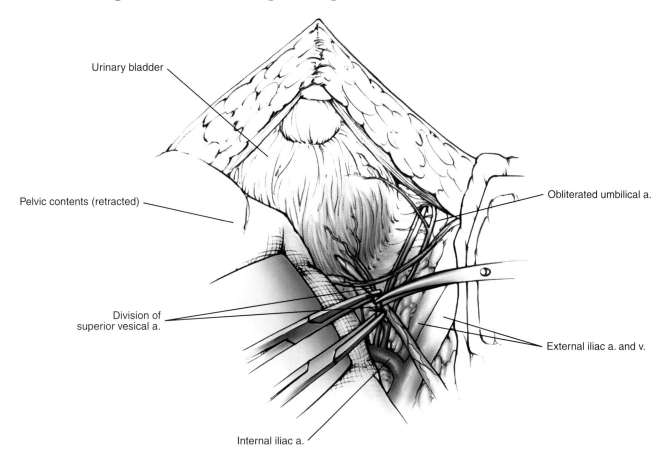

After the rectus abdominis muscles are divided in the midline, the peritoneum is opened in the midline. The patient is then placed in the Trendelenburg position, and the abdominal contents are lifted out of the pelvis with laparotomy pads.

The peritoneum over the iliac vessels is incised, and bilateral pelvic lymph node dissection is performed. The obliterated umbilical artery is followed to the takeoff of the superior vesical artery, which is divided. The bladder is then freed posteriorly as needed, stay sutures are placed, and the bladder is opened.

Removal of the bladder tumor, including the perivesical fat and peritoneum, reimplantation of the ureters, closure of the bladder, management of urethral catheters, and perivesical drains and wound closure, are as described for extraperitoneal partial cystectomy.

KEY REFERENCES

Giuliani L, Giberti C, Martorana G, et al. Radical extensive surgery for renal cell carcinoma: Long-term results and prognostic factors. J Urol 143(3):468-473; discussion 473-474, 1990.

These authors discuss the long-term outcome for radical nephrectomy and lymphadenectomy.

Graham SD Jr, Glenn JF. Enucleative surgery for renal malignancy. J Urol 122:546-551, 1979.

Minimally invasive surgery for enucleation of localized kidney tumors is described in this article.

Prout GR Jr. The surgical management of bladder carcinoma. Urol Clin North Am 149:175, 1976.

This article discusses different approaches to the management of bladder tumors.

Resnick MI, Pounds DM, Boyce WH. Surgical anatomy of the human kidney and its applications. Urology 17:367, 1981.

This reference displays the anatomy of the renal vasculature.

Tanagho EA. Anatomy of the lower urinary tract. In Walsh PC, Retik AB, Stamey TA, et al., eds. Campbell's Urology, 6th ed., vol. 1. Philadelphia: WB Saunders, 1992, pp 40-69.

This chapter describes the anatomy of the bladder and ureters, and their relations to other pelvic structures.

SUGGESTED READINGS

Dandekar NP, Tongaonkar HB, Dalal AV, et al. Partial cystectomy for invasive bladder cancer. J Surg Oncol 60:24, 1995.

Ditonno P, Traficante A, Battaglia M, et al. Role of lymphadenectomy in renal cell carcinoma. Prog Clin Biol Res 378:169-174, 1992.

Eigner EB, Freiha FS. The fate of the remaining bladder following supravesical diversion. J Urol 144:31, 1990.

Freiha FS. Open bladder surgery. In Walsh PC, Retik AB, Stamey TA, et al., eds. Campbell's Urology, 6th ed. Philadelphia: WB Saunders, 1992, pp 2765-2768.

Giuliani L, Martorana G, Giberti C, et al. Results of radical nephrectomy with extensive lymphadenectomy for renal cell carcinoma. J Urol 130:664-668, 1983.

Herr HW. Partial nephrectomy for incidental renal cell carcinoma. Br J Urol 74:431-433, 1994.

Herr HW. Urachal carcinoma: The case for extended partial cystectomy. J Urol 151:365, 1994.

Herr HW, Scher HI. Neoadjuvant chemotherapy and partial cystectomy for invasive bladder cancer. J Clin Oncol 12:975, 1994.

Hicks BA, Hensle TW, Burbige KA, et al. Bladder management in children with genitourinary sarcoma. J Pediatr Surg 28:1019, 1993.

Keane TE, Graham SD Jr. Conservative renal surgery. Has it a role in renal cell carcinoma? Surg Oncol Clin North Am 4:295-306, 1995.

Kinouchi T, Hanafusa T, Kuroda M, et al. Ossified cystic metastasis of bladder tumor to abdominal wound after partial cystectomy. J Urol 153:1049, 1995.

Neves RJ, Zincke H, Taylor WF. Metastatic renal cell cancer and radical nephrectomy: Identification of prognostic factors and patient survival. J Urol 139:1173-1176, 1988.

Novick AC, Streem S, Montie JE. Conservative surgery for renal cell carcinoma: A single center experience with 100 patients. J Urol 141:835, 1989.

Parra RO, Worischek JH, Hagood PG. Laparoscopic simple cystectomy in a man. Surg Laparosc Endosc 5:161, 1995.

Ramon J, Goldwasser B, Raviv G, et al. Long-term results of simple and radical nephrectomy for renal cell carcinoma. Cancer 67(10):2506-2511, 1991.

Robey EL, Schellhammer PF. The adrenal gland and renal cell carcinoma: Is ipsilateral adrenalectomy a necessary component of radical nephrectomy. J Urol 135:453-455, 1986.

Robson CJ. Radical nephrectomy for renal cell carcinoma. J Urol 89:37, 1963.

Sampaio FJ, Aragao AH. Anatomical relationship between the intrarenal arteries and the kidney collecting system. J Urol 143:679, 1990.

Schlegel PN, Walsh PC. Neuroanatomical approach to radical cystoprostatectomy with preservation of sexual function. J Urol 138:1402-1406, 1986.

Sweeney P, Kursh ED, Resnick MI. Partial cystectomy. Urol Clin North Am 19:701, 1992.

Wishnow KI, Lorigan J, Charnsangavej CJ. Results of radical nephrectomy for peripheral well-circumscribed renal cell carcinoma. Urology 34:171-174, 1989.

Index